PREHOSPITAL EMERGENCY PHARMACOLOGY

SIXTH EDITION

BRYAN E. BLEDSOE, D.O., F.A.C.E.P., EMT-P

EMS Physician
Midlothian, Texas
*   and*
Clinical Associate Professor of Emergency Medicine
University of North Texas Health Sciences Center
Fort Worth, Texas

DWAYNE E. CLAYDEN, M.E.M., EMT-P

Assistant to the Medical Director
City of Calgary Emergency Medical Services
Calgary, Alberta, Canada

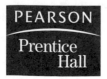

PEARSON

Prentice
Hall

Upper Saddle River, New Jersey 07458

Library of Congress Cataloging-in-Publication Data

Bledsoe, Bryan E.
   Prehospital emergency pharmacology / Bryan E. Bledsoe, Dwayne E. Clayden—6th ed.
     p. cm.
   Includes bibliographical references and index.
   ISBN 0-13-150711-7
    1. Medical emergencies. 2. Chemotherapy. 3. Drugs. I. Clayden, Dwayne E. II. Title
   [DNLM: 1. Emergency Treatment. 2. Drug Therapy. 3. Pharmaceutical Preparations.
   WB 105 B646p 2005]
RC86.7.B597 2005
616.02'5—dc22   2004055196

Publisher: Julie Levin Alexander
Publisher's Assistant: Regina Bruno
Executive Editor: Marlene McHugh Pratt
Senior Acquisitions Editor: Tiffany Price Salter
Senior Managing Editor for Development: Lois Berlowitz
Project Manager: Andrea Edwards, Triple S Press
Senior Marketing Manager: Katrin Beacom
Channel Marketing Manager: Rachele Strober
Marketing Coordinator: Michael Sirinides
Director of Production and Manufacturing: Bruce Johnson
Managing Editor for Production: Patrick Walsh
Production Liaison: Julie Li
Production Editor: Lynn Steines, Carlisle Publishers Services
Media Editor: John Jordan
Manager of Media Production: Amy Peltier
New Media Project Manager: Stephen J. Hartner
Manufacturing Manager: Ilene Sanford
Manufacturing Buyer: Pat Brown
Creative Director: Cheryl Asherman
Senior Design Coordinator: Christopher Weigand
Cover Designer: Michael Ginsberg
Composition: Carlisle Publishers Services
Printing and Binding: Courier Westford
Cover Printer: Phoenix Color

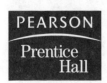

10 9 8 7 6 5 4 3
ISBN 0-13-150711-7

Dedication

The sixth edition of Prehospital Emergency Pharmacology *is dedicated to the memory of Dave Jackson. Dave and I attended the first paramedic program in Tarrant County, Texas, and worked together for years. Our careers took us in different directions, but we stayed in touch and shared stories and tales. Dave was an EMS intellectual before there was such a thing. My old coworkers and I miss Dave; we are much better human beings for having known him.*

Bryan E. Bledsoe, D.O., F.A.C.E.P., EMT-P,

CONTENTS

8 Drugs Used in the Treatment of Respiratory Emergencies 220

9 Drugs Used in the Treatment of Metabolic-Endocrine Emergencies 265

10 Drugs Used in the Treatment of Neurological Emergencies 283

PREFACE

Modern emergency medical service (EMS) is based on sound principles, practice, and research. The paramedic of today must be knowledgeable in all aspects of prehospital emergency medicine. Nowhere is this more important than when administering of medications. *Prehospital Emergency Pharmacology* is a complete guide to the most common medications used in prehospital emergency care. This comprehensive text is designed with two purposes in mind: First, it is a complete pharmacology teaching text. Second, it is a handy reference to the most common drugs and fluids used in prehospital care.

Welcome to the sixth edition of *Prehospital Emergency Pharmacology*. This text has been a cornerstone of EMS education for more than 20 years. The sixth edition has been extensively revised to reflect current trends in prehospital care. EMS is undergoing an essential evolutionary step in that modern prehospital practice must be based on sound scientific principles. We have been careful to ensure that the sixth edition reflects the trend toward evidenced-based practice. However, practices and formularies are different among regions and among countries. We have attempted to make the text as comprehensive as possible. We hope that *Prehospital Emergency Pharmacology* will prove a valuable aid to both the practicing paramedic and paramedic student.

It is the intent of the authors and publishers that this textbook be used as part of a formal paramedic education program taught by a qualified instructor and supervised by a licensed physician. The knowledge and skills outlined in this textbook are best learned in the classroom, skills laboratory, and then the clinical field setting. It is important to point out that this or any other text cannot teach skills. Care skills are only learned under the watchful eye of a paramedic instructor and perfected during clinical and field internships.

The care procedures presented here represent accepted practices in the United States and Canada. They are not offered as a standard of care. Paramedic-level care is to be performed only under the authority and guidance of a licensed physician. It is the reader's responsibility to know and follow local care protocols and standing orders as provided by medical advisers directing the system to which he or she belongs. Also, it is the reader's responsibility to stay informed of emergency care procedures and changes.

Bryan E. Bledsoe, D.O., F.A.C.E.P., EMT-P
Dwayne E. Clayden, M.E.M., EMT-P

ACKNOWLEDGMENTS

We wish to acknowledge the talents and efforts of the following people who contributed to *Prehospital Emergency Pharmacology.*

Chapter Authors

First, we would like to thank Alan Mikolaj for his outstanding chapter on drug calculations. His work on this chapter provides easy-to-use instructions for both the paramedic student and the seasoned veteran.

Second, we would like to thank Andy Anton, M.D., F.R.C.P.C., for his work on the toxicology chapter. He has written a chapter that provides the essential information for a paramedic dealing with complicated overdose and poisoning situations.

Revised Text Reviewers

We appreciate the dedication of the text reviewers to this profession and especially appreciate their efforts in reviewing the revision of this text. The quality of the reviews has been outstanding. The reviewers' comments and suggestions were invaluable as we revised this text. The assistance provided by these EMS experts is deeply appreciated.

Roy L. Alson, Ph.D., M.D., F.A.C.E.P.
Associate Professor of Emergency Medicine
Wake Forest University School of Medicine
Winston Salem, North Carolina
    and
Assistant Medical Director
NMRT-East (SORT)
Department of Homeland Security

JoAnn Cobble, Ed.D., NREMT-P, R.N.
Chair, Department of EMS
University of Arkansas for Medical Sciences
Little Rock, Arkansas

Richard A. Craven, M.D., F.A.C.E.P.
Clinical Director
East Coast Clinical Research
Virginia Beach, Virginia

R. Scott Crawford, NREMT-P, EMSI
Lead Instructor, Advance EMS Programs
Nebraska Methodist College
Omaha, Nebraska

James F. Gross, B.S., MICP
Hemer, California

Mike Pirie, EMT-P
Medical Education Coordinator
Airdrie Emergency Services
Airdrie, Alberta, Canada

John Eric Powell, M.S., NREMT-P
Paramedic Instructor
Roane State Community College
Knoxville, Tennessee

Katharine P. Rickey, NREMT-P; EMS I/C
New Hampshire Community Technical College
Laconia, New Hampshire

Regina Twisdale
Director, School of Paramedic Sciences
Camden County College
Blackwood, New Jersey

Development and Production

We would like to acknowledge the efforts and support of many talented individuals who assisted with the sixth edition.

First, we would like to thank Julie Alexander, publisher at Brady, for her ongoing support of this text and our other EMS projects. We would also like to thank the following editors, Tiffany Price Salter, Lois Berlowitz, and Marlene Pratt, who brought this project to completion. A special thank you to Monica Moosang, Editorial Assistant, for her help with reviewing the drug dosage calculations.

We would like to thank Lynn Steines of Carlisle Publishers Services for her persistence and hard work in seeing this project through to completion. Her attention to detail speaks well for her and Carlisle.

We would like to particularly thank Susan Simpfenderfer of Triple SSS Press Media Development for her tremendous work in developmental editing and production of the sixth edition. Susan is a consummate expert.

ABOUT THE AUTHORS

Bryan E. Bledsoe, D.O., F.A.C.E.P., EMT-P

Dr. Bryan Bledsoe is an emergency physician with special interest in prehospital care. He received his bachelor of science degree from the University of Texas at Arlington and received his medical degree from the University of North Texas Health Sciences Center/Texas College of Osteopathic Medicine. He completed his internship at Texas Tech University and residency training at Scott and White Memorial Hospital/Texas A&M College of Medicine. Dr. Bledsoe is board-certified in emergency medicine.

Prior to attending medical school, Dr. Bledsoe worked as an emergency medical technician (EMT), paramedic, and paramedic instructor. He completed EMT training in 1974 and paramedic training in 1976 and worked for 6 years as a field paramedic in Fort Worth, Texas. In 1979, he joined the faculty of the University of North Texas Health Sciences Center and served as coordinator of EMT and paramedic education programs at the university. Dr. Bledsoe is active in emergency medicine and serves as medical director for several emergency medical service (EMS) agencies and educational programs.

Dr. Bledsoe has authored several EMS books published by Brady including *Paramedic Care: Princples and Practice, Essentials of Paramedic Care, Atlas of Paramedic Skills, Prehospital Emergency Pharmacology,* and *Anatomy and Physiology for Emergency Care.* He is married to Emma Bledsoe. They have two children, Bryan and Andrea, and live in Midlothian, Texas, a suburb of Dallas. He enjoys saltwater fishing and listening to Jimmy Buffett.

Dwayne E. Clayden, M.E.M., EMT-P

Dwayne Clayden is the Assistant to the Medical Director for the City of Calgary Emergency Medical Services in Calgary, Alberta, Canada. He is responsible for prehospital research, quality care, the in-house paramedic program, and the tactical EMS team.

In 2000 Mr. Clayden received the Exemplary Service Medal from the governor general of Canada for his contributions to EMS in Canada. In 1998 the Alberta Prehospital Professions Association presented him with the Award of Excellence for his contributions to Emergency Medical Services in Alberta.

Mr. Clayden began his career as a police officer in Calgary. In 1980 he joined the Calgary Fire Department, Ambulance Division, as an emergency medical technician (EMT). Following his paramedic education at the

Southern Alberta Institute of Technology (SAIT), he became a member of the Staff Development Division of the City of Calgary Emergency Medical Services. In 1987 he began his teaching career at SAIT, first in the EMT program and then in 1988 in the paramedic program.

From 1991 to 1996, Mr. Clayden was the publisher and editor-in-chief of *ON SCENE,* and EMS periodical for Canadian EMS. He has coauthored two books with Dr. Bryan Bledsoe for Brady Publishing, *Prehospital Emergency Pharmacology* and *Pocket Reference for EMTs and Paramedics.* He also wrote the web-based companion version of *Prehospital Emergency Pharmacology.*

He lives in Airdrie, Alberta, with his wife Nancy and their four children.

NOTICES

NOTICE ON DRUGS AND DRUG DOSAGES

Every effort has been made to ensure that the drug dosages presented in the textbook are in accordance with nationally accepted standards. When applicable, the dosages and routes are taken from the American Heart Association's Advanced Cardiac Life Support Guidelines. The American Medical Association's publication *Drug Evaluations*, the *Physicians' Desk Reference*, and Appleton & Lange's *Health Professions Drug Guide 2004* are followed with regard to drug dosages not covered by the American Heart Association's guidelines. It is the responsibility of the reader to be familiar with the drugs used in his or her system, as well as the dosages specified by the medical director. The drugs presented in this text should only be administered by direct order, whether verbally or through accepted standing orders, by a licensed physician.

NOTICE ON GENDER USAGE

The English language has historically given preference to the male gender. Among many words, the pronouns "he" and "his" are commonly used to describe both genders. Society evolves faster than language and the male pronouns still predominate in our speech. The authors have made great effort to treat the two genders equally, recognizing that a significant percentage of paramedics and patients are female. However, in some instances, male pronouns may be used to describe both male and female paramedics and patients solely for the purpose of brevity. This is not intended to offend any readers.

Precautions on Bloodborne Pathogens and Infectious Diseases

Prehospital emergency personnel, like all health care workers, are at risk for exposure to bloodborne pathogens and infectious diseases. In emergency situations it is often difficult to take or enforce proper infection control measures. However, paramedics must recognize their high-risk status. Readers should study the following information on infection control before turning to the main portion of this book.

Infection control is designed to protect emergency personnel, their families, and their patients from unnecessary exposure to communicable diseases.

Laws, regulations, and standards regarding infection control include the following:

- *Centers for Disease Control and Prevention (CDC).* The CDC has published extensive guidelines regarding infection control. Proper equipment and techniques that should be used by emergency response personnel to prevent or minimize risk of exposure are defined.

- *The Ryan White Act.* The Ryan White Act of 1990 allows emergency personnel to find out if they were exposed to an infectious disease while rendering patient care. Employers are required to name a "designated officer" to coordinate communications with the treating hospital.

- *Americans with Disabilities Act.* This act prohibits discrimination against individuals with disabilities, including those with contagious diseases. It guarantees equal employment opportunities and job protection if the infected individual can perform essential job functions and does not pose a threat to the safety and health of patients and coworkers.

- *Health Insurance Portability and Accountability Act of 1996 (HIPAA).* HIPAA significantly increased patient confidentiality and restricted access to medical records. Despite this, provisions were made in the act that allow for access to information related to possible exposure to infectious diseases. Thus, HIPAA does not prohibit infectious disease exposure notification, testing, and follow-up for EMS personnel.

- *Occupational Safety and Health Administration (OSHA) Regulations.* OSHA enacted a regulation entitled Occupational

Exposure to Bloodborne Pathogens that classifies emergency response personnel as being at the greatest risk of occupational exposure to communicable diseases. This regulation requires employers to provide hepatitis B (HBV) vaccinations free of charge, maintain a written exposure control plan, and provide personal protective equipment. These requirements primarily apply to private employers. Applicability to local and state governmental employees varies by locality. Many states have developed their own OSHA plans.

- *National Fire Protection Association (NFPA) Guidelines.* This is a national organization that has established specific guidelines and requirements regarding infection control for emergency response agencies, particularly fire departments and emergency medical service agencies.

BODY SUBSTANCE ISOLATION PRECAUTIONS AND PERSONAL PROTECTIVE EQUIPMENT

Emergency response personnel should practice *body substance isolation (BSI)*, a strategy that considers *all* body substances potentially infectious. To avoid contact with body substances, all emergency personnel should utilize *personal protective equipment (PPE)*. Appropriate PPE should be available on every emergency vehicle. The minimum recommended PPE includes the following:

- *Gloves.* Disposable gloves should be donned by all emergency response personnel *before* initiating any emergency care. When an emergency incident involves more than one patient, paramedics should attempt to change gloves between patients. When gloves have been contaminated, they should be removed as soon as possible. To remove gloves, the gloved fingers of one hand are first hooked under the cuff of the other glove. Then that glove is pulled off without letting the gloved fingers come in contact with bare skin. Then the fingers of the ungloved hand are slid under the remaining glove's cuff. That glove is pushed off without contact between the glove's exterior and the bare hand. Hands should always be washed after gloves are removed, even when the gloves appear intact.

- *Masks and Protective Eyewear.* Masks and protective eyewear should be present on all emergency vehicles and used in accordance with the level of exposure encountered. Proper eyewear and masks prevent a patient's blood and body fluids from spraying into paramedics' eyes, nose, and mouth. Masks and protective eyewear should be worn together whenever blood spatter is likely to occur, such as during arterial bleeding, childbirth, endotracheal intubation, invasive procedures, oral suctioning, and cleanup of equipment that requires heavy scrubbing or brushing. Both the paramedic and the patient should wear masks whenever the potential for airborne transmission of disease exists.

- *High-Efficiency Particulate Air (HEPA) Respirators.* Due to the resurgence of tuberculosis (TB), prehospital personnel should protect themselves from TB infection through use of a HEPA respirator, a design approved by the National Institute of Occupational Safety and Health. It should fit snugly and be capable of filtering out the tuberculosis bacillus. The HEPA respirator should be worn when caring for patients with confirmed or suspected TB. This is especially true when performing "high hazard" procedures such as administration of nebulized medications, endotracheal intubation, or suctioning on such a patient.

- *Gowns.* Gowns protect clothing from blood splashes. If large splashes of blood are expected, such as with childbirth, impervious gowns should be worn.
- *Resuscitation Equipment.* Disposable resuscitation equipment should be the primary means of artificial ventilation in emergency care. Such items should be used once, then disposed of.

Remember, the proper use of PPE ensures effective infection control and minimizes risk. *All* protective equipment recommended for any particular situation should be used to ensure maximum protection.

All body substances should be considered potentially infectious, and body substance isolation should *always* be practiced.

HANDLING CONTAMINATED MATERIAL

Many of the materials associated with the emergency response become contaminated with possibly infectious body fluids and substances. These include soiled linen, patient clothing and dressings, and used care equipment, including intravenous needles. It is important that prehospital personnel collect these materials at the scene and dispose of them appropriately to ensure their safety as well as that of their patients, their family members, bystanders, and fellow caregivers. Contaminated materials should be disposed of according to the following recommendations:

- Handle contaminated materials only while wearing the appropriate PPE.
- Place all blood- or body-fluid-contaminated clothing, linen, dressings, and patient care equipment and supplies in properly marked biological hazard bags and ensure they are disposed of properly.
- Ensure that all used needles, scalpels, and other contaminated objects that have the potential to puncture the skin are properly secured in a puncture-resistant and clearly marked sharps container.
- Do not recap a needle after use, stick it into a seat cushion or other object, or leave it lying on the ground. These practices increase the risk of an accidental needle stick.
- Always scan the scene before leaving to ensure all equipment has been retrieved and all potentially infectious material has been bagged and removed.
- If prehospital personnel are exposed to an infectious disease, have contact with body substances with a route for system entry (such as an open wound on a hand when a glove tears while moving a soiled patient), or receive a needle stick with a used needle, the receiving hospital should be alerted and the service's infection control officer contacted immediately.

Following these recommendations will help protect paramedics and the people they care for from the dangers of disease transmission.

1

GENERAL INFORMATION

OBJECTIVES

After completing this chapter, the reader should be able to

1. Define the terms *pharmacology, pharmacologists,* and *pharmacognosy.*
2. List four drug sources and give examples of each source.
3. Understand common pharmacological terminology and abbreviations.
4. List four references for drug information and demonstrate how to find a medication in one of these references.
5. Describe the four phases of drug development.
6. Explain the legal regulations that apply to drugs, including the schedule of controlled drugs.
7. Identify drugs by their chemical name, generic name, trade name, and official name.
8. List several examples of both liquid and soild drugs.

INTRODUCTION

Drugs are chemical agents used in the diagnosis, treatment, or prevention of disease. The study of drugs and their actions on the body is called *pharmacology.* Scientists who study the effects of drugs on the body are called *pharmacologists.* It is through experimental pharmacology that medicine has made many of its most profound advances.

Historical Considerations

The use of herbs and minerals to treat various medical disorders is as old as the practice of medicine itself. Written records of drug use date back to early Egyptian times. Ancient Egyptians, Arabs, and Greeks probably passed formulations down through generations by word of mouth for centuries until they were recorded in pharmacopeias. Hippocrates, generally considered the father of modern medicine, wrote extensively on the use of drugs, although he rarely used them in the care of his patients. After the Renaissance, healers began to take a somewhat more scientific approach to disease and found that certain drugs were useful in treating some disorders but not others. Drug therapy was based largely on observation, and physicians were frequently unsure which body systems the drugs affected. Pharmacology had now become a distinct and growing discipline, separate from medicine.

One common additive to early medications was the purple foxglove plant. A common flowering plant, the purple foxglove was first described in A.D. 1250 by Welsh physicians. It was long thought to be a diuretic because of its role in the treatment of dropsy, an old term used to describe the generalized body edema associated with congestive heart failure. In 1785 William Withering described the use of the purple foxglove plant in the treatment of dropsy and other disorders. Although he did not associate the improvement seen in the treatment of dropsy with the foxglove's effect on the heart, he did note its effectiveness. He wrote, "It has a power over the motion of the heart to a degree yet unobserved in any other medicine." It was not until 1800 that the effect of foxglove specifically on the heart was actually described and its suspected action as a diuretic finally discarded.

Digitalis is the active agent in foxglove. Digitalis tends to increase myocardial contractile force. It is this increase in cardiac performance, with subsequently improved renal perfusion and filtration, that causes a reduction in the body swelling and not its diuretic effect as earlier thought. Even today digitalis remains one of the most commonly prescribed medications in the treatment of congestive heart failure and other cardiovascular disorders.

During the seventeenth and eighteenth centuries, tinctures of opium, coca, and digitalis were available. The related concept of vaccination from biologic extracts began in 1796 with Edward Jenner's smallpox inoculations. By the nineteenth century, atropine, chloroform, codeine, ether, and morphine were in use. The discoveries of animal insulin and penicillin in the early twentieth century dramatically changed the treatment of endocrine/ metabolic and infectious diseases. Now, at the start of the twenty-first century, recombinant DNA technology has produced human insulin and tissue plasminogen activator (tPA). These drugs have markedly changed the treatment of diabetes and cardiovascular disease.

Medicine changed dramatically in the early part of the twentieth century with the discovery of antibiotics. Prior to the introduction of the sulfa-class antibiotics in 1935, physicians had virtually no effective therapy for infections. Penicillin became widely available in the early 1940s, thus providing physicians a versatile yet inexpensive antibiotic. Additional antibiotics were subsequently developed. The introduction of antibiotic therapy resulted in a significant decrease in mortality and a resultant increase in life expectancy in the United States and other developed countries.

Pharmacognosy

Traditionally, *pharmacognosy* refers to the study of natural drug sources, such as plants, animals, or minerals and their products. Today, however, chemicals developed and used in the laboratory allow researchers to increase the number of drug sources. For example, oral contraceptives, which are synthetic analogues of human sex hormones, are manufactured chemically. Chemically developed drugs are free of the impurities found in natural substances.

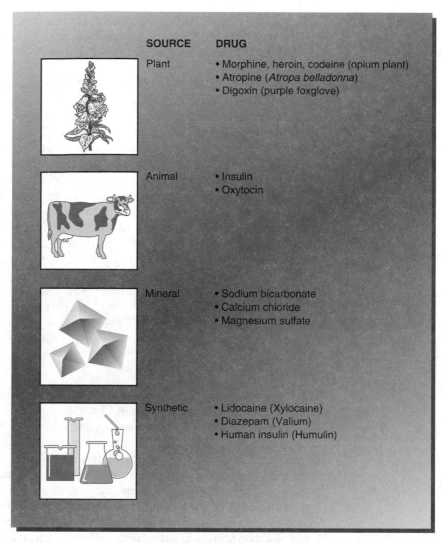

SOURCE	DRUG
Plant	• Morphine, heroin, codeine (opium plant) • Atropine (*Atropa belladonna*) • Digoxin (purple foxglove)
Animal	• Insulin • Oxytocin
Mineral	• Sodium bicarbonate • Calcium chloride • Magnesium sulfate
Synthetic	• Lidocaine (Xylocaine) • Diazepam (Valium) • Human insulin (Humulin)

FIGURE 1–1 Drug sources.

Researchers and drug developers also can now manipulate the molecular structure of substances, such as antibiotics, so that a slight change in chemical structure makes the drug effective against different organisms.

The hormone insulin, used to treat diabetes mellitus, was customarily obtained from the pancreas of slaughtered animals, mainly cattle and pigs. Although animal insulin is not chemically identical to human insulin, it is physiologically active in humans. Porcine insulin (insulin derived from pigs) most nearly resembles human insulin. The chemical alteration of three amino acids in porcine insulin makes it identical to human endogenous insulin. The chemically altered porcine insulin is marketed and usually referred to as "human insulin." Drug developers also can manufacture true human insulin from bacteria through recombinant deoxyribonucleic acid (DNA) technology.

The four main sources of drugs are plants, animals, minerals, and the laboratory (synthetic) (see Figure 1–1).

Plant Sources of Drugs

Plants may be the oldest source of medications. The earliest concoctions using plants as drug sources consisted of the entire plant, including leaves, roots, bulb, stem, seeds, buds, and blossoms. Some of the extra material was harmful to human tissues. As the understanding of plants as a drug source became more sophisticated, researchers sought to isolate the active components (the components that caused the drug's effect) and avoid the harmful material.

The active components consist of several types and vary in character and effect. The most important are alkaloids (one of the largest groups of active components), which act as alkali. The organic alkaloids react with acids to form a salt. This salt, a neutralized or partially neutralized form, is more readily soluble in body fluids. The names of alkaloids and their salts usually end in -ine; examples include atropine, caffeine, and nicotine. Atropine sulfate is used in the treatment of slow heart rates and in certain types of toxicological emergencies. Atropine is derived from the deadly nightshade plant (*Atropa belladonna*). This plant is native to central and southern Europe but cultivated widely in North America.

Another emergency medication derived from *plant sources* is morphine sulfate. Morphine is used to treat moderate to severe pain. It is made from parts of the opium plant, which is native to Turkey and other parts of the Middle East. In addition to morphine, heroin, codeine, and many other analgesic preparations are derived from the opium plant. However, because of their psychotropic effects, narcotic analgesics are subject to abuse. They also can result in physical and psychological dependence.

Animal Sources of Drugs

The body fluids or glands of animals can act as sources of drugs. The drugs obtained from animal sources include hormones, such as insulin (as previously discussed); oils and fats (usually mixed), such as cod-liver oil; and enzymes, produced by living cells, which act as catalysts. Enzymes include pancreatin and pepsin. Vaccines (suspensions of killed, modified, or attenuated microorganisms) also are obtained from animal sources. Examples of hormone drugs derived from *animal sources* include insulin and oxytocin. Both of these agents are extracted from the desiccated endocrine glands of mammals. Insulin is used in the treatment of diabetes mellitus, whereas oxytocin is used to induce labor and treat certain types of vaginal bleeding. Cod-liver oil is an example of an oil derived from animals.

Mineral Sources of Drugs

Metallic and nonmetallic minerals provide various inorganic material not available from plants or animals. The mineral sources are used as they occur in nature or are combined with other ingredients to yield acids, bases, or salts. Two emergency medications come from *mineral (inorganic) sources*. They are sodium bicarbonate ($NaHCO_3$) and magnesium sulfate ($MgSO_4$). Sodium bicarbonate is occasionally used to treat severe metabolic acidosis and is an adjunct in certain toxicological emergencies. Magnesium sulfate is used in the treatment of eclampsia, a life-threatening seizure disorder associated with pregnancy, and in some cardiac emergencies.

Laboratory-Produced Drug Sources

Researchers today produce an ever-increasing number of drugs in the laboratory. The new drugs may be natural (from animal or plant sources), *synthetic*, or a combination of the two. Examples of drugs produced in the laboratory include thyroid hormone (natural), cimetidine (synthetic), and anistreplase (combination of natural and synthetic). Recombinant DNA research has led to another chemical source of organic compounds: The reordering of genetic information enables scientists to develop bacteria that

TABLE 1–1

Sources of Drug Information

Pharmacopeia: Official

- *United States Pharmacopeia (USP)* and *National Formulary (NF)*
- *British Pharmacopeia (BP)*
- *British National Formulary (BF)*
- *Compendium of Pharmaceuticals and Specialties (CPS)*, Canada

Compendia: Nonofficial

- *Martindale: The Extra Pharmacopeia*
- *Drug Information/Hospital Formulary, American Hospital Formulary Service,* published by authority of the American Society of Hospital Pharmacists
- *Facts and Comparisons*
- *USP* dispensing information
- Pharmaceutical companies
- *Physicians' Desk Reference (PDR)*
- Package inserts: brochures required by law; content is approved by Food and Drug Administration

Journal

The Medical Letter on Drugs and Therapeutics

produce insulin for humans. This technology is used to manufacture insulin, hepatitis B vaccine, glucagon, and several other products. Insulin is manufactured by taking the genetic code for human insulin and placing it into the cells of selected bacteria. These bacteria can then be grown in large quantities, thus producing a large amount of insulin at relatively low cost.

Many drugs on the market today are synthetically derived. Common examples of emergency drugs that are synthetically manufactured include lidocaine (Xylocaine), bretylium tosylate (Bretylol), and diazepam (Valium). Lidocaine and bretylium tosylate are used to treat cardiac dysrhythmias. Valium is used to treat seizures, anxiety, and other neuropsychiatric disorders.

Sources of Drug Information

Obtaining information on drugs can be difficult. Using multiple sources of information about drugs is usually a good idea. Every book about drugs, including this one, has a disclaimer regarding doses and current uses, referring the reader to local medical direction for the final word. Using multiple sources and comparing the author's statements about a drug may lead you to the best available information. EMS providers generally like small, short guides that they can carry in a shirt pocket. These usually include important details about drugs that the prehospital providers administer along with a long list of commonly prescribed drugs and their classes. These EMS guides will be useful if you clearly understand the drugs used in your system and have a working knowledge of commonly prescribed drug classes.

Many sources of drug information are available to the prehospital provider (see Table 1–1).

DRUG RESEARCH AND BRINGING A DRUG TO MARKET

The pharmaceutical industry is highly motivated to bring profitable new drugs to market. Proving the safety and reliability of these new drugs, however, requires extensive research. While better understanding of biology is

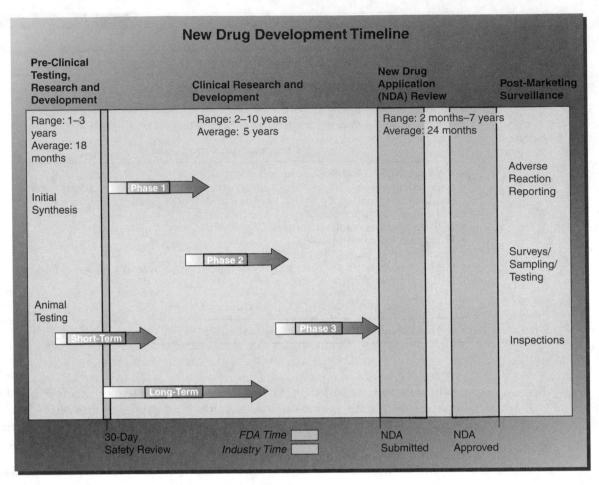

New Drug Development Timeline

Pre-Clinical Testing, Research and Development

Clinical Research and Development

New Drug Application (NDA) Review

Post-Marketing Surveillance

Range: 1–3 years
Average: 18 months

Initial Synthesis

Animal Testing

Range: 2–10 years
Average: 5 years

Phase 1

Phase 2

Phase 3

Range: 2 months–7 years
Average: 24 months

Adverse Reaction Reporting

Surveys/ Sampling/ Testing

Inspections

Short-Term

Long-Term

30-Day Safety Review

FDA Time
Industry Time

NDA Submitted

NDA Approved

CHART 1–1 New drug development timeline.

shortening the time needed to bring a new drug to market, the process still takes many years. To ensure the safety of new medications, the U.S. Food and Drug Administration (FDA) has developed a process for evaluating their safety and efficacy. The process, illustrated in Chart 1–1, adds even more time to the development cycle. Initial drug testing begins with the study of both male and female mammals. After testing a drug's toxicity, researchers evaluate its pharmacokinetics—it is absorbed, distributed, metabolized (biotransformed), and excreted—in animals. These animal studies also help determine the drug's therapeutic index (the ratio of its lethal dose to its effective dose). If the results of the animal testing are satisfactory, the FDA designates the drug as an Investigational New Drug (IND) and researchers can then test it in humans. Human studies take place in four phases.

Common Pharmacological Terminology and Abbreviations

It is common to use abbreviations in pharmacology. Abbreviations serve to expedite paperwork and promote efficiency. The abbreviations used in pharmacology are fairly standard. It is important to be familiar with these abbreviations and with some of the common terminology applicable to the field of emergency pharmacology (see Table 1–2).

TABLE 1–2

Common Abbreviations

Abbreviation	Meaning	Abbreviation	Meaning
ā	*ante* (before)	↑	increase
a.c.	*ante cibos* (before meals)	IC	intracardiac
ACh	acetylcholine	IM	intramuscular
ACLS	advanced cardiac life support	IO	intraosseous
ACS	acute coronary syndrome	IV	intravenous
admin.	administer	IVP	intravenous push
α	alpha	IVPB	intravenous piggyback
ALS	advanced life support	K^+	potassium
AMA	against medical advice	kg	kilogram
AMI	acute myocardial infarction	KO	keep open
Amp.	ampule	KVO	keep vein open
APAP	acetaminophen	LMA	laryngeal mask airway
ASA	aspirin	L	liter
β	beta	lb	pound
bid	*bis in die* (twice a day)	<	less than
c̄	*cum* (with)	LR	lactated Ringer's solution
Ca^{2+}	calcium ion	$MgSO_4$	magnesium sulfate
$CaCl_2$	calcium chloride	♂	male
caps	capsules	MAX	maximum
cc	cubic centimeter	MDI	metered-dose inhaler
CC	chief complaint	μ	micro
CHF	congestive heart failure	μgtt	microdrop
Cl^-	chloride ion	μg	microgram
cm	centimeter	mcg	microgram
cm^3	cubic centimeter	μm	micrometer
c/o	complains of	mEq	milliequivalent
CO	carbon monoxide	mg	milligram
CO_2	carbon dioxide	min	minute
COPD	chronic obstructive pulmonary disease	mL	milliliter
		mm	millimeter
CSM	carotid sinus massage	MS	morphine sulfate
CVA	cerebrovascular accident	MSO_4	morphine sulfate
°	degree	N_2O	nitrous oxide
°C	degrees Celsius	Na^+	sodium ion
°F	degrees Fahrenheit	$NaHCO_3$	sodium bicarbonate
D/C	discontinue	nitro	nitroglycerin
↓	decrease	NKA	no known allergies
D_5W	5 percent dextrose in water	NKDA	no known drug allergies
$D_{10}W$	10 percent dextrose in water	NTG	nitroglycerin
$D_{50}W$	50 percent dextrose in water	∅	null or none
dig	digitalis	O_2	oxygen
Dx	diagnosis	OD	overdose
ECG	electrocardiogram	OD	*oculus dexter* (right eye)
EKG	electrocardiogram (from German)	OS	*oculus sinister* (left eye)
elix	elixir	OU	*oculus utro* (both eyes)
EOA	esophageal obturator airway	oz	ounce
=	equal to	p	post (after)
et	and	pc	*post cibos* (after eating)
ET	endotracheal	PAC	premature atrial contraction
ETC	endotracheal Combitube	PEA	pulseless electrical activity
ETOH	alcohol (ethyl)	pedi	pediatric
♀	female	PJC	premature junctional contraction
g	gram	po	*per os* (by mouth)
gr	grain	pr	*per rectus* (by rectum)
>	greater than	prn	*pro re nata* (when necessary)
gtt	*gutta* (drop)	PSVT	paroxysmal supraventricular tachycardia
gtts	*guttae* (drops)		
HHN	handheld nebulizer	q	*quisque* (every)
hs	*hora somni* (at bedtime)	qd	*quisque die* (every day)

(continued)

TABLE 1–2 (continued)

Common Abbreviations

Abbreviation	Meaning	Abbreviation	Meaning
qh	*quisque hora* (every hour)	SpO$_2$	oxygen saturation (oximetry)
qid	*quarter in die* (four times a day)	SQ or SC	subcutaneous
qod	*tertio quoque die* (every other day)	stat	*statim* (now or immediately)
qt	quart	STEMI	ST elevation myocardial infarction
®	registered trademark	SVN	small-volume nebulizer
RL	Ringer's lactate solution	tid	*ter in die* (three times a day)
Rx	treatment	tPA	tissue plasminogen activator
s̄	*sine* (without)	TKO	to keep open
SC	subcutaneous	u	unit
SK	streptokinase	ut dict	*ut dictum* (as directed)
sol	solution	y/o	year old

FDA CLASSIFICATION OF NEWLY APPROVED DRUGS

The FDA has developed a method for immediately classifying new drugs. This method of drug classification utilizes a number and a letter for each new drug in the IND phase or upon New Drug Application (NDA) review by the FDA. The manufacturer has a right to contest this classification and have it changed before the final classification is established.

Numerical Classification (Chemical)

1. A new molecular drug

2. A new salt of a marketed drug

3. A new formulation or dosage form not previously marketed

4. A new combination not previously marketed

5. A drug that is already on the market, a generic duplication

6. A product already marketed by the same company (This designation is used for new indications for a marketed drug.)

7. A drug product on the market without NDA approval (drug was marketed prior to 1938)

Letter Classification (Treatment or Therapeutic Potential)

A. Drug offers an important therapeutic gain (P-priority)

B. Drug that is similar to drugs already on the market (S-similar)

Other Classifications

A. Drugs indicated for AIDS and HIV-related disease

B. Drugs developed to treat life-threatening or severely debilitating illness

I. An orphan drug

NEW DRUG DEVELOPMENT

In the past, drugs were found by trial and error. Now they are developed primarily by systematic research. Scientists still search for new organic and inorganic sources; however, they now focus most of their attention on the laboratory to discover needed drugs.

The FDA carefully monitors new drug development, which can take many years to complete. Testing of new drugs begins with animals to evaluate a drug's pharmacological use, dosage ranges, and possible toxic effects. Only after reviewing extensive animal studies and data on the safety and effectiveness of the proposed drug will the FDA approve the application for an investigational new drug.

Four phases of clinical evaluation involving human subjects follow approval of the IND. The clinical studies are intended to provide information on purity, bioavailability, potency, efficacy, safety, and toxicity. Depending on the results of testing, the studies can be stopped at any phase.

Phase I

The primary purposes of phase I testing are to determine the drug's pharmacokinetics, toxicity, and safe dose in humans.

In phase I, a clinical pharmacologist supervises studies involving a small number of healthy volunteers. All effects of the drug on the volunteers are recorded. The recorded clinical data determine the need for further testing.

Phase II

The primary purpose of phase II testing is to find the therapeutic drug level and watch carefully for toxic and side effects.

A small number of individuals who have the disease for which the drug is purported to be diagnostic or therapeutic are then given the drug. Supervisors carefully document toxic effects and adverse reactions to determine the drug's proper dosage. Researchers then review and compare data from the animal studies and human studies, closely monitoring effects on animal and human fertility and reproduction.

Phase III

The main purpose of phase III testing is to refine the usual therapeutic dose and to collect relevant data on side effects.

In phase III, large numbers of patients in medical research centers receive the drug. This larger sampling provides information about infrequent or rare adverse effects. Information collected during this phase helps determine risks associated with the new drug. Researchers also must perform various tests that take into account those patients who are so emotionally involved that they experience relief of symptoms based on suggestion. The administration of a placebo, a medically inert substance, to some patients provides control for such psychological responses. In one frequently used procedure, one-half of the patients receive the drug and one-half receive the placebo. To remove all bias, neither the patient nor the physician knows who has received the drug and who has received the placebo until completion of the study; this type of study is known as a double-blind study. In another type of study (crossover study) patients receive the drug for part of the time and a placebo for the rest of the time.

After the three phases, the FDA evaluates the results. If the FDA announces a favorable evaluation, the company developing the drug then completes a New Drug Application. FDA approval of the company's NDA means that the new drug has been accepted and can be marketed exclusively by its sponsoring company.

Phase IV

Phase IV testing involves post-marketing analysis during conditional approval. Once the drug is being used in the general population, the FDA requires the drug's maker to monitor its performance.

Phase IV is voluntary. After the NDA is approved, the drug company begins surveillance or post-market surveillance. It receives reports about the therapeutic results of the drug from physicians. The company must communicate adequately with the FDA and with the public during the drug's use. Some medications, such as benoxaprofen (Oraflex), have been found to be toxic and have been removed from the market after their initial release. At times, manufacturers have contended that a drug's benefits for a certain segment of the population outweigh its risks. Such was the manufacturer's response when the antidepressant tranylcypromine was withdrawn from the market. Eventually, but with certain restrictions, the FDA reinstated tranylcypromine in the market for use by patients with severe depression.

Expedited Drug Approval

Although most INDs undergo all four phases of clinical evaluation, a few can receive expedited approval. For example, because of the public health threat posed by acquired immunodeficiency syndrome (AIDS), the FDA and drug companies have agreed to shorten the IND approval process, allowing physicians to give qualified AIDS patients so-called Treatment INDs not yet approved by the FDA. Sponsors of drugs that reach phase II or III clinical trials can apply for FDA approval of Treatment IND status. When the IND is approved, the sponsor supplies the drug to physicians whose patients meet appropriate criteria.

Orphan Drugs

Some drugs useful for treating various diseases never reach the market. Drug companies do not adopt and develop these medications, appropriately referred to as orphan drugs. The reasons vary. Some orphan drugs useful for rare diseases have a limited market; others produce high-risk adverse reactions that make insurance costs prohibitive. Many useful drugs remain orphans because manufacturers cannot hope to recover the huge amounts of money spent in developing a new drug.

In 1983, Congress signed the Orphan Drug Act, which offers substantial tax credits to companies that develop orphan drugs. Small companies may receive federal financial grants to help them research and develop orphan drugs. As a result, thousands of patients may now use drugs that until recently were unavailable. Despite legislation, many orphan drugs remain without developers.

Black Box Warnings

When a special problem arises with a drug that may lead to death or serious injury, the FDA may require the manufacturer to post those warnings in a prominently displayed "black box" in the labeling material. The FDA reserves boxed warnings for risks that can be minimized by conveying the information to health care personnel in this highlighted manner. *Black box warnings* must be considered when determining whether a medication should be a part of an emergency medical service (EMS) formulary.

UNLABELED USES OF DRUGS

When approving a new drug, the FDA accepts it only for the indications for which phase II and phase III clinical studies have shown it to be safe and effective. These indications are approved (labeled); all others are not approved (unlabeled).

For example, the FDA may approve a new drug to treat hypertension if phase II and phase III studies showed that it was safe and effective for use in patients with hypertension. If the drug also works as an antianginal agent, the FDA cannot approve it for this indication unless formal studies in patients with angina pectoris are completed successfully. Such a drug is unapproved for treatment of angina pectoris, yet it may be used for this unlabeled indication, based on empirical evidence.

After prescribing a new drug approved to treat hypertension, a physician may discover that it also decreases the patient's angina. Then the physician may share this finding with colleagues in medical journals or at meetings, and they, too, may prescribe it for unlabeled uses.

The FDA recognizes that a drug's labeling does not always contain the most current information about its usage. Therefore, after the FDA approves a drug for one indication, a physician legally may prescribe it, a pharmacist may dispense it, and a nurse or paramedic may administer it for any labeled—or unlabeled—indication.

Although clinicians are not prohibited from prescribing, dispensing, or administering a drug for an unlabeled use, the FDA forbids the manufacturer from promoting a drug for any unlabeled indications. That is why drug package inserts and the *Physicians' Desk Reference* (a collection of drug manufacturers' product labeling) contain no information about unlabeled uses, and pharmaceutical sales representatives cannot discuss such uses. Nevertheless, many drugs commonly are prescribed for unlabeled uses.

MEDICAL OVERSIGHT

Prehospital care has evolved as an extension of health care provided within the hospital setting. As such, all aspects of prehospital care have traditionally fallen under the supervision of physicians. This role is referred to as medical oversight and is currently enforced by legislation throughout Canada and the United States. Although the specifics of this legislation vary from province to province and state to state, it is based on a common theme involving all prehospital care providers acting under the direction and control of a physician. The prehospital care provider is acting as a delegate for the physician and is, in essence, working under the medical license of the physician providing medical control.

The Medical Director

The individual physician who assumes the medical oversight role described in the previous section is designated the *medical director*. The medical director is typically a licensed physician active in emergency medicine with an understanding of, and experience in, prehospital care. The specific duties of the medical director include development and implementation of medical control guidelines, education, quality assurance, equipment, and medication review, and assessment of competency. The role of the medical director has also evolved in recent years to include some scene response and field triage at mass casualty incidents. The medical director is responsible for the actions of care providers working under his or her medical control and, as such, is the ultimate authority with respect to all medical control and competency issues. Because prehospital care providers work under the license of the medical director, the medical director can be found medicolegally liable in cases of litigation involving prehospital care. In some systems, the medical director receives input from a medical control or medical advisory board, which generally has physician representation from the various institutions served by the EMS system. The roles and authority of these types of committees are system specific. Although the level of involvement of the medical director within an EMS system varies, ideally that individual should have ongoing exposure to activities in the field as a means of staying abreast of medical and operational issues. Care providers should view the medical director as a resource who can provide constructive feedback and answer questions as they arise. At the same time, the medical director must serve as a patient advocate, ensuring that patient care is the foremost priority.

Medical Control

Medical control constitutes one of the components of medical oversight and can be further subdivided into direct (on-line) and indirect (off-line) medical control.

Direct Medical Control

Direct medical control refers to orders given directly to prehospital care providers by a physician, generally via radio or telephone. Typically the prehospital care provider speaks to a physician in the emergency department to which the patient is being transported. Also known as a "base" physician, this individual is generally well acquainted with local medical control guidelines and the overall capabilities of the local EMS system and personnel.

Indirect Medical Control

Indirect medical control essentially includes all aspects of medical oversight that do not involve direct medical control, including system design, protocol development, education, and quality improvement. To be effective, medical control must have the authority to discipline or limit the activities of those who deviate from an established standard of care. As an advancing field, prehospital care demands a commitment to lifelong learning, and it is the responsibility of both the care provider and the medical director to ensure that this process is ongoing. The education component of prehospital care is becoming increasingly important as the complexity of care, including medications and equipment, increases. The importance of training and education can be demonstrated by the ever-increasing number of medications and interventions provided in the field that have lethal potential if used inappropriately.

Medical Control Protocols and Guidelines

All treatments and interventions in the prehospital field are provided under the direct or indirect orders of a physician. Many of these orders are provided in the form of medical protocols that provide an algorithm for treating patients in the field. Many systems provide *standing orders* or standing protocols that allow the care provider to treat patients without speaking to a physician. These *treatment protocols* are designed to facilitate management of specific presenting signs and symptoms rather than a specific diagnosis. Certain treatments and presenting problems may require base physician contact prior to implementation. Recently some EMS systems have implemented treat-and-release protocols that allow staff to release patients who respond to treatment and meet certain preestablished criteria. This is an example of the ever-increasing responsibility that prehospital care providers face, and it emphasizes the importance of education, judgment, and critical-thinking skills.

Legal Regulations, Standards, and Legislation

As a society develops and uses drugs, it needs to establish controls regulating the manufacture, distribution, and use of those drugs. In many cases a society's attitude and values, rather than formal controls, determine the acceptable limits of drug use. Formal drug controls range from individual institutional policies to governmental legislation.

International Controls

The United Nations, through its World Health Organization, attempts to influence international health by providing technical assistance and encouraging research for drug use. One committee has been established to cope with the problems associated with habit-forming drugs. Drug enforcement agencies in various nations cooperate, but no administrative or judicial structures enforce controls. As a result, control of international drug trade depends largely on the voluntary cooperation of nations.

Controls in the United States

Before a drug can be marketed, it must undergo extensive testing. This testing generally involves two phases, animal studies and clinical patient studies. Only after these extensive tests, and with governmental approval, can drugs be placed on the market. Even after clinical usage, the effectiveness of the drugs must be closely monitored. The FDA is the federal agency responsible for approval of drugs before they are made available to the general public.

Legislative control in the United States began in 1906, when Congress enacted the Pure Food and Drug Act. In addition to establishing the FDA, this act prohibited the sale of medicinal preparations that had little or no use and restricted the sale of drugs with a potential for abuse. The Pure Food and Drug Act named the *United States Pharmacopeia (USP)* and the *National Formulary (NF)* as official drug standards. Any drug bearing the official title *USP* or *NF* must conform to rigid standards regarding purity, preparation, and dosage.

The Pure Food and Drug Act was not as all-encompassing as its planners had envisioned it to be. For several years stronger drug laws were debated in both Congress and state legislatures. In the 1930s more than 100 people died from ingesting sulfanilamide, an antibacterial drug. Researchers discovered that the sulfanilamide had been prepared with a previously uninvestigated toxic substance called diethylene glycol. Finally in 1938, Congress enacted the Federal Food, Drug, and Cosmetic Act. Among the most important features of this act was the truth-in-labeling clause. The act required the following:

1. A statement accurately describing the package's contents
2. The usual names of the drugs, for official drugs (preparations listed in the pharmacopeia and adopted by the government as meeting pharmaceutical standards) and nonofficial drugs (drugs not listed in the pharmacopeia)

3. Indication of the presence, quantity, and proportion of certain drugs (such as alcohol, atropine, and bromides)

4. Warning of habit-forming drugs in the product and of their effects

5. The names of the manufacturer, packager, and distributor

6. Directions for use and warnings against unsafe use, including recommendations for dosage levels and frequency

Narcotics

A problem almost as old as medicine itself is abuse and addiction to certain drugs. Narcotics are among the drugs most frequently abused. Recognizing the need to control the sale of narcotics, the federal government enacted the Harrison Narcotic Act in 1914. This act served to control the importation, manufacture, and sale of the opium plant and its derivatives. It also controlled the derivatives of the coca plant. The primary drug derived from the coca plant is cocaine. As a result of this act, these drugs, as well as other drugs added to the list later, could be obtained only with special prescriptions. Only physicians who qualified and attained a special narcotic license could prescribe this class of drugs.

In 1970 major revisions were made in the use and control of narcotics and other drugs. This law, the Comprehensive Drug Abuse Prevention and Control Act of 1970 (commonly called the Controlled Substances Act of 1970), classifies the drugs used in medicine into five different schedules. A summary of the five schedules is found in Table 1–3.

The Controlled Substances Act

The Controlled Substances Act mandates that prescriptions for Schedule II drugs cannot be refilled. Moreover, it requires that prescriptions for Schedule II drugs be filled within 72 hours. Prescriptions for drugs in this class cannot be called into the pharmacy over the telephone (except in special situations). Prescriptions for drugs in Schedules III and IV may be refilled up to five times within 6 months. Prescriptions for Schedule V drugs may be refilled at the discretion of the physician.

Responsibility for enforcing the Controlled Substances Act rests with the U.S. Drug Enforcement Administration (DEA). Only physicians approved by the DEA may write prescriptions for scheduled drugs. The physician must indicate his or her DEA number on the prescription. Many states have enacted laws further regulating controlled substances.

Canadian Drug Legislation

Drug control in Canada falls under the direct supervision of the Department of National Health and Welfare. The Food and Drug Act, passed in 1941, empowers the governor-in-council to prescribe drug standards and limit variation in any food or drug. The 1953 Canadian Food and Drug Act (amended yearly) provides regulations for drug manufacture and sale. A comparison of the drug schedules in the United States and Canada is found in Table 1–3.

Canadian Narcotic Control Act and Regulations

In 1965, the Canadian Narcotic Control Act restricted the sale, possession, and use of narcotics. It further restricted narcotics to authorized personnel.

TABLE 1–3

Schedule of Controlled Drugs

United States		Canada	
Category	*Examples*	**Category**	*Examples*

Schedule I
No recognized medical
   use
High abuse potential
Research use only
	Opiates
	Heroin
	Hallucinogens
	LSD
	Mescaline
	Depressants
	Methaqualone
		Schedule H
		Restricted drugs
		No recognized medicinal
		   properties
			Hallucinogens
			Peyote
			LSD
			Mescaline

Schedule II
Written prescriptions
   required
No telephone renewals
In an emergency, a
   prescription may be
   renewed by telephone
	Opiates
	Codeine
	Morphine
	Meperidine
	Stimulants
	Amphetamines
	Phenmetrazine
	Depressants
	Secobarbital
		Narcotics schedule
		Stringently restricted
		   drugs
		The letter *N* must appear
		   on all labels and
		   professional
		   advertisements
			Coca leaf derivatives
			Cocaine
			Opiates and opiate
			   derivatives
			Morphine
			Codeine
			Methadone
			Hydromorphone
			Meperidine
			Other drugs
			Phencyclidine
			Cannabis

Schedule III
Prescriptions required
   to be rewritten after
   6 months or five refills
Prescriptions may be
   ordered by telephone
	Opiates
	Codeine of less than
	   1.8 g/dL
	Opium of less than
	   25 mg/5 mL
	Stimulants
	Benzphetamine
	Mazindol
	Depressants
	Butabarbital
	Glutethimide
	Talbutal
	Anabolic steroids
	Ethylestrenol
	Fluoxymesterone
	Methyltestosterone
	Nandrolone decanoate
		Schedule G
		Controlled drugs
		Prescriptions are
		   controlled because of
		   the abuse potential of
		   these drugs
			Narcotic analgesics
			Nalbuphine
			Butorphanol
			Stimulants
			Amphetamines
			Barbiturates
			Phenobarbital
			Amobarbital
			Secobarbital

Schedule IV
Prescriptions required
   to be rewritten after
   6 months or five refills
	Opiates
	Pentazocine
	Propoxyphene
	Stimulants
	Fenfluramine
	Phentermine
	Depressants
	Benzodiazepines
	Chloral hydrate
		Schedule F
		Prescription drugs
		Although not controlled
		   drugs, agents in this
		   category include some
		   with a relatively low
		   abuse potential
		The symbol *Pr* must
		   appear on their labels
			Anxiolytics
			Benzodiazepines

Schedule V
Dispenses as any
   (nonnarcotic)
   prescription
Some may be dispensed
   without prescription
   unless additional state
   regulations apply
	Primarily small amounts
	   of opiates, such as
	   opium, dihydrocodeine,
	   and diphenoxylate,
	   when used as
	   antitussives or
	   antidiarrheals in
	   combination products
		Nonprescription drug
		   schedule (group 3)
		Drugs available only in
		   the pharmacy and
		   used only on a
		   physician's
		   recommendation
		Limited public access
			Analgesics
			Low-dose codeine
			   preparations
			Other drugs
			Insulin
			Nitroglycerin
			Muscle relaxants

This act defines who may prescribe a narcotic drug, such as physicians, dentists, research personnel, and their agents, and places conditions on the recipient of a narcotic prescription, requiring disclosure of all previous narcotics received within the past 30 days. In addition, the act describes procedures for record keeping and dispensing by pharmacists. Hospital regulations are also outlined.

Methadone is covered individually in this act, which sets requirements for authorized practitioners who prescribe and dispense this drug.

Drug Standards

The federal government establishes and enforces drug standards to ensure the uniform quality of drugs. Because some generic drugs affect patients differently than their brand name counterparts, standardization of drugs is necessary. Despite FDA standards, drugs sold or distributed by various manufacturers may have biological or therapeutic differences. An assay determines the amount of purity of a given chemical in a preparation in the laboratory (*in vitro*). While two generically equivalent preparations may contain the same amount of a given chemical (drug), they may have different therapeutic effects. This relative therapeutic effectiveness is determined by a bioassay, which attempts to ascertain their bioequivalence. The *United States Pharmacopeia* is the official standard for the United States. These standards pertain to the following drug properties:

Purity   refers to the uncontaminated state of a drug containing only one active component. In reality, a drug consisting of only one active compound rarely exists because manufacturers usually must add other ingredients to facilitate drug formation and to determine absorption rate. As a result, standards of purity do not demand 100 percent pure active ingredients but specify the type and acceptable amount of extraneous material.

Bioavailability   describes the degree to which a drug becomes absorbed and reaches general circulation. Factors affecting bioavailability include the particle size, crystalline structure, solubility, and polarity of the compound. The blood or tissue concentration of a drug at a specified time after administration usually determines bioavailability.

Potency   of a drug refers to its strength or its power to produce the desired effect. Potency standards are set by testing laboratory animals to determine the definite measurable effect of an administered drug.

Efficacy   refers to the effectiveness of a drug used in treatment. Objective clinical trials attempt to determine efficacy, but absolute measurement remains difficult.

Safety and toxicity   are determined by the incidence and severity of reported adverse reactions to the use of a drug. Some harmful effects may not appear for a considerable time. Safety and toxicity standards are being refined constantly as past experiences illuminate deficiencies in the standards.

Drug Names

Drugs are identified by four different names: chemical, generic, trade, and official. A drug's chemical name precisely describes its atomic and molecular structure. Because drugs are usually chemically complex in nature, so too are the chemical names. When a manufacturer decides to market a new drug, the United States Adopted Names (USAN) Council selects a generic name. The *generic name,* usually an abbreviated version of the chemical name, is frequently used. Manufacturers of pharmaceuticals rarely refer to drugs by their generic names. Instead, they select a name for a drug that is based on its chemical name or on the type of problem it is used to treat. This is referred to as the *trade name.* Trade names are always capitalized, whereas generic names are not. Trade names are protected by copyright. The symbol ® after the trade name means it is registered by and restricted to the drug manufacturer. The fourth method of naming a drug is the *official name.* The official name is followed by the initials *USP* or *NF,* which are official publications that list drugs conforming to standards set forth by the publication. The official name is usually the same as the generic name. Following is an example of the four names of a specific drug:

Chemical name: *Ethyl 1-methyl-4-phenylisonipecotate hydrochloride*
Generic name: Meperidine hydrochloride
Trade name: Demerol Hydrochloride
Official name: Meperidine hydrochloride, *USP*

Proprietary (Trade) Names

In recent years, controversy has developed regarding generic and nongeneric drugs. When writing a prescription, a physician can order the drug by either the trade name or the generic name. Until recently, the pharmacist had to fill the prescription as written. Now, in many states, the pharmacist may substitute a less expensive generic drug for the prescription. As a rule, generic drugs are not inferior in quality. They are usually cheaper because lesser known companies with minimal advertising and production costs manufacture them.

Most pharmaceutical houses market their drugs primarily under trade names rather than under generic names. Today a single drug may be sold under a number of trade names. The practice of using these trade names is often confusing to the medical provider and sometimes even to the physician, to say nothing of the inconvenience to the pharmacist, who must stock four or five different brands of the same drug. Currently, there is a trend to return to the use of official or generic names on prescriptions. When a physician orders a specific trade name, however, the pharmacist must dispense it. No other brand, even if the product is exactly the same as the one ordered, may be substituted without the physician's knowledge and consent.

Drugs that share similar characteristics are grouped together as a pharmacological class (family), such as beta-blockers. A second grouping is the therapeutic classification, which groups drugs by therapeutic use, such as antihypertensives. Thiazides and beta-blockers are both antihypertensives, but they share few characteristics.

COMPONENTS OF A DRUG PROFILE

A drug's profile describes its various properties. As a paramedic or paramedic student, you will become familiar with drug profiles as you study specific medications. A typical drug profile will contain the following information:

Names.   These most frequently include the generic and trade names, although the occasional reference will include chemical names.

Classification. This is the broad group to which the drug belongs. Knowing classifications is essential to understanding the properties of drugs.

Mechanism of action. The way in which a drug caused its effects; its pharmacodynamics.

Indications. Conditions that made administration of the drug appropriate (as approved by the Food and Drug Administration).

Pharmacokinetics. How the drug is absorbed, distributed, and eliminated; typically includes onset and duration of action.

Side effects/adverse reactions. The drug's untoward or undesired effects.

Routes of administration. How the drug is given.

Contraindications. Conditions that make it inappropriate to give the drug. Unlike when the drug is simply not indicated, a contraindication means that a predictable harmful event will occur if the drug is given in this situation.

Dosage. The amount of the drug that should be given.

How supplied. This typically includes the common concentrations of the available preparations; many drugs come in different concentrations.

Special considerations. How the drug may affect pediatric, geriatric, or pregnant patients.

Drug profiles may also include other components, such as its interactions with other drugs or with foods, when appropriate.

Drug Forms

Drugs come in many forms and are packaged in numerous styles. Each form and each style has advantages and disadvantages. For example, drugs taken by mouth tend to have a slow and unpredictable rate of absorption and thus a slower rate of onset of effect. Drugs given intravenously, although rapidly acting, are much more difficult to administer. Drugs may be packaged in unit-dose form, in which one dose of a drug comes in a labeled container or wrapper. They may also be packaged in bulk form, in which multiple doses of a drug are packaged in a container, bottle, or wrapper.

Drugs are manufactured in many different forms including liquids, solids, suppositories, inhalants, sprays, creams, lotions, patches, and lozenges. To administer drugs safely, you must be knowledgeable about the different effects of the many drug forms. For example, nitroglycerin administered sublingually (allowing it to dissolve under the tongue) can relieve anginal pain in less than 1 minute. The same drug administered as an ointment applied to the chest wall may not relieve acute pain at all; however, it may be used prophylactically for anginal pain. Common drug preparations are described in the following sections.

Liquid Drugs

Liquid drugs usually consist of a powder dissolved in a liquid. The drug is referred to as the *solute.* The liquid into which it is dissolved is called the *solvent.* In liquid drug preparations, the primary difference between one preparation and another is the solvent.

Solutions. Solutions are preparations that contain the drug dissolved in a solvent, usually water (for example, 5 percent dextrose in water).

Tinctures. Tinctures are drug preparations whereby the drug was extracted chemically with alcohol. They usually contain some dilute alcohol (for example, tincture of iodine).

Suspensions. Suspensions are drugs that do not remain dissolved. After sitting for even short periods, these drugs tend to separate. They must always be shaken well before use (for example, penicillin preparations).

Spirits. Spirit solutions contain volatile chemicals dissolved in alcohol (for example, spirit of ammonia).

Emulsions. Emulsions are preparations in which an oily substance is mixed with a solvent into which it does not dissolve. When mixed, it forms globules of fat floating in the solvent. An example of a common emulsion outside of medicine is oil and vinegar salad dressing.

Elixirs. Elixirs are preparations that contain the drug in an alcohol solvent. Flavoring, often cherry, is added to improve the taste (for example, Tylenol Elixir).

Syrups. Often drugs are suspended in sugar and water to improve the taste. These are referred to as syrups (for example, cough syrup).

Liquid drugs administered into the body through intramuscular, subcutaneous, or intravenous routes are called *parenteral drugs.* Most drugs used in emergency medicine are parenteral. Because they are introduced into the body, they must be sterile.

Liquid drugs given parenterally are available in four packaging styles: vials, ampules, self-contained systems or syringes, and nebules. Sterile parenteral containers designed to carry a single patient dose are called *ampules* (see Figure 1–2). An ampule is a glass container with a thin neck, which usually is scored so it can be snapped off. After the tops are broken, the drug is drawn into a syringe for administration.

In emergency medicine many drugs given parenterally are in self-contained systems or *prefilled syringes* (see Figures 1–3 and 1–4). These preparations save time by avoiding the problems inherent with ampules. Self-contained systems or prefilled syringes contain a single dose of a drug in a plastic bag or in a prefilled syringe with an attached needle. Prefilled

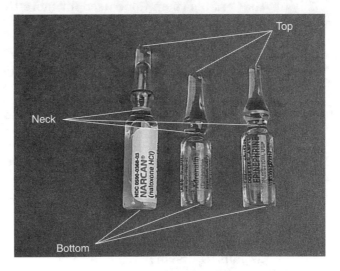

FIGURE 1–2 Ampules.

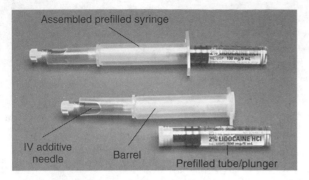

FIGURE 1–3 Prefilled syringes.

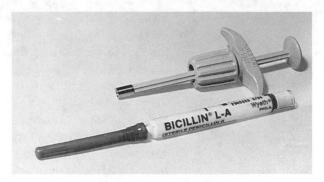

FIGURE 1–4 Tubex syringes.

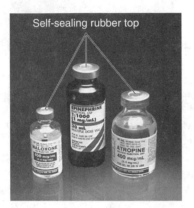

FIGURE 1–5 Multidose vials.

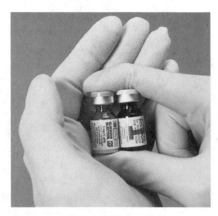

FIGURE 1–6 Single-dose vials.

syringes are often used during cardiopulmonary resuscitation and other advanced life support activities.

Vials are another type of container for parenteral drugs (see Figures 1–5 and 1–6). Vials are bottles sealed with a rubber diaphragm and may contain a single or multiple doses. Multidose vials contain preservatives that enable them to be used for more than one dose, whereas single-dose vials do not contain such agents. Many drugs used in emergency medicine are supplied in vials.

Nebules are used for medications that are premixed. For example, salbutamol (Ventolin) and ipratropium bromide (Atrovent) are both administered to the patient by nebulizer. Each nebule is filled with the amount of medication generally administered to an adult patient.

Solid Drugs

Solid drugs are usually administered orally, although many can be administered rectally. They include the following:

Pills. Pills are drugs that are shaped into a form that makes them easy to swallow.

Powders. Powders are drugs in powdered form. They are not as popular as pills, but some are still in use (for example, B.C. powder).

Capsules. Capsules consist of gelatin containers into which a powder is placed. The gelatin dissolves, liberating the powder (for example, Dalmane capsules) into the gastrointestinal tract.

Tablets. Tablets are similar to pills. They are composed of a powder that has been compressed into an easily swallowed form and are often covered with a sugar coating to improve taste.

Suppositories

Administered rectally and vaginally, suppositories carry medications in a solid base that melts at body temperature. Suppositories produce local (analgesic, laxative, and anti-infective) and systemic (antiemetic, antipyretic, and analgesic) effects. Usually bullet shaped, most suppositories are about 1 inch (2.5 cm) long and require lubrication for insertion. Because they melt at body temperature, suppositories require refrigeration until administration. When placed into the body, either rectally or vaginally, they dissolve and are then absorbed into the surrounding tissue.

Inhalants

Inhalants are powered or liquid forms of a drug that are given using the respiratory route and are absorbed rapidly by the rich supply of capillaries in the lungs. Several frequently used methods of inhalation are nebulizers, metercd-dose aerosol, or turbo inhalers or vaporizers.

IMPORTANT PHARMACOLOGICAL TERMINOLOGY

Important pharmacological terminology includes the following:

Antagonism. Antagonism signifies the opposition between two or more medications (for example, between Naloxone and morphine).

Bolus. A bolus is a single, oftentimes large dose of mcdication (for example, lidocaine bolus, which is often followed by a lidocaine infusion).

Contraindications. Contraindications are the medical or physiological conditions present in a patient that would make it harmful to administer a medication of otherwise known therapeutic value.

Cumulative action. A cumulative action occurs when a drug is administered in several doses, causing an increased effect. This increased effect is usually due to a quantitative buildup of the drug in the blood.

Depressant. A depressant is a medication that decreases or lessens a body function or activity.

Habituation. Habituation is physical or psychological dependence on a drug.

Hypersensitivity. Hypersensitivity is a reaction to a substance that is normally more profound than seen in a population not sensitive to the substance (for example, an allergic reaction to penicillin).

Idiosyncrasy. An idiosyncrasy is an individual reaction to a drug that is unusually different from that seen in the rest of the population.

Indication. An indication refers to the medical condition or conditions in which the drug has proven to be of therapeutic value.

Potentiation.   Potentiation is the enhancement of one drug's effects by another (for example, barbiturates and alcohol).

Refractory.   Patients or conditions that do not respond to a drug are said to be refractory to the drug (for example, a patient with premature ventricular contractions who does not respond to lidocaine).

Side effects.   Side effects are the unavoidable, undesired effects frequently seen even in therapeutic drug dosages.

Stimulant.   A stimulant is a drug that enhances or increases a bodily function (for example, caffeine in coffee).

Synergism.   Synergism is the combined action of two drugs. The action is much stronger than the effects of either drug administered separately.

Therapeutic action.   A therapeutic action is the desired, intended action of a drug given in the appropriate medical condition.

Tolerance.   When patients are receiving drugs on a long-term basis, they may require larger and larger dosages of the drug to achieve a therapeutic effect. This increased requirement is termed *tolerance.*

Untoward effect.   An untoward effect is a side effect that proves harmful to the patient.

SUMMARY

Drugs are chemical agents used in the diagnosis, treatment, or prevention of disease. They are necessary for successful emergency care. It is important to be familiar with the commonly used emergency medications and with the terminology and abbreviations used in medicine so that communication with other medical personnel will be efficient and professional. Overall, it is essential to appreciate the inherent danger of any and all drugs and to use them properly. The rule to remember is, *When in doubt, do no harm.*

KEY WORDS

assay.   A test that determines the amount and purity of a given chemical in a preparation in the laboratory.

bioassay.   Test to ascertain a drug's availability in a biological model.

bioequivalence.   Relative therapeutic effectiveness of chemically equivalent drugs.

black box warning.   Special warning placed on a drug label listing any special problems that may lead to death or serious injury.

controlled drug.   Federal, state, and local laws control the use of a drug that may lead to drug abuse or drug dependence.

drug.   Any substance introduced into the body that changes a body function.

drug abuse.   The self-directed use of drugs for nontherapeutic purposes, a practice that does not comply with a culture's sociocultural norms.

drug dependence.   Condition in which a person cannot control drug intake; may be physiological, psychological, or both.

Drug Enforcement Administration (DEA).   Federal agency with responsibility for enforcing the Controlled Substances Act.

empirical. Skill or knowledge based entirely on experience.

enteral. Administration of a drug via the gastrointestinal tract.

Food and Drug Administration (FDA). The federal agency responsible for approval of drugs before they are made available to the general public.

genetic engineering. Also called recombinant DNA technology; involves taking genetic material (DNA) from one organism and placing it into another.

medical director. A licensed physician who serves as the chief medical officer of an EMS or educational program system. Each paramedic functions under the license of the system medical director.

National Formulary. The Pure Food and Drug Act named the *National Formulary (NF)* and the *United States Pharmacopeia (USP)* as official drug standards. Any drug bearing the official title *NF* or *USP* must conform to a rigid set of standards regarding purity, preparation, and dosage.

off-line medical control. Also known as *indirect medical control;* the establishment of system policies and procedures, such as training, chart review, protocol development, audit, and quality improvement.

on-line medical control. Also known as *direct medical control;* communication between field personnel and a medical control physician, with the medical control physician providing immediate direction for on-scene care.

parenteral. Routes of administering drugs into the body without going through the digestive tract.

pharmacologist. Scientist who studies the effects of drugs on the body.

pharmacology. The study of drugs and their actions on the body.

recombinant DNA technology. Also called genetic engineering; involves taking genetic material (DNA) from one organism and placing it into another.

solute. A powder (drug) that is dissolved in a liquid (solvent).

solvent. The liquid into which a drug (solute) is dissolved.

standing orders. Written directives that may be carried out without, or prior to, contacting medical control.

synthetic. Substance made by combining two or more simpler compounds.

treatment protocols. Treatment guidelines for prehospital care. They may incorporate standing orders or may require contact with medical control prior to initiating advanced life support therapy.

United States Pharmacopeia. The Pure Food and Drug Act named the *United States Pharmacopeia (USP)* and the *National Formulary (NF)* as official drug standards. Any drug bearing the official title *USP* or *NF* must conform to a rigid set of standards regarding purity, preparation, and dosage.

PHARMACOKINETICS AND PHARMACODYNAMICS

OBJECTIVES

After completing this chapter, the reader should be able to:

1. Define pharmacokinetics and pharmacodynamics.
2. Define drug absorption and explain the factors involved in drug absorption.
3. Explain the factors that can affect drug distribution.
4. Explain biotransformation.
5. Explain how a drug is eliminated from the body and list factors that affect elimination.
6. Understand the mechanisms of action of drugs.
7. Explain the special considerations in drug therapy.

INTRODUCTION

To exert its desired biochemical and physiological effects on the body, a drug must reach its targeted tissues in a suitable form and in a sufficient concentration. The study of how drugs enter the body, reach their site of action, and eventually become eliminated is termed *pharmacokinetics*. Once drugs reach their targeted tissues, they begin a chain of biochemical events that ultimately leads to the physiological changes desired. These biochemical and physiological events are called the drug's *mechanism of action*.

After describing pharmacokinetics this chapter describes *pharmacodynamics*, or the mechanisms by which drugs produce biochemical or physiological changes in the body. It describes the interaction between drugs and receptors as well as drug action and drug effect. Pharmacotherapeutics addresses the different types of therapy and identifies factors that influence the choice of drug therapy and the patient's response to drugs during therapy.

This chapter addresses the fundamentals of pharmacokinetics, pharmacodynamics, and pharmacotherapeutics as they apply to prehospital emergency care.

PHARMACOLOGY

Pharmacology is the study of drugs and their interaction with the body. Drugs do not confer any new properties on cells or tissues; they only modify or exploit existing conditions. They may be given for their local action (in which case systemic absorption of the drug is discouraged) or for systemic action. Although generally given for a specific effect, drugs tend to have multiple actions at multiple sites, so they must be thought of in terms of their systemic effects rather than in terms of an isolated single effect. Pharmacology's two major divisions are pharmacokinetics and pharmacodynamics. Pharmacokinetics addresses how drugs are transported into and out of the body. Pharmacodynamics deals with their effects once they reach the target tissues.

PHARMACOKINETICS

Strictly defined, pharmacokinetics is the study of the basic processes that determine the duration and intensity of a drug's effect. These four processes are absorption, distribution, biotransformation, and elimination.

To produce its desired effects, a drug must be present in the appropriate concentration at its various sites of action. Lidocaine, a drug commonly used in the treatment of life-threatening ventricular dysrhythmias, must reach its target—cardiac tissue—rapidly and in a sufficient concentration to suppress the dysrhythmia. Several factors influence the concentration of a drug at its site of action. These factors include *absorption* of the drug into the circulatory system; *distribution* of the drug throughout the body; *biotransformation* of the drug into its active form, if required; and, finally, *elimination* of the drug from the body. All of these factors do not play a role in every medication used in prehospital care, but a fundamental understanding of each of these factors is essential.

REVIEW OF PHYSIOLOGY OF TRANSPORT

Pharmacokinetics is dependent on the body's various physiological mechanisms that move substances across the body's compartments. These mechanisms can be broken down into two broad categories based on their energy requirements and then further classified. A mechanism is referred to as *active transport* if it requires the use of energy to move a substance. This energy is achieved by the breakdown of high-energy chemical bonds found in chemicals such as ATP (adenosine triphosphate). ATP is broken down into ADP (adenosine diphosphate) liberating a considerable amount of biochemical energy. A common example of an active transport mechanism is the sodium-potassium (Na^+-K^+) pump. This is a protein pump that actively moves sodium ions into the cell and potassium ions out of the cell. Because this movement goes against the ion's concentration gradients, it must use energy.

Large molecules, such as glucose and most of the amino acids, do not readily pass through the cell membrane because of their size. These molecules are moved across the cell membrane with the help of special "carrier" proteins found on the surface of the target cells. These large molecules are "carried" across the cell membrane in a special transport process called carrier-mediated diffusion or facilitated diffusion. Once the molecule to be transported binds with the carrier protein, the configuration of the cell membrane changes, allowing the large molecule to enter the target cell. Insulin, an important hormone secreted by the endocrine pancreas, can increase the rate of carrier-mediated glucose transport from 10- to 20-fold. This is the principal mechanism by which insulin controls glucose use in the body.

Most drugs travel through the body by means of passive transport, the movement of a substance without the use of energy. This requires the presence of concentration gradients in a solution. Diffusion and osmosis are forms of passive transport. Diffusion involves the movement of solute in the solution, whereas osmosis involves the movement of the solvent (usually water). In diffusion, the solute's molecules or ions move down their concentration gradients from an area of higher concentration to an area of lower concentration. Conversely, in osmosis the solvent's molecules move up the concentration gradient to an area of higher concentration. Another way of looking at this is to think of osmosis as simply the diffusion of solvent from an area of high solvent concentration to an area of low solvent concentration. A final type of passive transport is filtration. This is simply the movement of molecules across a membrane down a pressure gradient, from an area of high pressure to an area of low pressure. This pressure typically results from the hydrostatic force of blood pressure.

Drug Absorption

Drug absorption encompasses a drug's progress from its pharmaceutical dosage form to a biologically available substance that can then pass through or across tissues. The transformation from dosage form to a biologically available substance must occur before the active drug ingredient reaches the systemic circulation. After a tablet or capsule disintegrates in the stomach or small intestine, enough liquid must be available for the active drug ingredients to dissolve before systemic absorption can occur. The body requires a solution of the drug's active ingredients to dissolve before systemic absorption can occur because tissues cannot absorb dry powders or dry crystals. Because syrups and suspensions occur in dosage form as solutions, their progress from drug administration to drug absorption is more rapid, leading to a quicker onset of drug action.

Absorption is the process of movement of a drug from the site of application into the body and into the extracellular compartment. The duration and intensity of a drug's action are directly related to the rate of absorption of the drug. Many factors affect drug absorption, including:

1. Solubility of the drug
2. Concentration of the drug
3. pH of the drug
4. Site of absorption
5. Absorbing surface area
6. Blood supply to the site of absorption
7. Bioavailability

The *solubility* is the tendency of a drug to dissolve. To facilitate drug absorption, the solubility of the administered drug must match the cellular constituents of the absorption site. Lipid-soluble (fat-soluble) drugs can penetrate lipoid (fat-containing) cells; water-soluble drugs cannot. For example, a water-soluble drug such as penicillin cannot penetrate the highly lipoid cells that act as barriers between the blood and brain. However a highly lipoid-soluble drug such as thiopental can penetrate the lipoid cells, cross into the brain, and induce an effect such as anesthesia. The human body is approximately 60 percent water. Thus, drugs given in water solutions are more rapidly absorbed than those given in oil-based solutions, suspensions, or solid forms.

The *concentration* of a drug also affects the rate of absorption. Drugs administered in high concentrations are absorbed much more rapidly than drugs administered in low concentrations.

Another factor that affects drug absorption is the *pH* of a drug. The pH refers to how acidic or how basic (alkaline) the drug is. Most drugs are either weak acids or weak bases. Acidic drugs tend to be more rapidly absorbed when placed into an acidic environment (such as the stomach). Alkaline drugs, on the other hand, are more rapidly absorbed when placed into an alkaline environment (such as the kidneys).

The *site of absorption* directly affects the rate of drug absorption. Once administered, drugs must pass through the various biological membranes until they reach the circulation. Drugs placed on the skin (transdermal route) must pass through several cell layers before reaching the circulatory system. On the other hand, drugs placed on mucous membranes (intranasal route) have many fewer cell layers through which to pass. Thus, drug absorption through mucous membranes is faster than drug absorption through the skin. It is sometimes useful to have slow absorption of a drug. A common emergency drug for which prolonged absorption is desired is nitroglycerin; nitroglycerin can be placed on the skin, where it is slowly absorbed over a prolonged period.

The *surface area* of the absorbing surface is an important determinant of the rate of drug absorption. Drugs are absorbed quite rapidly from large surface areas. Inhaled medications are quickly distributed across the vast pulmonary epithelium. Drugs administered by this route are rapidly absorbed into the circulation. In fact, some studies have shown that the rate of drug absorption through the inhaled route is nearly as rapid as administration by the intravenous route.

Finally, drug absorption is related to *blood supply* to the site of absorption. Some areas of the body have very rich blood supplies, whereas other areas do not. Medications placed in areas with rich blood supplies, such as the tissues under the tongue (sublingual), are absorbed rapidly. Medications placed in areas with poor blood supply, such as the fatty tissues (subcutaneous), are absorbed slowly. Muscle, as a rule, is more richly supplied with blood vessels than is subcutaneous tissue. Therefore, one would expect a drug to be absorbed more rapidly from muscle than from subcutaneous tissue (see Figure 2–1).

Knowledge of the various rates of drug absorption from each of the various routes is essential. (Routes of drug administration are discussed in detail in Chapter 3.) Epinephrine 1:1000, a drug commonly used in the management of acute allergic reactions, is generally given by the subcutaneous route. The reasons for choosing this site are many. First, epinephrine 1:1000 is a potent and concentrated drug. Rapid absorption

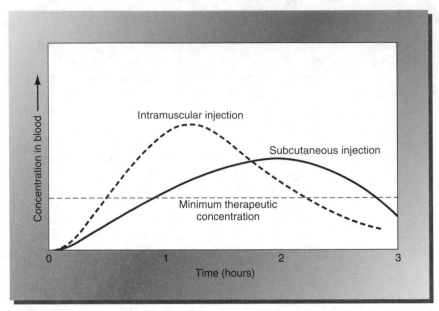

FIGURE 2–1 Comparision of drug levels following intramuscular and subcutaneous injections.

of a large quantity of this drug into the circulation would certainly accentuate epinephrine's side effects such as tachycardia, trembling, and elevated blood pressure. Second, the therapeutic effects of epinephrine are fairly brief. The slower absorption obtained with subcutaneous injection allows prolonged release of the drug into the circulation, thus maintaining the desired effects for a longer period (see Table 2–1).

Systemic blood flow can also affect drug absorption. Factors that may *delay* absorption from parenteral sites include shock, acidosis, and peripheral vasoconstriction secondary to such things as hypothermia. Factors such as peripheral vasodilation, which can occur in hyperthermia and fever, may *increase* the rate of drug absorption.

Drug absorption time may be minimized by injecting the medication directly into the circulatory system by the intravenous (IV) route. The desired effects are seen much sooner, and the eventual blood levels of the

TABLE 2–1	
Comparison of Rates of Drug Absorption of Various Routes of Administration	
Route	*Rate of Absorption*
Oral	Slow
Subcutaneous	Slow
Topical	Moderate
Intramuscular	Moderate
Intralingual	Rapid
Rectal	Rapid
Sublingual	Rapid
Endotracheal	Rapid
Inhalation	Rapid
Intraosseous	Immediate
Intravenous	Immediate
Intracardiac	Immediate

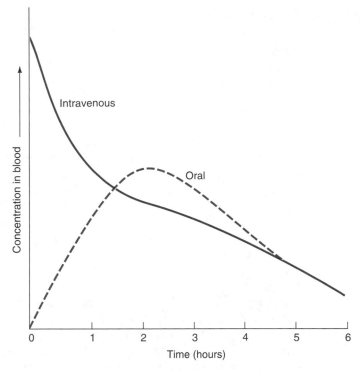

FIGURE 2–2 Comparison of drug levels following IV and oral drug administration.

drug are much more predictable. Consequently, most critical-care medications are given intravenously (see Figure 2–2).

Bioavailability is the measure of the amount of a drug that is still active after it reaches its target tissue. This is the bottom line as far as absorption is concerned. The goal of administering a drug is to assure sufficient bioavailability of the drug at the target tissue in order to produce the desired effect, after considering all of the absorption factors.

Distribution

Once a drug has entered the bloodstream, it must be distributed throughout the body. Most drugs will pass easily from the bloodstream, through the interstitial spaces, into the target cells. Distribution is the process whereby a drug is transported from the site of absorption to the site of action.

Several factors can affect drug distribution:

1. Cardiovascular function
2. Regional blood flow
3. Drug storage reservoirs
4. Physiological barriers

As with drug absorption, drug distribution depends on *cardiovascular function*. Following administration and absorption, the drug is initially distributed to highly perfused body areas such as the brain, heart, kidneys, and liver. Delivery of the drug to the gastrointestinal system, skin, muscles, and fat is generally much slower. In certain conditions, such as shock and congestive heart failure, cardiac output will fall. When it does, drug distribution becomes much slower and much more unpredictable. When cardiac output is markedly diminished, some body areas are minimally perfused, and drug delivery to these areas is negligible.

Variances in *regional blood flow* can also affect drug distribution. For example, in cardiogenic shock, blood flow to the kidneys is often diminished. Medications that act specifically on the kidneys, such as diuretics, may not reach the kidneys in an adequate concentration to be effective.

In the body, a drug may be stored in various sites known as *drug reservoirs.* These reservoirs store drugs by binding the drugs to proteins present within the tissue in question. This action tends to delay the drug's onset of action and prolongs its duration of effect. There are two types of storage reservoirs: *plasma reservoirs* and *tissue reservoirs.*

During drug distribution through the vascular or lymphatic system, the drug comes in contact with proteins and remains free or binds to plasma carrier protein, storage tissue protein, or receptor protein. The portion of the drug that is bound to plasma proteins is called the *bound drug,* and the unbound portion is often referred to as the *free drug.* As soon as a drug binds to plasma carrier protein or storage tissue protein, it becomes inactive, rendering it unavailable for binding to a receptor protein and incapable of exerting therapeutic activity. However, a bound drug can free itself rapidly to maintain a balance between the amounts of free and bound drug. Only the free, or unbound, percentage of the drug remains active.

The percentage of drug that remains free and available for activity depends on the amount of plasma protein available for binding. The most common plasma protein involved in drug binding is *albumin.* However, other plasma proteins, such as hemoglobin and globulins, are utilized as well. This binding of drug to protein is usually reversible. The extent of binding depends on the physical properties of the drug itself. Some drugs are highly bound, whereas others have limited binding. The degree to which a drug is bound is referred to as the *binding capacity.* Binding of a drug to plasma proteins tends to limit its concentration in the tissues.

Drugs can also accumulate in the various tissues of the body. Common tissue reservoirs include fat, bone, and muscle tissue. Once in these compartments, the drug binds to proteins and similar substances. As with plasma protein binding, tissue binding is usually reversible. Some body compartments, such as the muscle tissue, can represent a sizable drug reservoir. Many drugs are lipid soluble (fat soluble). These drugs concentrate in the fatty tissues of the body, resulting in a prolonged drug effect.

Physiological barriers also affect drug distribution. Physiological barriers inhibit the movement of certain substances while permitting the passage of others. One of the most important physiological barriers is the *blood–brain barrier.* The blood–brain barrier refers to a network of capillary endothelial cells in the brain. These cells have no pores and are surrounded by a sheath of glial connective tissue that makes them impermeable to water-soluble drugs. The network excludes most ionized drug molecules, such as dopamine, from the brain. However, it allows nonionized, unbound drug molecules, such as barbiturates, to pass readily and enter the brain. The blood–brain barrier is an effective boundary between the central nervous system and the peripheral nervous system. Delivery of drugs and other substances to the brain is limited by the blood–brain barrier. It allows entry of certain drugs and is considered a protective mechanism of the brain.

The so-called *placental barrier* can likewise prevent drugs from reaching a fetus, although it is not the solid barrier that its name implies. The fetus is exposed to almost every drug that the mother takes. But because any drug must traverse the maternal blood supply and cross the capillary membranes into the placenta (fetal) circulation, delivering drugs to a fetus requires them to be lipid soluble, nonionized, and non-protein-bound. This may slow some drugs or reduce their placental transfer to benign levels.

Biotransformation

Like other chemicals that enter the body, drugs are metabolized, or broken down into different chemicals (metabolites). The special name given to the *metabolism* of drugs is *biotransformation*. Biotransformation has one of two effects on most drugs: (1) it can transform the drug into a more or less active metabolite, or (2) it can make the drug more water soluble (or less lipid soluble) to facilitate elimination. Some drugs, such as lidocaine, are totally metabolized before elimination, others only partially, and still others not at all. The body will transform some molecules of most drugs and eliminate others without transformation. Protein-bound drugs are not available for biotransformation. Some so-called *prodrugs* (or parent drugs) are not active when administered, but biotransformation converts them into active metabolites.

Many biotransformation processes occur in the liver. The endoplasmic reticula of hepatocytes (liver cells) contain microsomal enzymes that perform much of the metabolizing. (Smaller quantities of the enzymes are also found in the kidney, lung, and GI tract.) Because the blood supply from the GI tract passes through the liver via the portal vein, all drugs absorbed in the GI tract pass through the liver before moving on through the systemic circulation. The first pass through the liver may partially or completely inactivate many drugs. This *first-pass effect* is why some drugs cannot be given orally but instead must be given intravenously to bypass the GI tract and prevent first-pass hepatic metabolism. It is also why drugs that can be given either orally or intravenously may require a much higher oral dose than IV dose. Because we can observe the extent of first-pass metabolism, we can predict how much to increase a dose of an oral medication to deliver an effective amount of the drug into the general circulation.

Through biotransformation, the body detoxifies and disposes of foreign substances. Because drugs are unnatural to the body, they are disposed of, as are other toxins. In most cases, the enzyme system increases the water solubility of a drug so that the renal system can excrete it. The lipid solubility of some drugs may be altered enzymatically so that the end products enter into and are excreted through the biliary system. Using the renal or the biliary pathway for disposal, the body usually transforms the drug into a readily eliminated, pharmacologically inactive product.

Biotransformation begins immediately following introduction of the drug into the body. Certain drugs are rapidly biotransformed, and others are not. For example, the emergency drug epinephrine is active as administered. However, it is very rapidly metabolized to inactive forms before elimination. Because of this rapid biotransformation, epinephrine must be readministered approximately every 3 to 5 minutes if still required.

Some drugs are inactive when administered. Once they have been absorbed, they must be converted to an active form, either in the blood or by the target tissue. The inactive precursor is referred to as a *prodrug*. Several

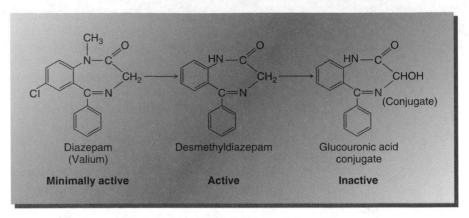

FIGURE 2-3 Metabolites of diazepam.

drugs used in prehospital care must be converted into an active form before they can exert their desired effects. Diazepam (Valium), a drug used in the treatment of seizures, is relatively inactive as administered. Once in the body it is converted to its active metabolite, *desmethyldiazepam,* which then induces the desired effects (see Figure 2–3).

Elimination

Drugs are eventually eliminated from the body in either their original form or as metabolites. Drug *excretion* refers to movement of a drug or its metabolites from the tissues back into the circulation and from the circulation into the organs of excretion. Drugs may be excreted by the kidneys into the urine, by the liver into the bile, by the intestines into the feces, or by the lungs with the expired air. Additionally, drugs may be excreted through sweat, saliva, and breast milk. Excretion through sweat glands is rarely a significant mechanism for elimination. Excretion through mammary glands becomes a concern when nursing mothers take medications. Drugs may also be removed artificially by direct interventions, such as peritoneal dialysis or hemodialysis. The rate of elimination varies with the medication and the state of the body. During shock states, the kidneys are poorly perfused. In such cases, drugs that are primarily eliminated by the kidneys remain present in the body for longer periods. The slower the rate of elimination, the longer the drug stays in the body.

Elimination can be affected by the following:

1. Drug half-life
2. Accumulation
3. Clearance
4. Onset, peak, and duration

Drug Half-Life

To predict the frequency of the drug dosage schedule, the physician must determine how long a drug will remain in the body. Usually the rate of drug loss from the body can be estimated by determining the drug's *half-life.* Drug half-life is the time required for the total amount of a drug in the body to diminish by one-half. If a patient receives a single dose of a drug with a half-life of 5 hours, the total amount of the drug in the patient's body would diminish by one-half after 5 hours. The drug amount would continue to decrease accordingly with each subsequent half-life. Most drugs are essentially eliminated after five half-lives because the amount remaining is too low to exert a beneficial or adverse effect. This concept is useful in many situations. For example, if a drug overdose occurs and the excretion rate of the drug is not compromised, about 97 percent of the original dose will be eliminated after five half-lives.

Accumulation

Drug half-life is also useful when assessing drug accumulation. A drug that is not readministered is eliminated almost completely after five half-lives, but a regularly administered drug reaches a constant total body amount, or steady state, after about five half-lives.

Having reached a steady state, the drug's concentration in the blood fluctuates above and below the average concentration. Thus, although the drug was once at steady state, its concentration does not remain uniform; rather, it increases, peaks, and declines, although within a constant range.

For some drugs, the time required to reach therapeutic blood concentration may be too long. For example, when using digoxin, with a half-life of about 1.6 days, the physician would not be able to wait 8 days (1.6 days times five half-lives) to achieve steady-state blood concentration levels to control a life-threatening arrhythmia, such as atrial fibrillation. Therefore, an initial large dose, called a *loading dose,* would be administered to reach the desired therapeutic blood concentration level. Consequently, smaller *maintenance doses* would be given daily to replace the amount of drug eliminated since the last dose. These dosages maintain a therapeutic blood concentration in the body at all times.

Clearance

Drug clearance refers to the removal of a drug from the body. A drug with a slow clearance rate is removed from the body slowly; one with a high clearance rate is removed rapidly. A drug with a high clearance rate may require more frequent administration and higher doses than a comparable drug with a low clearance rate. A drug with a low clearance rate can accumulate to a toxic concentration in the body unless it is administered less frequently or at lower doses.

Onset, Peak, and Duration

Besides absorption, distribution, metabolism, and excretion, three other factors play an important role in a drug's pharmacokinetics:

1. Onset of action
2. Peak concentration
3. Duration of action

The onset of action refers to the time when the drug is sufficiently absorbed to reach an effective blood level and sufficiently distributed to its site of action to elicit a therapeutic response.

As the body absorbs more of the drug, the drug concentration in the blood rises, more drug reaches the site of action, and the therapeutic response increases. These occurrences characterize the peak concentration level for the drug dose administered.

As soon as the drug begins to circulate in the blood, it also begins to be eliminated. Eventually drug elimination exceeds its absorption rate because less of the drug dose remains to be absorbed. At this point, the drug concentration in the blood and the drug's effect begin to decline. When the blood concentration falls below the minimum needed to produce an effect, drug action ceases, although some drug remains in the blood. Therefore, the duration of action is the length of time that drug concentration is sufficient in the blood to produce a therapeutic response.

A drug's onset, peak, and duration are determined primarily by its bioavailability (the extent to which a drug's active ingredient is absorbed and transported to its site of action) and drug concentration in the blood.

PHARMACODYNAMICS

Pharmacodynamics is the study of the mechanisms by which specific drug dosages act to produce biochemical or physiological changes in the body.

Mechanisms of Action of Drugs

Drugs can act in four different ways. They may bind to a receptor site, change the physical properties of cells, chemically combine with other chemicals, or alter a normal metabolic pathway. Each of these actions involves a physiochemical interaction between the drug and a functionally important molecule in the body.

Drugs That Act by Binding to a Receptor Site

Most drugs operate by binding to a receptor. Almost all drug receptors are protein molecules on the surfaces of cells. They are part of the body's normal regulatory stimulation/inhibition function, and can be stimulated or inhibited by chemicals. Each different receptor's name generally corresponds to the drug that stimulates it. For example, if an opiate stimulates the receptor, then the receptor is an *opioid receptor.* When multiple drugs stimulate the same receptor, standard practice is to use the generic name.

The force of attraction between a drug and a receptor is called their *affinity.* The greater the affinity, the stronger the bond. Different drugs may bind to the same type of receptor site, but the strength of their bonds may vary. The binding site's shape determines its receptivity to other chemicals, whether they are drugs or endogenous substances. These binding sites are relatively specific—a nonopiate drug generally will not affect an opiate binding site, although occasionally a drug with a similar receptor binding site will unexpectedly cross-react. Receptors can also have subtypes. At least five subtypes of adrenergic receptors, for example, are important to prehospital practice.

A drug's pharmacodynamics also involves its ability to cause the expected response, called its *efficacy.* Just as different drugs may have different affinities for a site, they may also have different efficacies; that is, drug A may cause a stronger response than drug B. Affinity and efficacy are not directly related. Drug A may cause a stronger response than drug B, even though drug B binds to the receptor site more strongly than drug A.

When a drug binds with its specific type of receptor, a chemical change occurs that ultimately leads to the drug having its desired effect on the body. In most cases, drugs will either stimulate or inhibit the cell's normal biochemical actions. In fact, a drug cannot impart a new function to a cell. Some drugs may interact with a receptor and directly result in the desired effect. Other drugs, however, may interact with a receptor and cause the release or production of a second compound. This secondary compound, or second messenger, includes such compounds as calcium or cyclic adenosine monophosphate (cAMP). Cyclic AMP is the most common second messenger. It has a multitude of effects inside the cell. These secondary messengers are particularly important in the endocrine system, because they principally occur in endocrine glands. Once cAMP is formed inside the cell, it activates still other enzymes, usually in a cascading action. That is, the first enzyme activates another enzyme, which activates a third enzyme, and so forth. This is important in that it amplifies the action so that even a small amount of a drug (or hormone) acting on the cell surface can initiate a powerful, cascading, activating force for the entire cell.

The number of receptors on a target cell usually does not remain constant on a daily basis or even from minute to minute. This is because the receptor proteins are often destroyed during the course of their function. At other times, they are either reactivated or remanufactured by the protein-manufacturing mechanism of the cell. Binding of a drug (or hormone) to a target cell receptor causes the number of receptors to decrease. This process is termed downregulation of the receptors. It results in a decreased responsiveness of the target cell to the drug or hormone as the number of available active receptors decreases. In other cases, but less commonly, a drug (or hormone) can cause the formation of more receptors than normal. This process, upregulation, increases the target tissue's sensitivity to the particular drug or hormone.

Chemicals that stimulate a receptor site generally fall into two broad categories, *agonists* and *antagonists.* Agonists bind to the receptor and cause it to initiate the expected response. Antagonists bind to a site but do not cause the receptor to initiate the expected response. Some drugs, agonist-antagonists (also called partial agonists), may do both. Nalbuphine (Nubain), for instance, stimulates some of the opioid agonists' analgesic properties, but partially blocks others such as respiratory depression.

Receptor-mediated drug actions work like a lock (the receptor) and key (the agonist). If you put the key in the lock and turn it, the lock will open. An antagonist is like a key that fits into the lock, but will not turn and cannot open the lock. Target tissues generally have many receptors, so to take the analogy another step, imagine that to get maximal effect a single key (agonist) must move around and open many doors (trigger many biochemical responses). An agonist-antagonist would be a key that unlocks and opens a door but gets stuck in the lock. That is, the drug will cause the expected effect, but that drug will also block another drug from triggering the same receptor. This competitive antagonism is considered surmountable because a sufficiently large dose of the agonist can overcome the antagonism.

Noncompetitive antagonism can also occur. Continuing the lock, key, and door analogy, imagine the door is barred. This antagonism would be insurmountable; no amount of agonist could overcome it. Noncompetitive antagonism occurs because the binding of the antagonist at a different site causes a deformity of the binding site that actually prevents the agonist from fitting and binding. Irreversible antagonism may also occur when a competitive antagonist permanently binds with a receptor site. When this occurs, no amount of agonist will stimulate the receptor. For the effects of such an antagonist to wear off, the body must create new receptors.

Two drugs may appear to be antagonists while actually acting independently. This physiological antagonism can occur when one drug's effects counteract another's. Although neither agent chemically affects the other, their net effect is antagonistic. An example of a receptor, agonist, antagonist, and agonist-antagonist can be described using an opiate receptor. These receptors occur naturally in the brain and respond to natural endorphins. Morphine sulfate acts as an agonist. It binds to the opiate receptor and causes the expected response of pain relief. Naloxone (Narcan) acts as an antagonist. It will bind to the opiate receptor, but will not initiate the pain relief. It will prevent morphine sulfate from binding to the site and thus effectively blocks the morphine and its response. If the patient is given nalbuphine (Nubain), an agonist-antagonist, it will bind to the opiate receptor and relieve pain, but it is less efficacious than morphine. The nalbuphine blocks morphine from the receptor like an antagonist, but stimulates the receptor on its own like an agonist, although to a lesser extent.

Drugs That Act by Changing Physical Properties

Some drugs change the physical properties of a part of the body. Drugs that change the osmotic balance across membranes are good examples of this type of drug action. The osmotic diuretic mannitol (Osmotrol), for instance, increases urine output by increasing the blood's osmolarity, or osmotic "pull." This increased osmolarity triggers the normal regulatory systems to decrease water reabsorption in the renal tubules, thereby reducing the total amount of water in the body.

Drugs That Act by Chemically Combining with Other Substances

Drugs that participate in chemical reactions that change the chemical nature of their substrates (the chemical or substance on which a drug acts) play a large role in prehospital practice. For example, isopropyl alcohol, which is often used to disinfect skin before percutaneous needle insertion for phlebotomy or IV cannulation, denatures the proteins on the surface of bacterial cells. This ruptures the cells, destroying the bacteria. The antacids are another example. They act by chemically neutralizing the hydrochloric acid in the stomach. Sodium bicarbonate given intravenously chemically neutralizes some of the acids in the bloodstream, effectively making the blood more alkalotic.

Drugs That Act by Altering a Normal Metabolic Pathway

Some anticancer and antiviral drugs are chemical analogs of normal metabolic substrates. In a process that has been dubbed a counterfeit incorporation mechanism, these drugs can be incorporated into the products of metabolism of cancer cells. Because these drugs are not really the expected substrate, the anticipated product either will not form or, if formed, will be substantially or completely inactive.

Drug Potency and Efficacy

Drug potency refers to the relative amount of a drug required to produce the desired response. Comparing the drug potency of one drug with that of another drug can reveal which is the more potent drug. The power of a drug to produce a therapeutic effect is called the drug's *efficacy*. Drugs that are agonists have both affinity and efficacy. Drugs that are antagonists have affinity but not efficacy, because they do not produce a physiological response. Classic illustrations of this principle are the drugs epinephrine and propranolol (Inderal). Epinephrine, once administered, is transported to its various target tissues—namely, the heart, the lungs, and the peripheral blood vessels. Once at these target tissues, it finds and binds to its receptors, which are called *beta-receptors*. If the drug is able to bind to these beta-receptors, then the desired physiological response will be seen. Several drugs themselves are inactive but can bind to beta-receptors in much the same manner as epinephrine. These drugs are referred to as *beta-blockers*, and the prototype drug of this group is propranolol. If a beta-blocker has already bound to the receptor, then epinephrine cannot bind, and the desired effect is effectively blocked (see Figures 2–4 and 2–5). A more detailed discussion of beta-receptors and beta-blockers can be found in Chapter 6.

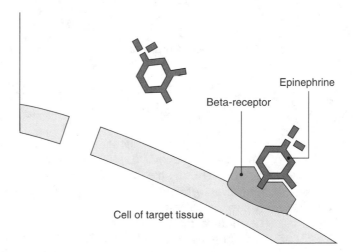

FIGURE 2–4 Epinephrine interacting with beta-receptor.

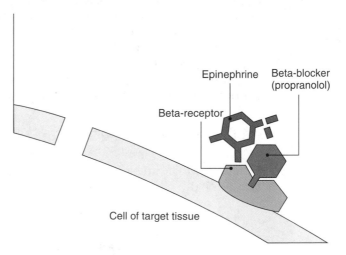

FIGURE 2–5 Beta-receptor blocked by propranolol.

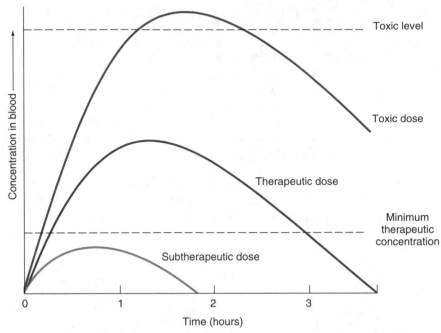

FIGURE 2–6 Comparison of blood levels following subtherapeutic, therapeutic, and toxic doses of the same drug.

Therapeutic Index

Once again, for a medication to be effective it must reach a certain concentration at the target tissue. The minimal concentration of a drug necessary to cause the desired response is referred to as the *therapeutic threshold*, or *minimum effective concentration*. A concentration below this therapeutic threshold will not induce a clinical response. There is also a point at which the drug concentration can get high enough to be toxic or even fatal. The general goal of drug therapy is to give the minimum concentration of a drug necessary to obtain the desired response (see Figure 2–6).

The difference between the minimum effective concentration and the toxic level varies significantly from drug to drug. The difference between these two concentrations is referred to as the *therapeutic index* and is usually obtained in the laboratory. Certain drugs, such as digitalis, have very little difference between the effective dose and the toxic dose. Such drugs are said to have a low therapeutic index. Drugs such as naloxone (Narcan), the narcotic antagonist, have a significant margin between the effective dose and the toxic dose and are said to have a high therapeutic index. Prehospital care providers should be familiar with the therapeutic indexes of the medications they use.

Factors Altering Drug Response

Different individuals may have different responses to the same drug. Factors that alter the standard drug–response relationship include the following:

- *Age.* The liver and kidney functions of infants are not yet fully developed, so their response to drugs may be altered. Likewise, as we age, the functions of these organs begins to deteriorate. As a result, infants and the elderly are most susceptible to having an altered response to a drug.

- *Body mass.* The more body mass a person has, the more fluid that is potentially available to dilute a drug. A given amount of drug will have a higher concentration in a person with little body mass than in a much larger person. Thus, most drug dosages are stated in terms of body mass. For example, the standard dose of lidocaine for a patient in cardiac arrest is a .5 mg/kg. A 100-kg patient will receive 150 mg of lidocaine, whereas a 50-kg patient will receive only 75 mg.

- *Gender.* Most differences in drug response due to gender result from the relative body masses of men and women. The different distribution and amounts of body fat also affect the amounts of drug available at any given time.

- *Environmental milieu.* Various stimuli in a patient's environment affect his response to a given drug. This is most clearly seen with drugs affecting mood or behavior. The same dose of an antianxiety medication such as diazepam (Valium) will have different effects on different patients, depending on the patients' moods or surroundings. For example, if a patient is afraid of heights, his usual dose of diazepam would not be likely to help him remain calm while rappelling from the top of a tall building. Surrounding conditions may also affect the distribution or elimination of a drug. Heat, for example, causes vasodilation and increases perspiration, both of which may alter the rate at which the body distributes and eliminates a drug.

- *Time of administration.* If a patient takes a drug immediately after eating, its absorption will be different than if he took the same drug before breakfast in the morning. Some drugs may cause nausea if taken on an empty stomach and must therefore be taken only after eating.

- *Pathologic state.* Several disease states alter the drug–response relationship. Most notable are renal and hepatic dysfunctions, both of which may lead to excess accumulation of a drug in the body. Renal failure is likely to decrease elimination of drugs, and hepatic failure may decrease or inhibit their metabolism, prolonging their duration of action. Acid–base disturbances may alter a drug's solubility or the extent to which it ionizes, thus changing its absorption rate.

- *Genetic factors.* Genetic traits such as a lack of specific enzymes or a lowered basal metabolic rate alter drug absorption or biotransformation and thus modify the patient's response.

- *Psychological factors.* A patient's mental state can also affect his response to a drug. The best known example of this is the placebo effect. Essentially, if a patient believes that a drug will have a given effect, then he is much more likely to perceive that the effect has occurred.

Special Considerations in Drug Therapy

Age, pregnancy, and lactation are important considerations in drug therapy. Both children and the elderly are particularly susceptible to the adverse effects of drugs. Consequently, drug dosages often must be modified for persons in these age groups. Likewise, special precautions must be taken when administering medications to a pregnant patient, because many medications will also affect the fetus. Certain drugs are excreted into the breast milk, which becomes a particular concern in mothers who are breast-feeding their infants. The following sections discuss these special considerations in drug therapy.

Pediatric Patients

Children are typically smaller than adults, and drug dosages must be reduced accordingly. Pediatric drug dosages are typically based on the child's body weight or body surface area (BSA). Thus, it is essential that prehospital personnel determine or approximate a child's weight before administering a medication. Often, the parents can provide an approximate weight from a recent doctor's visit. In emergencies the child's body weight can be estimated by determining the child's age and finding the average body weight for that age on a reference table.

Neonates (infants from birth to 4 weeks) are a special concern. Common sites of drug metabolism and elimination, such as the liver and kidneys, are not well developed in neonates. Thus both drug metabolism and excretion may be impaired. Drug dosages for neonates must often be modified to reflect these factors.

The American Heart Association (AHA) and the American Academy of Pediatrics (AAP) publish recommended drug dosages for most emergency medications. Often, the doses of common emergency drugs are listed on easy-to-use reference cards. To use these, prehospital care providers simply look up the child's age or weight. Below the age or weight are the recommended dosages for common emergency drugs.

Another popular device for determining pediatric drug dosages is the Broselow tape (see Figure 2–7). The Broselow tape is simply unfolded and placed alongside the supine child to measure the child from the top of the head to the bottom of the feet. The tape is divided into various color-coded drug dosage charts based on the child's length (which is directly related to the child's weight and body surface area). Prehospital care providers simply use the dosage chart that corresponds to the child's length. In addition to drug dosages, the Broselow tape contains recommended endotracheal tube sizes, defibrillator settings, and other important emergency information.

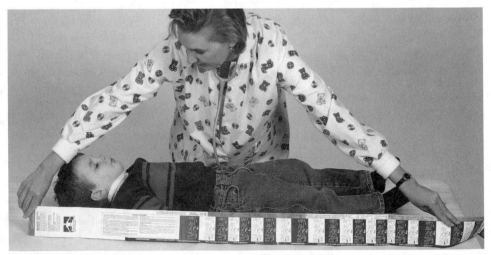

FIGURE 2–7 A Broselow tape is useful for calculating drug dosages for pediatric patients.

Geriatric Patients

The elderly age group is the fastest growing segment of the U.S. population, and older adults are frequent users of the emergency medical services (EMS) system. The aging process begins at the cellular level and affects virtually every body system. Common physiological effects of aging include the following:

1. Decreased cardiac output
2. Decreased renal function
3. Decreased brain mass
4. Decreased total body water
5. Decreased body fat
6. Decreased serum albumin
7. Decreased respiratory capacity

These changes can lead to altered pharmacodynamics and pharmacokinetics for many medications. With aging, the rate of metabolism and the excretion of medications can be significantly decreased. In addition, there is often decreased protein binding because the level of serum albumin decreases. These factors combine to increase the relative potency of a drug. Consequently, the dosages of many medications must be reduced when administered to an elderly patient.

The elderly are more apt to suffer from more than one disease process at a time. In addition, they may be on chronic medications, which may affect the emergency medications paramedics need to administer in the prehospital setting. Multiple medical problems make drug dosing much more difficult. For example, treating a patient with congestive heart failure may be more difficult if the patient also has renal failure. In this case, the dosage of furosemide (Lasix) may need to be increased, and the dosage of morphine may need to be decreased. All factors must be considered before administering medications to the elderly.

Pregnancy and Lactation

Pregnancy presents two pharmacological problems. First, pregnancy causes a number of anatomical and physiological changes in the mother, including:

1. Increased cardiac output
2. Increased heart rate
3. Increased blood volume (by up to 45 percent)
4. Decreased protein binding
5. Decreased hepatic metabolism
6. Decreased blood pressure

These anatomical and physiological changes must be considered prior to administering medications or fluids to a pregnant patient.

The second consideration associated with pregnancy is that any medication administered to the mother has the potential to cross the placenta and affect the fetus. Some drugs cross the placenta rapidly, but others do not. Thus, drugs should only be administered in pregnancy when the potential benefits outweigh the risks. The U.S. Food and Drug

TABLE 2–2

FDA Pregnancy Categories

Category	Description
A	Adequate studies in pregnant women have not demonstrated a risk to the fetus in the first trimester or later trimesters.
B	Animal studies have not demonstrated a risk to the fetus, but there are no adequate studies in pregnant women.
	OR
	Adequate studies in pregnant women have not demonstrated a risk to the fetus in the first trimester and there is no risk in the last trimester, but animal studies have demonstrated adverse effects.
C	Animal studies have demonstrated adverse effects, but there are no adequate studies in pregnant women; however, benefits may be acceptable despite the potential risk.
	OR
	No adequate animal studies or adequate studies of pregnant women have been done.
D	Fetal risk has been demonstrated. In certain circumstances, benefits could outweigh the risks.
X	Fetal risk has been demonstrated. This risk outweighs any possible benefit to the mother. Avoid using in pregnant or potentially pregnant patients.

Administration (FDA) categorizes most drugs based on their safety in pregnancy (see Table 2–2).

As with pregnancy, drug therapy can affect a breast-feeding infant. Many medications are excreted readily into the breast milk. If the mother continues to breast-feed while receiving these medications, the medications can be excreted into the breast milk and be ingested by the baby. If a breast-feeding mother is to receive medications, she should be instructed to stop breast-feeding and pump her breasts. She should dispose of the expressed milk until she is certain that the drug has been cleared from her system. During the time she is pumping her breasts, she should switch the infant to a commercial formula.

SUMMARY

A basic understanding of pharmacokinetics and pharmacodynamics is essential for prehospital personnel to anticipate the desired therapeutic effects as well as any possible side effects of the medications they administer. Such factors as rate of absorption, elimination, minimum therapeutic concentration, and toxic levels should be considered in all drugs.

KEY WORDS

absorption. The process whereby a drug is moved from the site of application into the body and into the extracellular fluid compartment.

affinity. The tendency of a drug to combine with a specific drug receptor.

agonist. A drug or other substance that binds with a specific drug receptor and causes a physiological response.

albumin. Protein found in almost all animal tissue. It constitutes one of the major proteins in human blood.

antagonist. A drug or other substance that blocks a physiological response or that blocks the action of another drug or substance.

binding capacity. The degree to which a drug is bound to tissue or plasma proteins.

biotransformation. Biotransformation, also called metabolism, is the process of changing a drug into a different form, either active or inactive, by the body.

blood–brain barrier. Protective mechanism that selectively allows the entry of specific compounds into the brain. It is an effective boundary between the central nervous system and the peripheral nervous system.

cumulative effect. A phenomenon that occurs when a drug is administered in several doses, causing an increased effect. It is usually due to a buildup of a drug in the blood.

distribution. The process whereby a drug is transported from the site of absorption to the site of action.

efficacy. The power of a drug to produce a therapeutic effect.

elimination. The process whereby a drug is removed from the body by excretion into the urine, feces, bile, saliva, sweat, breast milk, or expired air.

excretion. The elimination of waste products from the body. *Excretion* is often used interchangeably with the term *elimination.*

globulin. One of a broad category of simple proteins found in the body.

half-life. The time required for a level of a drug in the blood to be reduced by 50 percent of its beginning level.

hemoglobin. An iron-containing compound found within the blood cell that is responsible for the transport and delivery of oxygen to the body cells.

loading dose. The initial dose of a drug given in a sufficient amount to achieve a therapeutic plasma level.

maintenance dose. The dose of a drug necessary to maintain a constant therapeutic plasma level.

metabolism. The sum total of all physical and chemical changes that occur within the body. In pharmacology it is often used interchangeably with the term *biotransformation.*

minimum effective concentration. The minimum amount of drug needed in the bloodstream to cause the desired therapeutic effect.

onset of action. The time interval between the administration of a drug and the first sign of its onset; onset of action is influenced by the physical and chemical properties of a drug as well as by its route of administration.

pH. A scientific method of expressing the acidity or alkalinity of a solution, which is the logarithm of the hydrogen ion concentration divided by 1. The higher the pH, the more alkaline the solution; the lower the pH, the more acidic the solution.

pharmacodynamics. The study of a drug's action on the body.

pharmacokinetics. The study of how drugs enter the body, reach their site of action, and eventually are eliminated.

plasma (serum) level. The amount of the drug present in the plasma. The peak plasma level refers to the highest concentration produced by a specific dose.

solubility. The tendency of a drug to dissolve.

therapeutic index. An index of the drug's safety profile, which is determined by calculating the difference between the drug's therapeutic threshold and toxic level. It is typically determined in the laboratory.

therapeutic range. The difference between the minimal therapeutic and toxic concentrations of a drug. Drugs with a low therapeutic range present a higher risk of toxicity than do drugs with a high therapeutic range. The therapeutic range is also referred to as the margin of safety.

therapeutic threshold. The minimum amount of drug needed in the bloodstream to cause a desired therapeutic effect.

toxicity. The degree to which a substance is poisonous. At high doses drugs can produce toxic effects that are not seen at low doses.

toxic level. The plasma level at which severe adverse reactions are expected or likely.

3

ADMINISTRATION OF DRUGS

OBJECTIVES

After completing this chapter, the reader should be able to:

1. State the necessary components of a verbal or standing medication order.
2. Explain the six rights of drug administration.
3. Explain the advantages and disadvantages of enteral versus parenteral administration.
4. List and explain five enteral tract routes.
5. List and explain 13 parenteral routes.
6. Briefly explain the following routes of drug administration:
   a. Transdermal
   b. Sublingual
   c. Subcutaneous route
   d. Intramuscular route
   e. Intravenous bolus
   f. Intravenous piggyback
   g. Via the endotracheal tube
   h. Via an intraosseous infusion
7. Describe the different methods of administering medications through inhalation therapy.
8. Describe the special considerations in administering medications to a pediatric patient.
9. Briefly explain the following pediatric routes of drug administration:
   a. Intramuscular route
   b. Subcutaneous route
   c. Intravenous route
   d. Rectal

INTRODUCTION

In the field of emergency medicine, medications must be administered promptly, in the correct dose, and by the correct route. Many drugs with a therapeutic value when given by the appropriate route can be fatal when given by an inappropriate route. Norepinephrine, for example, is a potent drug used to treat severe hypotension. It is designed to be given by slow, intravenous infusion. If given in an intravenous bolus, however, it may be fatal. This admonition applies to most medications used in emergency medicine.

The emergency scene is often hectic. Paramedics must often prepare and administer medications in the worst of environments. Consequently, it is essential that all prehospital personnel develop safe habits regarding drug preparation and drug administration. These safe habits serve to protect both the patient and the paramedic.

This chapter presents the procedures for medication preparation and administration of medications used in emergency medical practice.

PATIENT CARE USING MEDICATIONS

Paramedics are responsible for the standard of care for patients in their charge. They are, therefore, personally responsible—legally, morally, and ethically—for the safe and effective administration of medications. The following guidelines will help you to meet that responsibility:

- Know the precautions and contraindications for all medications you administer.
- Practice proper technique.
- Know how to observe and document drug effects.
- Maintain a current knowledge in pharmacology.
- Establish and maintain professional relationships with other health care providers.
- Understand the pharmacokinetics and pharmacodynamics.
- Have current medication references available.
- Take careful drug histories including:
  - Name, strength, and daily dose of prescribed drugs
  - Over-the-counter drugs
  - Vitamins
  - Herbal medications
  - Folk medicine or folk remedies
  - Allergies
- Evaluate the compliance, dosage, and adverse reactions.
- Consult with medical direction when appropriate.

THE MEDICATION ORDER

Prehospital personnel are responsible for preparing and administering many emergency drugs and fluids. The selection and administration of a particular medication depends on an accurate and complete patient assessment. The results of this assessment must be relayed to medical control or applied to prehospital treatment protocols or standing orders. An inaccurate or incomplete patient assessment may lead to administration of the wrong drug.

The first step in medication administration is the medication order. The order may be in the form of a direct verbal order or through written standing treatment orders. The order generally specifies the following:

1. Medication desired
2. Dose desired
3. Administration route
4. Administration rate

If possible, verbal medication orders should be written down as soon as they are received. After receiving the order, the paramedic should repeat the entire order back to the medical control physician. Doing so ensures that there is no misunderstanding related to the medication order. A typical medication order interchange is as follows:

Medical Control: Start an IV of lactated Ringer's solution at 125 mL per hour and administer 5 mg of diazepam intravenously over 1 minute.

Medic 1: Confirming an IV of lactated Ringer's solution at 125 mL per hour and 5 mg of diazepam intravenously over 1 minute.

Medical Control: Affirmative Medic 1.

In systems that utilize standing orders, paramedics first review the appropriate standing order. They then confirm the ordered medication, dosage, route, and rate of medication administration and, if possible, have another crew member review and double-check the standing order. Finally, paramedics prepare and administer the medication as detailed in the standing order.

It is essential to use good judgment regarding medication administration. Paramedics should always carefully evaluate the orders they receive. Occasionally, orders will be received that differ from accepted local prehospital protocols. In these cases, paramedics must contact the medical control physician and advise him or her of the discrepancy. If, after discussion of the discrepancy, the medical control physician does not change the order, paramedics should follow the order. The exceptions to this rule, of course, are orders that paramedics believe will harm the patient. If paramedics believe a particular medication or dose will harm the patient, they should notify the medical control physician that they are withholding the drug and give the reason for doing so. Paramedics must document well the circumstances surrounding the controversy and submit documentation to the system medical director for resolution. Although prehospital care providers are responsible to the medical control physician, they have a higher duty to protect the health and well-being of their patients.

SIX RIGHTS OF MEDICATION ADMINISTRATION

After paramedics have received the medication or fluid order, they should then administer the drug in question. In performing drug administration, prehospital care providers adhere to the *six rights of medication administration:*

1. Right patient
2. Right medication

3. Right dose
4. Right route
5. Right time
6. Right documentation

Right Patient

Ensuring that the right patient receives the right drug is usually not a problem in prehospital care because typically only one patient is being treated. However, in some circumstances more than one patient may be undergoing treatment, especially in multiple casualty incidents in which many patients are involved. In cases with multiple patients, it is prudent to use some label to distinguish patients. Some systems prefer to use the patient's last name. However, it is not uncommon for several members of one family to be involved in an emergency. Each family member usually has the same last name, and some have the same first name (e.g., William and William Jr.). In these cases, it is best to assign numbers (e.g., Patient 1 and Patient 2) or letters of the alphabet (e.g., Patient A and Patient B) to each patient to avoid confusion.

Confusion regarding multiple patients is more of a problem for medical control than for individual paramedics. A multiple casualty incident may utilize several ambulances, often with similar call signs. Personnel in each ambulance will contact medical control regarding the patient or patients they are transporting. Care should be taken to distinguish the patients and units to avoid confusion and possible medication error. Errors can be minimized by using effective scene management techniques such as the incident command system. In this system, each patient is designated with a number or letter at the time of triage. Radio communications, both initial and subsequent, should refer to the patient by this designation to help avoid confusion both in the field and at medical control.

Right Medication

A common error in prehospital drug administration is selection of the wrong medication. Most emergency medications are supplied in ampules, vials, or prefilled syringes. Many look very similar. To ensure that the right drug is selected, paramedics should carefully read the label. If the drug is supplied in a box, they should check the label on the box and compare it with the label on the vial or ampule itself after removing it from the box. Paramedics can never assume that a medication is correct simply because it is in the correct place in the drug box. They must always read and check the label three times.

Drug preparations and concentrations can vary. In addition to checking the drug name, paramedics should always check to ensure that the drug concentration is the one desired. This check is especially important for drugs that are carried in differing concentrations (e.g., epinephrine 1:1000 and epinephrine 1:10 000 or lidocaine 100 mg for intravenous bolus and lidocaine 1 g for intravenous infusion).

When following a physician's verbal order, repeat the order back to confirm that you both intend the same thing for the patient. Inspect the label on the drug at least three times before giving the medication to the patient: first as you remove the medication from the drug box or cabinet; second, as you draw the medication into the syringe; and third, immediately before you administer the medication. The expiration date of a drug should always be checked prior to administration. The medication should be held up to the light and inspected for discoloration or particles in the solution. Expired and discolored medications should be discarded. Routine (preferably daily) drug box inspections should detect any expired medications. However, paramedics should always double-check the medication prior to administration.

Failure to confirm the medication name is one of the most common medication administration errors. If you have any question about a drug, do not administer it without confirmation. Showing the medication container to your partner and asking for confirmation is an easy way to further ensure that you are giving the right drug.

Right Dose

Administration of the correct drug dose is crucial. Errors in dosage occur in either calculating the correct dose or preparing the correct dose. Most drug orders are fairly straightforward, and many medications are supplied in unit-dose forms. In these cases, drug dosage calculation and drug preparation are easy. However, many medications, especially those administered by intravenous infusion, are much more difficult to dose. For these medications, paramedics should refer to standardized dosage charts to assist with preparation and administration of the desired dose.

Right Route

Most medications used in prehospital care are designed to be given by the intravenous route. However, certain medications can be given by other routes depending on the physician's orders. It is the paramedic's responsibility to know the various routes by which a particular drug can be administered. For example, the drugs hydroxyzine (Vistaril) and promethazine (Phenergan) are frequently used in the treatment of nausea. Promethazine can be administered both intravenously and intramuscularly. Hydroxyzine, in comparison, can be administered only by the intramuscular route.

Right Time

Most medication orders for prehospital care call for immediate (*stat*) administration of the drug. These orders are generally one-time orders. However, certain drugs may be administered repeatedly, especially in cardiac arrest situations, in which drugs are administered at specific time intervals.

An important consideration is the rate at which a drug should be administered. The rate is usually expressed as the period of time over which the drug in question should be administered. Many drugs can be administered rapidly as an intravenous bolus. Others must be administered at a specific rate. Diazepam, for example, should never be administered faster than 1 mL/min (5 mg/min). The rate of drug administration is particularly crucial for intravenous infusion medications (e.g., lidocaine, dopamine, and norepinephrine).

Right Documentation

The drugs you administer in the field do not stop affecting your patient when he/s enters the hospital. As a result, you must completely document all of your care, especially any drugs you have administered, so that long after you have gone on to your next call, other providers will know what drugs your patient has been given.

GENERAL ADMINISTRATION ROUTES

The two primary channels for getting medications into the body are enteral [through the *alimentary canal*, or gastrointestinal (GI) tract] and parenteral routes. The GI tract provides a fairly safe but relatively slow-acting site for drug absorption. Oral, sublingual, and rectal preparations are given via the GI tract. Administration by the parenteral route can involve all routes other than the GI tract. This chapter deals primarily with medications given by injection. Paramedics use the parenteral route to provide a rapid onset of action and to ensure high blood levels of the drug. The parenteral route also is used when the GI route would inactivate the drug, in unconscious patients, and in unstable or seriously ill patients who require precise administration and monitoring. In acute care medicine, administration is almost always parenteral because the onset of action is much quicker and usually more predictable.

Table 3–1 compares the relative advantages and disadvantages of enteral versus parenteral administration.

Enteral Tract Routes

The common enteral routes of administration used in general medical practice are as follows:

Oral (PO). The best, and most convenient, way of administering drugs is by mouth. Most medical drugs are available in oral preparations. The effects of oral administration are often not seen until 30 to 45 minutes after administration.

TABLE 3–1

Comparison of Enteral vs Parenteral Routes

Enteral Route	
Advantages	*Disadvantages*
Simple	Slow rate of onset
Safe	Cannot be given to unconscious or nauseated
Generally less expensive	patients
Low potential for infection	Absorbed dosage may vary significantly because of actions of digestive enzymes and the condition of the intestinal tract

Parenteral Route	
Rapid onset	Administration often difficult and painful
Can be given to unconscious and nauseated patients	Usually more expensive
Absorbed dosage and action are more predictable	Side effects usually more severe
	Potential for infection

Orogastric/nasogastric tube (OG/NG). This route is generally used for oral medications when the patient already has the tube in place for other reasons.

Sublingual (SL). Some drugs can be administered sublingually (i.e., under the tongue). When administered in this fashion, the drug is placed under the tongue, where it quickly dissolves. The drug is then absorbed into the vast capillary network present in the mucous membranes. Nitroglycerin, a drug frequently used in the management of angina pectoris, is administered by this route.

Buccal. Absorption through this route between the cheek and gum is similar to sublingual absorption.

Rectal (PR). Rectal administration may have both *local* and *systemic* effects. It may be necessary to administer some medications rectally, especially if the patient is nauseated. The rectal route is frequently used in infants and children, who may not be able to swallow oral medications. Absorption of rectally administered drugs is generally somewhat slower than by the oral route.

Parenteral Routes

Any method of administration that does not involve passage through the digestive tract is termed parenteral. Parenteral routes include the following:

Topical. Certain drugs can be placed on the skin, where they are slowly absorbed into the capillary network underneath the skin. The rate of onset varies, but the duration of action is prolonged. This route is often used to administer nitroglycerin in the emergency setting.

Intradermal. Drugs can be injected into the dermal layer of the skin. The amount of medication that can be given via this route is limited, and systemic absorption (into the bloodstream) is very slow. Generally, this route is reserved for diagnostic skin tests, such as allergy testing.

Intranasal. Intranasal administration of selected drugs has become a popular route of prehospital drug administration. The drug is aerosolized and instilled in the nose, whereby the drug is rapidly absorbed through the massive vascular network in the nasal tissues. This route is often considerably more comfortable for the patient than other routes.

Subcutaneous. With subcutaneous administration, medications are injected into fatty, subcutaneous tissue under the skin and overlying the muscle. The rate of absorption is slower than that seen with intramuscular and intravenous administration. Epinephrine 1:1000, which is used in the treatment of acute asthma and other respiratory emergencies, is almost always administered subcutaneously. A maximum of 2 mL of a drug can be given subcutaneously.

Intramuscular. The most commonly used route of parenteral medication administration is the intramuscular route. The drug is injected into muscle tissue, from which it is absorbed into the bloodstream. This method of administration has a predictable rate of absorption but is considerably slower than intravenous administration.

Intravenous. Most medications used in emergency medicine are designed to be administered intravenously. These can be in the form of an intravenous (IV) *bolus* or as a slow *IV infusion*, sometimes referred to as a *piggyback infusion*. The rate of absorption is rapid and predictable.

Of all the routes frequently employed, however, IV administration of drugs has the most potential for causing adverse reactions.

Endotracheal. When an IV line cannot be started, it is sometimes possible to administer emergency medications down an endotracheal tube, which permits absorption into the capillaries of the lungs. It has been shown that this route has a rate of absorption as fast as the IV route. Drugs that can be administered endotracheally include epinephrine, lidocaine, naloxone, and atropine.

Sublingual injection. In the rare instance in which neither an IV line can be started nor an endotracheal tube inserted, certain drugs can be injected into the vast capillary network immediately under the tongue. Lidocaine is the agent most frequently given by this route.

Intracardiac. Injection of a medication directly into the ventricle of the heart is referred to as intracardiac administration. Because of the many complications associated with this procedure, it is reserved exclusively for life-threatening situations, such as cardiac arrest, when an IV line cannot be established nor an endotracheal tube placed. This is not a paramedic skill.

Intraosseous. When an IV line cannot be started in children under 6 years of age, many emergency medications can be administered intraosseously. A needle can be placed in the anterior aspect of the proximal tibia, through which medications and fluids can be administered. The onset of action is similar to that for IV administration.

Inhalational. Medications can be administered directly into the respiratory tree in cases of respiratory distress resulting from reversible airway disease including asthma and certain types of chronic obstructive pulmonary disease. These medications are usually nebulized into a water vapor and breathed with normal respiration.

Umbilical. Both the umbilical vein and umbilical artery can provide an alternative to IV administration in newborns.

Vaginal. Medications can be placed into the vagina, where they are absorbed into surrounding tissues. Most vaginal medications are supplied in creams or vaginal suppositories. The onset of action is slow, and the effects are generally limited to the lower female genital tract.

DRUG ADMINISTRATION AND PREPARATION

Preparation

Medications can be injected into several body spaces, and the type of injection depends on the body space that is used. The techniques and equipment used for each injection type vary. All injections require a liquid form of the prescribed drug and some type of syringe and needle. The paramedic must know and use the correct type of needle and syringe for the different kinds of injections. For example, an intramuscular (IM) injection requires a long IM needle. A short subcutaneous needle would not reach the muscle, and pain or tissue damage could result.

Dead Space

Manufacturers calibrate syringes so that dead space compensation (amount of drug left behind when syringe is emptied) is not necessary.

Reconstitution and Withdrawal from a Vial

Liquid and powdered medications for parenteral administration are packaged in *sterile* vials. The paramedic can withdraw liquid medication into the syringe, but powdered forms must be reconstituted first. The paramedic must use sterile technique during all medication preparation and injection procedures to decrease the risk of infection.

Small air bubbles may adhere to the interior surface of the syringe when medication is withdrawn from a vial. This small amount of air would not harm the patient if injected, but it could change the dose of medication actually administered. Therefore, the paramedic should remove the air bubbles. To do so, he or she holds the syringe with the needle pointed upward, taps the side of the syringe until the bubbles accumulate at the hub, then slowly pushes the plunger until the air is expelled. If the amount of medication is not accurate after this procedure, the paramedic withdraws more of the drug to complete the prescribed dose.

Withdrawal from an Ampule

Liquid medications for parenteral administration also can be packaged in sterile ampules. Powdered ones rarely are packaged in ampules. Before administering medication from an ampule, the paramedic must withdraw it carefully.

Mixing Drugs

On occasion, the paramedic must mix drugs in one syringe. In prehospital care, mixing may be necessary to administer a narcotic, such as morphine, and an antiemetic, such as promethazine.

Skin Preparation

After filling the syringe, the paramedic must prepare the patient's skin for injection. If the skin is soiled, it should be washed and dried thoroughly if possible. Then an alcohol swab is used to clean the skin. An iodine (Betadine) swab may be used as well. Alcohol swabs should only be used with patients allergic to iodine.

Care should be taken not to touch the patient's skin with anything except the sterile swab. When using a disinfectant, the paramedic should always begin at the point where the needle will be inserted and wipe in a spiral pattern from the center outward. Cleaning from the puncture site outward carries bacteria away from the site.

Before injecting the medication, the disinfected area should be allowed to dry for about 1 minute, if possible. Blowing on or fanning the area to hasten the drying process is discouraged because these activities increase the risk of contamination. Injecting while the skin is still moist can introduce alcohol or iodine into the tissues and causes irritation. Allowing the skin to dry before injection in many cases reduces injection pain.

MEDICAL DIRECTION

Paramedics do not practice autonomously. You will operate under the license of a medical director who is responsible for all of your actions; this responsibility extends to the administration of medication.

The medical director determines which medications you will use and the routes by which you will deliver them. Some states have a "state drug list" whereby the medications a service may carry is dictated by law or legislation or a regulatory agency. While some medications can be administered via off-line medical direction (written standing orders), you will need specific authorization for others after consulting on-line or direct medical direction. You must strictly abide by all of your medical director's guidelines.

Knowing all drug administration protocols is essential, especially which drugs to administer under standing orders and which to deliver only after authorization from medical direction. You can ill afford to waste valuable time looking up procedures and directives for the critical patient who requires immediate drug therapy. Furthermore, because inappropriate drug delivery can have serious consequences, you may face severe legal ramifications even if your patient suffers no harm.

Body Substance Isolation

Establishing routes for drug delivery presents the constant potential for exposure to blood and other body fluids. Always take appropriate body substance isolation (BSI) measures to decrease your risk of exposure. The type of BSI you use will vary according to the delivery route and your patient's condition. At a minimum, you should wear gloves and goggles. Optimally you will also wear a mask. Remarkably, the simplest form of BSI is often the most neglected: hand washing. Washing your hands before and after patient contact is one of the most effective ways to decrease your exposure to infectious material.

MEDICAL ASEPSIS

Medical *asepsis* describes a medical environment free of pathogens. Many paramedical procedures, especially those related to drug administration, place the patient at increased risk for inflection. The external environment is full of microorganisms, many of them pathogenic. Techniques such as intravenous access or endotracheal intubation can allow pathogens to enter the patient's body, where they may cause local or systemic complications.

Sterilization

The most aseptic environment is a sterile one. A sterile environment is free of all forms of life. Generally, environments are sterilized with extensive heat or chemicals. A sterile environment is difficult to attain in the prehospital setting. Consequently, you must practice *medically clean techniques* to minimize your patient's risk of infection. Medically clean techniques involve the careful handling of sterile equipment to prevent contamination. For example, much of the equipment used for drug administration is in sterile packaging. Once you open the package, you must use a medically clean technique to keep the equipment clean and uncontaminated until you use it. If you drop a piece of equipment on a dirty surface, you must discard it and obtain a new piece. Other medically clean techniques, including hand washing, glove changing, and discarding equipment in opened packages, help to prevent equipment and patient contamination. Remember, too, that many patients have lowered immunity levels or carry infectious diseases. Thus, keeping the ambulance and equipment clean is another essential medically clean procedure.

Disinfectants and Antiseptics

When administering medications you must use disinfectants and antiseptics to ensure local cleanliness. Do not confuse disinfectants and antiseptics; the distinction is important. *Disinfectants* are toxic to living tissue. You will therefore use them only on nonliving surfaces or objects such as the inside of an ambulance or laryngoscope blades after use. Never use disinfectants on living tissue.

Antiseptics are not toxic to living tissue. They destroy or inhibit pathogenic microorganisms already living on surfaces and are generally used to cleanse the local area before needle puncture. Common antiseptics include alcohol and iodine preparations used either alone or together. Frequently, antiseptics are diluted disinfectants.

DISPOSAL OF CONTAMINATED EQUIPMENT AND SHARPS

Blood and body fluid can harbor infectious material that endangers the health care provider, family, bystanders, or the patient himself. Many times the patient is infected with pathogenic organisms long before signs and symptoms appear. Therefore, you must treat all blood and body fluids as potentially infectious.

Drug administration commonly involves needles in direct contact with the patient's blood and body fluid. Once used, a needle represents a significant risk. Inadvertent needle sticks, the most common accident in health care as a whole, can transmit diseases between the patient and paramedic. Properly handling needles and other sharps before and after patient use can prevent many of these accidental needle sticks. To minimize or eliminate the risk of an accidental needle stick, take these precautions:

- *Minimize the tasks you perform in a moving ambulance.* Use needles as sparingly as possible in the back of a moving ambulance. When appropriate, perform all interventions involving needles on scene. If en route, it may be occasionally necessary to have the driver pull the ambulance over to the side of the road and stop briefly if you have to use a needle.
- *Immediately dispose of used sharps in a sharps container.* You should dispose all sharps, including needles and prefilled syringes, directly into the sharps container without removing or bending a needle. You should also dispose of items such as used ampules in the sharps container. Avoid dropping sharps onto the floor for later disposal. In the heat of the moment, you may forget the sharp or misplace it.
- *Recap needles only as a last resort.* If you absolutely must recap a needle, never use two hands to do so. Place the sharp on a stationary surface and replace the cap with one hand. Although the one-hand method is still hazardous, it at least reduces the chance for accidental needle stick.

MEDICATION ROUTES USED IN EMERGENCY MEDICINE

Emergency medications are administered parenterally by either the transdermal, sublingual, subcutaneous, intramuscular, intravenous, endotracheal, intraosseous, or inhalational route. Paramedics must always use universal precautions in patient care, particularly with drug administration. This section outlines the procedure for administration by each of these routes. Prior to the administration of any medication, the following steps should be completed:

Administration of Medication

1. Identify any patient allergies prior to base hospital contact.
2. Take and record vital signs.
3. Determine if the order is consistent with training and scope of practice.
4. Confirm order by repeating:
   a. Medication
   b. Dosage, volume, and concentration
   c. Route of administration
5. Write down the order and time of order.
6. Select proper medication and check the name of the medication:
   a. When the medication is first selected
   b. When drawing up the medication
   c. Prior to administering to patient
   d. When replacing medication in storage or disposing of ampule
7. Check for cloudiness, particles, discoloration, and expiration date.
8. Confirm order and medication with partner.
9. Prior to administration of any medication, check the six rights:
   a. Right patient
   b. Right medication
   c. Right dose or amount
   d. Right route
   e. Right time
   f. Right documentation
10. Record drug, dose and volume, route, and time and check and record patient vital signs.
11. Properly dispose of needles in an approved sharps container.

All drug administration skill checklists are given in Appendix H.

Transdermal Administration

Medications given by the transdermal route promote slow, steady absorption. Nitroglycerin, hormones, and analgesics are commonly administered transdermally. Transdermal delivery can also produce localized effects, as with anti-inflammatories and other bacteriostatic and softening agents. Applying medication locally avoids passing larger quantities of the medication throughout the entire body, where it is not needed. Transdermal medications include lotions, ointments, creams, foams, wet dressings, adhesive-backed applications, and suppositories.

Sublingual

Sublingual drugs are absorbed through the mucous membranes beneath the tongue. The sublingual region is extremely vascular and permits rapid absorption with systemic delivery. These medications are generally dissolvable tablets or sprays. One commonly administered sublingual medication is nitroglycerin.

Subcutaneous Injection

Subcutaneous (SC) injections provide a slow, sustained release of medication and a longer duration of action and are used when the total volume injected is no more than 1 mL of liquid. Many medications, including insulin, heparin, and epinephrine, are given by the SC route.

SC injection sites, all areas relatively distant from bones and major blood vessels, include the area over the scapula, the lateral aspects of the upper arm and thigh, and the abdomen. At least 1 inch (2.5 cm) pinched fold of skin and tissue is necessary for administering SC injections. Burned, edematous, or scarred skin should not be used as a SC injection site, nor should the area 2 inches (5 cm) in diameter around the umbilicus or belt line.

Aspiration is not necessary with SC injection because subcutaneous tissue usually contains only small blood vessels. Therefore, the danger of unintended IV injection is minimal. In fact, aspirating SC injections may cause tissue damage that could affect drug absorption adversely.

Intramuscular Injection

Intramuscular injection is useful when drug action faster than that provided by SC injection is desired but rapid effects are not required. The onset of action usually occurs within 10 to 15 minutes after an IM injection. However, the blood flow to the injection site affects the absorption rate. The most common muscles into which drugs are administered are the deltoid and the gluteus. In general, 5 mL of fluid can be administered with an IM injection, but a maximum of 1 mL of medication can be given into the deltoid, whereas 10 mL can be given into the gluteus. Accurate identification of injection sites is important because major blood vessels and nerves traverse the muscle groups used for IM injections. Therefore, using an inappropriate injection site could result in permanent damage to the patient. The technique for administering an IM injection is the same for both adult and pediatric patients.

It is important to note that, as a rule, patients presenting with a chief complaint of chest pain should not receive medications by the IM route. Intramuscular injection of medication may cause an elevation of certain muscle enzymes that routinely circulate in the blood. In the emergency department these enzymes are frequently measured to determine whether the chest pain is of myocardial origin. An intramuscular injection in the prehospital phase of emergency medical care can cause a false elevation of these enzymes, which can subsequently confuse the emergency physician as he or she attempts to determine the etiology of the chest pain. On some occasions, however, the medical control physician may permit intramuscular injections when no other immediate route is available and administration of the medication is essential.

Intravenous Administration

Medications are administered intravenously to obtain an immediate onset of action, to obtain the highest possible blood concentration of a drug, and to treat conditions that require the constant titration of medication. In many cases, life-threatening situations such as shock require such constant titration.

Sites used for IV administration include the veins on the hand and wrist, the forearm veins that traverse the antecubital fossa, the veins on the scalp and umbilical vessels (for infants), and the superficial veins of the leg and foot when other sites cannot be used.

As mentioned previously, there are two distinct methods of IV medication administration: (1) the IV bolus and (2) slow IV infusion (sometimes called "piggyback"). Emergency medications administered by the IV bolus technique are usually administered with prefilled syringes. Many medications, however, are still available only in ampule or vial form.

In all but a few cases, it is essential that an IV be established before administering medications intravenously. Establishing an IV line makes the repeated administration of medications less traumatic.

Endotracheal Administration

The endotracheal route is very effective and often forgotten in the emergency setting. When an IV cannot be established, and the patient is in dire need of lidocaine, naloxone, atropine, or epinephrine, which may be the case in cardiac arrest, these drugs may be instilled via the endotracheal tube. The rate of absorption is as fast as with IV administration. When administering a medication via the endotracheal tube, the dose should be increased to 2 to 2.5 times the intravenous dose.

A common situation follows: A patient is encountered in ventricular fibrillation and is immediately countershocked. The patient converts to an improved rhythm with a fair pulse. An IV line cannot be immediately established, however. The patient begins to have frequent multifocal premature ventricular contractions. Lidocaine can now be administered down the endotracheal tube to stabilize the rhythm until a peripheral line can be established.

Intraosseous Injection

It is often difficult to establish an IV line in children younger than 6 years of age. In instances in which an IV cannot be established and the child needs emergency medications or fluids, an intraosseous line can be established. A needle is placed into the proximal tibia, approximately 1 to 3 cm below the tibial tuberosity, on the anterior surface. The needle is advanced through the cortex of the bone into the bone marrow cavity. Entry into the marrow cavity is evidenced by a lack of resistance after penetrating the bony cortex, the needle standing upright without support, the ability to aspirate bone marrow into a syringe connected to the needle, or the free flow of the infusion without significant subcutaneous infiltration. Fluids and drugs administered into the marrow cavity quickly enter the circulatory system. The onset of action of drugs administered by this route is similar to that found with IV injection. Drugs that can be administered by this route include the catecholamines, lidocaine, atropine, and sodium bicarbonate, as well as fluids. Intraosseous infusion is only indicated in children younger than 6 years of age and only when an IV line cannot be established.

Inhalational Administration

Many medications used in the treatment of respiratory emergencies are administered by inhalation. The most common example is oxygen. In addition, some medications are designed to be administered into the respiratory tree. The most common of these are the bronchodilators, including metaproterenol (Alupent), racemic epinephrine, isoetharine (Bronkosol), ipratropium (Atrovent), and salbutamol (Ventolin). If these drugs are administered directly into the respiratory tree, they can quickly reach their site of action with minimal absorption delays. Following are three common methods for administering these medications:

Metered-dose inhalers. Metered-dose inhalers are aerosolized forms of the medication in a small canister. Most bronchodilators are supplied in this form. Many patients have inhalers at home and use them routinely. The canister is attached to a mouthpiece. The patient places his or her lips around the mouthpiece, begins to inhale, and presses the canister. When the canister is pressed, a metered amount of the drug is delivered in aerosol form. The amount of drug delivered is accurate and limited. Metered-dose inhalers are designed for single-patient use (see Figure 3–1). Some metered-dose inhalers come equipped with a spacer. The spacer is a

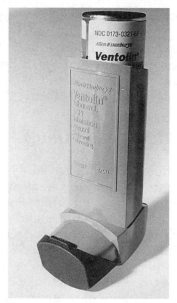

FIGURE 3–1 Metered-dose inhaler.

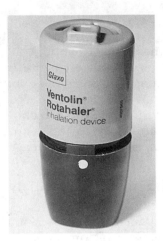

FIGURE 3–2 Spinhaler (Ventolin Rotohaler).

cylindrical canister between the inhaler and the mouthpiece. Prior to administration, the patient will depress the inhaler sending a measured dose of drug into the spacer. The patient will then breathe in and out of the spacer through the mouthpiece, thus inhaling the drug into the lungs. The system is particularly useful for patients who have a hard time operating and inhaling the metered-dose inhaler. This is common in the elderly and in young children. The spacer, when used in conjunction with a metered-dose inhaler, is very effective.

Spinhaler, rotahaler. These commercial devices are designed for patients who have difficulty operating the metered-dose inhalers. Special capsules are placed in the device. When inhaled, the capsules release medication that is delivered to the respiratory tree (see Figure 3–2).

Small-volume nebulizer. Small-volume nebulizers, also called updraft or handheld nebulizers, are the most commonly used method of administering inhaled medications in the emergency setting. The nebulizer has a chamber into which a solution of the medication, usually diluted with 2 to 3 mL of sterile saline, is placed. Oxygen or compressed air is blown past the chamber, causing the medication to be aerosolized. The patient inhales the aerosolized medication with each breath. This method of bronchodilator administration is advantageous because it delivers supplemental oxygen, delivers the medication over a 5- to 10-minute interval, and is supplied in single-dose ampules (see Figure 3–3).

PEDIATRIC ADMINISTRATION TECHNIQUES

Administering drugs safely to a child requires special attention to the six rights because any medication error can have a much greater impact on a child than on an adult. For each route of administration, the paramedic must modify adult administration techniques for a pediatric patient. No matter which route is used, the paramedic should attempt to elicit the child's cooperation to make medication administration as easy as possible. If the child is unable to cooperate, the paramedic may need to ask a parent to assist and hold the child during administration.

Although absorption from the GI tract is less predictable than from other routes, oral administration may be used. In prehospital care, the ad-

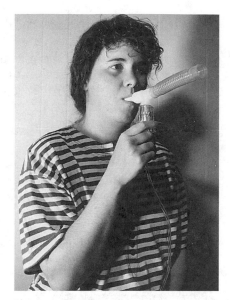

FIGURE 3–3 Small-volume nebulizer.

ministration of Tylenol may be required in febrile patients. Administering medications to a child may be a challenge.

If an infant or small child must be restrained for medication administration, the paramedic should use a syringe without a needle to administer small, controlled doses. To minimize the risk of choking or aspirating, the paramedic should hold the child's head upright or to the side.

The paramedic then slides the syringe into the child's mouth about halfway back between the gums and cheeks and squirts a small amount of medication. This administration technique offers several advantages. Placing the medication deep in the side of the mouth makes it difficult for the child to lose the medication by spitting or drooling. Although medication administration may take longer because the drug is given in small amounts, this technique reduces the risk of choking, coughing, and vomiting because it does not stimulate the gag reflex.

Intramuscular Injection

For an IM injection the paramedic should use the smallest gauge needle appropriate for the medication, usually a needle that is 25 to 22 gauge. The needle length should not exceed 1 inch (2.5 cm), except in the adult-sized adolescent, who may require a 1.5-inch (3.8-cm) needle.

The recommended injection sites vary with age. The vastus lateralis and rectus femoris muscles are the recommended sites for an infant or toddler. For a child who has been walking for about 1 year, the paramedic can give the injection in the ventrogluteal or dorsogluteal area. Walking develops muscles and thus reduces the risk of sciatic nerve damage during an IM injection. For an older child, an injection site such as the deltoid, gluteus maximus, ventrogluteus, vastus lateralis, or rectus femoris may be used. The same injection technique used in an adult is used in a child. If necessary, the child's parent or the paramedic's partner may be asked to hold the child still during injection.

Subcutaneous Administration

Subcutaneous administration is the same in a child as in an adult. Injection sites include the abdomen and the middle third of the upper arm or thigh. The needle should be 27 to 23 gauge and 3/8 to 5/8 inch (1 to 1.5 cm) long.

Intravenous Administration

Pediatric IV administration poses several challenges for the paramedic. Pediatric IV administration is the same as for an adult, with the caution that any medication error can have a much greater impact on a child than on an adult.

Rectal Administration

Drug absorption from the rectum may be unpredictable. Nevertheless, medications may be administered rectally when oral administration or other routes are not available. For example, in a febrile patient having a seizure, administration of medications by other routes would be difficult. In this situation, the rectal administration of diazepam (Valium) or lorazepam (Ativan) may be indicated.

SUMMARY

It is essential that acute-care personnel be competent with all of the medication routes used in emergency medicine. These skills can be developed only after repeated practice in the classroom and the clinical setting. It is important for paramedics to be familiar with all of the medications used in routine prehospital care in their system and the routes by which the medications are administered. If there is any doubt concerning an order or an administration route, the medical control physician or a drug reference source should be consulted. Each time a medication is administered, the paramedic should ensure he or she has met each of the six rights of medication administration: right patient, right medication, right dose, right route, right time, and right documentation.

This book is not a substitute for a rigorous classroom instruction session on medication administration. It is designed purely as a teaching aid for the student and as a reference source for others.

KEY WORDS

alimentary canal.   The digestive tract.

antiseptic.   Cleaning agent that is not toxic to living tissue.

asepsis.   A condition free of pathogens.

bolus.   A method of intravenous medication administration by which a drug is rapidly administered rather than infused over a period of time.

disinfectant.   Cleansing agent that is toxic to living tissue.

endotracheal.   A route of medication administration by which drugs are administered down an endotracheal tube.

inhalational route. Route via which a medication is introduced into the body through the respiratory tract.

intracardiac. Administration of medications directly into the heart. This route is not recommended for prehospital care.

intradermal. A parenteral route of medication administration by which a drug is injected into the dermal layer of the skin.

intramuscular. A common parenteral route of medication administration by which a drug is injected into the skeletal muscle.

intraosseous. A route of fluid and drug administration in which select medications or fluids are injected into the bone marrow. This route is considered an alternative to venous access in children under the age of 6 years.

intravenous. A commonly used parenteral route of medication administration by which a drug is injected directly into venous circulation.

intravenous infusion. A method of medication administration by which a drug or fluid is given over time.

local. Limited to one area of the body.

medically clean technique. Careful handling to prevent contamination.

metered-dose inhaler. A device for administering medication by inhalation; it consists of a canister containing a liquid that, when activated, delivers the medication via a fine mist.

piggyback. A method of administering a medication by slow IV infusion.

rectal. An enteral route of medication administration by which a drug is instilled in the rectum.

stat. Latin abbreviation meaning "immediately."

sterile. Free of all forms of life.

subcutaneous. A common parenteral route of medication administration by which a drug is injected into the loose connective tissue between the dermis and the muscle.

sublingual. A route of medication administration by which a drug is absorbed across the rich blood supply of the tongue.

systemic. Throughout the body.

4

DRUG DOSAGE CALCULATIONS

OBJECTIVES

After completing this chapter, the reader should be able to:

1. Define the metric system.
2. Identify and utilize the common metric prefixes, multiples, and submultiples.
3. Convert between units of the metric system.
4. Convert between units of the metric system and the customary or apothecary system.
5. Utilize the rules of the metric system.
6. Solve a basic order word problem using either the ratio and proportion, cross multiplication, or formula method.
7. Recognize an order based on patient's weight.
8. Solve an order problem based on patient weight using the simple three-step method.
9. Recognize the two basic types of concentration problems.
10. Define and recognize a weight/volume percentage solution.
11. Find the amount of solute in a weight/volume percentage solution using either the formula method or the ratio and proportion method.
12. Find the concentration of a solution using either the formula method or the ratio and proportion method.
13. Recognize an intravenous drip problem.
14. Organize the information from an intravenous drip problem.
15. Recognize and be familiar with the dimensional analysis method of solving intravenous drip problems.
16. Recognize and be familiar with the rule of fours method of solving intravenous drip problems.

17. Solve an intravenous drip problem using either the dimensional analysis or the intravenous rule of fours method.

18. Recognize an intravenous drip problem based on patient weight.

19. Organize the information from an intravenous drip problem that is based on patient weight.

20. Solve an intravenous drip problem based on patient weight using either the dimensional analysis or rule of fours method.

21. Recognize an intravenous order of milliliters per hour that needs to be converted to drops per minute.

22. Utilize the formula method to solve a conversion from milliliters per hour to drops per minute.

INTRODUCTION

Administration of the correct drug dosage is essential to proper prehospital medical care. This skill will be tested in written exams, practical skill stations, and on a daily basis in the prehospital environment. Medications used in emergency medicine are available from many different manufacturers. They also vary in concentration, volume, and packaging. The importance of being familiar with the common emergency drug preparations and calculating correct dosages cannot be overemphasized. All prehospital personnel should be able to prepare the correct medication dose quickly and accurately from available ampules, vials, pills, tablets, or other prepackaged medications regardless of drug concentration, volume, or packaging. This responsibility requires knowledge, skill, and practice. This chapter will help paramedics prepare to meet that responsibility.

Familiarity with the systems of measurement frequently used in medicine, especially the metric system, is essential to meet this responsibility. Conversion from one system to another is often required.

In this chapter a review of the metric system, common mathematical operations, and dosage calculations are presented. The practice problems at the end of this chapter provide an opportunity to hone the skills learned.

SECTION 1: THE METRIC SYSTEM

The International System of Units (SI), or the metric system, is an international system of measurement that originated in France during the period of the French Revolution. It has been internationally developed and is approved for use in the United States with some minor modifications. The metric system is the standard system of weights and measures used worldwide in the sciences, including medicine and pharmacology. However, tradition has caused some apothecary and household weights and measures, known as the customary system, to endure in the United States.

The metric system is a decimal system based on multiples or submultiples of the number 10. All units are either 10 times larger or 1/10 as large as the next unit. Because the metric system is based on 10, the conversion from one unit to another is simple. To change from one multiple or submultiple to another requires moving only a decimal point. Greek prefixes are used to express these multiples and submultiples. Different prefixes produce units that are of an appropriate size for the application that is needed.

Units of the Metric System

There are many units in the metric system. The following units of the metric system are approved for use in the United States and are the units most commonly used in the prehospital environment:

- Meter (m) for length
- Degrees Celsius (°C) for temperature
- Gram (g) for mass
- Liter (L) for volume

The liter (L) is not an SI unit. That is why the abbreviation, or symbol, is capitalized. The SI unit for volume is the cubic meter (m^3). However, the liter (L) is an approved and preferred unit of volume in Europe, Canada, and the United States. Other nonmetric units that are acceptable to use in the United States include the minute, the hour, and the nautical mile.

Multiples, Submultiples, and Prefixes of the Metric System

Units are used like home bases. Very large numbers or very small numbers can be difficult to manage. The metric system answers this problem with an easy solution: Multiples or submultiples are used in a decimal system and each is given a prefix to attach to the base unit. Although Table 4–1 does not list all of them, it lists some of the common multiples, submultiples, and prefixes of the metric system. Symbols over 1 million are capitalized; all others are lowercase.

Instead of using a large number of zeros, a person making metric conversions can simply change the prefix. A quantity of 1000 g of something is much easier to work with mathematically if it is converted to 1 kg.

Metric Conversions

Converting within the metric system is logical and simple. The most common multiples or prefixes used in the prehospital setting are the *kilo-*, the *milli-*, and the *micro-*. One can convert between these multiples by a factor

TABLE 4–1

Common Multiples, Submultiples, and Prefixes of the Metric System

Multiples and Submultiples	Prefix Name	Prefix Symbol
$1\,000\,000\,000 = 10^9$	*giga-*	G
$1\,000\,000 = 10^6$	*mega-*	M
$1\,000 = 10^3$	*kilo-*	k
$100 = 10^2$	*hecto-*	h
$10 = 10^1$	*deka-*	da
	Base unit	
$0.1 = 10^{-1}$	*deci-*	d
$0.01 = 10^{-2}$	*centi-*	c
$0.001 = 10^{-3}$	*milli-*	m
$0.000\,001 = 10^{-6}$	*micro-*	μ
$0.000\,000\,001 = 10^{-9}$	*nano-*	n

of 1000 by either multiplying or dividing by 1000 depending on the need. Examples of common metric conversions follow:

$$1 \text{ kg} = 1000 \text{ g}$$
$$1 \text{ g} = 1000 \text{ mg}$$
$$1 \text{ mg} = 1000 \text{ } \mu\text{g}$$
$$1 \text{ L} = 1000 \text{ mL}$$

Let us say we have 1 mg of a drug and we need to divide it up to work with it more effectively. Rather than deal with fractions, we can simply convert it to 1000 μg. Now, it will be easier to divide and work with.

Some conversions between the customary and the metric systems may still be necessary. Just ask anyone in the United States how much he weighs. What unit will he respond? Pounds. Because prehospital medicine uses the metric system, common conversion factors between the two systems are provided in Table 4–2.

The following temperature conversion formulas may also prove helpful:

$$°C = (°F - 32) \times \frac{5}{9}$$

$$°F = (°C \times \frac{9}{5}) + 32$$

Rules of the Metric System

Units

The written names of all metric units start with lowercase letters unless they begin a sentence. The units *meter, gram, liter,* and so on begin with lowercase letters. The one exception, however, is degrees Celsius. The unit *degrees* is lowercase, but the word *Celsius* is capitalized. Normal body temperature would be written as

37 degrees Celsius

Symbols (Abbreviations)

Generally, the metric symbols or the abbreviations are written in lowercase letters. For example:

km for kilometer
mg for milligram

TABLE 4–2

Common Conversion Factors between the Metric and Customary Systems

Metric		Customary
5 mL	=	1 tsp
15 mL	=	1 T (tablespoon)
30 mL	=	1 fl oz
950 mL	=	1 qt
3.8 L	=	1 gal
2.54 cm	=	1 inch
65 mg	=	1 gr
0.45 kg	=	1 lb
1 kg	=	2.2 lb

The liter is not an SI unit, but it is approved for use in the United States and Europe. So, to set it apart, the symbol for liter is generally capitalized. Also, if a unit name is derived from a person's name, it is also capitalized:

L for liter
Pa for pascal
mL for milliliter

Plurals

The full written names of units (e.g., meter, gram, and liter) are only made plural when the numerical value that precedes them is more than 1. One exception to this rule is 0 degrees Celsius.

0 degrees Celsius
2 liters
0.25 liter, *not* 0.25 liters

Symbols for units are not made plural:

50 mL = 50 milliliters
50 mL, *not* 50 mL's

Spacing

A space is used between the number and the symbol (abbreviation) to which it refers:

5 km
10 mg
40° C

Hyphens

Hyphens between a number and a metric unit are not necessary when used as a one-thought modifier. If a hyphen is used, the name of the metric value should be written out. Hyphens should not be used with symbols (abbreviations).

1-liter bag, *not* 1-L bag
5-kilometer run, *not* 5-km run

Spaces

Spaces are used in place of commas when writing metric values that contain five or more digits. For values with four digits, either a space or no space is acceptable. The spaces are added on either side of the decimal point.

1 234 567 km, *not* 1,234,567 km
2000 mL or 2 000 mL
0.123 456 kg

Period

A period is not used with metric unit names and symbols (abbreviations) except at the end of a sentence.

50 cm, *not* 50 cm.

Decimal Point

A period is used as a decimal point within numbers to designate decimal fractions. When the number is less than 1 (a decimal fraction), a 0 is written before the decimal point. This leading 0 is especially important in drug calculations because it draws attention to the decimal point and prevents drug dosage errors. Common fractions are not used in the metric system.

0.5 mg, *not* .5 mg

SECTION 2: FIND THE ORDERED DOSE

The ordered dose is the most simple dosage calculation for the prehospital care provider. In this type of problem, the paramedic is given an order to administer a medication to a patient. There are three components to locate in this type of problem: the doctor's order, the concentration of the drug on hand, and what unit to administer.

The Doctor's Order

The order from the physician includes the amount of the medication and should also include the route of administration. The routes of administration include subcutaneous, intramuscular, intravenous (IV), endotracheal, sublingual, intraosseous, intralingual, transdermal, oral, and rectal. Orders can be verbal or written as a standing order or protocol. The order in the example that follows is known as a *basic order.*

Concentration

The second item to identify is the concentration or "what's on hand," as referred to by some texts. The paramedic is given the concentration of either a vial, an ampule, a prefilled syringe, or a tablet. Concentrations can be listed as common fractions, ratio percentages, percentage solutions, or by mass (e.g., grams and milligrams).

Unit to Administer

It is essential to look at the doctor's order and identify the unit of measurement that will be administered to the patient. Some texts refer to the unit to administer as "what you are looking for."

All three components can be identified in the following example.

EXAMPLE PROBLEM

A physician orders 2.5 mg of morphine to be administered IV to a patient with substernal chest pain. You have a 1 mL vial that contains 10 mg of morphine (10 mg/mL). How many milliliters are you going to have to draw into a syringe and push IV into your patient?

Note: Some problems may not ask, "How many milliliters?" They may simply ask, "How much are you going to administer?" You will have to deduce "milliliters" from the context of the problem.

To solve dosage calculation problems consistently and accurately you must be organized. Developing the habit of organization early will make drug dosage problems seem easier. So, before starting any calculations, write down all of the components to the problem.

Doctor's order	2.5 mg of morphine IV
Concentration	10 mg/mL or 10 mg per 1 mL
Unit to administer	mL

Now that you have identified the three components, you will need to solve the problem. There are three methods that can be used. The first two methods are basic algebraic equations and the third is a formula.

Ratio and Proportion Method

1. On the left side of the proportion, put the ratio that is known:

$$10 \text{ mg} : 1 \text{ mL} ::$$

2. On the right side of the proportion, put the ratio that is unknown (usually the ratio composed of the order). It is essential that you put the *units* on both sides of the equation in the same sequence:

$$10 \text{ mg} : 1 \text{ mL} :: 2.5 \text{ mg} : x \text{ mL}$$

3. Now put the proportion in the form of a basic algebraic equation. The extremes can be placed to the left of an equal sign and the means to the right.

$$10x = 2.5 \times 1$$

4. Multiply the right side:

$$10x = 2.5$$

5. Divide both sides by the number in front of x and check to see if the answer's unit matches what you are looking for:

$$x = 0.25 \text{ mL}$$

Cross Multiplication Method

The cross multiplication method is very similar to the ratio and proportion method. It simply sets up the problem using common fractions. The first fraction can be the concentration. The second fraction is the doctor's order over what is to be administered.

$$\frac{10 \text{ mg}}{1 \text{ mL}} = \frac{2.5 \text{ mg}}{x \text{ mL}}$$

Cross multiply the fractions by multiplying the numerators by the opposite denominators. The resulting algebraic equation is exactly the same as from the preceding equation:

$$10x = 2.5 \times 1$$
$$10x = 2.5$$
$$x = 0.25 \text{ mL}$$

In both methods, remember to place the unit to administer, or "what you are looking for," into the answer.

Formula Method

Some people prefer to memorize a formula to solve this type of problem. The following formula will be helpful if you prefer this method:

$$\text{Volume to be administered } (x) = \frac{\text{Volume on hand} \times \text{Ordered dose}}{\text{Concentration on hand}}$$

Using the preceding example, place each of the components in their proper places in the formula, as illustrated in the following example.

EXAMPLE PROBLEM

A physician orders 2.5 mg of morphine to be administered IV to a patient with substernal chest pain. You have a 1 mL vial that contains 10 mg of morphine (10 mg/mL). How many milliliters are you going to have to draw into a syringe and push IV into your patient?

1. Fill in the formula:

$$x = \frac{(1 \text{ mL}) (2.5 \text{ mg})}{10 \text{ mg}}$$

2. Cancel any like units (mg):

$$x = \frac{(1 \text{ mL}) (2.5 \text{ mg})}{10 \text{ mg}}$$

3. Work the algebra:

$$x = \frac{2.5}{10} \text{ mL}$$

$$x = 0.25 \text{ mL}$$

SECTION 3: FIND THE UNITS PER KILOGRAM

Finding the units per kilogram adds a new dimension to the problems in the previous section. Instead of a basic order, the doctor will order a certain number of units (e.g., grams and milligrams) of a drug to be administered based on the patient's weight, almost always in kilograms. This is referred to as an order based on patient's weight. Look at the following example.

EXAMPLE PROBLEM

The doctor orders 5 mg/kg of bretylium IV to be administered to your patient. You have premixed syringes with 500 mg/10 mL. Your patient weights 220 lb. How many milliliters will you administer?

You can see that the order of 5 mg/kg of bretylium is a little different than a basic order. Start by writing down all of the key information. In this type of problem, add a patient weight category. Always begin with organizing the information:

Doctor's order	5 mg/kg bretylium IV
Concentration	500 mg/mL
Unit to administer	mL
Patient's weight	220 lb

Look at the order. It is directly tied to the patient's weight. Put another way, the order is saying, "For every kilogram of patient, give 5 mg of bretylium."

In the following three-step method, only step 2 is new. The other steps have been covered in previous sections.

Three-Step Method

1. Convert the patient's weight from pounds to kilograms.
2. Convert the ordered dose based on patient's weight to a basic order.
3. Find the ordered dose.

Step 1: Convert pounds to kilograms.

$$220 \text{ lb} \div 2.2 = 100 \text{ kg}$$

or

$$220 \text{ lb} \times 0.45 = 99 \text{ kg}$$

Note: For ease of computation, 99 kg could then be approximated to 100 kg without compromising patient care.

Step 2: Convert the order by weight to a basic order.

This step can be calculated by using a formula or by using the ratio and proportion method.

Formula Method

$$x = \frac{\text{Ordered dose} \times \text{Weight (kg)}}{1 \text{ kg}}$$

Set up the formula.

$$x = \frac{5 \text{ mg} \times 100 \text{ kg}}{1 \text{ kg}}$$

The unit of kilogram in the numerator cancels out the unit of kilogram in the denominator, leaving milligrams. Now, work the math:

$$x = 500 \text{ mg}$$

This is the basic ordered dose. You can now proceed to step 3 or look at the ratio and proportion method.

Ratio and Proportion Method

$$5 \text{ mg} : 1 \text{ kg} :: x \text{ mg} : 100 \text{ kg}$$

$$x = 5 \times 100$$

$$x = 500 \text{ mg}$$

Either way, this is now a basic order that can be worked with. Draw a line through the order based on patient weight and write in the new basic order of 500 mg over it. This habit will help keep information organized. Now, the ordered dose must be calculated.

Step 3: Find the ordered dose.

Because you now have a basic order, find the ordered dose using the method that you prefer from Section 2.

Answer: 10 mL

SECTION 4: CONCENTRATION PROBLEMS

Prehospital care providers encounter two types of concentration problems. The first type of concentration problem, amount of solute problems, tests knowledge of the solutions that paramedics work with. The second type not only helps in finding the concentration in an IV bag but is also a major step used when solving IV drip problems (Sections 5 and 6).

Amount of Solute

Concentration problems dealing with amount of solute are seen more often on tests than in practical applications. They involve searching for the amount of solute in a weight/volume percentage solution. Weight/volume percentage is a commonly used percentage concentration with prehospital solutions. It always expresses the number of grams of solute in a total of 100 mL of solution.

For example, 50 percent dextrose in water, or $D_{50}W$, is a common prehospital drug. This expression means that there are 50 g of dextrose in every 100 mL of solution. The fraction expression of the weight/volume percentage solution is as follows:

$$\frac{50 \text{ g}}{100 \text{ mL}} \text{ of dextrose in water}$$

Knowing this, it is obvious that when there are 50 mL of this solution, there are 25 g of dextrose. Following are a couple of examples of how this type of problem could be worded.

EXAMPLE PROBLEM

You have a 250 mL bag of D_5W. How many grams of dextrose are in the bag?

Formula Method

Number of grams (x) = Percentage of solution × Volume of solution

Filling in the formula and working the problem solves the preceding example:

$$x = \frac{5 \text{ g}}{100 \text{ mL}} \times 250 \text{ mL}$$

$$x = \frac{1250}{100} \text{ g}$$

$$x = 12.5 \text{ g}$$

Hint: If the problem had asked for answers in milligrams, the grams would need to be converted to milligrams to find the correct answer.

Ratio and Proportion or Cross Multiplication Method

This problem could also be worked using either the ratio and proportion or cross multiplication methods:

$$5 \text{ g} : 100 \text{ mL} :: x \text{ g} : 250 \text{ mL} \quad or \quad \frac{5 \text{ g}}{100 \text{ mL}} = \frac{x \text{ g}}{250 \text{ mL}}$$

$$100x = 5 \times 250$$

$$100x = 1250$$

$$x = 12.5 \text{ g}$$

These same types of problems can be twisted around. What if the number of grams to be administered and the percentage were given and the amount to be infused was the unknown? Look at the following example.

EXAMPLE PROBLEM

The doctor orders 12.5 g of 5 percent dextrose to be infused. How many milliliters will be infused?

A formula, the ratio and proportion method, or cross multiplication may be used to solve this type of problem.

Formula Method

$$\text{Volume } (x) = \frac{\text{Amount ordered (g)}}{\text{Percentage}}$$

$$x = \frac{12.5 \text{ g}}{5 \text{ percent}}$$

or mathematically the same:

$$x = 12.5 \text{ g} \times \frac{5 \text{ g}}{100 \text{ mL}}$$

$$x = 12.5 \text{ g} \times \frac{100 \text{ mL}}{5 \text{ g}}$$

$$x = \frac{1250}{5} \text{ mL}$$

$$x = 250 \text{ mL}$$

Ratio and Proportion Method

Still using the preceding example, we can use the ratio and proportion method to find the answer:

$$5 \text{ g} : 100 \text{ mL} :: 12.5 \text{ g} : x \text{ mL}$$

$$5x = 1250$$

$$x = 250 \text{ mL}$$

Find the Concentration of a Solution

In most facilities and EMS systems, the pharmacy or drug manufacturer prepares solutions for IV use. However, in small hospitals, rural EMS systems, and other settings (such as testing sites), paramedics are required to measure, prepare, and administer these solutions.

The second type of concentration problem is used to find the concentration of a particular premixed IV solution (or syringe, vial, or the like). It is also used as a major step in solving IV drip problems. It is important to know the answer to the question "What do they mean by concentration?" The usual answer is how many milligrams or micrograms of a drug are contained per 1 mL of a given solution. There are other ways to express concentration, but when prehospital care workers are referring to an IV solution's concentration they usually mean a per milliliter concentration.

EXAMPLE PROBLEM

One gram of lidocaine has been added to a 250 mL bag of D_5W. What is the concentration?

Formula Method

A standard formula is used to express concentration. Once it is set up, it is simply a matter of reducing the fraction to a denominator of 1.

$$x = \frac{\text{Solute (grams or milligrams of drug)}}{\text{Solvent (liters or milliliters of volume)}}$$

Set up the formula:

$$x = \frac{1 \text{ g lidocaine}}{250 \text{ mL } D_5W}$$

Convert grams to milligrams (lidocaine is ordered in milligrams):

$$x = \frac{1000 \text{ mg lidocaine}}{250 \text{ mL D}_5\text{W}}$$

Reduce the fraction to a denominator of 1:

$$x = \frac{1000 \text{ mg lidocaine}}{250 \text{ mL D}_5\text{W}} \div \frac{250}{250}$$

$$x = \frac{4 \text{ mg lidocaine}}{1 \text{ mL D}_5\text{W}}$$

This result can be expressed verbally as "The concentration is 4 milligrams per milliliter" or "4 to 1." This is the per milliliter concentration.

Ratio and Proportion Method

$$1000 \text{ mg} : 250 \text{ mL} :: x \text{ mg} : 1 \text{ mL}$$

$$250x = 1000$$

$$x = 4 \text{ mg/mL}$$

Both of these methods can be used to find the per milliliter concentration of any solution.

SECTION 5: CALCULATE AN IV DRIP

Calculating IV drips has been a quandary for many prehospital care providers for a long time. Asking any paramedic, nurse, or doctor to set up an IV drip without a calculator, reference, electric pump, or computerized device is likely to produce all kinds of moans and excuses. But that is exactly what paramedics are expected to do at test stations and in the prehospital environment. There is an easy way to solve drip problems. This section will examine both the dimensional analysis and the rule of fours methods. Paramedics may choose the method that works best for them.

IV Drip

In some cases, patients require medication to be infused on a continual basis. Paramedics will receive orders to administer a certain number of units (usually milligrams or micrograms) of a medication per minute to a patient through an IV. Known as an infusion, it is also referred to as an IV drip because it involves calculating the number of drops that "drip" and are delivered intravenously each minute to deliver the amount of drug the doctor is ordering.

Even though most of these IV infusions are commercially available already premixed, paramedics will be tested on mixing the medication and starting the infusion correctly. If an occasion occurs in which paramedics do not have a premixed bag, they will know what to do. This process involves drawing medication from a vial or ampule into a syringe and mixing it into an IV bag. Then, paramedics will be required to set a drip rate based on the doctor's order and the administration set that is available. The solution is the number of drops that fall each minute (gtt/min).

Formula Method (Dimensional Analysis)

If paramedics have a chemistry or algebra background, they will understand the formula method and probably prefer it. It very systematically and mathematically calculates the IV drip rate. If they do not like math or chemistry, they may not like this method. They do need to understand it, however. This method shows how a drip rate is calculated and answers a lot of questions that may arise later. Organization of the material is still the key to success.

EXAMPLE PROBLEM

A doctor orders 2 mg/min of lidocaine to be administered to a patient who was experiencing an arrhythmia. You have a vial that contains 1 g of lidocaine in 5 mL. Your ambulance carries only 250 mL bags of D_5W. Your administration set is a microdrip set (60 gtt/mL). At how many drops per minute will you adjust your administration set to drip?

Before starting any calculations, organize the information just as you were doing in Section 2. There are a couple of new categories in this type of problem.

Order	2 mg lidocaine IV
On hand	1 g lidocaine/5 mL
Bag	250 mL D_5W
Administration set	60 gtt/mL
Unit to administer	gtt/min

Formula (Dimensional Analysis) Method

$$x = \frac{\text{IV bag volume (mL)}}{\text{Amount of drug in bag}} \times \frac{\text{Unit ordered}}{1 \text{ min}} \times \frac{\text{Administration set (gtt)}}{1 \text{ mL}}$$

1. Fill in the formula:

$$x = \frac{250 \text{ mL}}{1 \text{ g}} \times \frac{2 \text{ mg}}{1 \text{ min}} \times \frac{60 \text{ gtt}}{1 \text{ mL}}$$

Note: The 5 mL in the vial on hand is not figured into the equation.

2. Convert the grams in the bag to match the milligrams in the doctor's order:

$$x = \frac{250 \text{ mL}}{1000 \text{ mg}} \times \frac{2 \text{ mg}}{1 \text{ min}} \times \frac{60 \text{ gtt}}{1 \text{ mL}}$$

3. Cancel out like units and zeros. Confirm that the remaining units are what you are looking for:

$$x = \frac{25}{10} \times \frac{2}{1 \text{ min}} \times \frac{6 \text{ gtt}}{1}$$

4. Multiply and reduce the fraction:

$$x = \frac{300 \text{ gtt}}{10 \text{ min}}$$

$$x = \frac{30 \text{ gtt}}{1 \text{ min}} \quad \text{or} \quad 30 \text{ gtt/min}$$

You can now set your drip rate on the IV administration set. Remember, in most ambulances and test centers, an electric or computerized IV pump will not be available and you will have to set the rate by hand.

Rule of Fours Method

This method is called the rule of fours because it is based on multiples of the number 4. This is also known as the "easy" way. Many people find it far simpler than the formula method or dimensional analysis. It requires the memorization of a process, not a formula, and requires only simple logic and very little math. Look at the same example problem from earlier:

EXAMPLE PROBLEM

A doctor orders 2 mg/min of lidocaine to be administered to a patient who was experiencing an arrhythmia. You have a vial that contains 1 g of lidocaine in 5 mL. Your ambulance carries only 250 mL bags of D_5W. Your administration set is a microdrip set (60 gtt/mL). At how many drops per minute will you adjust your administration set to drip?

We begin by organizing the information from the problem similarly to how it was done in the previous example. However, this time we add a new category: the concentration of the IV solution (1 g into 250 mL).

Note: Finding the concentration in the bag is the *key* to solving IV drip problems when using this method. Refer to Section 4 to review this process.

Order	2 mg lidocaine IV
On hand	1 g lidocaine/5 mL
Bag	250 mL D_5W
Concentration	4 mg/mL
Administration set	60 gtt/mL
Unit to administer	gtt/min

1. *Compare.* Now that the information is organized, a logical comparison can be made between the concentration and the administration set. Looking at the concentration we could say that in every 1 mL there are 4 mg of lidocaine. We could also say that there are 60 drops in each milliliter. Therefore, in every 60 drops there are 4 mg or 60 gtt/4 mL.

2. *Set up.* Set up the rule of fours "clock" based on step 1. Drops go on the inside of the clock, and milligrams go on the outside. The relationship between the 4 mg and the 60 gtt becomes the 12 o'clock position. Halfway around the clock is the logical half of that relationship. So, 30 gtt equals 2 mg and so on around the clock.

$$4 \text{ mg/mL CLOCK}$$

$$1 \text{ gram into 250 mL yields 4 mg/mL}$$

3. *Look.* Find the doctor's order on the outside of the "clock" and compare it with the drops per minute on the inside. This is the rate at which the administration set is to drip.

$$x = 30 \text{ gtt/min}$$

It is that easy. Different "clocks" can be set up depending on the concentration in the IV bag and/or the administration set available. These parameters can change. The process of setting up the "clock" will be the same and work every time. You will find that there are just a few "clocks" that you will use regularly.

SECTION 6: CALCULATE AN IV DRIP BASED ON PATIENT WEIGHT

This section takes the calculation in the previous section just one step further. It adds the dimension of patient weight. IV drip medication orders can be based on patient weight just as basic orders can.

EXAMPLE PROBLEM

An order is received to administer 10 µg/kg/min of dopamine IV. You have a vial that contains 200 mg of dopamine in 10 mL (200 mg/10 mL). You also have 250 mL bags of D_5W with a microdrip administration set. Your patient weighs 176 pounds. At how many drops per minute will you adjust your administration set to drip?

Organize the material as before. This time the category of patient weight is added. Remember that finding the concentration in the bag is still the key to solving drip problems.

Order	10 µg/kg/min
On hand	200 mg dopamine/10 mL
Bag	250 mL D_5W
Administration set	60 gtt/mL
Concentration	800 µg/mL
Patient's weight	176 lb
Unit to administer	gtt/min

1. Convert the patient's weight to kilograms.
   176 lb ÷ 2.2 = 80 kg

2. Convert the doctor's order from micrograms per kilogram per minute to micrograms per minute.
   10 µg × 80 kg = 800 µg/min

3. You now have the ordered dose. Find the concentration in the bag and use the "clock" or use the dimensional analysis method to solve.

$$200 \text{ milligrams into } 250 \text{ mL yields } 800 \text{ } \mu g/mL$$

Answer: 60 gtt/min

The dimensional analysis method may also be used to solve this type of problem. After converting the patient's weight and the doctor's order, use the formula from Section 5.

SECTION 7: MILLILITERS PER HOUR TO DROPS PER MINUTE

Sometimes, doctors order IVs to be infused in milliliters per hour or over a specific period of time. To set an IV's administration set, the order must be converted to drops per minute. This section shows how to convert that type of order. A simple conversion formula is all that is needed.

EXAMPLE PROBLEM

The doctor orders you to start an IV of normal saline to run at 100 mL/hr. You have a macrodrip set of 15 gtt/mL. At how many drips per minute will you set your administration set to drip?

Note: Macrodrip administration sets can vary in size.

Formula Method

$$x = \frac{\text{Order amount (mL)}}{\text{Order time (min)}} \times \frac{\text{Administration set (gtt)}}{1 \text{ mL}}$$

1. Fill in the formula. Convert the doctor's order in hours to minutes when you enter the ordered time:

$$x = \frac{100 \text{ mL}}{60 \text{ min}} \times \frac{15 \text{ gtt}}{1 \text{ mL}}$$

2. Cancel units, zeros, and multiply:

$$x = \frac{150 \text{ mL}}{6 \text{ min}}$$

3. Simplify the fraction:

$$x = \frac{25 \text{ gtt}}{1 \text{ min}} \qquad \text{or} \qquad 25 \text{ gtt/min}$$

PRACTICE PROBLEMS

Section 1

Solve the following conversion problems. Answers may be found in Appendix J.

1. 1 g   = _____ mg
2. 1 mg   = _____ μg
3. 1 mg   = _____ g
4. 0.8 mg   = _____ μg
5. 1.5 L   = _____ mL
6. 400 000 mg = _____ g
7. 800 mg   = _____ g
8. 500 mL = _____ L
9. 37 °C   = _____ °F
10. 104 °F   = _____ °C
11. 1/4 gr   = _____ mg
12. 2 Tbsp = _____ mL
13. 180 lb   = _____ kg
14. 7 lb   = _____ kg
15. 25 kg   = _____ lb

Section 2

Solve the following dosage calculation problems. Answers may be found in Appendix J.

1. The doctor orders 1 mg of epinephrine IV for a pulseless and apneic patient in ventricular fibrillation. Epinephrine is supplied as 0.1 mg/mL. How many milliliters will you give?
2. Medical control orders 200 mg of lidocaine IV for your patient in ventricular tachycardia. The prefilled syringe reads 50 mg/mL. How many milliliters will you administer?
3. Your patient meets the criteria for the standing order of 0.5 mg of atropine IV. It comes supplied in your ambulance as 1 mg/10 mL. How many milliliters will you give?
4. You receive an order in the emergency center to administer 100 mEq of sodium bicarbonate IV. Your prefilled syringe label reads 50 mEq/50 mL. How many milliliters will you administer?
5. A radio order is received from medical control to administer 10 mg of Valium IV push to your patient experiencing seizures; 5 mg/mL is printed on the vial of Valium. How many milliliters will you administer?
6. You are assessing a patient in severe congestive heart failure and medical control orders 5 mg of morphine IV. The prefilled syringe reads 15 mg/mL. How many milliliters will you administer?

7. Your patient is bradycardic and you are ordered to administer 0.6 mg of atropine IV. The prefilled syringe reads 0.4 mg/mL. How many milliliters will you administer?

8. Your patient is exhibiting paroxysmal supraventricular tachycardia (PSVT). Vagal maneuvers are ineffective and medical control orders 6 mg of adenosine rapid IV push. The vial reads 3 mg/mL. How many milliliters will you administer?

9. A patient's ventricular fibrillation (v-fib) is refractory to lidocaine and defibrillation attempts. Medical control orders 400 mg of bretylium over 1 minute IV. The prefilled syringe reads 50 mg/mL, 10 mL total volume. How many milliliters will you administer?

10. A patient's Dextro-stix reads approximately 40 mg/dL and she is unconscious. Medical control orders 25 g of dextrose IV bolus. The prefilled syringe reads 0.5 g/mL. How many milliliters will you administer?

Section 3

Solve the following dosage calculation problems. Answers may be found in Appendix J.

1. Your 150 lb patient is experiencing multifocal PVCs and complains of chest pain. Your standing orders state to administer 1 mg/kg of lidocaine. The vial reads 100 mg/5 mL. How many milliliters will you administer?

2. Your patient from problem 1 does not respond to the lidocaine, and medical control orders 5 mg/kg of bretylium IV. Bretylium is supplied in prefilled syringes containing 500 mg/10 mL. How many milliliters will you administer?

3. The doctor orders 0.01 mg/kg of atropine IV for your bradycardic patient who weighs 130 lb. The atropine in your ambulance reads 1 mg/mL. How many milliliters will you administer?

4. You are ordered to administer sodium bicarbonate at 1 mEq/kg to a patient who weighs 160 lb. It is supplied by the emergency center's medication cabinet in prefilled syringes that read 50 mEq/50 mL. How many milliliters will you administer?

5. A severely bradycardic 44 lb pediatric patient does not respond to your initial treatments. Standing orders tell you to administer 0.01 mg/kg epinephrine IV. Your ampule reads 10 mg/10 mL. How many milliliters will you administer?

Section 4

Solve the following concentration problems. Answers may be found in Appendix J.

1. The doctor orders 200 mg of dopamine to be added to a 250 mL bag of D_5W. What is the per milliliter concentration? *Hint:* Dopamine is ordered in micrograms.

2. How many grams of sodium chloride are in a 1000 mL bag of 0.9 percent normal saline?

3. The doctor orders 0.5 g of aminophylline to be placed in a 100 mL bag of D_5W for an IV piggyback. What is the per milliliter concentration?

4. There is a prefilled syringe of 1 percent lidocaine in your ambulance. It contains 5 mL. How many milligrams does it contain?

5. There is another prefilled syringe in your ambulance. It contains 2 percent lidocaine. It also contains 5 mL. How many milligrams does it contain?

6. You are ordered to prepare a lidocaine drip; 1 g is ordered to be placed into a 250 mL bag of D_5W. What is the per milliliter concentration?

7. You are reading the label on a 250 mL bag in the ICU. The label reads 400 mg dopamine added. The bag now has 150 mL left in it. What is the per milliliter concentration in the bag now?

8. Your patient has accidentally overdosed on Cardizem. The doctor orders 300 mg of a 10 percent solution of calcium chloride IV. How many milliliters will you administer?

9. 1 mg of epinephrine has been added to a 250 mL bag of D_5W. What is the per milliliter concentration?

10. The label on a 500 mL bag hanging in the ICU reads 1 g lidocaine added. What is the per milliliter concentration?

Section 5

Solve the following IV drip problems. Answers may be found in Appendix J.

1. The doctor orders 400 µg/min of dopamine to be administered IV. You have a vial that contains 200 mg of dopamine in 10 mL (200 mg/10 mL). Your ambulance has 250 mL bags of D_5W, and you choose a microdrip administration set (60 gtt/mL). At how many drops per minute will you adjust your administration set to drip?

2. You are ordered to administer an Isuprel drip at 4 µg/min. You are ordered to place 1 mg into a 250 mL bag of D_5W. At what rate will you set your microdrip (60 gtt/mL) administration set?

3. Your patient's blood pressure is critically low following conversion from ventricular fibrillation. Medical control orders you to mix 400 mg of dopamine into a 250 mL bag of D_5W and infuse it at 800 µg/min. What is the drip rate with a microdrip administration set (60 gtt/mL)?

4. The doctor orders a starting dose of 2 µg/min of epinephrine. Your assistant has mixed 1 mg of epinephrine into a 250 mL bag of normal saline. What is the drip rate with a microdrip administration set (60 gtt/mL)?

5. You are ordered to administer a lidocaine drip at 2 mg/min. You have 2 g of lidocaine added to a 500 mL bag. What is the drip rate with a microdrip administration set (60 gtt/mL)?

6. Solve problem 5 using a macrodrip administration set (10 gtt/mL).

7. You receive orders to initiate a Bretylol drip following conversion of multifocal premature ventricular contractions (PVCs). The order is for 1 mg/min. You have 1 g of Bretylol added to a 250 mL bag of D_5W and a microdrip administration set (60 gtt/mL). What is the drip rate?

8. You receive an order to start a dopamine drip at 600 μg/min. You place 800 mg of dopamine into a 500 mL bag of normal saline. What is the drip rate with a microdrip administration set (60 gtt/mL)?

9. Solve problem 5 using a macrodrip administration set (15 gtt/mL).

10. You have an order to administer lidocaine at 4 mg/min. The 1 L bag of normal saline has had 4 g of lidocaine added. What is the drip rate with a microdrip administration set (60 gtt/mL)?

Section 6

Solve the following IV drip problems based on patient weight. Answers may be found in Appendix J.

1. You receive an order to administer dopamine to a 176 lb patient at 5 μg/kg/min; 200 mg of dopamine have been added to a 250 mL bag of D_5W. What is the drip rate with a microdrip administration set (60 gtt/mL)?

2. A 22 lb pediatric patient requires an epinephrine drip at 0.1 μg/kg/min. You place 1 mg of epinephrine in a 250 mL bag of D_5W. What is the drip rate with a microdrip administration set (60 gtt/mL)?

3. Your patient in problem 2 does not significantly improve and the doctor doubles the order to 0.2 μg/kg/min. What is the drip rate?

4. A 132 lb cardiac patient is in cardiogenic shock. The doctor orders a dopamine drip at 10 μg/kg/min. Your partner has just placed 400 mg of Intropin into a 500 mL bag of normal saline. At how many drops per minute will you adjust your microdrip administration set to drip?

5. You are transporting a 66 lb pediatric patient with a congenital heart defect. The doctor orders 20 μg/kg/min of lidocaine to be infused. Your partner hands you a 250 mL bag of D_5W that she has labeled "200 mg lidocaine added." What is the drip rate with a microdrip administration set (60 gtt/mL)?

6. The patient in problem 5 does not significantly improve. You are told to increase the current infusion to 40 μg/kg/min. Now what is the drip rate?

7. Your cardiac patient is exhibiting the signs and symptoms of cardiogenic shock. Among other procedures, standing orders call for a dopamine drip at 3 μg/kg/min. The patient's wife states that her husband weighs 150 lb. The vial of dopamine

to be added is labeled 200 mg/5 mL. You have a 250 mL bag of D_5W and a microdrip set. What is the drip rate to be?

8. You are setting up an Isuprel drip for your 75 lb pediatric patient suffering from refractory bronchospasm. The doctor has ordered 0.1 μg/kg/min. The vial is labeled 1 mg/5 mL. You have a 250 mL bag of D_5W and a microdrip set (60 gtt/mL). What is the drip rate to be?

9. You are completing your report after delivering a patient to the emergency center, and you notice that the dopamine dose ordered by medical control is missing from your notes. To avoid any problems, you decide to determine the ordered dose based on the information available. The patient weighs 176 lb and the IV infusion is flowing through a microdrip administration set at 30 gtt/min. The label you put on the 500 mL bag of normal saline reads "800 mg dopamine added." What was the doctor's original dose per kilogram per minute order?

10. You are in the same situation as you were in problem 9. The patient weighs 220 lb. The infusion set is a microdrip set and is flowing at 30 gtt/min. The label on the 250 mL bag of D_5W reads "200 mg dopamine added." What was the doctor's original dose per kilogram per minute order?

Section 7

Solve the following problems of converting milliliters per hour to drops per minute. Answers may be found in Appendix J.

1. The doctor orders you to start an IV of normal saline to run at 100 mL/hr. You have a microdrip administration set (60 gtt/min). What is the drip rate?

2. While doing internship hours at the emergency center, you are asked to start an IV of D_5W to run at 200 mL/hr. You have a macrodrip set (15 gtt/mL). What is the drip rate?

3. Your standing order is to start an IV of normal saline to run at 90 mL/hr. Now you have a macrodrip administration set of 10 gtt/mL. What is the drip rate?

4. A 6-week-old pediatric patient is admitted to the emergency center severely dehydrated. The order reads to infuse 100 mL of 0.45 percent sodium chloride in 2.5 percent D_5W over 1 hour. This is to be followed with 200 mL/hr of the same fluid over 8 hours. What are the two drip rates using a microdrip set?

5. The order on the patient's chart in a busy emergency center reads 1500 mL Plasmanate IV over 10 hours. You choose a 15 gtt/mL administration set. What is the drip rate?

5
FLUIDS, ELECTROLYTES, AND INTRAVENOUS THERAPY

OBJECTIVES

After completing this chapter, the reader should be able to:

1. Identify the body's major fluid compartments and the proportion of total body water they contain.

2. List the major electrolytes and discuss the role they play in maintaining a fluid balance within the human body.

3. Define the following cell physiology terms and explain the role each process plays in human fluid dynamics:
   a. Diffusion
   b. Osmosis
   c. Active transport
   d. Facilitated diffusion

4. Identify the major elements of blood and describe their purposes.

5. Define hypotonic, hypertonic, and isotonic solutions.

6. List the various fluid replacement products and describe the advantages and disadvantages of field use.

7. State the size and type of intravenous catheter to be used for particular applications.

8. Explain the different types of intravenous fluids that can be used.

9. State which intravenous administration sets should be used and in what circumstances.

10. List the possible sites an intravenous tube can be inserted and the rationale for each.

11. Demonstrate the procedure for inserting an intravenous tube.

12. Describe the procedure for collecting blood samples from an intravenous tube.

INTRODUCTION

One of the most important aspects of prehospital care is the administration of intravenous (IV) fluids and electrolytes. There are two major reasons for administering intravenous fluids during the prehospital phase of emergency medical care. The first is to immediately replace intravascular blood volume, and the second is to provide an easily accessible route for the administration of lifesaving emergency drugs.

FLUIDS

Water is the most abundant substance in the human body. Approximately 60 percent of the total body weight is water, which is located within two fluid compartments, or spaces. The largest of these fluid compartments is the *intracellular fluid (ICF) compartment,* which includes all fluids found within the cells. Three-fourths of all body water is within the intracellular compartment. The remaining water can be found outside of the cell membrane in the *extracellular fluid (ECF) compartment.* There are two major components of the ECF: *intravascular fluid,* which is found within the blood vessels and outside of the cell membranes; and the *interstitial fluid,* that fluid found outside the cell membrane yet not within any defined blood vessels. The relationship of the various fluid compartments is illustrated as follows:

Extracellular Fluid	15 percent of total body weight
(Interstitial fluid	10.5 percent of total body weight)
(Intravascular fluid	4.5 percent of total body weight)
Intracellular Fluid	45 percent of total body weight
Total Body Water	60 percent of total body weight

Internal Environment

The internal environment is the extracellular fluid, which bathes each body cell. An important balance must be maintained regarding the internal environment. Whenever one aspect of the internal environment deviates from normal, as frequently occurs in injury and illness, the body immediately responds and attempts to return to normal. The body's tendency to maintain all of its physiological activities in proper balance, including the internal environment, is called *homeostasis.*

ELECTROLYTES

In addition to the body fluids, some important chemicals are also required for life. These chemicals are divided into two main classes: *electrolytes* and *nonelectrolytes.* Chemicals that take on an electrical charge when placed in water are called electrolytes; chemicals that do not take on an electrical charge are called nonelectrolytes. All electrolytes are measured in quantities called *milliequivalents (mEq).* Sodium bicarbonate, a common emergency drug, is an electrolyte. When placed in water, it quickly divides into charged particles, or ions. All dosages of sodium bicarbonate are calculated in milliequivalents. Certain electrolytes, when dissolved in water, take on a positive charge. These are called *cations.* The major cations—sodium (Na^+), calcium (Ca^{2+}) potassium (K^+), and magnesium (Mg^{2+})—have a special significance. Sodium (Na^+) and calcium (Ca^{2+}) have their greatest concentration in the extracellular fluid, and potassium (K^+) and magnesium (Mg^{2+}) are more concentrated in intracellular space. Imbalances in any one of these electrolytes can result in major problems.

Sodium (Na^+)

Sodium is the most abundant extracellular cation and is especially important in the regulation of body water. Sodium is also important in nerve impulse transmission and in the transfer of calcium into the cell. The most common source of sodium is sodium chloride, or table salt. Sodium is often found in conjunction with chloride (Cl^-) or bicarbonate (HCO^{3-}).

Regulation of sodium occurs in the kidney, primarily through reabsorption in the tubules. Aldosterone is the hormonal regulator. Secreted by the kidney, aldosterone increases renal absorption of sodium. Because of sodium's high attraction for water, alterations in sodium and water balance are closely related. An imbalance in one leads to an imbalance in the other. Hypernatremia, or too much sodium, may be due to either an acute gain in sodium or a loss of water without corresponding loss of sodium.

Calcium (Ca^{2+})

Calcium is necessary for the structure of bone and teeth. It also functions as an enzyme cofactor for blood clotting and is required for hormone secretion, membrane stability and permeability, and muscle contraction. One common source of calcium is dairy products.

Most calcium in the body is located in bone tissue, with the remainder found in the plasma and body cells. Inside the cells, calcium is necessary for energy used by muscle fibers to contract. The strength of the contraction is directly related to the concentration of calcium. Calcium is often found in conjunction with phosphate (HPO_4^-).

Blood levels of calcium are closely regulated by parathyroid hormone (PTH), vitamin D, and calcitonin (from the thyroid gland). Renal regulation of calcium requires PTH, which is secreted in response to low plasma levels.

Potassium (K^+)

Potassium is necessary in the transmission and conduction of nerve impulses, maintenance of normal cardiac rhythms, and skeletal smooth muscle contraction. It is also required for glycogen deposits in the liver and skeletal muscles. In this capacity, potassium works closely with sodium, momentarily trading places with sodium across the cellular membranes to maintain electrical neutrality. This action conducts nerve impulses from one end of the cell to the other. It becomes extremely important in the conduction of cardiac rhythms and the movement of calcium into the cell for muscle contraction.

Magnesium (Mg^{2+})

Approximately 40 to 60 percent of magnesium is stored in muscle and bone. Most of the remainder is stored intracellularly and appears to be related to potassium and calcium. Magnesium activates the enzyme (ATPase) that is essential for normal cell membrane function and is the energy source for the sodium-potassium pump. Physiological effects include relaxing smooth muscle and increasing the stability of cardiac cells, thus reducing the potential for dysrhythmias.

Electrolytes that take on a negative charge are called *anions*. Examples of anions found within the body include chlorine (Cl$^-$), bicarbonate (HCO$_3^-$), phosphate (HPO$_4^-$), and most of the organic (carbon-based) molecules. In addition to the fluid balance mentioned earlier, electrical neutrality must be carefully maintained between cations and anions.

CELL PHYSIOLOGY

To maintain physiological homeostasis, there must be an exchange of electrolytes and water materials across the membrane of the cell. The cell membrane is very complex. It is said to be *semipermeable*, meaning that it allows certain compounds to pass readily across it while restricting the passage of others. Many materials must pass across the cell membrane including oxygen, carbon dioxide, nutrients, fluids, and electrolytes. There are three major ways to move substances across the cell membrane: *diffusion*, *facilitated diffusion*, and *active transport*. Diffusion is a passive process, whereas facilitated diffusion and active transport require energy expenditure by the cell (see Figure 5–1).

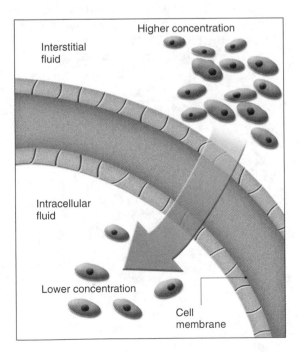

FIGURE 5–1 Diffusion.

Diffusion

Diffusion occurs when concentrations of various substances become higher on one side of the semipermeable cell membrane. When this difference occurs, an *osmotic gradient* is created. The side of the cell membrane with the higher concentration is said to be *hypertonic* with respect to the other side. Conversely, the side of the membrane with the lower concentration is said to be *hypotonic* in relation to the other (see Figure 5–2). When both sides of the cell membrane have an equal concentration of the substance in question, the system is said to be *isotonic.* These concepts underpin the rationale for IV therapy. IV fluids with a solute concentration less than that of blood are said to be hypotonic solutions. An example of a hypotonic solution is 0.45 percent sodium chloride (one-half normal saline).

Substances that have a solute concentration equal to that of blood are said to be isotonic. Lactated Ringer's solution and 0.9 percent sodium chloride are examples of isotonic fluids. An example of a hypertonic solution is 50 percent dextrose in water. Although not a classical IV fluid, it plays a major role in prehospital care. One of the most important substances that passes across the cell membrane is water. Water diffuses readily across the cell membrane from an area of higher water concentration to an area of lesser water concentration. The diffusion of water in this manner is called *osmosis* (see Figure 5–3).

Facilitated Diffusion

Certain molecules can move across the cell membrane by a process known as *facilitated diffusion.* Glucose is an example of such a molecule. Facilitated diffusion requires the assistance of "helper proteins" on the surface of the cell membrane. These proteins, once activated, bind to the glucose molecule. After binding, the protein changes its configuration and transports the glucose molecule into the cell, where it is released. The transport protein is then ready for another glucose molecule. Depending on the substance being transported, facilitated diffusion may or may not require energy.

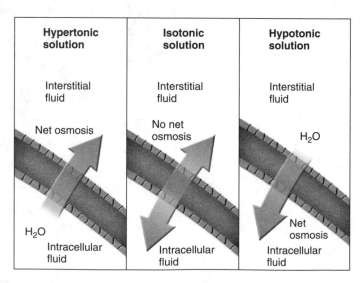

FIGURE 5–2   Relationships and effects of hypertonic, isotonic, and hypotonic solutions.

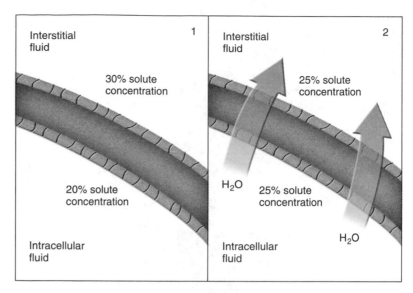

FIGURE 5–3 Osmosis.

Active Transport

Sometimes it is desirable for the body to maintain a gradient along a cell membrane. This is especially true regarding the ions sodium (Na^+) and potassium (K^+). To sustain life, the concentration of sodium outside the cell membrane must be significantly higher than that inside the cell. Also, the concentration of potassium must be maintained at a much higher level within the cell. To maintain the gradient, the sodium must be pumped out of the cell and potassium must be pumped into the cell. Both of these processes require energy. This is an example of active transport.

BLOOD

One of the most important aspects of the extracellular fluid, and thus the internal environment, is blood. Blood is the main element involved in the oxygenation of body cells, transport of nutrients, transport of control maintenance factors (hormones), waste removal, and temperature regulation. Blood is a complex substance divided into two basic components: plasma and formed elements.

Plasma

Plasma is the complex fluid portion of blood. Plasma communicates continually through pores in the capillaries with the fluid that is circulating between the cells (interstitial fluid). Plasma is approximately 92 percent water and contains a number of formed elements (see Figure 5–4).

Formed Elements

Formed elements consist of plasma proteins, plasma lipids, electrolytes, nutrients, and cellular elements such as red blood cells, white blood cells,

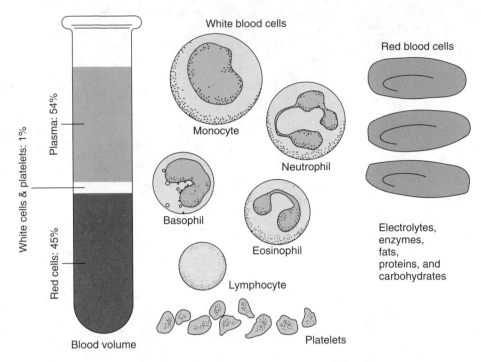

FIGURE 5–4 Various components of blood.

and platelets. The formed elements make up approximately 45 to 50 percent of blood volume. The continuous movement of blood keeps the formed elements dispersed throughout the plasma, where they are available to carry out the following functions:

1. Respiratory: delivery of oxygen to the cells and exchange of carbon dioxide
2. Nutritional: delivery of other substances needed for cellular metabolism (glucose and other carbohydrates, amino acids, fatty acids, vitamins, minerals, and trace elements)
3. Regulatory: delivery of substances such as electrolytes and hormones
4. Excretory: removal of cellular debris and waste products such as those of cellular metabolism (carbon dioxide, water, and acids)
5. Protective: defense against injury and invading microorganisms

There are three major classes of blood cells. The first are the red blood cells, or *erythrocytes* (see Figure 5–5). Erythrocytes have an important iron-containing protein called *hemoglobin*. Hemoglobin is responsible for the transport of oxygen and carbon dioxide. A significant percentage of blood, approximately 45 percent, is red blood cells. The percentage of red blood cells present is referred to as the *hematocrit*. White blood cells, or *leukocytes*, are the second type of cells found in the blood. The leukocytes are responsible for combating infection. The last type of blood cells present is platelets, or *thrombocytes*, which are responsible for blood clotting.

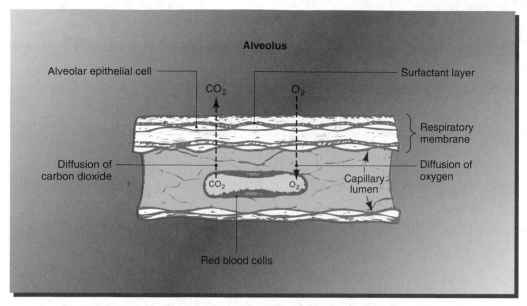

FIGURE 5–5 The red blood cell.

Blood Types

An antigen is the protein identifier in most cells. The presence or absence of a particular antigen identifies that cell as either "self" or "foreign." Once a cell is identified as foreign, specific antibodies to that cell are formed. Subsequently, all antigens (cells with that specific foreign identifier) are attacked and destroyed. This is termed an antigen–antibody reaction. When the reaction occurs because two types of blood are mixed, it is called a *transfusion reaction.* At least two commonly occurring antigens, each of which can trigger antigen–antibody reaction, have been found in human blood cells, especially on the cell membrane surfaces. There are two types of antigens in the blood that are more likely than others to cause reactions: the ABO system of antigens and the Rh system.

ABO Types

The ABO group consists of two major antigens, labeled A and B, that are found on the surfaces of red blood cells (RBCs). These antigens can appear by themselves or together or be entirely absent. The result of their presence or absence is one of the four blood types:

Type A. Individuals with blood type A carry the A antigen on the RBCs.
Type B. Individuals with blood type B carry the B antigen on the RBCs.
Type AB. Individuals with blood type AB carry the A and B antigens on the RBCs.
Type O. Individuals with blood type O carry neither antigen on the RBCs.

In the ABO system, the body spontaneously develops antibodies to the other blood types. This system determines which blood type or types each person can receive without triggering a transfusion reaction (see Table 5–1).

TABLE 5–1

ABO Blood Types

Blood Types	Antibodies	Can Receive	Can Donate to
Type A	B antibodies	Type A or O	Type A, AB
Type B	A antibodies	Type B or O	Type B, AB
Type AB	No antibodies	Type AB, A, B, O	Type A, B, AB
Type O	A and B antibodies	Type O	Type A, B, AB, O

Rh Factor

The second important system in blood transfusion is the Rh system. The Rh antigen, type D, is widely prevalent. People with this type of antigen are said to be Rh positive; those without the type D antigen are said to be Rh negative. Approximately 85 to 95 percent of Americans are Rh positive.

Antibodies to the Rh factor do not occur naturally and must be acquired through exposure to Rh-positive blood. This process is most evident in Rh-positive babies born to Rh-negative mothers. The mother must be given a vaccine after each birth to prevent the formation of antibodies to any subsequent Rh-positive fetuses. In adult Rh-negative patients, a similar but delayed reaction can occur if Rh-positive blood is received. On receiving the second Rh-positive transfusion, a severe and potentially life-threatening reaction may occur in the patient.

IV THERAPY

As mentioned earlier, there are two major indications for IV therapy. The first is to replace fluid losses, which may occur as a result of hemorrhage caused by trauma or from severe diarrhea, vomiting, heat exhaustion, or burns. It is best to replace the fluid losses with intravenous fluids of similar isotonicity. The second is to provide a route for the administration of drugs.

There are two major classes of IV fluids: colloids and crystalloids. *Colloids* contain compounds of high molecular weight, usually proteins, which do not readily diffuse across the cell membrane. In addition, they exert *colloid osmotic pressure*, which means they tend to attract water into the intravascular space. Thus, a small amount of a colloid can be administered to a patient with a greater than expected increase in intravascular volume. This is because the colloid will draw water from the interstitial space and the intracellular compartment to increase the intravascular volume. Common examples of colloids include the following:

Plasma protein fraction (Plasmanate). Plasmanate is a protein-containing colloid. The principal protein present is albumin, which is suspended, along with other proteins, in a saline solvent.

Salt-poor albumin. Salt-poor albumin contains only human albumin. Each gram of albumin holds approximately 18 mL of water in the bloodstream.

Dextran. Dextran is not a protein but a large sugar molecule with osmotic properties similar to those of albumin. It comes in two molecular weights (40,000 and 70,000 Da). Dextran 40 has 2 to 2.5 times the colloid osmotic pressure of albumin.

Hetastarch (Hespan).   Hetastarch, like dextran, is a sugar molecule with osmotic properties similar to those of protein. It does not appear to share many of dextran's side effects.

Polygeline (Haemaccel).   Haemaccel is a gelatinous colloid with osmotic properties similar to albumin. It is relatively free of side effects and is temperature stable with an excellent shelf life.

Colloid replacement therapy, at present, does not have a role in prehospital care except under rare circumstances. Colloid products are expensive and most of them have a short shelf life.

Crystalloids contain only water and electrolytes. These substances all readily diffuse across the cell membrane. Crystalloids are the primary solutions used in prehospital intravenous fluid therapy. Because there are multiple fluid preparations, it is often helpful to classify them according to the *tonicity* related to plasma:

Isotonic solutions.   Isotonic solutions have an electrolyte composition similar to that of blood plasma. When placed into a normally hydrated patient, they do not cause a significant fluid or electrolyte shift.

Hypertonic solutions.   Hypertonic solutions have a higher solute concentration than does plasma. These fluids tend to cause a fluid shift out of the intracellular compartment into the extracellular compartment when administered to a normally hydrated patient. Later, there is a diffusion of solutes in the opposite direction.

Hypotonic solutions.   Hypotonic solutions have less of a solute concentration than does plasma. When administered to a normally hydrated patient, they cause a movement of fluid from the extracellular compartment into the intracellular compartment. Later, solutes move in an opposite direction.

Hemoglobin-based oxygen-carrying solutions (HBOCs).   Considerable research has been devoted to creating IV solutions that can carry oxygen in much the same manner as blood. Two compounds have been developed and are being used in some countries while clinical testing continues in other countries. Both solutions use modified hemoglobin derived from either expired human blood or bovine (cattle) blood. The hemoglobin is extracted from the blood and filtered to remove any antigens or foreign substances. The hemoglobin is then chemically joined in a process called polymerization. The polymerized hemoglobin is a long chain of hemoglobin molecules (not located in red blood cells) that can be administered to a patient. These products have longer shelf lives and appear to be as effective as standard human blood products. They are packaged so that a unit of HBOC will have the same oxygen-carrying capacity of a unit of human packed red blood cells. The human blood-based product is called PolyHeme®, and the bovine-based product is called HemoPure®.

Paramedics choose replacement fluids based on patient needs and the patient's underlying problem. As a rule, hemorrhage occurs so fast that there is not time for a significant fluid shift between the extracellular and intracellular space. Consequently, replacement fluids are most commonly isotonic; lactated Ringer's solution and normal saline are used most often. If the patient is dehydrated because of fluid loss from diarrhea or fever, then there is a greater deficit of water than sodium. In this case, the paramedic may be asked to use hypotonic fluids such as one-half normal saline.

Some replacement fluids contain a single element, such as sodium chloride or dextrose, whereas others contain multiple elements. Solutions such as lactated Ringer's are designed so that the concentration of electrolytes is very similar to that of the plasma; they are thus referred to as *balanced salt solutions.*

Three of the most commonly used solutions in prehospital care are lactated Ringer's solution, 0.9 percent sodium chloride (normal saline), and 5 percent dextrose in water (D_5W).

Lactated Ringer's solution. Lactated Ringer's solution is an isotonic electrolyte solution. It contains sodium chloride, potassium chloride, calcium chloride, and sodium lactate in water.

Normal saline. Normal saline is an electrolyte solution containing sodium chloride in water that is isotonic with extracellular fluid.

5 percent dextrose in water. D_5W is a hypotonic glucose solution used to keep a vein open and to supply the calories necessary for cell metabolism. Although it has an initial effect of increasing the circulatory volume, glucose molecules rapidly move across the vascular membrane. The resultant free water follows almost immediately, leaving little effect on circulating blood volume.

Both lactated Ringer's solution and normal saline are used to replace fluid volume because their administration causes an immediate expansion of the circulatory volume. However, as was noted earlier, due to the movement of the electrolytes and water, two-thirds of either of these solutions is lost to the interstitial space within 1 hour. Lactated Ringer's solution is a better IV fluid than normal saline for the patient who is losing blood. However, it is not compatible with whole blood, which will most likely be given when the patient arrives at the emergency department. In aggressive fluid resuscitation, it is recommended that paramedics initiate two IV lines, one with lactated Ringer's solution and one with normal saline.

The second reason for initiating an IV infusion in the field is to provide a route for the administration of drugs. The following IV fluids are most frequently used in prehospital emergency care (see Table 5–2).

PLASMA PROTEIN FRACTION (PLASMANATE)

Class: Natural colloid

Description

Plasma protein fraction is a protein-containing colloid that is suspended in a saline solvent. The principal protein in plasma protein fraction is serum human albumin. Other proteins present include globulin and gamma globulin. Plasma protein fraction is prepared from large pools of human plasma. It is quite expensive and has a very short shelf life. Although rarely used in the prehospital phase of emergency medical care, plasma protein fraction is preferred by some emergency specialists in the management of hypovolemic states, especially burn shock. After a patient sustains a severe burn, fluid is

TABLE 5–2

Approximate Ionic Concentrations (mEq/L) and Calories per Liter

	Ionic Concentrations (mEq/L)							
	Sodium	Potassium	Calcium	Chloride	Lactate	Calories per liter	Osmolarity[a] (mOsm/L)	pH Range[b]
5% Dextrose Injection, USP	0	0		0	0	170	252	3.5–6.5
10% Dextrose Injection, USP	0	0	0	0	0	340	505	3.5–6.5
0.9% Sodium Chloride Injection, USP	154	0	0	154	0	0	308	4.5–7.0
Sodium Lactate Injection, USP (M/6 Sodium Lactate)	167	0	0	0	167	54	334	6.0–7.3
2.5% Dextrose & 0.45% Sodium Chloride Injection, USP	77	0	0	77	0	85	280	3.5–6.0
5% Dextrose & 0.2% Sodium Chloride Injection, USP	34	0	0	34	0	170	321	3.5–6.0
5% Dextrose & 0.33% Sodium Chloride Injection, USP	56	0	0	56	0	170	365	3.5–6.0
5% Dextrose & 0.45% Sodium Chloride Injection, USP	77	0	0	77	0	170	406	3.5–6.0
5% Dextrose & 0.9% Sodium Chloride Injection, USP	154	0	0	154	0	170	560	3.5–6.0
10% Dextrose & 0.9% Sodium Chloride Injection, USP	154	0	0	154	0	340	813	3.5–6.0
Ringer's Injection, USP	147.5	4	4.5	156	0	0	309	5.0–7.5
Lactated Ringer's Injection	130	4	3	109	28	9	273	6.0–7.5
5% Dextrose in Ringer's Injection	147.5	4	4.5	156	0	170	561	3.5–6.5
Lactated Ringer's with 5% Dextrose	130	4	3	109	28	180	525	4.0–6.5

[a]Normal physiological isotonicity range is approximately 280–310 mOsm/L. Administration of substantially hypotonic solutions may cause hemolysis, and administration of substantially hypertonic solutions may cause vein damage.

[b]pH ranges are USP for applicable solution; corporate specification for non-USP solutions.

lost from the blood into the surrounding tissue. Plasma protein fraction, because it remains in the circulating blood volume, is effective in maintaining adequate blood volume and blood pressure. It is usually used in combination with lactated Ringer's solution or normal saline.

Mechanism of Action

Plasmanate is a protein-containing colloid that remains in the intravascular compartment. It increases intravascular volume by attracting water from other fluid compartments by virtue of its colloid osmotic pressure.

Indications

Hypovolemic shock, especially burn shock
Hypoproteinemia (low protein states)

Contraindications

There are no major contraindications to plasma protein fraction when used in the treatment of life-threatening hypovolemic states.

Precautions

It is important to monitor constantly the response of the patient and adjust the rate of infusion accordingly. The patient should be monitored for elevated blood pressure and pulmonary edema during and following plasmanate administration.

Side Effects

Chills, fever, urticaria (hives), nausea, and vomiting have all been reported with plasma protein fraction use.

Dosage

The plasma protein fraction infusion rate should be titrated according to the patient's hemodynamic response. In the management of shock secondary to burns, the physician's orders regarding the rate of administration must be closely followed. Standard formulas for IV fluid administration have been developed. The medical control physician will use these formulas in judging the correct rate of intravenous administration.

Interactions

Solutions should not be mixed with or administered through the same administration sets as other intravenous fluids.

Route

Intravenous infusion

How Supplied

Plasma protein fraction is supplied in 250 mL and 500 mL bottles of a 5 percent solution. An administration set is usually attached.

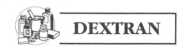

DEXTRAN

Class: Artificial colloid

Description

Dextran is a colloid that differs significantly from plasma protein fraction. Instead of proteins, dextran contains chains of sugars that are approximately the same molecular weight as serum albumin. Thus, because of their large molecular size, they remain within the circulating blood volume for an extended period. Although not as effective as plasma protein fraction, dextran has proved effective as an adjunctive aid in the management of hypovolemic shock. Dextran is supplied in two molecular weights. Dextran 40 has an average molecular weight of approximately 40,000 Da. Dextran 40 is secreted by the kidneys much more readily than the higher molecular weight form, dextran 70 (molecular weight of 70,000 Da). The higher molecular weight form tends to be broken down into glucose instead of being secreted in the dextran form, as occurs with dextran 40. The decision on which type of dextran to use in prehospital care rests with the system medical director. Because dextran is excreted through the urine, urine output is usually maintained with the administration of dextran.

Mechanism of Action

Dextran is a sugar-containing colloid used as an intravascular volume expander. It remains in the intravascular compartment for approximately 12 hours. It increases intravascular volume by attracting water from other fluid compartments by virtue of its colloid osmotic pressure.

Indication

Hypovolemic shock

Contraindications

Dextran should not be administered to patients who have a known hypersensitivity to the drug. It should not be administered to patients with congestive heart failure, renal failure, or known bleeding disorders.

Precautions

A major drawback to the use of dextran is that it coats the red blood cells, thus preventing accurate blood typing and possibly hindering administration of whole blood if required. A tube of blood should be drawn before administering dextran for blood typing at the hospital.

Allergic reactions, ranging from mild to severe anaphylaxis, have been known to occur following the administration of dextran. If these occur, therapy should be immediately discontinued. In the case of mild reactions, the patient should be closely monitored, and emergency resuscitative drugs should be readily available. Severe allergic reactions may require the administration of epinephrine, diphenhydramine (Benadryl), and possibly corticosteroids. It is usually preferable to use crystalloid solutions, such as lactated Ringer's solution, rather than dextran, in the management of profound hypovolemic shock.

Side Effects

Rash, itching, dyspnea, chest tightness, and mild hypotension have all been reported with dextran use. The incidence of these side effects is very low, however, and reactions are generally mild.

Increased bleeding time has also been reported with dextran use due to its interference with platelet function.

Interactions

Dextran should not be administered to patients who are receiving anticoagulants because it significantly retards blood clotting.

Dosage

The dosage of dextran is titrated according to the patient's physiological response. In the management of burn shock, it is especially important to follow standard fluid resuscitation regimens to prevent possible circulatory overload.

Route

Intravenous infusion

How Supplied

Dextran 40 and dextran 70 are supplied in 250 and 500 mL bottles.

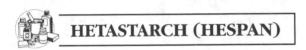

HETASTARCH (HESPAN)

Class: Artificial colloid

Description

Hetastarch is an artificial colloid differing from both plasma protein fraction and dextran. Hetastarch is derived from amylopectin and chemically resembles glycogen. The average molecular weight is approximately 450,000 Da, which gives it colloidal properties similar to those of human albumin. Intravenous infusion of hetastarch results in plasma volume expansion slightly greater than the amount infused.

Because the colloidal properties of hetastarch are quite similar to those of human albumin, it has proved effective in the management of hypovolemic shock, especially burn shock. It does not appear to share the blood-typing problems seen with dextran.

Mechanism of Action

Hetastarch is a starch-containing colloid used as an intravascular volume expander. Following administration, the plasma volume is expanded slightly in excess of the volume of hetastarch administered. This effect has been observed for up to 24 to 36 hours. Hetastarch increases intravascular volume by virtue of its colloid osmotic pressure.

Indications

Hypovolemic shock, especially burn shock
Septic shock

Contraindications

There are no major contraindications to hetastarch when used in the management of life-threatening hypovolemic states.

Precautions

It is important to constantly monitor the response of the patient and adjust the rate of infusion accordingly. The patient should be monitored for signs of pulmonary edema and elevated blood pressure during and following hetastarch administration.

Large volumes of hetastarch may alter the body's coagulation mechanism. Hetastarch should be used with caution in patients who are receiving anticoagulants.

Side Effects

Nausea, vomiting, mild febrile reactions, chills, itching, and urticaria (hives) have been reported with hetastarch administration. Severe anaphylactic reactions have been rarely reported.

Interactions

Hetastarch should not be administered to patients who are receiving anticoagulants.

Dosage

The hetastarch infusion rate should be titrated according to the patient's hemodynamic response. In the management of burn shock, the physician's orders regarding the rate of administration must be closely followed. Standard formulas for colloid administration to burn patients have been developed. It is important to remember that a fall in blood pressure in burn shock occurs much later than with hemorrhagic causes.

Route

Intravenous infusion

How Supplied

Sterile 6 percent hetastarch in 0.9 percent sodium chloride is supplied in 500 mL bottles.

POLYGELINE (HAEMACCEL)*

Class: Artificial colloid

Description

Haemaccel, although not used in North America, is utilized by EMS systems throughout the rest of the world. Haemaccel is a manufactured protein derived from gelatin obtained from cattle in the United States. It is

---

*Not currently used in North America.

sterile, pyrogen free, and contains no preservatives. Furthermore, studies have shown that it remains effective after freezing and thawing. The molecular weight of Haemaccel is approximately 35,000 Da. In addition to polygeline, Haemaccel contains Na^+ (145 mEq), K^+ (5.1 mEq), Ca^{2+} (6.25 mEq), and Cl^- (145 mEq). The pH is approximately 7.3. Following administration of 1 L, the colloidal osmotic pressure of Haemaccel draws an additional 500 mL or so of fluid into the intravascular space.

Mechanism of Action

Haemaccel is a gelatinous colloid used as an intravascular volume expander. The half-life of Haemaccel is approximately 8 hours. It increases intravascular fluid volume by attracting water from other fluid compartments by virtue of its colloid osmotic pressure.

Indications

Hypovolemic shock

Contraindications

Haemaccel is contraindicated in patients with known hypersensitivity to any of its components. It should be used with caution in patients with a history of anaphylaxis.

Precautions

Although rare, be alert for allergic reactions and possible anaphylaxis.

Side Effects

Transient skin reactions (wheals, urticaria), tachycardia, bradycardia, nausea, vomiting, dyspnea, hypotension, fall in temperature, and shivering have been reported with Haemaccel administration. If these occur, the infusion should be stopped.

Interactions

None reported

Dosage

The dosage of Haemaccel is titrated according to the patient's physiological response. In the management of burn shock, it is especially important to follow standard fluid resuscitation regimens to prevent possible circulatory overload.

Route

Intravenous infusion

How Supplied

Haemaccel, 3.5 percent, is supplied in 500 mL plastic infusion bottles.

LACTATED RINGER'S SOLUTION (HARTMANN'S SOLUTION)

Class: Isotonic crystalloid solution

Description

Lactated Ringer's solution is one of the most frequently used IV fluids in the management of hypovolemic shock. It is an isotonic crystalloid solution containing electrolytes in the following concentrations:

Sodium (Na^+) 130 mEq/L
Potassium (K^+) 4 mEq/L
Calcium (Ca^{2+}) 3 mEq/L
Chloride (Cl^-) 109 mEq/L

In addition to the electrolytes mentioned earlier, lactated Ringer's solution contains 28 mEq of lactate (lactic acid), which acts as a buffer.

Mechanism of Action

Lactated Ringer's solution replaces water and electrolytes.

Indications

Hypovolemic shock
Keep open IV

Contraindications

Lactated Ringer's solution should not be used in patients with congestive heart failure or renal failure.

Precautions

Patients receiving lactated Ringer's solution should be monitored to prevent circulatory overload.

Side Effects

Rare in therapeutic dosages

Interactions

Few in the emergency setting

Dosage

Crystalloids, such as lactated Ringer's solution, diffuse out of the intravascular space and into the surrounding tissues in less than an hour. Thus, it is often necessary to replace 1 L of lost blood with 3 to 4 L of lactated Ringer's solution.

In severe hypovolemic shock, lactated Ringer's solution should be infused through large-bore (14- or 16-gauge) IV cannulas. These infusions should be administered "wide open" until a systolic blood pressure of approximately 100 mmHg is achieved. When this blood pressure is attained, the infusion should be reduced to about 100 mL/hr. If the blood pressure falls again, then the infusion rate should be increased and adjusted accordingly. Adjunctive devices, such as the pneumatic anti-shock garment (PASG) and extremity elevation, may be used in the management of severe hypovolemic shock.

Route

Intravenous infusion

How Supplied

Lactated Ringer's solution is supplied in 250, 500, and 1000 mL bags and bottles.

5 PERCENT DEXTROSE IN WATER (D₅W)

Class: Hypotonic dextrose-containing solution

Description

When vigorous fluid replacement is not indicated, 5 percent dextrose in water (D_5W) may be used. D_5W can be used for the administration of intravenous drugs. D_5W is hypotonic, which prevents circulatory overload in patients with congestive heart failure.

Mechanism of Action

D_5W provides nutrients in the form of dextrose as well as free water.

Indications

IV access for emergency drugs
For dilution of concentrated drugs for intravenous infusion

Contraindications

D_5W should not be used as a fluid replacement for hypovolemic states.

Precautions

Dextrose-containing solutions are acidic and may produce local venous irritation. Subcutaneous administration from extravasation may result in tissue necrosis.

As with any IV fluid, it is important to watch for signs of circulatory overload when administering D_5W.

When treating hypoglycemia, it is imperative that a tube of blood be drawn before administering D_5W or 50 percent dextrose ($D_{50}W$).

Side Effects

Rare in therapeutic dosages

Interactions

D_5W should not be used with phenytoin (Dilantin) or amrinone (Inocor).

Dosage

D_5W is usually administered through a minidrip (60 drops/mL) set at a rate of "to keep open" (TKO).

Route

Intravenous infusion

How Supplied

D_5W is supplied in bags and bottles of 50, 100, 150, 250, 500, and 1000 mL.

10 PERCENT DEXTROSE IN WATER ($D_{10}W$)

Class: Hypertonic dextrose-containing solution

Description

Ten percent dextrose in water ($D_{10}W$) is a hypertonic solution. Like D_5W, $D_{10}W$ is used only when vigorous fluid replacement is not indicated. $D_{10}W$ has twice as much carbohydrate as does D_5W, which makes it of use in the management of hypoglycemia.

Mechanism of Action

$D_{10}W$ provides nutrients in the form of dextrose as well as free water.

Indications

Neonatal resuscitation
Hypoglycemia

Contraindications

$D_{10}W$ should not be used as a fluid replacement for hypovolemic states.

Precautions

Dextrose-containing solutions are acidic and may produce local venous irritation. Subcutaneous administration from extravasation may result in tissue necrosis.

   As with any IV fluid, it is important to be alert for signs of circulatory overload.

   When treating hypoglycemia, it is imperative that a tube of blood be drawn before administering $D_{10}W$ or 50 percent dextrose ($D_{50}W$).

Side Effects

Rare in therapeutic dosages

Interactions

$D_{10}W$ should not be used with phenytoin (Dilantin) or amrinone (Inocor).

Dosage

The administration rate of $D_{10}W$ usually depends on the patient's condition.

Route

Intravenous infusion

How Supplied

$D_{10}W$ is supplied in bottles and bags of 50, 100, 150, 250, 500, and 1000 mL.

0.9 PERCENT SODIUM CHLORIDE (NORMAL SALINE)

Class: Isotonic crystalloid solution

Description

The use of 0.9 percent sodium chloride, or normal saline (as it is often called), has several applications in emergency medicine. Normal saline contains 154 mEq/L of sodium ions (Na^+) and approximately 154 mEq/L of chloride (Cl^-) ions. Because the concentration of sodium is near that of blood, the solution is considered isotonic. Normal saline is especially useful in heat stroke, heat exhaustion, and diabetic ketoacidosis.

Mechanism of Action

Normal saline replaces water and electrolytes.

Indications

Heat-related problems (heat exhaustion, heat stroke)
Freshwater drowning
Hypovolemia
Diabetic ketoacidosis
Keep open IV

Contraindications

The use of 0.9 percent sodium chloride should not be considered in patients with congestive heart failure because circulatory overload can be easily induced.

Precautions

Normal saline contains only sodium and chloride. When large amounts of normal saline are administered, it is quite possible for other important physiological electrolytes to become depleted. In cases in which large amounts of fluids may have to be administered, it might be prudent to use lactated Ringer's solution.

Side Effects

Rare in therapeutic dosages

Interactions

Few in the emergency setting

Dosage

The specific situation being treated dictates the rate at which normal saline is administered. In severe heat stroke, diabetic ketoacidosis, and freshwater drowning, it is quite likely that paramedics will be called on to administer the fluid quite rapidly. In other cases, it is advisable to administer the fluid at a moderate rate (e.g., 100 mL/hr).

Route

Intravenous infusion

How Supplied

Normal saline is supplied in 250, 500, and 1000 mL bags and bottles. Sterile normal saline for irrigation should not be confused with that designed for intravenous administration.

0.45 PERCENT SODIUM CHLORIDE (ONE-HALF NORMAL SALINE)

Class: Hypotonic crystalloid solution

Description

One-half normal saline (0.45 percent sodium chloride) solution is a hypotonic crystalloid solution containing approximately one-half the concentration of sodium and chloride as does blood plasma.

Mechanism of Action

One-half normal saline replaces free water and electrolytes.

Indication

Patients with diminished renal or cardiovascular function for whom rapid rehydration is not indicated

Contraindications

Cases in which rapid rehydration is indicated

Precautions

One-half normal saline contains only sodium and chloride. When large amounts of one-half normal saline are administered, it is possible for other important physiological electrolytes to become depleted. In cases in which large amounts of fluids must be administered, it might be prudent to use lactated Ringer's solution.

Side Effects

Rare in therapeutic dosages

Interactions

Few in the emergency setting

Dosage

The specific situation and patient condition dictate the rate at which one-half normal saline is administered.

Route

Intravenous infusion

How Supplied

One-half normal saline is supplied in 250, 500, and 1000 mL bags and bottles.

5 PERCENT DEXTROSE IN 0.45 PERCENT SODIUM CHLORIDE (D₅1/2NS)

Class: Hypertonic dextrose-containing crystalloid solution

Description

Five percent dextrose in 0.45 percent sodium chloride ($D_5$1/2NS) is a versatile fluid. It contains the same amount of sodium and chloride as does one-half normal saline. Dextrose has been added for its nutrient properties, providing 80 calories per liter.

Mechanism of Action

$D_5$1/2NS replaces free water and electrolytes and provides nutrients in the form of dextrose.

Indications

Heat exhaustion
Diabetic disorders
For use as a TKO solution in patients with impaired renal or cardiovascular function

Contraindication

$D_5$1/2NS should not be used when rapid fluid resuscitation is indicated.

Precautions

Dextrose-containing solutions are acidic and may produce local venous irritation. Subcutaneous administration from extravasation may result in tissue necrosis.

As with any IV fluid, it is important to watch for signs of circulatory overload when administering $D_5 1/2NS$.

When treating hypoglycemia, it is imperative that a tube of blood be drawn before administering $D_5 1/2NS$ or 50 percent dextrose ($D_{50}W$).

Side Effects

Rare in therapeutic dosages

Interactions

$D_5 1/2NS$ should not be used with phenytoin (Dilantin) or amrinone (Inocor).

Dosage

The specific situation and patient condition dictate the rate at which $D_5 1/2NS$ should be administered.

Route

Intravenous infusion

How Supplied

$D_5 1/2NS$ is supplied in bottles and bags containing 250, 500, and 1000 mL of the fluid.

5 PERCENT DEXTROSE IN 0.9 PERCENT SODIUM CHLORIDE (D_5NS)

Class: Hypertonic dextrose-containing crystalloid solution

Description

Five percent dextrose in 0.9 percent normal saline is a hypertonic crystalloid to which 5 g of dextrose per 100 mL of fluid has been added for its nutrient properties (80 calories per liter).

Mechanism of Action

D_5NS replaces free water and electrolytes and provides nutrients in the form of dextrose.

Indications

Heat-related disorders
Freshwater drowning
Hypovolemia
Peritonitis

Contraindications

D_5NS should not be administered to patients with impaired cardiac or renal function.

Precautions

Dextrose-containing solutions are acidic and may produce local venous irritation. Subcutaneous administration from extravasation may result in tissue necrosis.

D_5NS contains only the electrolytes sodium and chloride. When large amounts of fluids must be administered, it might be prudent to use lactated Ringer's solution to prevent depletion of the other physiological electrolytes.

When treating hypoglycemia, it is imperative that a tube of blood be drawn before administering D_5NS or 50 percent dextrose ($D_{50}W$).

Side Effects

Rare in therapeutic dosages

Interactions

D_5NS should not be used with phenytoin (Dilantin) or amrinone (Inocor).

Dosage

The specific situation and patient condition dictate the rate at which D_5NS is given.

Route

Intravenous infusion

How Supplied

D_5NS is supplied in bags and bottles containing 250, 500, and 1000 mL of the solution.

5 PERCENT DEXTROSE IN LACTATED RINGER'S SOLUTION (D_5LR)

Class: Hypertonic dextrose-containing crystalloid solution

Description

Five percent dextrose in lactated Ringer's solution (D_5LR) contains the same concentration of electrolytes as does lactated Ringer's solution. In addition to the electrolytes, however, 5 g of dextrose per 100 mL of fluid has been added for nutrient properties. This added dextrose causes the solution to be hypertonic and adds 80 calories per liter.

Mechanism of Action

D_5LR replaces water and electrolytes and provides nutrients in the form of dextrose.

Indications

Hypovolemic shock
Hemorrhagic shock
Certain cases of acidosis

Contraindications

D$_5$LR should not be administered to patients with decreased renal or cardiovascular function.

Precautions

Patients receiving D$_5$LR should be constantly monitored for signs of circulatory overload. It is essential that a blood sample be drawn before administering D$_5$LR to patients with hypoglycemia.

Dextrose-containing solutions are acidic and may produce local venous irritation. Subcutaneous administration from extravasation may result in tissue necrosis.

Side Effects

Rare in therapeutic dosages

Interactions

D$_5$LR should not be used with phenytoin (Dilantin) or amrinone (Inocor).

Dosage

In severe hypovolemic shock, D$_5$LR should be infused through a large-bore catheter (14 or 16 gauge). This infusion should be administered "wide open" until a blood pressure of 100 mmHg is achieved. When the blood pressure is attained, the infusions should be reduced to 100 mL/hr. In other cases, the specific situation and patient condition dictate the rate of administration.

Route

Intravenous infusion

How Supplied

D$_5$LR is supplied in bags and bottles containing 250, 500, and 1000 mL of the fluid.

INSERTION OF INDWELLING IV CATHETER

One of the earliest stages in the management of an acutely ill or injured patient is the placement of an IV catheter. In trauma cases an IV catheter provides access for fluid resuscitation, whereas in medical disorders it provides a route for drugs that must be given intravenously.

Before inserting an IV catheter, several decisions must be made to ensure the best possible care for the patient. They are as follows:

1. What Size Catheter Should Be Inserted?

When managing patients with trauma who require rapid fluid administration, it is imperative that a large catheter, 16 gauge, be inserted. It is important to remember that patients who are likely to need whole blood on arrival at the hospital require a large-bore catheter (18 gauge or larger). Medical patients may receive an 18- or 20-gauge catheter.

2. What Type of IV Catheter Should Be Inserted?

As a rule, an over-the-needle catheter is all that should be used in the pre-hospital setting. Butterfly catheters are usually too small to administer large amounts of fluids rapidly. Butterfly catheters should be carried for use in children, however. Occasionally, an adult with exceptionally small veins may be encountered, and, in this case, a butterfly catheter may be inserted if one of the other types of catheters cannot be placed.

3. What Type of IV Fluid Should Be Used?

Usually, the decision of what type of IV fluid to use is left up to the base station physician or written in the protocols. It is important to be familiar with the types of fluids that have been discussed in this chapter.

4. What Type of Administration Set Should Be Used?

There are two general types of IV administration sets. The macrodrip, or standard, set delivers in the neighborhood of 10 to 20 gtt/mL, depending on the manufacturer. Minidrip, or microdrip, sets deliver anywhere from 50 to 60 gtt/mL, depending on the manufacturer. If a large quantity of fluids will be administered, then a macrodrip set should be used. Whenever a paramedic is going to administer a drug, he or she should use a minidrip set. This is especially true for piggyback drug infusions. Many systems also use Buretrol or Volutrol sets for administering aminophylline and similar drugs. If these sets are used, paramedics should remember them when preparing to administer drugs such as aminophylline.

5. Where Should the IV Be Inserted?

Routinely, IV infusions should be started in the larger veins of the forearm. These are usually the most accessible and the least painful for the patient. When these veins are not available, as often occurs in shock and trauma, then any of the other peripheral sites should be attempted.

The veins of the leg and the external jugular in the neck are considered peripheral veins. When treating medical or traumatic emergencies, the rule of thumb for starting an intravenous infusion is "any port in a storm." In a cardiac/traumatic arrest, the antecubital vein is a preferred site.

Procedure for Intravenous Cannulation

Once the preceding five decisions have been made, then the actual procedure of inserting the IV can begin. The procedure is as follows:

1. Observe body substance isolation precautions.
2. Receive the order.
3. Confirm the order and write it down.

4. Prepare the equipment and don gloves and protective eyewear:
   a. Appropriate IV fluid
   b. Appropriate administration set
   c. Appropriate indwelling catheter
   d. Extension IV tubing
   e. Tourniquet
   f. Antibiotic swab
   g. 2 × 2 gauze pad
   h. 1-inch tape
   i. Antibiotic ointment
   j. Short arm board
5. Remove the envelope from the IV fluid.
6. Inspect the fluid, making sure that it is not discolored and does not contain any particulate matter; check that it contains the amount of fluid it should have. Do not administer if discolored, if particles are present, or if less than the indicated quantity of fluid is present.
7. Open and inspect the IV tubing.
8. Attach the extension tubing.
9. Close the clamp on the tubing.
10. Remove the sterile cover from the IV fluid and the administration set.
11. Insert the administration set into the IV fluid.
12. Squeeze the drip chamber to fill it with fluid.
13. Bleed all of the air out of the IV tubing.
14. Hang the bag on an IV pole (or have a bystander hold it) at the appropriate height.
15. Place the tourniquet on the patient to occlude venous flow only.
16. Select a suitable vein and palpate it (see Figures 5–6 and 5–7).
17. Prepare the site by cleansing it with an antibiotic swab.
18. Make the puncture using appropriate sterile technique, enter the vein, observe flashback, and advance the catheter (see Figures 5–8 through 5–10).
19. Connect the IV tubing and remove tourniquet.
20. Slowly open the valve.
21. Confirm that the fluid is flowing appropriately without any evidence of infiltration.
22. Apply an antibiotic ointment over the puncture and cover with a sterile 2 × 2 gauze pad or adhesive bandage.
23. Securely tape the IV catheter and tubing down.
24. Adjust the flow rate.

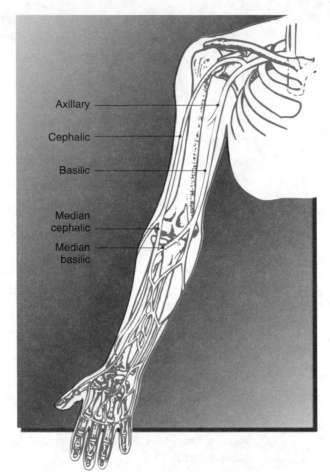

Axillary

Cephalic

Basilic

Median
cephalic

Median
basilic

FIGURE 5–6 Veins of the arm.

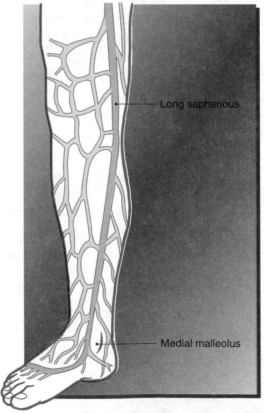

Long saphenous

Medial malleolus

114

FIGURE 5–7 Veins of the leg.

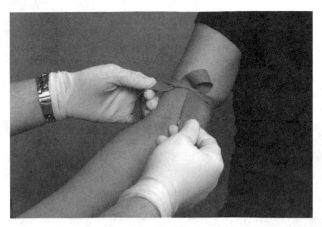

FIGURE 5-8 Apply the tourniquet.

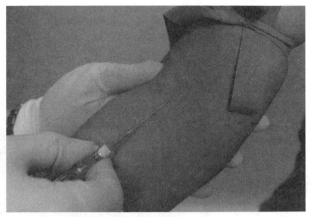

FIGURE 5-9 Puncture the skin.

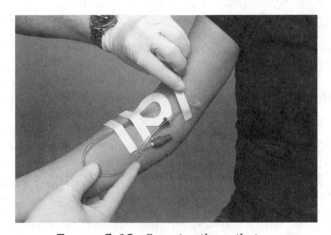

FIGURE 5-10 Securing the catheter.

25. Apply a short arm board.

26. Label the IV bag with the patient's name, date, time the IV was initiated, gauge of the catheter, and your initials.

27. Confirm with medical control the successful completion of the IV.

28. Monitor the patient for the desired effects and any undesired ones as well.

COLLECTION OF BLOOD SAMPLES FOR LABORATORY ANALYSIS

Prehospital personnel may be required to obtain blood samples in the field for later laboratory analysis. Although this practice was more common in the past, there are still instances in which this practice is important. There are several advantages to obtaining blood samples in the field.

First, it provides the emergency physician with information about the patient before medical intervention. This information is especially important in cases of suspected hypoglycemia when 50 percent dextrose is administered (although electronic glucometers are very accurate and thus the need for blood samples prior to glucose administration is diminishing). In situations in which a patient may be trapped or transport to the hospital is otherwise delayed, blood samples can be taken to the hospital before the patient so that blood can be typed, cross-matched, and ready when the patient eventually arrives in the emergency department. Whenever a prehospital intervention might affect the subsequent care of the patient (e.g., administering dextran, which may inhibit blood typing), the paramedic should always draw a blood sample according to local protocol.

Most commonly, blood samples are taken when an IV is started. The paramedic should always follow universal precautions when caring for a patient and especially when handling a blood sample. Gloves and goggles should be worn. After placing the IV catheter and before connecting the IV line, a 10 mL syringe can be attached to the catheter and blood gently withdrawn from the vein. The syringe can be removed and the IV line connected. It is important to withdraw the blood from the syringe slowly. Withdrawing it rapidly can damage the blood cells, causing them to rupture and leak their contents, which in turn can erroneously alter the blood chemistries and render the sample useless.

Once blood is withdrawn from a patient, it is usually placed into evacuated blood collection tubes (Vacutainer). These tubes have a vacuum that allows the tube to fill with a predetermined amount of blood. Most tubes contain a chemical to keep the blood from clotting. Each tube has a different colored rubber top, depending on its use and contents. The type of tube a paramedic may be asked to draw may vary from region to region. After withdrawing the blood as described earlier, an 18-gauge needle is placed on the syringe. The needle is inserted into the rubber top and the tube is allowed to fill with blood. The paramedic should not attempt to overfill the tube or press on the plunger of the syringe, but allow the vacuum to fill the vial.

After the vials are filled, they should be inverted several times to mix the blood and the anticoagulant. The patient's name, date, time drawn, paramedic's name, and incident number (if any) are immediately written on the vial. The tubes are given to the appropriate emergency department personnel on arrival. The paramedic documents on the patient report form the time the blood was drawn and to whom it was given. At critical scenes, labeling tubes may be difficult. As an alternative until tubes can be labeled, tape the tubes to the IV bag.

BLOOD TRANSFUSIONS

When mismatched blood is transfused, the donor's antibodies can bind to antigens on the recipient's red blood cells (RBCs). This reaction, known as a transfusion reaction, causes clumping of RBCs in the blood (agglutination) and subsequent hemolysis (RBCs breaking apart). Transfusion reaction can only be prevented by complete and careful type matching between donor and recipient.

Paramedics occasionally transport a patient receiving blood. These patients need careful monitoring for signs and symptoms of transfusion reaction. The severity of the reaction depends on the degree of incompatibility, the amount of blood given, and the rate of administration. Onset is usually rapid, either during or immediately after a transfusion. More rarely, it occurs later. Signs and symptoms include anxiety; facial flushing; pain in the neck, chest, and lumbar area; tachycardia; cold, clammy skin; hypotension; nausea or vomiting; dizziness; hives; headaches; and fever.

When signs and symptoms of transfusion reaction appear, the transfusion should be discontinued immediately. A physician should be consulted as soon as possible and a crystalloid infusion for drug administrations maintained. A diuretic such as mannitol (Osmitrol) and an antihistamine such as diphenhydramine (Benadryl) may be indicated. One of the most lethal effects of transfusion reaction is kidney shutdown, which can begin within a few minutes to a few hours and may progress to lethal renal failure.

SUMMARY

As with the skills of medication administration, the insertion of an IV requires vigorous mannequin, classroom, and clinical training under the supervision of a qualified instructor.

KEY WORDS

colloid. A substance of high molecular weight, such as plasma proteins. Colloids tend to remain in the intravascular space, as opposed to crystalloids, which tend to diffuse out.

crystalloid. A solution containing crystalline substances, such as normal saline.

diffusion. The movement of solute (substances dissolved in a solution) from an area of greater concentration to an area of lesser concentration.

electrolytes. A chemical substance that dissociates into charged particles when placed in water.

erythrocytes. Red blood cells; responsible for transport of oxygen.

extracellular. The space outside the cell membrane.

hematocrit. A measure of the number of red blood cells found in the blood, stated as a percentage of the total blood volume.

homeostasis. The body's natural tendency to keep the natural environment constant.

hypertonic. A state in which a solution has a higher solute concentration on one side of a semipermeable membrane than on the other side.

hypotonic. A state in which a solution has a lower solute concentration on one side of a semipermeable membrane than on the other side.

intracellular. The space and materials within the cell membrane.

intravascular. The space within the blood vessels.

isotonic. A state in which solutions on opposite sides of a semipermeable membrane are equal in concentration.

leukocytes. White blood cells; responsible for fighting infection.

osmosis. The movement of a solvent (water) across a semipermeable membrane from an area of lesser (solute) concentration to an area of greater (solute) concentration; osmosis is a form of diffusion.

semipermeable membrane. A specialized biological membrane, such as that which encloses the body's cells, that allows passage of certain substances and restricts the passage of others.

6

THE AUTONOMIC NERVOUS SYSTEM

OBJECTIVES

After completing this chapter, the reader should be able to:

1. Describe the anatomy and physiology of the autonomic nervous system.
2. Compare sympathetic and parasympathetic actions.
3. Explain the function of the sympathetic nervous system.
4. List the four adrenergic receptors and explain the effect of each one on body organs.
5. Explain the function of the parasympathetic nervous system.

INTRODUCTION

The autonomic nervous system is a part of the peripheral nervous system and is responsible for control of involuntary, or visceral, bodily functions. It controls crucial cardiovascular, respiratory, digestive, urinary, and reproductive functions. It also plays a key role in the body's response to stress.

Many of the medications used in emergency care act directly or indirectly on the autonomic nervous system. Thus, it is essential that prehospital personnel have a good understanding of the structure and function of the autonomic nervous system. This chapter discusses the anatomy and physiology of the autonomic nervous system as it applies to emergency pharmacological therapy.

THE AUTONOMIC NERVOUS SYSTEM

The *nervous system* is the body's principal control system. It regulates virtually all bodily functions via electrical impulses transmitted through nerves. Closely related to the nervous system is the *endocrine system*. Like the nervous system, the endocrine system is an important control system.

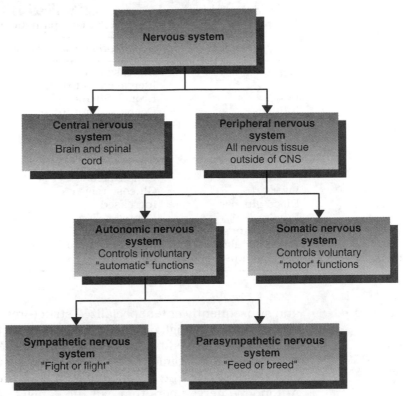

FIGURE 6–1 Functional organization of the nervous system.

However, unlike the nervous system, it exerts its effect on the body through the release of specialized chemical substances called *hormones.*

The nervous system is customarily divided into the central nervous system and the peripheral nervous system. The *central nervous system (CNS)* consists of the brain and spinal cord. In contrast, the *peripheral nervous system (PNS)* is composed of the cranial nerves and the peripheral nerves. The peripheral nervous system can be further divided into the somatic nervous system and the autonomic nervous system. The *somatic nervous system (SNS)* controls voluntary motor functions such as movement. The *autonomic nervous system (ANS)* controls involuntary automatic functions (see Figure 6–1).

The two functional divisions of the autonomic nervous system are the sympathetic nervous system and the parasympathetic nervous system. The *sympathetic nervous system* allows the body to function under stress. It is often referred to as the *fight-or-flight* aspect of the nervous system. The *parasympathetic nervous system,* on the other hand, primarily controls vegetative functions such as digestion of food. It is often referred to as the *feed-or-breed* or *rest-and-repose* aspect of the autonomic nervous system. The parasympathetic nervous system is in constant opposition to the sympathetic nervous system (see Table 6–1).

Autonomic Nervous System Anatomy and Physiology

Although the autonomic nervous system is primarily located outside of the central nervous system, it arises from the central nervous system. The nerves of the autonomic nervous system exit the central nervous system

TABLE 6–1

Comparison of Sympathetic and Parasympathetic Actions

Organ	Sympathetic stimulation	Parasympathetic stimulation
Heart	Increased rate	Decreased rate
	Increased contractile force	Decreased contractile force
Lungs	Bronchodilation	Bronchoconstriction
Kidneys	Decreased output	No change
Systemic blood vessels		
Abdominal	Constricted	None
Muscle	Constricted α	None
	Dilated β	None
Skin	Constricted	None
Liver	Glucose release	Slight glycogen synthesis
Blood glucose	Increased	None
Pupils	Dilated	Constricted
Sweat glands	Copious sweating	None
Basal metabolism	Increased up to 100%	None
Skeletal muscle	Increased strength	None

and subsequently enter specialized structures called *autonomic ganglia*. In the autonomic ganglia, the nerve fibers from the central nervous system interact with nerve fibers that extend from the ganglia to the various target organs. Autonomic nerve fibers that exit the central nervous system and terminate in the autonomic ganglia are called *preganglionic nerves.* Autonomic nerve fibers that exit the ganglia and terminate in the various target tissues are called *postganglionic nerves.* The ganglia of the sympathetic nervous system are located close to the spinal cord, whereas the ganglia of the parasympathetic nervous system are located close to the target organs (see Figure 6–2).

No actual physical connection exists between two nerve cells or between a nerve cell and the organ it innervates. Instead, there is a space between nerve cells called a *synapse.* The space between a nerve cell and the target organ is called a *neuroeffector junction.* Specialized chemicals called *neurotransmitters* are used to conduct the nervous impulse between nerve cells or between a nerve cell and its target organ. Neurotransmitters are released from presynaptic neurons and subsequently act on postsynaptic neurons or on the designated target organ. When released by the nerve ending, the neurotransmitter travels across the synapse and activates membrane receptors on the adjoining nerve or target tissue. The neurotransmitter is then either deactivated or taken back up into the presynaptic neuron. The primary neurotransmitters of the autonomic nervous system are *acetylcholine* (ACh) and *norepinephrine.* Acetylcholine is utilized in the preganglionic nerves of the sympathetic nervous system and in both the preganglionic and postganglionic nerves of the parasympathetic nervous system. Norepinephrine is the primary postganglionic neurotransmitter of the sympathetic nervous system. Synapses that use ACh as the neurotransmitter are called *cholinergic* synapses. Synapses that use norepinephrine as the neurotransmitter are called *adrenergic* synapses.

The Sympathetic Nervous System

The sympathetic nervous system arises from the thoracic and lumbar region of the spinal cord. Preganglionic nerves leave the spinal cord through the spinal nerves and end in the sympathetic ganglia. There are two types

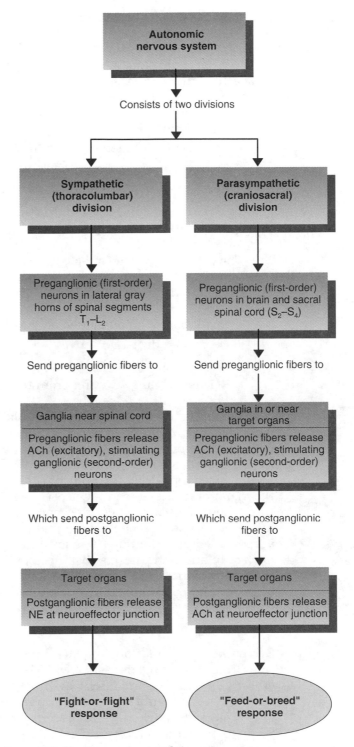

FIGURE 6–2 Components of the autonomic nervous system.

of sympathetic ganglia: sympathetic chain ganglia and collateral ganglia (see Figure 6–3). In addition, special preganglionic sympathetic nerve fibers innervate the adrenal medulla. Postganglionic nerves that exit the *sympathetic chain ganglia* extend to several peripheral target tissues of the sympathetic nervous system. When stimulated, these fibers have several effects, including the following:

- Stimulation of secretion by sweat glands
- Constriction of blood vessels in the skin
- Increase in blood flow to skeletal muscles
- Increase in heart rate and in the force of cardiac contractions
- Bronchodilation
- Stimulation of energy production

The *collateral ganglia* are located in the abdominal cavity. Nerves leaving the collateral ganglia innervate many of the organs of the abdomen. Stimulation of these fibers causes the following:

- Reduction of blood flow to abdominal organs
- Decreased digestive activity
- Relaxation of smooth muscle in the wall of the urinary bladder
- Release of glucose stores from the liver

Sympathetic nervous system stimulation also results in direct stimulation of the *adrenal medulla*. The adrenal medulla in turn releases the hormones *norepinephrine* (noradrenalin) and *epinephrine* (adrenalin) into the circulatory system. Approximately 80 percent of the hormones released by the adrenal medulla are epinephrine, with norepinephrine constituting the remaining 20 percent. Once released, these hormones are carried throughout the body, where they cause their intended effects by acting on hormone receptors. The release of norepinephrine and epinephrine by the adrenal medulla stimulates tissues that are not innervated by sympathetic nerves. In addition, these substances prolong the effects of direct sympathetic stimulation. All of these effects serve to prepare the body to deal with stressful and potentially dangerous situations.

Adrenergic Receptors

Sympathetic stimulation ultimately results in the release of norepinephrine from postganglionic nerves. The nervous impulse subsequently crosses the synapse and interacts with adrenergic receptors. Shortly thereafter, the norepinephrine is taken up by the presynaptic neuron for reuse or is broken down by enzymes present within the synapse (see Figure 6–4). Sympathetic stimulation also results in the release of epinephrine and norepinephrine from the adrenal medulla. Both epinephrine and norepinephrine also interact with specialized receptors on the membranes of the target organs. These receptors, called *adrenergic receptors,* are located throughout the body. Once stimulated by the appropriate hormone, they cause a response in the organ or organs they control.

The two known types of sympathetic receptors are the adrenergic receptors and the dopaminergic receptors. The adrenergic receptors are generally divided into four types. These four receptors are designated *alpha*$_1$ (α_1), *alpha*$_2$

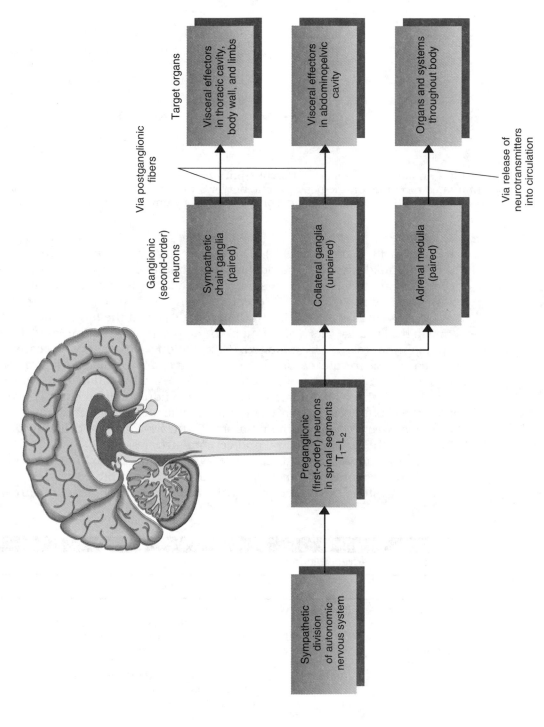

Figure 6-3 Organization of the sympathetic division of the autonomic nervous system.

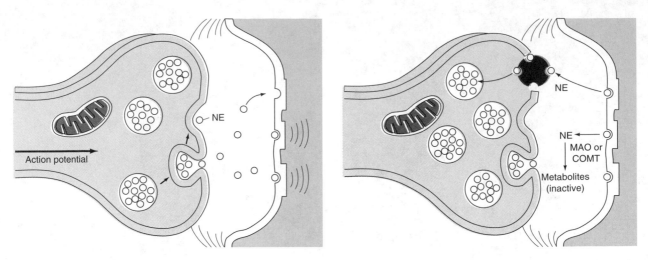

FIGURE 6–4 Physiology of an adrenergic synapse. Norepinephrine is released from the presynaptic nerve and stimulates receptors on the postsynaptic nerve. Subsequently, the norepinephrine is either taken up by the presynaptic nerve or deactivated by enzymes present in the synapse.

(α_2), *beta*$_1$ (β_1), and *beta*$_2$ (β_2). The α_1-receptors cause peripheral vasoconstriction, mild bronchoconstriction, and stimulation of metabolism. The α_2-receptors are found on the *presynaptic* surfaces of sympathetic neuroeffector junctions. Stimulation of α_2-receptors is inhibitory. They serve to prevent overrelease of norepinephrine in the synapse. When the level of norepinephrine in the synapse gets high enough, the α_2-receptors are stimulated and norepinephrine release is inhibited. Stimulation of β_1-receptors causes an increase in heart rate, cardiac contractile force, and cardiac automaticity and conduction. Stimulation of β_2-receptors causes vasodilation and bronchodilation (see Table 6–2). Additional types of beta adrenergic receptors have been identified, but their role in emergency medication usage remains unclear. *Dopaminergic receptors,* although not fully understood, are believed to cause dilation of the renal, coronary, and cerebral arteries.

Medications that stimulate the sympathetic nervous system are referred to as *sympathomimetics.* Medications that inhibit the sympathetic nervous system are called *sympatholytics.* Some medications are pure

---

TABLE 6–2

Actions of the Adrenergic Receptors

Receptor	Actions
alpha$_1$ (α_1)	Peripheral vasoconstriction
	Increased contractile force (positive inotropic effect)
	Decreased heart rate (negative chronotropic effect)
alpha$_2$ (α_2)	Peripheral vasoconstriction (by limiting norepinephrine release)
beta$_1$ (β_1)	Increased heart rate (positive chronotropic effect)
	Increased contractile force (positive inotropic effect)
	Increased automaticity (positive dromotropic effect)
beta$_2$ (β_2)	Peripheral vasodilation
	Bronchodilation
	Uterine smooth muscle relaxation
	Gastrointestinal smooth muscle relaxation
Dopaminergic	Renal vasodilation
	Mesenteric vasodilation

α-*agonists*, whereas others are pure α-*antagonists*. Some medications are pure β-agonists, whereas others are pure β-antagonists. Medications such as epinephrine stimulate both α- and β-receptors. Medications such as the *bronchodilators* are termed β selective, because they act more on β_2-receptors than on β_1-receptors.

The Parasympathetic Nervous System

The parasympathetic nervous system arises from the brain stem and the sacral segments of the spinal cord. The preganglionic neurons are typically much longer than those of the sympathetic nervous system because the ganglia are located close to the target tissues. Parasympathetic nerve fibers that leave the brain stem travel within four of the cranial nerves including the oculomotor nerve (III), the facial nerve (VII), the glossopharyngeal nerve (IX), and the vagus nerve (X). These fibers synapse in the *parasympathetic ganglia* with short postganglionic fibers, which then continue to their target tissues. Postsynaptic fibers innervate much of the body including the intrinsic eye muscles, the salivary glands, the heart, the lungs, and most of the organs of the abdominal cavity. The sacral segment of the parasympathetic nervous system forms distinct pelvic nerves that innervate ganglia in the kidneys, bladder, sex organs, and terminal portions of the large intestine (see Figure 6–5). Stimulation of the parasympathetic nervous system results in the following:

- Pupillary constriction
- Secretion by digestive glands
- Increased smooth muscle activity along the digestive tract
- Bronchoconstriction
- Reduction in heart rate and cardiac contractile force

Through these and other functions, the processing of food, energy absorption, relaxation, and reproduction are facilitated.

All preganglionic and postganglionic parasympathetic nerve fibers use *acetylcholine* as a neurotransmitter. Acetylcholine, when released by presynaptic neurons, crosses the synaptic cleft and activates receptors on the postsynaptic neuron or on the neuroeffector junction. Acetylcholine is also the neurotransmitter for the somatic nervous system and is present in the *neuromuscular junction*. Acetylcholine is very short lived. Within a fraction of a second after its release, acetylcholine is deactivated by another chemical called *acetylcholinesterase*. *Acetic acid* and *choline*, which are produced when acetylcholine is deactivated, are taken back up by the presynaptic neuron (see Figure 6–6).

The parasympathetic system has two main types of ACh receptors, nicotinic and muscarinic. Knowing these receptors' locations and functions will greatly simplify learning the functions of drugs in this class. Nicotinic$_N$ (neuron) receptors are found in all autonomic ganglia, where acetylcholine serves as the presynaptic neurotransmitter of both the parasympathetic and sympathetic nervous systems. Nicotinic$_M$ (muscle) receptors are found at the neuromuscular junction and initiate muscular contraction as part of the somatic nervous system. Muscarinic receptors are found in many organs thoughout the body and are primarily responsible for promoting the

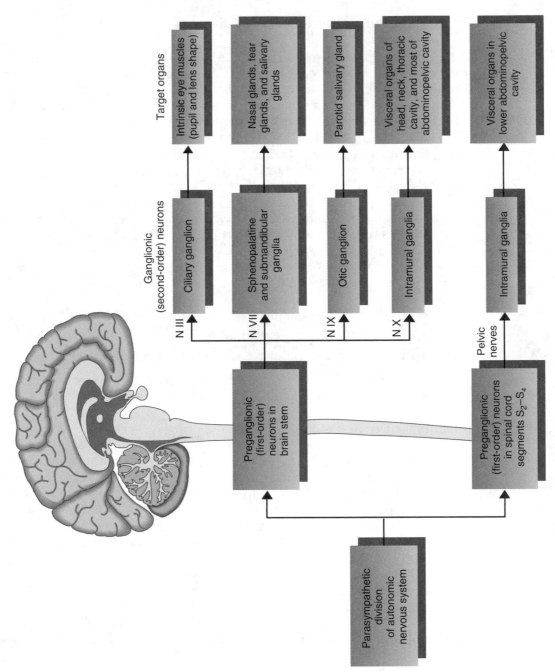

FIGURE 6-5 Organization of the parasympathetic division of the autonomic nervous system.

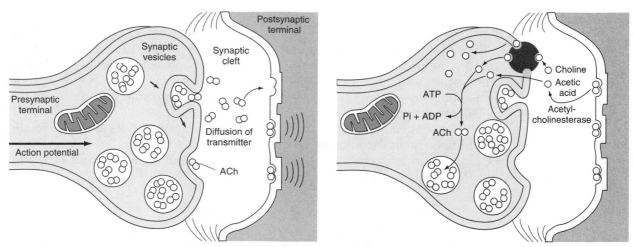

FIGURE 6–6 Physiology of a cholinergic synapse. Acetylcholine is released from the presynaptic nerve and stimulates receptors on the postsynaptic nerve. Subsequently, the acetylcholine is broken down by acetylcholinesterase and the products are taken up by the presynaptic nerve fiber.

parasympathetic response. Table 6–3 summarizes the locations and actions of the muscarinic receptors.

The emergency medication atropine is an antagonist to the parasympathetic nervous system and is used to increase heart rate. Atropine binds with ACh receptors, thus preventing ACh from exerting its effect. Medications such as atropine, which block the actions of the parasympathetic nervous system, are referred to as *parasympatholytics* or anticholinergics. Medications that stimulate the parasympathetic nervous system are referred to as *parasympathomimetics*.

TABLE 6–3

Location and Effect of Muscarinic Receptors

Organ	Functions	Location
Heart	Decreased heart rate	Sinoatrial node
	Decreased conduction rate	Atrioventricular node
Arterioles	Dilation	Coronary
	Dilation	Skin and mucosa
	Dilation	Cerebral
GI tract	Relaxed	Sphincters
	Increased	Motility
	Increased salivation	Salivary glands
	Increased secretion	Exocrine glands
Lungs	Bronchoconstriction	Bronchiole smooth muscle
	Increased mucous production	Bronchial glands
Gallbladder	Contraction	
Urinary bladder	Relaxation	Urinary sphincter
	Contraction	Detrusor muscle
Liver	Glycogen synthesis	
Lacrimal glands	Secretion (increased tearing)	Eye
Eye	Contraction for near vision	Ciliary muscle
	Constriction	Pupil
Penis	Erection	

The autonomic nervous system is a part of the peripheral nervous system and is responsible for control of involuntary, or visceral, bodily functions. It maintains the body's internal environment by controlling crucial cardiovascular, respiratory, digestive, urinary, and reproductive functions. It also plays a key role in the body's response to stress.

Because many of the medications used in prehospital care act directly or indirectly on the autonomic nervous system, it is essential that prehospital personnel have a good understanding of the structure and function of the autonomic nervous system.

KEY WORDS

acetylcholine (ACh). Chemical neurotransmitter found in all autonomic preganglionic synapses and in parasympathetic postganglionic synapses.

adrenal medulla. An endocrine gland, located atop the kidney, that manufactures and secretes epinephrine and norepinephrine.

adrenergic. Related to or pertaining to the sympathetic nervous system.

alpha$_1$ adrenergic receptor. A type of adrenergic receptor that, when stimulated, causes peripheral vasoconstriction, mild bronchoconstriction, and stimulation of metabolism.

alpha$_2$ adrenergic receptor. A type of adrenergic receptor that, when stimulated, inhibits parts of the sympathetic nervous system. It serves to prevent the overrelease of norepinephrine in the synapse.

autonomic nervous system (ANS). Part of the peripheral nervous system responsible for control of involuntary, or visceral, bodily functions.

beta$_1$ adrenergic receptor. A type of adrenergic receptor that, when stimulated, causes an increase in heart rate, cardiac contractile force, and cardiac automaticity and conduction.

beta$_2$ adrenergic receptor. A type of adrenergic receptor that, when stimulated, causes vasodilation and bronchodilation.

bronchodilator. A drug that helps to improve breathing by relaxing the smooth muscle of the bronchioles, causing bronchodilation.

central nervous system (CNS). The central portion of the nervous system, consisting of the brain and spinal cord.

cholinergic. Related to or pertaining to the parasympathetic nervous system.

chronotrope. A drug or other substance that affects heart rate.

dromotrope. A drug or other substance that affects nerve conduction.

epinephrine. A naturally occurring hormone that stimulates the adrenal glands, increases cardiac output, and causes bronchodilation.

ganglia. A mass of nerve cells.

inotrope. A drug or other substance that affects the strength of the cardiac contraction.

neurotransmitter. A substance that is released from the axon terminal of a presynaptic neuron. On excitation it travels across the synaptic cleft to either excite or inhibit the target cell. Examples include acetylcholine, norepinephrine, and dopamine.

norepinephrine.   A naturally occurring hormone that also serves as a sympathetic neurotransmitter. It is found in most postganglionic synapses.

parasympathetic nervous system.   The division of the autonomic nervous system that is responsible for controlling vegetative functions.

peripheral nervous system.   The portion of the nervous system outside the brain and spinal cord. It is composed of the cranial nerves and peripheral nerves.

somatic nervous system (SNS).   The portion of the nervous system that controls voluntary motor functions such as movement.

sympathetic nervous system.   The division of the autonomic nervous system that prepares the body for stressful situations.

sympatholytic (or antiadrenergic).   Drugs that block beta adrenergic receptors and slow the heart rate.

sympathomimetic.   A drug or other substance that causes effects such as those of the sympathetic nervous system (also called adrenergic).

7

DRUGS USED IN THE TREATMENT OF CARDIOVASCULAR EMERGENCIES

OBJECTIVES

After completing this chapter, the reader should be able to:

1. Describe and list the pharmacokinetics, indications, contraindications, and dosages for the sympathomimetics epinephrine, norepinephrine, isoproterenol, dopamine, dobutamine, metaraminol, amrinone, and vasopressin.

2. Discuss the pharmacology of vasopressin and its role in cardiac arrest management.

3. Explain the class of drugs known as sympathetic blockers.

4. Describe and list the pharmacokinetics, indications, contraindications, and dosages for the sympathetic blockers propranolol, sotalol, metoprolol, labetalol, and esmolol.

5. Discuss the use of antidysrhythmic medications.

6. Describe and list the pharmacokinetics indications, contraindications, and dosages for the antidysrhythmics lidocaine, procainamide, bretylium tosylate, adenosine, verapamil, diltiazem, amiodarone, phenytoin, edrophonium chloride, and magnesium sulfate.

7. Explain the role of the parasympatholytic atropine and list the pharmacokinetics, indications, contraindications, and dosages for its use.

8. Describe digitalis and list the pharmacokinetics, indications, contraindications, and dosages for its use.

9. Describe the indications for anticoagulant therapy in emergency care.

10. Discuss the use of fibrinolytics and aspirin in the treatment of myocardial infarction.

11. Describe and list the pharmacokinetics, indications, contraindications, and dosages for aspirin and the fibrinolytic agents streptokinase, anistreplase, tissue plasminogen activator, and retaplase recombinant.

12. List the pharmacokinetics, indications, contraindications, and dosages for sodium bicarbonate.

13. Explain the pharmacokinetics, indications, contraindications, and dosages for morphine and nitrous oxide in the treatment of cardiac chest pain.

14. Discuss the use of diuretics in the management of congestive heart failure.

15. List the pharmacokinetics, indications, contraindications, and dosages for the diuretics furosemide and bumetanide.

16. Discuss the use of the natriuretic peptide nesiritide for the management of congestive heart failure.

17. Describe the action of nitroglycerin in cardiac chest pain.

18. List the pharmacokinetics, indications, contraindications, and dosages for the antianginal agents nitroglycerin, nitroglycerin spray, and nitroglycerin paste.

19. Define and explain a hypertensive crisis.

20. List the pharmacokinetics, indications, contraindications, and dosages for the antihypertensives nifedipine, sodium nitroprusside, and hydralazine.

21. List the pharmacokinetics, indications, contraindications, and dosages for calcium chloride.

INTRODUCTION

Most prehospital emergency drugs are used in the treatment of cardiac emergencies. These drugs, because of the nature of their actions, may be accompanied by many side effects. Some general classifications follow for our discussion of the emergency cardiovascular drugs:

Gases
Oxygen

Sympathomimetics
Epinephrine
Norepinephrine (Levophed)
Isoproterenol (Isuprel)
Dopamine HCl (Intropin)
Dobutamine (Dobutrex)
Metaraminol (Aramine)
Amrinone (Inocor)
Vasopressin (Pitressin)

Sympathetic Blockers
Propranolol (Inderal)
Sotalol HCl (Sotacor, Betapace)
Metoprolol (Lopressor)
Labetalol (Trandate, Normodyne)
Esmolol (Brevibloc)

Antidysrhythmics
Lidocaine (Xylocaine)
Procainamide (Pronestyl)

Bretylium tosylate (Bretylol)

Adenosine (Adenocard)

Verapamil (Isoptin, Calan)

Diltiazem (Cardizem)

Amiodarone HCl (Cordarone)

Phenytoin (Dilantin)

Edrophonium chloride (Tensilon)

Magnesium sulfate

Propranolol (Inderal)

Parasympatholytics

Atropine sulfate

Cardiac Glycosides

Digoxin (Lanoxin)

Anticoagulants

Heparin

Enoxaparin (Lovenox)

Fibrinolytics

Aspirin

Streptokinase (Streptase)

Anistreplase (Eminase, Apsac)

Alteplase, tissue plasminogen activator (TPA) (Activase)

Retaplase Recombinant (Retavase)

Alkalinizing Agents

Sodium bicarbonate

Analgesics

Morphine sulfate

Nitrous oxide (Nitronox, Entonox)

Diuretics

Furosemide (Lasix)

Bumetanide (Bumex)

Natriuretic Agents

Nesiritide (Natrecor)

Antianginal Agents

Nitroglycerin (Nitrostat)

Nitroglycerin paste (Nitroglycerin Ointment)

Nitroglycerin spray (Nitroglycerin Spray)

Antihypertensives

Nifedipine (Procardia, Adalat)

Sodium nitroprusside (Nitropress, Nipride)

Hydralazine (Apresoline)

Other Cardiovascular Drugs

Calcium chloride

OXYGEN

Oxygen is one of the most important drugs used in prehospital care. It is required by the body's cells to facilitate the breakdown of glucose into usable energy forms. Without oxygen, the breakdown of glucose is ineffective and incomplete. This breakdown without oxygen is termed *anaerobic metabolism.* Anaerobic metabolism yields *lactic acid,* a strong acid, as its end product. This acid, in conjunction with an increased carbon dioxide level, leads to systemic acidosis.

Oxygen is an odorless, tasteless, colorless gas that vigorously supports combustion. It is present in room air at a concentration of approximately 21 percent. This concentration is adequate for our daily activities. In injury and illness, however, the body needs increased levels of oxygen to maintain homeostasis.

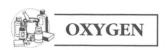 **OXYGEN**

Class: Gas

Description

Oxygen is an odorless, tasteless, colorless gas necessary for life.

Mechanism of Action

Oxygen enters the body through the respiratory system and is transported to the cells by hemoglobin, found in the red blood cells. Oxygen is required for the efficient breakdown of glucose into a usable energy form. Its onset of action following administration is immediate. The administration of enriched oxygen increases the oxygen concentration in the alveoli, which subsequently increases the oxygen saturation of available hemoglobin.

Pharmacokinetics

Onset: Immediate
Peak Effects: <1 minute
Duration: <2 minutes
Half-Life: N/A

Indication

Hypoxia. Oxygen is indicated whenever hypoxia is suspected or possible, including for all forms of trauma, medical emergencies, chest pain that may be due to cardiac ischemia, any respiratory difficulty, during labor and delivery, and in any critical patient.

Contraindications

There are no contraindications to oxygen. *Hypoxic patients should never be deprived of oxygen for fear of respiratory depression.*

Precautions

Oxygen should be used cautiously in patients with chronic obstructive pulmonary disease (COPD). In these patients respirations are often regulated by the level of oxygen in the blood (*hypoxic drive*) instead of carbon dioxide. In some cases COPD patients may suffer respiratory depression if high concentrations of oxygen are delivered. The administration of high concentrations of oxygen to neonates for a prolonged period of time can damage the infant's eyes (*retrolental fibroplasia*). Although this is rarely a problem in prehospital care, it is a consideration in long-distance and prolonged transport. Oxygen delivered at a flow rate of 6 lpm or greater should be humidified to prevent drying of the mucous membranes of the upper respiratory system. When possible, oxygen administration should be monitored by use of pulse oximetry. *Pulse oximetry* is a noninvasive method for accurately measuring the oxygen saturation of hemoglobin. It is relatively inexpensive, easy to use, and quite accurate in detecting oxygen delivery problems.

Side Effects

There are few, if any, side effects associated with oxygen administration. Prolonged administration of high-flow, nonhumidified oxygen may cause drying of the mucous membranes, resulting in irritation and possibly nosebleeds.

Interactions

There are no interactions associated with oxygen administration. However, oxygen may increase the toxicity of certain herbicides (e.g., paraquat and diaquat) in patients who have ingested these poisons. These chemicals are sometimes sprayed on illicit agricultural products such as marijuana. Poisoning by these agents is uncommon.

Dosage

The dosage of oxygen is based on the patient's underlying problems. In the prehospital setting oxygen should be administered at the highest concentration available (see Table 7–1). Pulse oximetry, if available, should be used to guide care. General guidelines follow:

Cardiac arrest and other critical patients—100 percent oxygen concentration

Chronic obstructive pulmonary disease—35 percent oxygen concentration (increase as needed)

How Supplied

Oxygen is supplied in pressurized cylinders of varying size (see Table 7–2). Liquid oxygen is becoming more common in prehospital care. The sizes and types of liquid oxygen containers vary.

TABLE 7–1		
Oxygen Delivery by Device		
Oxygen delivery device	*Flow rate (lpm)*	*Percentage delivered*
Nasal cannula	1–6	24–44
Simple face mask	8–10	40–60
Venturi mask	4–12	24–50
Partial rebreathing mask	6–10	35–60
Nonrebreathing mask	6–10	60–95
Bag, valve, and mask with reservoir	10–15	40–90
Demand valve	10–15	100

TABLE 7–2	
Capacity of Common Oxygen Cylinders	
Cylinder name	Volume (L)
D	400
E	660
M	3000

SYMPATHOMIMETICS

The term *sympathomimetic* means to mimic the actions of the sympathetic nervous system. Drugs in this group do exactly that. They either act directly on receptors of the sympathetic nervous system or act indirectly by stimulating the release of *endogenous* catecholamines. *Catecholamine* is the name used to describe several drugs that are chemically similar. These drugs are epinephrine, norepinephrine (Levophed), dopamine (Intropin), isoproterenol (Isuprel), dobutamine (Dobutrex), metaraminol (Aramine), amrinone (Inocor), and vasopressin (Pitressin). All of these agents, except isoproterenol and dobutamine, can be found naturally in the body. Isoproterenol and dobutamine are synthetic catecholamines. All sympathomimetics, monoamine oxidase inhibitors (MAOIs), and tricyclic antidepressants (TCAs) may increase blood pressure. To understand and appreciate the actions and roles of the sympathomimetics fully, it is essential to first review the sympathetic nervous system.

Sympathetic Nervous System

The *sympathetic nervous system* is sometimes called the fight-or-flight system. It is this part of the nervous system that prepares the body to deal with various stresses, whether real or imagined. Sometimes it is referred to as the *adrenergic system*. Both it and the other aspect of the autonomic nervous system, the parasympathetic nervous system, functionally oppose each other to maintain *homeostasis*. The *parasympathetic system* is sometimes called the *cholinergic system*.

As indicated by Table 7–3, the sympathetic nervous system tends to stimulate those organs needed to deal with stressful situations. It also tends to inhibit the use of organs not needed, such as the digestive tract.

The sympathetic nervous system uses the hormone *norepinephrine* to transmit impulses from the nerve to the effector cell. Chemicals that propagate the nervous impulse, such as norepinephrine, are called *neurotransmitters*. In emergency situations the norepinephrine released by the nerve endings may be augmented with epinephrine and norepinephrine secreted from the adrenal medulla. Like the adrenergic nerves, the adrenal medulla secretes norepinephrine. About 20 percent of the catecholamines secreted by the adrenals are in the form of norepinephrine. The remaining 80 percent are in the form of epinephrine (adrenalin).

When released, norepinephrine acts on specialized chemical receptors. These receptors are located at various points throughout the body. Once stimulated by the appropriate catecholamine, they cause a response in the organ or organs they control. There are two types of receptors, the *adrenergic receptors* and the *dopaminergic receptors*. The adrenergic receptors are further divided into four different types. These

TABLE 7–3

Comparison of Sympathetic and Parasympathetic Actions

Organ	Sympathetic stimulation	Parasympathetic stimulation
Heart	Increased rate	Decreased rate
	Increased contractile force	Decreased contractile force
Lungs	Bronchodilation	Bronchoconstriction
Kidneys	Decreased output	No change
Systemic blood vessels		
Abdominal	Constricted	None
Muscle	Constricted (α)	None
	Dilated (β)	None
Skin	Constricted	None
Liver	Glucose release	Slight glycogen synthesis
Blood glucose	Increased	None
Pupils	Dilated	Constricted
Sweat glands	Copious sweating	None
Basal metabolism	Increased up to 100%	None
Skeletal muscle	Increased strength	None

four types of receptors are designated *alpha*$_1$ (α_1), *alpha*$_2$ (α_2), *beta*$_1$ (β_1), and *beta*$_2$ (β_2). The α_1-receptors cause peripheral vasoconstriction and occasionally mild bronchoconstriction. The α_2-receptors, when stimulated, inhibit the release of norepinephrine. This effect is antagonistic to the actions of α_1-receptors and over time can cause peripheral vasodilation. The β_1-receptors, once stimulated, cause an increase in cardiac rate, cardiac force, and cardiac automaticity and conduction. The β_2-receptors cause vasodilation and bronchodilation. Dopaminergic receptors, though not totally understood, are believed to cause dilatation of the renal, coronary, and cerebral arteries. See Chapter 6 for a more detailed discussion of the autonomic nervous system.

Catecholamines

Certain drugs stimulate certain receptors to one degree or another. Norepinephrine, for example, has an effect on both α- and β-receptors. However, its effects are considerably stronger on α-receptors than on β-receptors. Consequently, norepinephrine is primarily regarded as an α-receptor-stimulating agent. Epinephrine, like norepinephrine, acts on both α- and β-receptors. However, unlike norepinephrine, epinephrine has a much greater effect on β-receptors and is considered a β-receptor-stimulating agent. Isoproterenol, the synthetic catecholamine occasionally used in emergency medicine, acts entirely on β-receptors with no α effects noted. Dopamine acts on both α- and β-receptors depending on the dosage. In addition, when used in certain doses, it acts on the dopaminergic receptors. This dopaminergic effect is quite useful because it tends to keep blood flowing to the renal arteries, even in emergency situations. One of the long-term major complications of severe medical emergencies such as cardiac arrest is renal failure. Using such agents as dopamine, which will maintain renal perfusion, helps in the long-term survival of the patient.

Drugs that cause an increase in the cardiac rate are called *positive chronotropic agents.* Drugs that cause an increase in cardiac force are referred to as *positive inotropic agents.* Drugs that cause an increase in contractility are referred to as *positive dromotropic agents.*

The primary use of the sympathomimetics in emergency medicine is to increase the blood pressure in cardiogenic shock. These drugs raise the blood pressure by one of two different methods. Drugs that stimulate α-receptors elevate blood pressure merely by peripheral vasoconstriction. Vasoconstriction reduces the size of the vascular pool, thus increasing the blood pressure. Drugs that act on β-receptors elevate blood pressure by causing an increase in cardiac output. Cardiac output can be defined as follows:

$$\text{Cardiac output} = \text{Stroke volume} \times \text{Heart rate}$$

Thus,

$$\text{Blood pressure} = \text{Cardiac output} \times \text{Peripheral vascular resistance}$$

The β-receptor-stimulating drugs, including epinephrine and dopamine, cause an increase in both heart rate (positive chronotropic) and stroke volume (positive inotropic). The different receptor effects are summarized in Table 7–4. Table 7–5 lists many of the sympathomimetic drugs used in emergency care, including their adrenergic effects and arrhythmia potential.

TABLE 7–4

Comparison of Effects of α- and β-Adrenergic Receptor Activity on Selected Organs

Organ	α-adrenergic receptors	β-adrenergic receptors
Heart	No cardiac effect	Increased heart rate (β_1) Increased contractile force (β_1) Increased automaticity (β_1)
Systemic blood vessels	Vasoconstriction	Vasodilation (β_2)
Lungs	Mild bronchoconstriction	Bronchodilation (β_2)

TABLE 7–5

Listing of Sympathomimetic Drugs with Adrenergic Actions

Drug	Adrenergic effects		Dysrhythmia potential
	α	β	
Epinephrine			
Low dose	+	++	+++
High dose	++	+++	+++
Norepinephrine			
Low dose	++	+	++
High dose	+++	++	++
Isoproterenol	0	+++	+++
Dopamine			
Low dose	+	+	++
High dose	+++	++	++
Dobutamine	0	+++	+
Amrinone	0	0	+

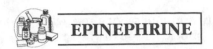

EPINEPHRINE

Class: Sympathetic agonist

Description

Epinephrine is a naturally occurring catecholamine. It is a potent α- and β-adrenergic stimulant; however, its effect on β-receptors is more profound.

Mechanism of Action

Epinephrine acts directly on α- and β-adrenergic receptors. Its effect on β-receptors is much more profound than its effect on α-receptors. The effects of epinephrine include the following:

Increased heart rate
Increased cardiac contractile force
Increased electrical activity in the myocardium
Increased systemic vascular resistance
Increased blood pressure
Increased automaticity

Epinephrine can stimulate spontaneous firing of myocardial conductive cells. In the emergency setting it is used to convert fine ventricular fibrillation to coarse ventricular fibrillation. This change significantly increases the chances of successful electrical defibrillation. In asystole it is used to initiate electrical activity in the myocardium. Once initiated, electrical defibrillation may be attempted.

Epinephrine's effects usually appear within 90 seconds of administration, and they are usually of short duration. Therefore, it must be administered every 3 to 5 minutes to maintain therapeutic levels.

Pharmacokinetics

> **Onset:**   <2 minutes [intravenous/endotracheal tube (IV/ET)]
> **Peak Effects:**   <5 minutes (IV/ET)
> **Duration:**   5–10 minutes (IV/ET)
> **Half-Life:**   5 minutes

Indications

Epinephrine is used in cardiac arrest (asystole, ventricular fibrillation, pulseless ventricular tachycardia, pulseless electrical activity), severe anaphylaxis, and severe reactive airway disease.

Contraindications

Epinephrine 1:10 000 is contraindicated in patients who do not require extensive cardiopulmonary resuscitative efforts. With simple allergic reactions and asthma, the 1:1000 dilution should be used and is administered subcutaneously.

Precautions

Epinephrine, like all catecholamines, should be protected from light. It can be deactivated by alkaline solutions such as sodium bicarbonate. Thus, it is essential that the IV line be adequately flushed between administrations of epinephrine and sodium bicarbonate.

Side Effects

Epinephrine can cause palpitations, anxiety, tremulousness, headache, dizziness, nausea, and vomiting. Because of its strong inotropic and chronotropic properties, epinephrine increases myocardial oxygen demand. Even in low doses it can cause myocardial ischemia. When administering epinephrine in the emergency setting, these effects should be kept in mind. Like most of the other drugs used in emergency medicine, epinephrine is only effective when the myocardium is adequately oxygenated.

Interactions

Epinephrine is pH dependent and can be deactivated when administered with highly alkaline solutions such as sodium bicarbonate. The effects of epinephrine can be intensified in patients who are taking antidepressants.

Dosage

Epinephrine 1:10 000 can be administered intravenously, intraosseously, or endotracheally. Common doses include the following:

Cardiac arrest (adults).   The dose of epinephrine in cardiac arrest is 1.0 mg of a 1:10 000 solution intravenously. This can be repeated every 3 to 5 minutes as required. Higher dosages may be ordered by medical control and are potentially helpful in the cardiac arrest setting. If an IV cannot be started, epinephrine can be administered endotracheally. The endotracheal dose should be increased to at least 2 to 2.5 times the intravenous dose.

Cardiac arrest (children).   The initial dose of epinephrine in pediatric cardiac arrest is 0.01 mg/kg of a 1:10 000 solution intravenously (0.1 mL/kg). Second and subsequent doses should be 0.1 mg/kg of a 1:1000 solution intravenously (0.1 mL/kg). The total volume of drug administered remains the same because epinephrine 1:1000 is used instead of epinephrine 1:10 000.

Severe anaphylaxis or severe asthma (adults).   Intravenous epinephrine should only be used for life-threatening, severe anaphylaxis and severe asthma. Less severe cases should be treated with epinephrine 1:1000 subcutaneously or with another β-agonist. In severe anaphylaxis or asthma, the initial dose should be 0.3 to 0.5 mg intravenously. The dose may be repeated every 5 to 15 minutes as required. An epinephrine drip may be required in severe cases.

Severe anaphylaxis or severe asthma (children).   Intravenous epinephrine should only be used for life-threatening, severe anaphylaxis and severe asthma. Less severe cases should be treated with epinephrine 1:1000 subcutaneously or with another β-agonist. In severe anaphylaxis or asthma the initial dose should be 0.01 mg/kg intravenously. The dose may be repeated every 5 to 15 minutes as required. An epinephrine drip may be required in severe cases.

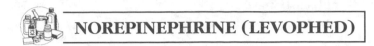

NOREPINEPHRINE (LEVOPHED)

Class: Sympathetic agonist

Description

Norepinephrine is a naturally occurring catecholamine. It acts on both α- and β-adrenergic receptors. However, its action on α-receptors is more profound.

Mechanism of Action

Because of its action on α-receptors, norepinephrine is a potent peripheral vasoconstrictor. This vasoconstriction serves to increase blood pressure in cardiogenic shock and other hypotensive emergencies. Because norepinephrine also tends to constrict the renal and mesenteric blood vessels, it is reserved for emergencies in which dopamine may not be effective. As a rule, dopamine, which maintains renal and mesenteric perfusion, is the preferred vasopressor for treating cardiogenic shock.

Pharmacokinetics

Onset: Immediate
Peak Effects: <1 minute
Duration: 1–2 minutes
Half-Life: 3 minutes

Indications

Norepinephrine is used in hypotension (systolic blood pressure <70 mmHg) refractory to other sympathomimetics and not related to hypovolemia, and in neurogenic shock.

Contraindications

Norepinephrine should not be given to patients who are hypotensive from hypovolemia.

Precautions

Because of the powerful effects of norepinephrine, it is essential to measure the blood pressure every 5 to 10 minutes to prevent dangerously high blood pressures. Fluid replacement should be initiated prior to administration of norepinephrine. Norepinephrine should be given through the largest vein readily available because it may cause local tissue necrosis if it extravasates. Phentolamine (Regitine) can be diluted in saline and infiltrated into the area of extravasation to help minimize necrosis and sloughing. Like the other sympathomimetics, norepinephrine can increase myocardial oxygen demand. It should be used with caution in persons with cardiac ischemia.

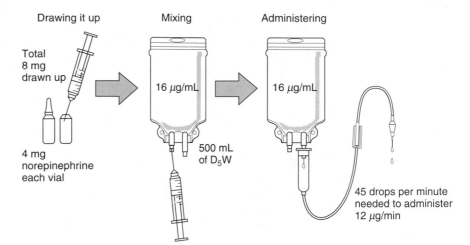

Drawing it up   Mixing   Administering

Total
8 mg
drawn up

16 µg/mL   16 µg/mL

4 mg
norepinephrine
each vial

500 mL
of D₅W

45 drops per minute
needed to administer
12 µg/min

FIGURE 7–1 Preparation of norepinephrine infusion.

Side Effects

Norepinephrine can cause anxiety, tremulousness, headache, dizziness, nausea, and vomiting. It can also cause bradycardia as a reflex response to increased peripheral vasoconstriction. Because of its inotropic and chronotropic properties, norepinephrine increases myocardial oxygen demand. Even in low doses it can cause myocardial ischemia. When administering norepinephrine in the emergency setting, these effects should be kept in mind.

Interactions

Norepinephrine can be deactivated by alkaline solutions such as sodium bicarbonate. Concomitant administration with β-blockers can result in markedly elevated blood pressure.

Dosage

The current dosage recommended by the American Heart Association for norepinephrine is 0.5 to 1.0 µg/minute (maximum of 30.0 µg/minute). Higher doses may be required to maintain adequate blood pressure. The best dilution is obtained by placing 8 mg in 500 mL of D₅W. This will give a concentration of 16 µg/mL. The same concentration can be attained by placing 4 mg in 250 mL of D₅W (see Figure 7–1).

Because of its potency, norepinephrine is given only in extremely diluted IV infusions. To control its administration, it should be piggybacked into an already established IV line.

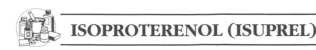 **ISOPROTERENOL (ISUPREL)**

Class: Sympathetic agonist

Description

Isoproterenol is a synthetic catecholamine. It acts primarily on β-adrenergic receptors.

Mechanism of Action

Isoproterenol is a potent, synthetic catecholamine that acts almost exclusively on β-receptors. Because it has no significant α-receptor-stimulating capabilities, its actions are primarily on the heart and lungs. In cardiac emergencies it may be used to increase heart rate in bradycardias that are refractory to atropine. With the advent of transcutaneous pacing, isoproterenol is seldom used by paramedics.

Pharmacokinetics

Onset: Immediate
Peak Effects: <1 minute
Duration: Varies
Half-Life: <1.5 minutes

Indications

Isoproterenol is used in bradycardias refractory to atropine (when transcutaneous pacing is unavailable) such as denervated hearts (transplants) and beta blocker overdoses. It is also useful in high degree heart blocks (Mobitz II and third-degree blocks) when transcutaneous pacing is unavailable, severe status asthmaticus and occasionally for refractory torsades de pointes.

Contraindications

Isoproterenol is not used to increase blood pressure in cardiogenic shock. It should only be used in shock resulting from bradycardias. Other sympathomimetics, such as dopamine and norepinephrine, should be used in cases of cardiogenic shock.

Precautions

When administering isoproterenol, the patient must be monitored for signs of ventricular irritability. These signs may take the form of premature ventricular contractions, ventricular tachycardia, or even ventricular fibrillation. Lidocaine should be readily available whenever isoproterenol is administered. It is important to be careful when administering isoproterenol. Like epinephrine, it significantly increases myocardial oxygen demand. The increase in myocardial oxygen uptake may increase myocardial infarction size. In patients who have not suffered a myocardial infarction, isoproterenol may cause myocardial ischemia. External pacing, if available, should be used instead of isoproterenol.

Side Effects

Isoproterenol can cause nervousness, headache, tremor, dysrhythmias, hypertension, angina, nausea, and vomiting. Many of these side effects are dose related.

Interactions

Isoproterenol can be deactivated by alkaline solutions such as sodium bicarbonate. It should be used with caution in patients with digitalis toxicity because it may aggravate tachydysrhythmias.

Dosage

The usual dosage of isoproterenol is 1 mg diluted in 500 mL of D$_5$W; this will give a concentration of 2 μg/mL. It should be titrated until the desired heart rate is attained or until signs of ventricular irritability, such as premature ventricular contractions, occur. The recommended infusion rate is 2 to 10 μg/min. Because of its potency, isoproterenol should only be given by IV infusion. An established IV line, into which the isoproterenol is piggybacked, should be maintained.

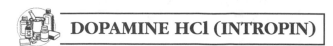 **DOPAMINE HCl (INTROPIN)**

Class: Sympathetic agonist

Description

Dopamine is a naturally occurring catecholamine. It is a chemical precursor of norepinephrine. It acts on α, β$_1$, and dopaminergic adrenergic receptors. Its effect on α-receptors is dose dependent.

Mechanism of Action

Dopamine is one of the most frequently used agents in the treatment of hypotension associated with cardiogenic shock. It is chemically related to both epinephrine and norepinephrine and increases blood pressure by acting on both α- and β$_1$-adrenergic receptors. Dopamine's effect on β$_1$-receptors causes a positive inotropic effect on the heart. It does not increase myocardial oxygen demand as much as isoproterenol and epinephrine do and does not have the same powerful chronotropic effects. Dopamine also acts on α-adrenergic receptors, causing peripheral vasoconstriction. Unlike norepinephrine, when used in therapeutic dosages, dopamine maintains renal and mesenteric blood flow because of its effect on the dopaminergic receptors. For these reasons, dopamine is the most commonly used vasopressor. Dopamine increases both the systolic blood pressure and the pulse pressure (the difference between the systolic and diastolic blood pressures), but, as a rule, there is usually less effect on the diastolic pressure.

Pharmacokinetics

Onset: <5 minutes
Peak Effects: 5–8 minutes
Duration: <10 minutes
Half-Life: 2 minutes

Indications

Dopamine is used in hemodynamically significant hypotension (systolic blood pressure of 70 to 100 mmHg) not resulting from hypovolemia, and in cardiogenic shock.

Contraindications

Dopamine should not be used as the sole agent in the management of hypovolemic shock unless fluid resuscitation is well under way. Dopamine should not be used in patients with known pheochromocytoma (a tumor of the adrenal gland).

Precautions

Dopamine increases the heart rate and can induce or worsen supraventricular and ventricular dysrhythmias. Whenever the dosage of dopamine surpasses 20 µg/kg/min, its α effects predominate and it functions very much like norepinephrine. Dopamine, like the other catecholamines, should not be administered in the presence of tachydysrhythmias or ventricular fibrillation.

Side Effects

Dopamine can cause nervousness, headache, dysrhythmias, palpitations, chest pain, dyspnea, nausea, and vomiting. Many of these side effects are dose related.

Interactions

Like all of the catecholamines, dopamine can be deactivated by alkaline solutions such as sodium bicarbonate. If the patient is taking MAOIs (a type of antidepressant), the dose should be reduced. Dopamine may cause hypotension when used concomitantly with phenytoin (Dilantin).

Dosage

The standard method of preparing a dopamine infusion is to place 800 mg in 500 mL of D_5W or by adding 400 mg to 250 mL of D_5W; this gives a concentration of 1600 µg/mL. The effects of dopamine are dose dependent. Table 7–6 illustrates effects based on common dosages.

The initial infusion is from 2–5 µg/kg/min. This rate may be increased until the blood pressure improves (see Figure 7–2) or until a maximum of 20 µg/kg/min. Dopamine is administered only by IV drip, which should be piggybacked into an already established IV infusion.

TABLE 7–6

Dopamine Hydrochloride (Intropin®) Dosage Phenomena

Physiological effect	2–5 µg/kg/min	5–20 µg/kg/min	More than 20 µg/kg/min
Cardiac output	No change	Increase	Increase
Stroke volume	No change	Increase	Increase
Heart rate	No change	Initial increase followed by a decrease toward normal rates as infusion continues	
Myocardial contractility	No change	Increase	Increase
Potential for excessive myocardial oxygen demands	Low[a] Coronary blood flow increased	Low[a] Coronary blood flow increased	Data unavailable
Potential for tachydysrhythmias	Low[a]	Low[a]	Moderate
Total systemic vascular resistance	Slight decrease to no change	No change to slight increase	Increase
Renal blood flow	Increase	Increase	Decrease[b]
Urine output	Increase	Increase	Decrease[b]

[a]Low but needs monitoring.

[b]Relative to peak values achieved at lower dosages.

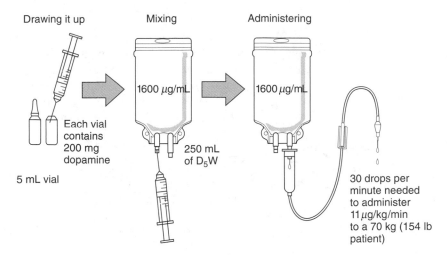

Drawing it up

Mixing

Administering

1600 μg/mL

1600 μg/mL

Each vial contains 200 mg dopamine

5 mL vial

250 mL of D$_5$W

30 drops per minute needed to administer 11 μg/kg/min to a 70 kg (154 lb patient)

FIGURE 7–2 Preparation of dopamine infusion.

 DOBUTAMINE (DOBUTREX)

Class: Sympathetic agonist

Description

Dobutamine is a synthetic catecholamine. It acts primarily on β_1-receptors but is a less potent β-agonist than is isoproterenol.

Mechanism of Action

Dobutamine increases the force of the systolic contraction (positive inotropic effect) with little chronotropic activity. For these reasons, it is useful in the management of congestive heart failure when an increase in heart rate is not desired.

Pharmacokinetics

Onset: 2–10 minutes
Peak Effects: 10–20 minutes
Duration: Varies
Half-Life: 2 minutes

Indication

Dobutamine is used for short-term management of congestive heart failure when an increased cardiac output, without an increased cardiac rate, is desired.

Contraindications

Dobutamine should not be used as the sole agent in hypovolemic shock unless fluid resuscitation is well under way. To increase cardiac output in severe emergencies, such as cardiogenic shock, dopamine is the preferred agent.

Precautions

Tachycardia and an increase in the systolic blood pressure are common following the administration of dobutamine. Increases in heart rate of more than 10 percent may induce or exacerbate myocardial ischemia. Premature ventricular contractions (PVCs) can occur in conjunction with dobutamine administration. Lidocaine should be readily available. As with any sympathomimetic, blood pressure should be monitored.

Side Effects

Dobutamine can cause nervousness, headache, hypertension, dysrhythmias, palpitations, chest pain, dyspnea, nausea, and vomiting. Many of these side effects are dose related.

Interactions

Dobutamine may be ineffective when administered to patients taking beta-blockers because these medications can block the beta-receptors on which dobutamine acts. Patients taking TCAs are at increased risk of hypertension with dobutamine administration.

Dosage

The desired dosage range for dobutamine is between 2 and 20 μg/kg/min. Dobutamine should be administered according to the patient's response (see Figure 7–3).

Dobutamine should be diluted in either 500 mL or 1 L of D_5W and administered via IV infusion.

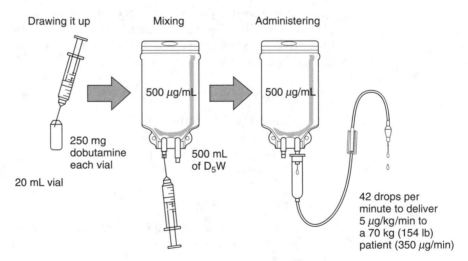

Drawing it up Mixing Administering

250 mg dobutamine each vial

20 mL vial

500 μg/mL

500 mL of D_5W

500 μg/mL

42 drops per minute to deliver 5 μg/kg/min to a 70 kg (154 lb) patient (350 μg/min)

FIGURE 7–3 Preparation of dobutamine infusion.

METARAMINOL (ARAMINE)

Class: Sympathetic agonist

Description

Metaraminol is a sympathetic agonist with effects similar to those of norepinephrine. It is much less potent than norepinephrine but has a more prolonged action.

Mechanism of Action

Although metaraminol is not a catecholamine, it is used in the treatment of hypotensive states. It is both an α- and β-agonist. Its vasopressor properties are primarily derived from its action on endogenous catecholamines. It causes the release of norepinephrine from sympathetic nerve endings. In recent years metaraminol has fallen into disuse, with dopamine being the preferred agent.

Pharmacokinetics

Onset: 1–2 minutes (IV), <10 minutes [intramuscular (IM)]
Peak Effects: Variable
Duration: 20–30 minutes
Half-Life: Variable

Indication

Metaraminol is used in hemodynamically significant hypotension not due to hypovolemia.

Contraindications

Metaraminol should not be used in hypovolemia unless fluid resuscitation is well under way.

Precautions

Rapid administration can cause hypertension. Ventricular ectopic activity has been known to occur with the administration of metaraminol. Lidocaine should be readily available.

Side Effects

Metaraminol can cause anxiety, tremulousness, headache, dizziness, nausea, and vomiting. It can also cause bradycardia as a reflex response to increased peripheral vasoconstriction.

Interactions

Metaraminol can be deactivated by alkaline solutions such as sodium bicarbonate. Concomitant administration with beta-blockers can result in markedly elevated blood pressure. Caution should be used when administering metaraminol to patients taking digitalis.

Dosage

The usual dosage of metaraminol is 200 mg in 500 mL of D_5W. This will give a dilution of 0.4 mg/mL. The infusion rate should be titrated according to the blood pressure response. An IV infusion should already be established, into which the metaraminol is piggybacked. Metaraminol can be administered intramuscularly when an IV cannot be established. The initial adult dose should be 5 to 10 mg for IM administration. Many agents, such as dopamine, are far superior to metaraminol and should be used initially.

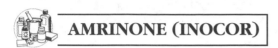

AMRINONE (INOCOR)

Class: Inotrope (phosphodiesterase inhibitor)

Description

Amrinone is a rapidly acting inotropic agent. It is a phosphodiesterase inhibitor and does not act on adrenergic receptors.

Mechanism of Action

Amrinone, like the other medications previously presented, increases cardiac output promptly following intravenous administration. It is a positive inotrope and has some vasodilatory properties. Unlike the other medications, however, it does not stimulate either α- or β-adrenergic receptors. The exact mechanism by which amrinone increases blood pressure is not well understood. It does not increase cardiac output in the same manner as the digitalis preparations. Clinically, amrinone resembles dobutamine in its effects. Because amrinone does not stimulate β-adrenergic receptors, it may be effective in cases of congestive heart failure that do not respond to dobutamine or one of the other inotropic agents.

Pharmacokinetics

> **Onset:** 2–5 minutes
> **Peak Effects:** 10 minutes
> **Duration:** 0.5–2.0 hours
> **Half-Life:** 4–6 hours

Indication

Amrinone is used in short-term management of severe congestive heart failure refractory to diuretics, vasodilators, and conventional inotropic agents.

Contraindications

Amrinone should not be administered to patients with a known hypersensitivity to the drug or to the bisulfite class of chemicals.

Precautions

Amrinone should not be used in cases of congestive heart failure occurring immediately after myocardial infarction. Like dobutamine, amrinone may increase myocardial ischemia. As with the other inotropic agents, the blood pressure, pulse, and electrocardiogram (ECG) should be constantly monitored. Amrinone should not be diluted in solutions containing dextrose (i.e., D_5W). Amrinone should be diluted with 0.9 percent sodium chloride (normal saline) or 0.45 percent sodium chloride (one-half normal saline).

Side Effects

Amrinone can cause dysrhythmias, hypotension, nausea, vomiting, abdominal pain, and decreased platelets (thrombocytopenia).

Interactions

Furosemide (Lasix) should not be administered into an intravenous line delivering amrinone. A chemical reaction occurs between these two drugs, resulting in the formation of a precipitate in the intravenous line. Amrinone should not be diluted in solutions containing dextrose.

Dosage

Therapy should be initiated with an IV bolus of 0.75 mg/kg given slowly during a 2- to 5-minute interval. This should be followed by a maintenance infusion of 2 to 15 µg/kg/min. This infusion can be prepared by placing one ampule (100 mg) in 500 mL of normal saline solution. This will give a concentration of 0.2 mg/mL (200 µg/mL).

An additional bolus of 0.75 mg/kg given slowly over 2 to 3 minutes can be given 30 minutes later if required.

The overall rate of amrinone administration must be carefully adjusted and based on the patient's clinical response.

Amrinone should only be administered by the IV route, either as a bolus or by infusion, as described earlier.

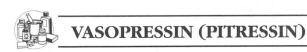

VASOPRESSIN (PITRESSIN)

Class: Hormone; vasopressor

Description

Vasopressin is a polypeptide hormone extracted from the posterior pituitaries of animals. It possesses pressor and antidiuretic hormone (ADH) properties. Conclusive evidence supporting the use of vasopressin in cardiac arrest is lacking.

Mechanism of Action

Vasopressin, in higher doses, acts as a non-alpha-adrenergic vasoconstrictor through direct stimulation of smooth muscle receptors. It can be used as an alternative to epinephrine during CPR.

Pharmacokinetics

 Onset: Variable
 Peak Effects: Variable
 Duration: 30–60 minutes
 Half-Life: 10–20 minutes

Indications

Vasopressin is used to increase peripheral vascular resistance during CPR (as an alternative to epinephrine or after epinephrine has been used).

Contraindications

Vasopressin is contraindicated in patients with a chronic nephritis, ischemic heart disease, PVCs, or advanced arteriosclerosis. When used in CPR, these contraindications may not apply.

Precautions

Vasopressin should be used with caution in patients with epilepsy, migraine, asthma, heart failure, and angina.

Side Effects

Side effects include blanching of the skin, abdominal cramps, nausea, hypertension, bradycardia, and minor dysrhythmias.

Interactions

None in advanced cardiac life support (ACLS) setting.

Dosage

Adult dose. 40 units IV (single dose only).
Pediatric dose. Usage in cardiac arrest not detailed.

SYMPATHETIC BLOCKERS

Sympathetic blockers are a unique class of drugs that antagonize adrenergic receptor sites. Certain drugs block only α-receptors, whereas others block only β-receptors. Some of the β-blockers are so selective that they block only β_1- or β_2-receptors. The drugs that block the β-receptors are receiving the most use. They are useful in the treatment of hypertension, cardiac dysrhythmias, and angina pectoris. The most popular sympathetic blocker is propranolol (Inderal), a nonselective beta-blocker that is both a β_1- and β_2-antagonist. Although used selectively in emergency medicine, propranolol does play a role in the treatment of certain cardiac dysrhythmias.

It is thought that some ventricular dysrhythmias, such as ventricular tachycardia and recurrent ventricular fibrillation, can be caused by excessive β-receptor stimulation. Administration of propranolol may inhibit these dysrhythmias. Propranolol should not be used in combination with verapamil. The *concomitant* blocking of slow calcium channels by verapamil, and the β-receptor antagonism caused by propranolol, may result in asystole.

PROPRANOLOL (INDERAL)

Class: Nonselective beta-blocker

Description

Propranolol is a nonselective β-antagonist. It inhibits the effects of circulating catecholamines.

Mechanism of Action

Propranolol nonselectively blocks both β_1- and β_2-adrenergic receptors. It causes a reduction in heart rate (negative chronotropic effect), cardiac contractile force (negative inotropic effect), blood pressure, and myocardial oxygen demand. It is useful in treating recurrent ventricular tachycardia and recurrent ventricular fibrillation that does not respond to lidocaine. It may also be of value in the treatment of tachydysrhythmias resulting from digitalis toxicity and selected supraventricular tachycardias.

Pharmacokinetics

Onset: <2 minutes
Peak Effects: 15 minutes
Duration: 2–6 hours
Half-Life: 2.3 hours

Indications

Propranolol is used in ventricular tachycardia refractory to lidocaine and bretylium, recurrent ventricular fibrillation refractory to lidocaine and bretylium, and selected supraventricular tachydysrhythmias.

Contraindications

Propranolol is contraindicated in patients with bradycardia, a history of asthma, COPD, and congestive heart failure.

Precautions

Because propranolol may decrease heart rate, atropine should be readily available. In bradycardia refractory to atropine, transcutaneous pacing should be utilized. Propranolol should be used with caution in diabetics because it may mask the signs and symptoms of hypoglycemia. Glucagon can be used in the management of severe beta-blocker overdose. It helps to maintain the heart rate and blood pressure.

Side Effects

Propranolol may cause bradycardia, hypotension, lethargy, congestive heart failure, dyspnea, wheezing, and weakness.

Interactions

Propranolol should not be administered to patients who have received intravenous verapamil. It should be used with caution in patients taking antihypertensive agents.

Dosage

Propranolol may produce significant, even life-threatening, side effects. When administered intravenously, care must be taken to dilute 1 mg in 10 mL of D_5W. The standard dosage is 1 to 3 mg, diluted in 10 to 30 mL of D_5W. Propranolol should be administered *slowly* (over 2 to 5 minutes). Propranolol should not be administered faster than 1 mg/min. Throughout administration, careful blood pressure monitoring is required. Like all drugs acting on the heart, it should only be administered to patients who are on cardiac monitors. The dosage may be repeated, again under careful monitoring, until a maximum of 3 to 5 mg has been administered. Propranolol should be administered intravenously in the treatment of life-threatening tachydysrhythmias.

SOTALOL HCL (SOTACOR, BETAPACE)

Class: Beta-blocker

Description

Sotalol is a nonselective beta-adrenergic blocking agent.

Mechanism of Action

Sotalol blocks stimulation of $beta_1$- (myocardial) and $beta_2$- (pulmonary, vascular, and uterine) adrenergic receptor sites.

Pharmacokinetics

Onset: Variable
Peak Effects: 2–3 hours
Duration: 24 hours
Half-Life: 7–18 hours

Indications

Sotalol is indicated for the treatment of documented life-threatening ventricular dysrhythmias such as sustained ventricular tachycardia. It may also be used for the treatment of patients with documented symptomatic ventricular dysrhythmias. Sotalol should be reserved for patients in whom the physician believes the benefit of treatment clearly outweighs the risks.

Contraindications

Sotalol is contraindicated in patients with bronchial asthma, allergic rhinitis, severe sinus node dysfunction, sinus bradycardia and second- and third-degree atrioventricular (AV) block (unless a functioning pacemaker is present), cardiogenic shock, severe or uncontrolled heart failure, and known hypersensitivity.

Precautions

Sotalol may cause new or worsen existing dysrhythmias. Such prodysrhythmic effects range from an increase in frequency of PVCs to the development of more severe ventricular tachycardia, ventricular fibrillation, and torsade de pointes.

Side Effects

Central nervous system effects include fatigue, weakness, anxiety, dizziness, drowsiness, insomnia, memory loss, mental status changes, nervousness, and nightmares. Respiratory effects include bronchospasm and wheezing. Cardiovascular effects include dysrhythmias, bradycardia, congestive heart failure, pulmonary edema, orthostatic hypotension, and peripheral vasoconstriction.

Interactions

General anesthesia, IV phenytoin, and verapamil may cause additive myocardial depression. Additive bradycardia may occur with digitalis glycosides. Additive hypotension may occur with other antihypertensives, acute ingestion of alcohol, or nitrates. Sotalol should be used cautiously within 14 days of MAOI therapy (may result in hypotension). Sotalol may interact with class IA antidysrhythmic drugs such as disopyramide, quinidine, and procainamide and class III drugs such as amiodarone.

Dosage

Oral administration of 80 mg twice daily may be gradually increased (usual maintenance dose is 160 to 320 mg/day in two to three divided doses, up to 480 to 640 mg/day).

METOPROLOL (LOPRESSOR)

Class: Selective beta-blocker

Description

Metoprolol is a β-antagonist that blocks both β_1- and β_2-adrenergic receptors. Unlike propranolol, however, metoprolol is selective for β_1-adrenergic receptors.

Mechanism of Action

Metoprolol causes a reduction in heart rate, systolic blood pressure, and cardiac output following administration because of its selective effects on β_1-adrenergic receptors. In addition, metoprolol appears to inhibit tachycardia, especially in the period following an acute myocardial infarction. Because of these effects, metoprolol is thought to be protective of the heart and is used to reduce potential complications in selected patients who have suffered an acute myocardial infarction. Metoprolol has proved effective in reducing the incidence of ventricular fibrillation and chest pain in these patients, thus reducing overall patient mortality in the post–myocardial infarction period.

Pharmacokinetics

Onset: Immediate
Peak Effects: 20 minutes
Duration: 13–19 hours
Half-Life: 3–4 hours

Indication

Metoprolol is used in patients with suspected or definite acute myocardial infarction who are hemodynamically stable.

Contraindications

Metoprolol is contraindicated in any patient with a heart rate of less than 45 beats per minute, a systolic blood pressure less than 100 mmHg, or congestive heart failure. In addition, metoprolol is contraindicated in patients with first-degree heart block with a PR interval greater than 0.24 second, second-degree heart block (either Mobitz I or Mobitz II), or third-degree block. It is also contraindicated in any patient showing either early or late signs of shock. Metoprolol should not be administered to any patient with a history of asthma or bronchospastic disease in the prehospital setting.

Precautions

The blood pressure, pulse rate, ECG, and respiratory status should be continuously monitored during metoprolol therapy. Prehospital personnel should be alert for signs and symptoms of congestive heart failure, bradycardia, shock, heart block, or bronchospasm when administering metoprolol. The presence of any of these signs or symptoms is an indication for discontinuing the medication.

Side Effects

Metoprolol may cause bradycardia, hypotension, lethargy, congestive heart failure, dyspnea, wheezing, and weakness.

Interactions

Metoprolol should not be administered to patients who have received intravenous verapamil. It should be administered with caution to patients taking antihypertensive agents.

Dosage

When administered following an acute myocardial infarction, an initial bolus of 5 mg metoprolol should be given by slow IV injection. If the vital signs remain stable, a second 5 mg bolus should be given 2 minutes after the first. Finally, if the first two boluses are well tolerated, a third 5 mg bolus should be administered 2 minutes after the second bolus. The total dose should not exceed 15 mg. As mentioned previously, the vital signs and ECG should be constantly monitored.

Metoprolol should only be administered by slow IV injection in the manner described earlier.

LABETALOL (TRANDATE, NORMODYNE)

Class: Nonselective beta-blocker

Description

Labetalol is a nonselective β-blocker and a selective α_1-blocker.

Mechanism of Action

Labetalol differs considerably in its action from the β-blockers previously presented. Like propranolol, labetalol is a nonselective β-adrenergic antagonist showing no preference for either β_1- or β_2-receptors. However, unlike the other β-blockers, labetalol also blocks α_1-adrenergic receptors. Blockage of α_1-receptors inhibits peripheral vasoconstriction, thus causing peripheral vasodilation. Because of these properties, labetalol is a potent agent for lowering blood pressure in cases of hypertensive crisis. It lowers blood pressure by decreasing cardiac output through its β_1-blocking properties and by causing peripheral vasodilation through its α_1-blocking properties.

Pharmacokinetics

Onset: 2–5 minutes
Peak Effects: 5–15 minutes
Duration: 2–4 hours
Half-Life: 3–8 hours

Indication

Labetalol is indicated for the acute management of hypertensive crisis.

Contraindications

Labetalol is contraindicated in patients with bronchial asthma, congestive heart failure, heart block, bradycardia, or cardiogenic shock.

Precautions

As with all β-blockers the blood pressure, pulse rate, ECG, and respiratory status should be continuously monitored. Prehospital personnel should be alert for signs and symptoms of congestive heart failure, bradycardia, shock, heart block, or bronchospasm when administering labetalol. The appearance of any of these signs or symptoms is an indication for discontinuing the drug. Because of the effects of labetalol on β_1-receptors, postural hypotension might occur and should be anticipated. The patient should be supine at all times during drug administration.

Side Effects

Labetalol may cause bradycardia, hypotension, lethargy, congestive heart failure, dyspnea, wheezing, and weakness.

Interactions

Labetalol should not be administered to patients who have received intravenous verapamil. It should be administered with caution to patients taking antihypertensive agents.

Dosage

The following are two accepted methods of administering labetalol in the treatment of hypertensive crisis:

1. Twenty milligrams of labetalol can be administered by slow IV injection over 2 minutes. Immediately before the injection and at 5 and 10 minutes after the injection, the supine blood pressure should be recorded. Additional injections of 40 mg can be given every 10 minutes until a desired supine blood pressure is achieved or 300 mg of the drug has been given.

2. Two ampules (200 mg) of labetalol can be added to 250 mL of D_5W. This gives a concentration of 0.8 mg/mL. This solution should be administered at a rate of 2 mg/min (2.5 mL/min). The blood pressure should be continuously monitored.

Labetalol should be administered by slow IV injection or infusion as described earlier.

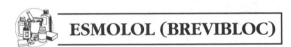

ESMOLOL (BREVIBLOC)

Class: Selective beta-blocker

Description

Esmolol is a β_1 selective (cardioselective) β-blocker with a very short half-life.

Mechanism of Action

Esmolol is a selective β_1-blocker. It has a very rapid onset and a short duration of action (9 minutes). Esmolol is used to slow rapid heart rates in patients with supraventricular tachycardia including atrial flutter and atrial fibrillation. Patients with extremely rapid heart rates can develop congestive heart failure or angina because the rapid heart rate may prevent adequate filling of the ventricles. The duration of action of esmolol is so brief that it should be administered by intravenous infusion.

Pharmacokinetics

Onset: <5 minutes
Peak Effects: 10–20 minutes
Duration: 10–30 minutes
Half-Life: 9 minutes

Indication

Esmolol is used in supraventricular tachycardia (including atrial fibrillation and atrial flutter) accompanied by a rapid ventricular rate.

Contraindications

Esmolol should not be used in patients with sinus bradycardia, heart block greater than first degree, cardiogenic shock, or overt congestive heart failure.

Precautions

A significant number of patients receiving esmolol may experience hypotension (systolic less than 90 mmHg). Hypotension can occur at any dose but primarily is dose related. If hypotension develops, the dosage should be reduced. Patients with congestive heart failure may have worsening of their symptoms with esmolol. Because esmolol may depress cardiac contractility, it should be used with extreme caution in patients prone to congestive heart failure. Patients with bronchospastic disease (e.g., asthma and COPD) should not receive β-blockers, including esmolol, unless the medical control physician deems that the benefits outweigh the risks.

Side Effects

Esmolol may cause bradycardia, dizziness, hypotension, lethargy, congestive heart failure, dyspnea, wheezing, and weakness.

Interactions

Esmolol should not be administered to patients who have received intravenous verapamil. It should be administered with caution to patients taking antihypertensive agents. Morphine can increase the blood levels of esmolol, requiring a reduction in dosage. Esmolol should not be used in cases of supraventricular tachycardia caused by epinephrine, dopamine, and norepinephrine.

Dosage

Esmolol therapy is started by administering a loading dose of 500 μg/kg/min for 1 minute. After 1 minute the dose should be reduced to a maintenance dose of 50 μg/kg/min for 4 minutes. If an adequate therapeutic effect is not seen, the loading dose should be repeated for 1 minute and then the maintenance dose is increased to 100 μg/kg/min. The dose can be titrated at 4-minute intervals by repeating the loading dose for 1 minute and increasing the maintenance dose by 50 μg/kg/min at 4-minute intervals until the desired effect is obtained. The maintenance dose should not exceed 200 μg/kg/min. In the event of an adverse reaction, the dose of esmolol can be reduced or discontinued immediately. The esmolol infusion is prepared by placing two 2.5 g ampules of esmolol in 500 mL of 5 percent dextrose, normal saline, or lactated Ringer's solution. An alternative method is to place one 2.5 g ampule in 250 mL of fluid. Either will provide a 10 mg/mL concentration. Esmolol should be administered intravenously.

ANTIDYSRHYTHMICS

Many different drugs are useful in the treatment and prevention of cardiac dysrhythmias. Some drugs are useful in the treatment of atrial dysrhythmias, whereas others are useful in the treatment of ventricular dysrhythmias. As a result, it is essential to distinguish between these two types of dysrhythmias. The common antidysrhythmic drugs are classified based on their action (see Table 7–7 and Figure 7–4).

TABLE 7–7

Antidysrhythmic Classifications and Examples

General action	Class	Prototype	ECG effects
Sodium channel blockers	IA	Quinidine, procainamide*, disopyramide	Widened QRS, prolonged QT
	IB	Lidocaine*, phenytoin, tocainide, mexiletine	Widened QRS, prolonged QT
	IC	Flecainide*, propafenone	Prolonged PR, widened QRS
	I (Miscellaneous)	Moricizine*	Prolonged PR, widened QRS
Beta blockers	II	Propranolol*, acebutolol, esmolol	Prolonged PR, bradycardias
Potassium channel blockers	III	Bretylium*, amiodarone	Prolonged QT
Calcium channel blockers	IV	Verapamil*, diltiazem	Prolonged PR, bradycardias
Miscellaneous		Adenosine, digoxin	Prolonged PR, bradycardias

*Prototype.

Class I effect
Sodium channel blockade

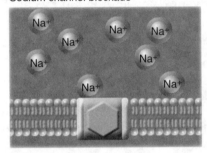

Class II effect
Noncompetitive alpha- and beta-blockade

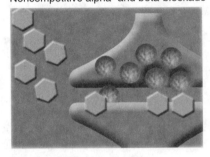

Class III effect
Potassium channel blockade

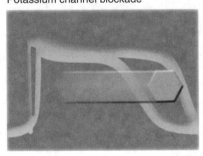

Class IV effect
Calcium channel blockade

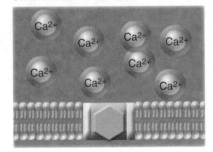

FIGURE 7–4   Vaughan Williams classification of antidysrhythmic drugs.

The most common antidysrhythmic drugs used in emergency medicine include the following:

Lidocaine (Xylocaine).   Lidocaine is the drug of choice in the treatment of ventricular tachycardia and malignant premature ventricular contractions.

Procainamide (Pronestyl).   Procainamide, like lidocaine, is useful in the suppression of ventricular dysrhythmias. It is generally not a first-line drug, and its use is reserved for dysrhythmias that do not respond to lidocaine.

Bretylium tosylate (Bretylol).   Bretylium is used in the treatment of ventricular fibrillation that is refractory to lidocaine.

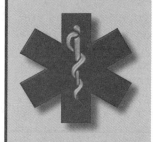

CASE PRESENTATION

EMS is dispatched to a residence to aid a man with chest pain. The patient is conscious and breathing and has a history of "heart attacks." On arrival paramedics are directed to a 63-year-old male (weight 80 kg) sitting on the couch in the living room. The patient is pale, cool, and diaphoretic.

On Examination

CNS: The patient is conscious, alert, and oriented × 4

Resp: Respirations are 24 and of normal depth; lung sounds clear bilaterally; trachea is midline; no signs of trauma

CVS: Carotid and radial pulses are strong and irregular; skin is pale, cool, and diaphoretic

ABD: Soft and nontender

Muscl/Skel: Patient able to move extremities on command; no weaknesses to hand grip

Vital Signs

Pulse: 72/min, irregular, strong

Resp: 24/min, shallow

BP: 122/72 mmHg

SpO$_2$: 95 percent

ECG: Regular sinus rhythm with multifocal PVCs at 10/min

Hx:
- **P** No provoking factors
- **Q** Crushing pain
- **R** Radiating to neck
- **S** 10/10, worst pain ever
- **T** Started suddenly 1/2 hour ago

Past Hx: The patient's wife states that her husband has had several episodes of chest pain brought on by exertion over the past few weeks. He was diagnosed with angina 6 years ago and had a "heart attack" last year. He has nitroglycerin spray, which he has used twice, prior to arrival of the ambulance. The patient takes nitroglycerin spray and ASA.

Treatment

Oxygen was administered by nonrebreather mask at 15 lpm. An IV was started with an 18-gauge catheter in the left arm and run TKO. The paramedics noticed a change on the ECG monitor to ventricular bigeminy. The patient was given nitroglycerin spray 0.4 mg with no relief; 2.5 mg of morphine was administered and provided slight relief of pain. Lidocaine 120 mg was given IV push, and a lidocaine drip was initiated at 2 mg/min, which converted the patient into a sinus rhythm.

ASA was not given because the patient already takes ASA daily. Transport to the hospital was initiated. The pain was rated at 8/10, and another nitroglycerin spray and 2.5 mg of morphine were given. A 12-lead ECG confirmed ST elevation in both the inferior and lateral leads. The destination hospital was informed of a potential candidate for thrombolytic therapy and a second 18-gauge IV was initiated and run TKO. On arrival at the hospital the patient was treated with a thrombolytic medication and then admitted to the CCU to recover.

Adenosine (Adenocard).   Adenosine is a naturally occurring nucleoside useful in the treatment of supraventricular tachycardias and is considered a first-line medication in emergency care of paroxysmal supraventricular tachycardia.

Verapamil (Isoptin, Calan).   Verapamil is a slow calcium channel blocker. It is used in the treatment of paroxysmal supraventricular tachycardia and other atrial dysrhythmias.

Diltiazem (Cardizem).   Diltiazem is a calcium channel blocker and is used to slow the rapid ventricular rate that often accompanies atrial flutter and atrial fibrillation.

Amiodarone HCl (Cordarone).   Amiodarone is a class III antidysrhythmic agent that decreases sinus automaticity, reduces the speed of conduction, and increases the refractory period of the AV node.

Phenytoin (Dilantin).   Phenytoin is infrequently used in the emergency setting as an antidysrhythmic agent. It has proven effectiveness, however, in the management of life-threatening dysrhythmias resulting from digitalis toxicity.

Edrophonium chloride (Tensilon).   Edrophonium chloride is an anticholinesterase agent that has proven effectiveness in terminating paroxysmal supraventricular tachycardias that do not respond to vagal maneuvers. Its usage is rapidly declining, with verapamil and adenosine being preferred.

Magnesium sulfate.   Magnesium is a cofactor in many of the chemical and enzyme reactions that occur in the body. Magnesium deficiency is associated with a high frequency of cardiac dysrhythmias and sudden death. Pharmacologically, it functions like a physiological calcium channel blocker.

Propranolol (Inderal).   Propranolol, discussed in the previous section, plays a role in the treatment of supraventricular dysrhythmias. Students are encouraged to review the section on propranolol and integrate the information with that on the drugs mentioned here.

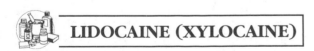

LIDOCAINE (XYLOCAINE)

Class: Antidysrhythmic

Description

Lidocaine is an amide-type local anesthetic. It is frequently used to treat life-threatening ventricular dysrhythmias.

Mechanism of Action

Lidocaine is probably the most frequently used antidysrhythmic agent in the treatment of life-threatening cardiac emergencies. Moreover, it has been shown to be effective in suppressing premature ventricular contractions, in treating ventricular tachycardia and some cases of ventricular fibrillation, and in increasing the fibrillation threshold in acute myocardial infarction. Lidocaine depresses depolarization and automaticity in the ventricles. It has very little effect on atrial tissues. In therapeutic doses it does not slow AV conduction and does not depress myocardial contractility. The most common cause of ventricular dysrhythmias is acute myocardial infarction. Lidocaine suppresses ventricular ectopy in the setting of myocardial infarction and increases the ventricular fibrillation threshold. This prevents PVCs from inducing ventricular fibrillation. After acute myocardial infarction, the ventricular fibrillation threshold is often significantly reduced. Moreover, because electrical defibrillation tends to cause ventricular irritability, patients who have been successfully defibrillated should be treated with lidocaine.

Lidocaine is most apt to suppress ventricular dysrhythmias when the level of the drug in the blood is between 1.5 and 6.0 µg/mL of blood. A 75 to 100 mg bolus of lidocaine will maintain adequate blood levels for only 20 minutes (see Figure 7–5). Therefore, once a dysrhythmia is suppressed, the lidocaine bolus should be followed by a 2 to 4 mg/min infusion to ensure therapeutic blood levels (see Figure 7–6). It is important to distinguish patterns of premature ventricular contractions that are likely to lead to serious dysrhythmias. Premature ventricular contractions that may lead to

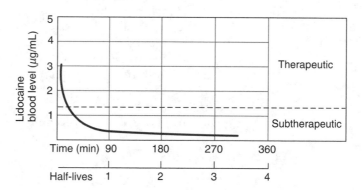

FIGURE 7–5 Blood levels of lidocaine following bolus without drip.

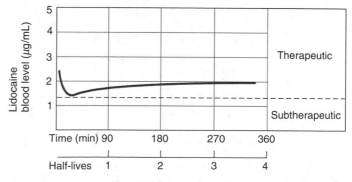

FIGURE 7–6 Blood levels of lidocaine following bolus with drip.

life-threatening dysrhythmias are called malignant premature ventricular contractions. These patterns include the following:

- More than six unifocal PVCs per minute
- PVCs that appear to be coming from more than one ectopic focus (i.e., multifocal PVCs)
- PVCs that occur in couplets (two PVCs together without a normal QRS complex in between)
- Runs of more than two PVCs or ventricular tachycardia PVCs falling in the vulnerable period of the preceding normal complex (R on T phenomena)

Pharmacokinetics

Onset: <3 minutes
Peak Effects: 5–7 minutes
Duration: 10–20 minutes
Half-Life: 1.5–2.0 hours

Indications

Lidocaine is used in ventricular tachycardia, ventricular fibrillation, and malignant premature ventricular contractions.

Contraindications

Lidocaine is usually contraindicated in second-degree Mobitz II and third-degree blocks. Lidocaine slows conduction of the electrical impulse from the atria to the ventricles. Decreased ventricular rates may accompany high-grade heart block, resulting in escape beats that are premature ventricular contractions. Whenever PVCs occur in conjunction with bradycardia (heart rate less than 60 beats per minute), the bradycardia should be treated first. The drug of choice is atropine sulfate, followed by transcutaneous pacing if atropine is not effective. If PVCs are still present after increasing the rate, lidocaine should be administered.

Precautions

Central nervous system depression may occur when the dosage exceeds 300 mg/hr. Symptoms of central nervous system depression include a decreased level of consciousness, irritability, confusion, muscle twitching, and eventually seizures. Exceedingly high doses can result in coma and death. Routine prophylactic lidocaine therapy in patients with acute myocardial infarction is no longer recommended. However, it may be used in conjunction with thrombolytic therapy to suppress expected reperfusion dysrhythmias.

Side Effects

Lidocaine may cause drowsiness, seizures, confusion, hypotension, bradycardia, heart blocks, nausea, vomiting, and respiratory and cardiac arrest.

Interactions

Lidocaine should be used with caution when administered concomitantly with procainamide, phenytoin, quinidine, and β-blockers because drug toxicity may result.

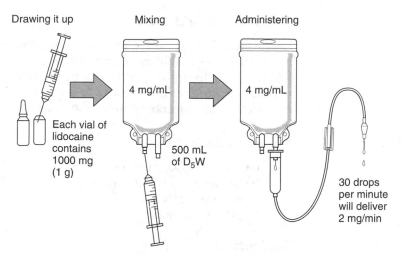

FIGURE 7–7 Preparation of lidocaine infusion.

Dosage

Refractory ventricular fibrillation and pulseless ventricular tachycardia. The initial dose of lidocaine should be 1.0 to 1.5 mg/kg body weight. Lidocaine can be repeated every 3 to 5 minutes at a dose of 0.5 to 0.75 mg/kg to a maximum of 3.0 mg/kg. A single bolus dose of 1.5 mg/kg in cardiac arrest is generally acceptable because plasma lidocaine levels will remain therapeutic as a result of reduced drug elimination during CPR. Only bolus therapy should be used during CPR. Once a patient has been resuscitated, IV infusion therapy can be started to maintain therapeutic blood levels of the drug.

Ventricular tachycardia with a pulse and/or malignant PVCs. The initial dose of lidocaine should be 1.0 to 1.5 mg/kg. Boluses of 0.5 to 0.75 mg/kg can be repeated every 5 to 10 minutes as required to a maximum dose of 3.0 mg/kg. Once the dysrhythmia has been suppressed, a lidocaine drip should be initiated at 2 to 4 mg/min.

The dosage of lidocaine should be reduced 50 percent in patients over 70 years of age and in patients with liver disease, heart failure, bradycardias, or conduction disturbances. Lidocaine is generally given in an IV bolus followed by an infusion (see Figure 7–7). It can also be given endotracheally, however, when an IV line cannot be established. The dose should be increased to 2 to 2.5 times the intravenous dose when administering it endotracheally. A preparation of lidocaine that can be given intramuscularly for ventricular dysrhythmias is also available. This usage should be reserved for times when an IV line cannot be established and the patient is not intubated.

 PROCAINAMIDE (PRONESTYL)

Class: Antidysrhythmic

Description

Procainamide is an ester-type local anesthetic. It is frequently used to treat life-threatening ventricular dysrhythmias refractory to lidocaine.

Mechanism of Action

Procainamide is effective in suppressing ventricular ectopy. It may be effective in cases in which lidocaine has not suppressed life-threatening ventricular dysrhythmias. Procainamide reduces the automaticity of the various pacemaker sites in the heart. Procainamide slows intraventricular conduction to a much greater degree than does lidocaine.

Pharmacokinetics

Onset: 10–30 minutes
Peak Effects: 15–20 minutes
Duration: 3–6 hours
Half-Life: 3 hours

Indications

Procainamide is used in persistent cardiac arrest due to ventricular fibrillation and refractory to lidocaine, premature ventricular contractions refractory to lidocaine, and ventricular tachycardia refractory to lidocaine.

Contraindications

Procainamide should not be administered to patients with severe conduction system disturbances, especially second- and third-degree heart blocks.

Precautions

Procainamide must not be administered to patients demonstrating PVCs in conjunction with bradycardia. The heart rate should first be increased with atropine or transcutaneous pacing. Only after increasing the heart rate can the PVCs be treated with lidocaine or procainamide if they persist. Hypotension is common with intravenous infusion. Constant blood pressure monitoring is essential.

Side Effects

Procainamide may cause drowsiness, seizures, confusion, hypotension, bradycardia, heart blocks, nausea, vomiting, and respiratory and cardiac arrest.

Interactions

The hypotensive effects of procainamide may be increased if administered with antihypertensive drugs. The chance of neurological toxicity by both lidocaine and procainamide increases when the medications are administered together.

Dosage

In treating PVCs or ventricular tachycardia, 100 mg should be administered every 5 minutes at a rate of 20 mg/min. This should be discontinued if any of the following occur:

1. Arrhythmia is suppressed.
2. Hypotension ensues.
3. QRS complex is widened by 50 percent of its original width.
4. A total of 17 mg/kg of the medication has been administered.

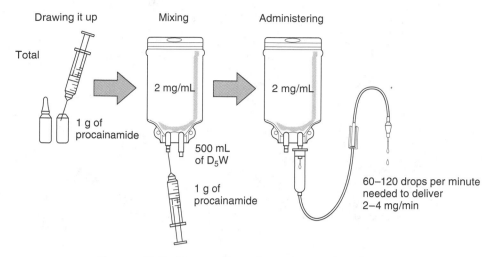

FIGURE 7–8 Preparation of procainamide infusion.

The maintenance infusion of procainamide is 1 to 4 mg/min. The duration of procainamide's effect is shorter than that of lidocaine, requiring a more rigorous approach. Procainamide should be administered by slow IV bolus (20 mg/min) followed by a maintenance infusion. Generally, 1 g of procainamide is placed in 500 mL of D$_5$W. This gives a final concentration of 2 mg/mL (see Figure 7–8).

BRETYLIUM TOSYLATE (BRETYLOL)

Class: Antidysrhythmic

Description

Bretylium is an antidysrhythmic that exhibits both adrenergic and direct myocardial effects.

Mechanism of Action

Bretylium tosylate causes two effects on adrenergic nerve endings. Once administered, bretylium causes release of norepinephrine from adrenergic nerve endings, which in turn causes a slight increase in heart rate, blood pressure, and cardiac output. These sympathomimetic effects last approximately 20 minutes in the noncardiac arrest setting. Then, norepinephrine re-uptake is inhibited, which results in an adrenergic blockade. At this time, hypotension may develop (particularly orthostatic hypotension). Adrenergic blockade usually begins 15 to 20 minutes after drug administration and lasts for several hours (see Figure 7–9). The antidysrhythmic effect of bretylium is poorly understood, but it appears that it elevates the ventricular fibrillation threshold much as lidocaine does. Bretylium sometimes converts ventricular fibrillation or ventricular tachycardia to a supraventricular rhythm. Because of this action, bretylium is sometimes referred to as a chemical defibrillator.

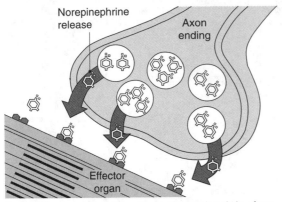

A. Bretylium provokes the release of norepinephrine from the axon ending.

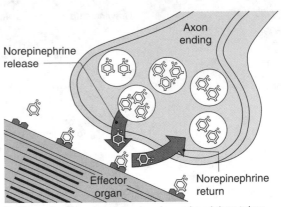

B. Normally, norepinephrine is released and then taken back up to the axon ending.

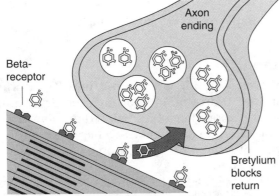

C. Bretylium blocks the return of norepinephrine to the axon ending.

FIGURE 7–9 The pharmacological effects of bretylium.

Pharmacokinetics

Onset: 1–2 minutes
Peak Effects: 1–2 minutes
Duration: 6–24 hours
Half-Life: 4–17 hours

Indications

Bretylium is used in ventricular fibrillation refractory to lidocaine and ventricular tachycardia refractory to lidocaine. At present, bretylium is not considered a first-line antidysrhythmic.

Contraindications

There are no contraindications to bretylium when used in the treatment of life-threatening ventricular dysrhythmias.

Precautions

Postural hypotension occurs in approximately 50 percent of patients receiving bretylium. This side effect should be anticipated, and the patient should be kept in a supine position.

Side Effects

Bretylium may cause dizziness, syncope, seizures, hypotension, hypertension, angina, nausea, and vomiting.

Interactions

Dysrhythmias caused by digitalis toxicity may be worsened by the initial release of norepinephrine that accompanies bretylium usage. Bretylium can interact with other antidysrhythmic agents, causing antagonistic or additive effects. The hypotensive effects of bretylium may be worsened if administered with class Ia antidysrhythmics such as procainamide, quinidine, or disopyramide.

Dosage

Bretylium should be administered at a dose of 5 mg/kg body weight. If the dysrhythmia persists, subsequent doses of 10 mg/kg can be administered at 5-minute intervals. The total dose should not exceed 30 mg/kg. Because bretylium is somewhat slow in its onset, it should be administered by IV bolus.

ADENOSINE (ADENOCARD)

Class: Antidysrhythmic

Description

Adenosine is a naturally occurring nucleoside that slows AV conduction through the AV node. It has an exceptionally short half-life and a relatively good safety profile.

Mechanism of Action

Adenosine is a naturally occurring substance (purine nucleoside) that is present in all body cells. Adenosine decreases conduction of the electrical impulse through the AV node and interrupts AV reentry pathways in paroxysmal supraventricular tachycardia (PSVT). It can effectively terminate rapid supraventricular arrhythmias such as PSVT. The half-life of adenosine is approximately 10 seconds. Because of its rapid onset of action and very short half-life, the administration of adenosine is sometimes referred to as chemical cardioversion. A single bolus of the drug was effective in converting PSVT to a normal sinus rhythm in a significant number (90 percent) of patients in the initial drug studies. Adenosine does not appear to cause hypotension to the same degree as does verapamil.

Pharmacokinetics

Onset: 20–30 seconds
Peak Effects: 20–30 seconds
Duration: 30 seconds
Half-Life: 10 seconds

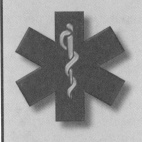

CASE PRESENTATION

At 1900 hours paramedics are dispatched to a residence to aid a 42-year-old female complaining of shortness of breath and chest pain. The patient is conscious and breathing. On arrival the paramedics are met by the patient's son, who directs the ambulance crew to the kitchen. They find the patient seated in a chair. The patient looks anxious, scared, and pale.

On Examination

CNS: The patient is conscious, alert, and oriented × 4; appears anxious

Resp: Respirations are 24 and shallow, with difficult, labored breathing; lung sounds clear bilaterally; trachea is midline; no signs of trauma

CVS: Carotid and radial pulses are present and rapid, pulse weaker radially; skin is pale and cool

ABD: Soft and nontender

Muscl/Skel: Patient able to move extremities on command; no weaknesses to hand grip

Vital Signs

Pulse: 220/min, regular, weak

Resp: 24/min, shallow, with difficulty breathing normally

BP: 110/60 mmHg

SpO$_2$: 97 percent

ECG: Supraventricular tachycardia

Hx:

    P   Was cooking at onset of symptoms

    Q   Palpitations, squeezing discomfort with a feeling of SOB

    R   Nonradiating

    S   3/10

    T   Started suddenly about 30 minutes ago

Past Hx: The patient states that this has never happened before. She was cooking dinner when it suddenly "hit" her. She thought it would go away if she sat down, but it seemed to just get worse. She states that her heart feels like it is going to "jump" out of her chest and that she is having a hard time catching her breath. She does not take any medication except vitamins and is not allergic to anything.

Treatment

Oxygen was administered by nonrebreather mask at 15 lpm and an 18-gauge IV was initiated in her left antecubital vein and run TKO. A 12-lead ECG confirmed the SVT, and paramedics had the patient attempt the Valsalva maneuver without successful conversion of the SVT.

They advised the patient about adenosine, explaining the potential side effects; 6 mg of adenosine was then administered by rapid IV push. Although the patient felt some of the side effects of the adenosine, the first dose did not convert the SVT. The paramedics then administered a second dose of adenosine, this time increasing the dose to 12 mg. After a 4-second interval of a second-degree heart block, the patient's rhythm converted to a regular sinus rhythm. The patient stated that she was free of symptoms. She was transported to the hospital for further assessment, and a 12-lead ECG done en route did not show any acute evidence of a myocardial infarction. The patient was released shortly after with no apparent lasting effects of the SVT.

Indication

Adenosine is used in PSVT (including that associated with Wolff-Parkinson-White syndrome) refractory to common vagal maneuvers.

Contraindications

Adenosine is contraindicated in patients with second- or third-degree heart block, sick sinus syndrome, or those with known hypersensitivity to the drug.

Precautions

Adenosine typically causes dysrhythmias at the time of cardioversion. These generally last a few seconds or less and may include PVCs, premature atrial contractions, sinus bradycardia, sinus tachycardia, and various degrees of AV block. In extreme cases, transient asystole may occur. If this occurs, appropriate therapy should be initiated. Adenosine should be used cautiously in patients with asthma.

Side Effects

Adenosine can cause facial flushing, headache, shortness of breath, dizziness, and nausea, among others. Because the half-life of adenosine is so brief, side effects are generally self-limited.

Interactions

Methylxanthines (e.g., aminophylline and theophylline) may decrease the effectiveness of adenosine, thus requiring larger doses. Dipyridamole (Persantine) can potentiate the effects of adenosine. The dosage of adenosine may need to be reduced in patients receiving dipyridamole.

Dosage

The initial dose of adenosine is 6 mg given as a rapid intravenous bolus over a 1- to 2-second period. To be certain that the drug rapidly reaches the central circulation, it should be given directly into a vein or into a proximal medication port of a functioning IV line. It should be followed immediately by a rapid saline flush. If the initial dose does not result in conversion of the PSVT within 1 to 2 minutes, a 12 mg dose may be given as a rapid IV bolus. The 12 mg dose may be repeated a second time if required. Doses greater than 12 mg should not be administered. Adenosine should only be given by rapid IV bolus, directly into the vein, or into the medication administration port closest to the patient.

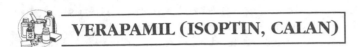

VERAPAMIL (ISOPTIN, CALAN)

Class: Calcium channel blocker

Description

Verapamil is a calcium ion antagonist (calcium channel blocker). Calcium channel blockers cause a relaxation of vascular smooth muscle and slow conduction through the AV node. Verapamil has a greater effect on conduction and a lesser effect on vascular smooth muscle than do other agents in the same class.

Mechanism of Action

Verapamil causes vascular dilation and slows conduction through the AV node. The advantages are twofold. First, verapamil inhibits dysrhythmias caused by a reentry mechanism such as with PSVT. Second, it decreases the rapid ventricular response seen with atrial tachydysrhythmias such as atrial flutter and fibrillation. Verapamil also reduces myocardial oxygen demand because of its negative inotropic effects and causes coronary and peripheral vasodilation.

Pharmacokinetics

Onset: 5 minutes
Peak Effects: 5–15 minutes
Duration: 10–60 minutes
Half-Life: 2–8 hours

Indication

Verapamil is used in PSVT refractory to adenosine.

Contraindications

Verapamil should not be administered to any patient with severe hypotension or cardiogenic shock. In addition, verapamil should not be administered to patients with ventricular tachycardia in the prehospital setting. Before attempting to treat a patient experiencing atrial flutter or atrial fibrillation, it is essential that the paramedic ensure that the patient does not have Wolff-Parkinson-White syndrome.

Precautions

Verapamil can cause systemic hypotension. Thus, it is essential that the blood pressure be constantly monitored following verapamil administration. Calcium chloride can be used to prevent the hypotensive effects of calcium channel blockers and in the management of calcium channel blocker overdosage.

Side Effects

Verapamil can cause nausea, vomiting, dizziness, headache, bradycardia, heart block, hypotension, and asystole.

Interactions

Verapamil should not be administered to patients receiving intravenous β-blockers because of an increased risk of congestive heart failure, bradycardia, and asystole.

Dosage

In the treatment of paroxysmal supraventricular tachycardia, a 2.5 to 5 mg IV dose should be given initially during a 2- to 3-minute interval. A repeat dose of 5 to 10 mg can be given in 15 to 30 minutes if PSVT persists and there have not been any adverse responses to the initial dose. The total dose of verapamil should not exceed 30 mg in 30 minutes.

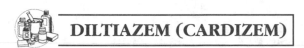

DILTIAZEM (CARDIZEM)

Class: Calcium channel blocker

Description

Diltiazem is a calcium-ion antagonist (calcium channel blocker). Calcium channel blockers cause a relaxation of vascular smooth muscle and slow conduction through the AV node. Diltiazem has a nearly equal effect on vascular smooth muscle and AV conduction.

Mechanism of Action

Diltiazem causes vascular dilation and slows conduction through the AV node. It slows the rapid ventricular rate associated with atrial fibrillation and atrial flutter. It is also used in the treatment of angina because of its negative inotropic effect and because it dilates the coronary arteries.

Pharmacokinetics

Onset: 3 minutes
Peak Effects: 7 minutes
Duration: 1–3 hours
Half-Life: 2 hours

Indications

Diltiazem is used to control rapid ventricular rates associated with atrial fibrillation and atrial flutter, for angina pectoris, and for PSVT refractory to adenosine.

Contraindications

Diltiazem should not be administered to any patient with severe hypotension or cardiogenic shock. In addition, diltiazem should not be administered to patients with ventricular tachycardia (wide-complex tachycardia) in the prehospital setting. Before attempting to treat a patient experiencing atrial flutter or atrial fibrillation, it is essential that the paramedic ensure that the patient does not have Wolff-Parkinson-White syndrome.

Precautions

Diltiazem can cause systemic hypotension. Thus, it is essential that the blood pressure be constantly monitored following diltiazem administration. Calcium chloride can be used to prevent the hypotensive effects of calcium channel blockers and in the management of calcium channel blocker overdosage. Diltiazem should be kept refrigerated; however, it can be kept at room temperature for 1 month but must be discarded if unused.

Side Effects

Diltiazem can cause nausea, vomiting, dizziness, headache, bradycardia, heart block, hypotension, and asystole.

Interactions

Diltiazem should not be administered to patients receiving intravenous β-blockers because of an increased risk of congestive heart failure, bradycardia, and asystole.

Dosage

In the treatment of rapid ventricular rates associated with atrial fibrillation and atrial flutter, a 0.25 mg/kg intravenous bolus (20 mg average adult dose) of diltiazem should be administered over 2 minutes. The bolus dose should be followed by a maintenance infusion of 5 to 15 mg/hr. For PSVT, a 0.25 mg/kg intravenous bolus should be administered over 2 minutes.

AMIODARONE HCL (CORDARONE)

Class: Antidysrhythmic agent

Description

Amiodarone is a class III antidysrhythmic agent used to treat ventricular dysrhythmias unresponsive to other antidysrythmics.

Mechanism of Action

Amiodarone prolongs the action potential duration in all cardiac tissues.

Pharmacokinetics

Onset: 2–3 days (oral)
Peak Effects: 3–7 hours (oral)
Duration: Varies
Half-Life: 40–55 days

Indications

Amiodarone is used in life-threatening cardiac dysrhythmias such as ventricular tachycardia and ventricular fibrillation.

Contraindications

Amiodarone is contraindicated in breast-feeding patients in cardiogenic shock and those with severe sinus node dysfunction resulting in marked sinus bradycardia, second- or third-degree AV block, symptomatic bradycardia, or known hypersensitivity.

Precautions

Amiodarone should be used with caution in patients with latent or manifest heart failure because failure may be worsened by its administration.

Side Effects

Paramedics should monitor the patient's ECG and be alert for hypotension, bradycardia, increased ventricular beats, prolonged PR interval, QRS complex, and QT interval. The patient should also be monitored for signs of pulmonary toxicity such as dyspnea and cough.

Interactions

Amiodarone may react with warfarin, digoxin, procainamide, quinidine, and phenytoin.

Dosage

Cardiac Arrest (V–Fib/V–Tach). 300 mg IV loading does followed by 150 mg in 3–5 minutes as needed.
Ventricular dysrhythmias (adults). Loading dose of 150 mg over 10 minutes (15 mg/min) IV or IO. May be repeated as necessary for recurrent or refractory dysrhythmias.
Maintenance dose. 1 mg/min for 6 hours. Then 0.5 mg/min.

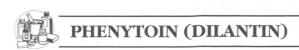 **PHENYTOIN (DILANTIN)**

Class: Antidysrhythmic and anticonvulsant

Description

Phenytoin is an anticonvulsant and antidysrhythmic that depresses spontaneous ventricular depolarization.

Mechanism of Action

Phenytoin (Dilantin) is used frequently in the treatment of epilepsy but also has antidysrhythmic properties. It has proved effective in the management of dysrhythmias caused by digitalis toxicity or tricyclic antidepressant drug overdoses. It depresses spontaneous depolarization of ventricular tissues and appears to improve atrioventricular conduction. Its use in the management of status epilepticus is discussed in Chapter 10.

Pharmacokinetics

Onset: 3–5 minutes
Peak Effects: 1–2 hours
Duration: Variable
Half-Life: 22 hours

Indication

Phenytoin is used in life-threatening dysrhythmias resulting from digitalis toxicity or tricyclic antidepressant overdose. Ventricular dysrhythmias in the setting of acute myocardial infarction should first be treated with lidocaine.

Contraindications

Phenytoin is contraindicated in cases of bradycardia and high-grade heart block. It should not be administered to patients who take the drug chronically for seizures until the blood level has been determined.

Precautions

Intravenous administration of phenytoin should not exceed 50 mg/min. Signs of central nervous system depression or hypotension may occur. Elderly patients are at increased risk of developing side effects from phenytoin administration. Extravasation should be avoided. Any patient receiving intravenous phenytoin should have continuous cardiac monitoring as well as frequent monitoring of vital signs.

Side Effects

Phenytoin can cause drowsiness, dizziness, headache, hypotension, dysrhythmias, itching, rash, nausea, and vomiting.

Interactions

Phenytoin must never be diluted in dextrose-containing solutions such as D_5W. It should be diluted in normal saline or other non-glucose-containing crystalloids.

Dosage

The recommended dose of phenytoin is 100 mg over 5 minutes to a maximum loading dose of 1000 mg, until the dysrhythmia is suppressed, or until symptoms of central nervous system depression appear. In the emergency setting, phenytoin should be given by slow IV bolus or IV infusion with constant ECG monitoring.

EDROPHONIUM CHLORIDE (TENSILON)

Class: Antidysrhythmic and cholinesterase inhibitor

Description

Edrophonium belongs to a class of drugs referred to as anticholinesterase agents. It is used in the treatment of paroxysmal supraventricular tachycardia refractory to first-line agents.

Mechanism of Action

Edrophonium inhibits the actions of the enzyme *acetylcholinesterase.* This enzyme plays an important role in neurophysiology because it deactivates the neurotransmitter of the parasympathetic nervous system, acetylcholine. Physostigmine, an emergency drug used in the management of atropine-type poisonings and tricyclic antidepressant overdoses, is chemically similar to edrophonium. The neurophysiology of the parasympathetic nervous system is discussed in more detail in the following section on parasympatholytics. Edrophonium has proven effectiveness in the management of PSVTs that do not respond to vagal maneuvers. The inhibition of acctylcholinesterase by edrophonium serves to enhance the acetylcholine secreted by the vagus nerve on the heart. This increased parasympathetic effect has been successful in slowing and eventually terminating PSVTs. With the introduction of adenosine and the calcium channel blockers (verapamil), edrophonium has fallen into relative disuse.

Pharmacokinetics

Onset: 30–60 seconds (IV), 2–10 minutes (IM)
Peak Effects: Variable
Duration: 5–10 minutes (IV), 5–30 minutes (IM)
Half-Life: 1–2 hours

Indication

Edrophonium is used for PSVT refractory to vagal maneuvers and adenosine.

Contraindications

Edrophonium should not be administered to patients with a history of hypersensitivity to the drug. It should not be used in patients who are hypotensive or bradycardic because it can worsen these conditions.

Precautions

The respiratory pattern should be carefully monitored during and following administration of edrophonium. Also, the patient should be constantly monitored for signs of bradycardia. Atropine sulfate should be readily available in those cases of bradycardia causing hemodynamic problems. Edrophonium should be used with caution in the elderly.

Side Effects

Edrophonium can cause dizziness, weakness, sweating, increased salivation, constricted pupils, hypotension, bradycardia, abdominal cramps, nausea, and vomiting.

Interactions

Edrophonium should not be administered in dextrose solutions because it tends to crystallize in the tubing. The chances of developing a significant bradycardia are enhanced when edrophonium is administered to patients taking digitalis.

Dosage

The standard dosage is 5 mg initially intravenously. If unsuccessful after 10 minutes or so, a second dose of 10 mg may be administered. Physicians frequently order the administration of a test dose of 0.1 to 0.5 mg, particularly to elderly patients, before the administration of the full dose. Edrophonium should be administered intravenously only.

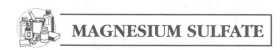

MAGNESIUM SULFATE

Class: Antidysrhythmic

Description

Magnesium sulfate is a salt that dissociates into the magnesium cation (Mg^{2+}) and the sulfate anion when administered. Magnesium is an essential element in numerous biochemical reactions that occur within the body.

Mechanism of Action

Magnesium is an essential element in many of the biochemical processes that occur in the body. It acts as a physiological calcium channel blocker and blocks neuromuscular transmission. A decreased magnesium level (hypomagnesemia) is associated with cardiac dysrhythmias, symptoms of cardiac insufficiency, and sudden death. Hypomagnesemia can cause refractory ventricular fibrillation. Administration of magnesium sulfate in the emergency setting appears to reduce the incidence of ventricular dysrhythmias that may follow an acute myocardial infarction. It also appears to decrease the complications associated with acute myocardial infarction. Magnesium sulfate has been used for years in the management of preterm labor and the hypertensive disorders of pregnancy (preeclampsia and eclampsia). Its usage in obstetrics is discussed in Chapter 11.

Pharmacokinetics

Onset: Immediate (IV), 1 hour (IM)
Peak Effects: Varies
Duration: 1 hour
Half-Life: Not applicable

Indications

Magnesium sulfate is used in severe refractory ventricular fibrillation or pulseless ventricular tachycardia, post–myocardial infarction for prophylaxis of dysrhythmias, and torsade de pointes (multiaxial ventricular tachycardia).

Contraindications

Magnesium sulfate should not be administered to patients who are in shock, who have persistent severe hypertension, who have third-degree AV block, who routinely undergo dialysis, or who are known to have a decreased calcium level (hypocalcemia).

Precautions

Magnesium sulfate should be administered slowly to minimize side effects. Any patient receiving intravenous magnesium sulfate should have continuous cardiac monitoring and frequent monitoring of vital signs. If possible, the knee and biceps deep tendon reflexes should be checked prior to beginning magnesium therapy. It should be used with caution in patients with known renal insufficiency. Hypermagnesemia (elevated magnesium level) can occur following magnesium sulfate administration. Calcium salts (calcium chloride or calcium gluconate) should be available as an antidote for magnesium sulfate in case serious side effects occur.

Side Effects

Magnesium sulfate can cause flushing, sweating, bradycardia, decreased deep tendon reflexes, drowsiness, respiratory depression, dysrhythmias, hypotension, hypothermia, itching, and rash.

Interactions

Magnesium sulfate can cause cardiac conduction abnormalities if administered in conjunction with digitalis.

Dosage

Ventricular fibrillation or ventricular tachycardia. 1 to 2 g of magnesium sulfate should be diluted in 10 mL of D_5W and administered by slow IV push over 1 to 2 minutes. Alternatively, 1 to 2 grams of magnesium sulfate can be diluted in 100 mL of D_5W and administered IV piggyback over 1 to 2 minutes.

Torsade de pointes. Higher doses are often required in the treatment of *torsade de pointes.* Typically, 5 to 10 g are diluted in 100 mL of D_5W and administered at a rate of 1 g/min until the dysrhythmia is suppressed or the maximum dose has been administered.

Post–myocardial infarction prophylaxis. 1 to 2 g of magnesium sulfate can be diluted in 100 mL of D_5W and administered over 5 to 30 minutes as an IV piggyback.

Magnesium should be administered intravenously in the prehospital setting. However, it can be administered intramuscularly if IV access cannot be obtained. Because of the volume of the drug (5 to 10 mL), the dose should be divided in half and each half administered intramuscularly at a separate site (usually each gluteus).

Drugs that inhibit the actions of the parasympathetic nervous system are referred to as *parasympatholytics*. Sometimes they are referred to as *anticholinergics*. To fully understand the role and actions of the parasympatholytics, we must first review the parasympathetic nervous system.

The parasympathetic, or *cholinergic*, system plays a major role in the maintenance of homeostasis. Parasympathetic stimulation induces peristalsis and causes pupillary constriction and a decrease in the heart rate. The primary nerve of the parasympathetic nervous system is the *vagus nerve*. The vagus nerve descends from the brain along the carotid arteries. It then innervates the heart and the digestive system. Paramedics should be familiar with the manual method of vagal stimulation, carotid sinus massage. Carotid sinus massage is used to slow the heart rate in paroxysmal supraventricular tachycardia.

When the vagus nerve is stimulated, it causes acetylcholine to be released from the presynaptic nerve endings. It then activates acetylcholine receptors on the target organs. These receptors cause the heart rate to slow. Then, after only a fraction of a second, cholinesterase is released, which deactivates acetylcholine. Several drugs act on these junctions. The primary drug of this type is atropine sulfate. Atropine binds to the acetylcholine receptors, thus inhibiting activation. Besides increasing the heart rate, atropine is used frequently as a preoperative medication because it decreases digestive secretions, especially salivation. Certain chemicals, especially the organophosphate insecticides, tend to block, in an irreversible manner, the action of cholinesterase. Excessive levels of acetylcholine can cause serious problems.

Research has shown that some cases of asystole can be caused by an increase in parasympathetic tone. The reason for the increase is not clear. Based on this information, however, the American Heart Association recommends administering 1 mg of atropine sulfate as soon as possible to any patient encountered in asystole.

It is important to remember that abdominal distension with air from CPR can increase parasympathetic tone. This can often go unrecognized and makes it difficult to restore a spontaneous rhythm from asystole. It should be a routine part of advanced life support (ALS) to decompress the stomach if distended. The use of proper CPR, Sellick's maneuver, and endotracheal intubation can help minimize abdominal distension.

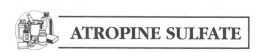

ATROPINE SULFATE

Class: Anticholinergic

Description

Atropine is a parasympatholytic (anticholinergic) that is derived from parts of the *Atropa belladonna* plant.

Mechanism of Action

Atropine sulfate is a potent parasympatholytic and is used to increase the heart rate in hemodynamically significant bradycardias. Hemodynamically significant bradycardias are those slow heart rates accompanied by hypotension, shortness of breath, chest pain, altered mental status, congestive heart failure, and shock. Atropine acts by blocking acetylcholine receptors, thus inhibiting parasympathetic stimulation. Although it has positive chronotropic properties, it has little or no inotropic effect. It plays an important role as an antidote in organophosphate poisonings. Atropine has been shown to be of some use in asystole, presumably because some cases of asystole may be caused by a sudden and tremendous increase in parasympathetic tone. The mechanism by which atropine is effective in asystole is not clear. However, despite no definite proof of its value in asystole, there is little evidence that its use is harmful in this setting.

Pharmacokinetics

Onset: Immediate
Peak Effects: 2–4 minutes
Duration: 4 hours
Half-Life: 2–3 hours

Indications

Atropine is used in hemodynamically significant bradycardia and asystole.

Contraindications

There are no contraindications in emergency situations.

Precautions

Atropine may actually worsen the bradycardia associated with second-degree Mobitz II and third-degree AV blocks. In these cases, the paramedic should go straight to transcutaneous pacing instead of trying atropine. A maximum dose of 0.04 mg/kg body weight of atropine should not be exceeded except in the setting of organophosphate poisoning. If the heart rate fails to increase after a total of 0.04 mg/kg has been given, then transcutaneous pacing is indicated.

Side Effects

Atropine sulfate can cause blurred vision, dilated pupils, dry mouth, tachycardia, drowsiness, and confusion.

Interactions

There are few interactions in the prehospital setting.

Dosage

Hemodynamically significant bradycardia. An initial dose of 0.5 mg should be administered intravenously. This dose can be repeated every 3 to 5 minutes until a maximum dose of 0.04 mg/kg has been administered.

Asystole. In the treatment of asystole, the dose should be increased to 1.0 mg. When an IV cannot be placed, atropine can be administered endotracheally. However, the dose should be increased to 2 to 2.5 times the intravenous dose.

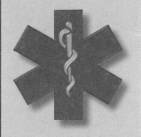

CASE PRESENTATION

Paramedics are called to a local shopping mall for a medical emergency. Reportedly, a patient collapsed and is unconscious, but breathing. On arrival the patient is found lying on the floor in the center court with a pillow under her head. The patient appears to be in her early 60s.

On Examination

CNS: The patient is conscious, slow to respond to verbal commands, and disoriented to person, place, and time

Resp: Respirations are 12 and shallow; lung sounds clear bilaterally; trachea is midline; no signs of trauma

CVS: Weak, regular, slow carotid pulse and radial pulses are present; skin is pale, cool, and diaphoretic; no complaint of chest pain

ABD: Soft and nontender

Muscl/Skel: Patient able to move extremities slightly, with delay, on command; weak bilateral hand grip; no obvious injuries

Vital Signs

Pulse: 36/min, regular, weak

Resp: 12/min, shallow

BP: 72/56 mmHg

SpO$_2$: 86 percent

ECG: Sinus bradycardia

Hx: Unknown; patient was in the mall alone and is unable to give a history or answer questions

Past Hx: Unknown; no Medic Alert

Treatment

Oxygen was administered by nonrebreather mask at 12 lpm and well tolerated by the patient. An IV of normal saline was established. The patient was given 0.5 mg of atropine. Following the atropine the patient's pulse rate increased slightly to 42/min and her blood pressure was 80/62. At this point the pacing pads were placed on the patient as a precautionary measure. A second dose of atropine 0.5 mg was given, and the heart rate improved to 68/min with a blood pressure of 108/82. The patient's level of consciousness improved. The patient was moved to the ambulance and transported to the hospital.

En route to the hospital the patient stated that she was shopping alone when she felt faint. She sat down to let the faintness pass. She does not remember what happened prior to fainting. She remembers waking and seeing the paramedics with her.

Atropine should be given as an IV bolus in emergency situations or endotracheally when an IV cannot be placed.

CARDIAC GLYCOSIDES

Digitalis, the principal drug in the cardiac glycoside class, is one of the oldest medications known to humans. For hundreds of years it has been used in the treatment of congestive heart failure. Digitalis and the related cardiac glycosides increase the force (inotropic effect) of the myocardial contraction. When given to patients in congestive heart failure, it significantly increases cardiac output, reducing left ventricular diameter; decreases venous pressure; and hastens reduction of peripheral and pulmonary edema. In recent years digitalis has also proved effective in the management of patients with atrial flutter and atrial fibrillation. In these patients rapid atrial rates produce accelerated ventricular rates, which can be reduced by digitalis therapy.

Several digitalis preparations are available:

Digitoxin.   Digitoxin is the longest acting cardiac glycoside. It must not be confused with the shorter acting digoxin.

Digoxin (Lanoxin).   Digoxin is the most commonly prescribed form of digitalis.

Ouabain.   Ouabain has a rapid rate of onset and a relatively short duration of effect. Its use is reserved for cases in which rapid digitalization is required.

Deslanoside (Cedilanid-D).   Deslanoside is the most rapidly acting digitalis preparation.

Cardiac glycosides have profound effects on cardiac function and rhythm. The therapeutic index (therapeutic dose/toxic dose) is low, which means that the possibility of digitalis toxicity should always be considered in patients with this medication. Signs of digitalis toxicity include cardiac dysrhythmias (PVCs, PSVT with 2:1 block, and so on), nausea, vomiting, headache, visual disturbances (yellow vision), and drowsiness. Almost any dysrhythmia can be associated with digitalis toxicity.

Digitalis is a potent and potentially toxic drug. Extreme care must be used whenever it is administered. Constant monitoring of vital signs and ECG is essential. In almost all cases digitalization should be deferred until the patient is in the emergency department and under the care of the emergency physician.

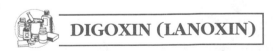 **DIGOXIN (LANOXIN)**

Class: Cardiac glycoside

Description

Digoxin is a moderately rapid-acting cardiac glycoside used in the management of congestive heart failure and to control the heart rate in atrial fibrillation and atrial flutter.

Mechanism of Action

Digoxin is a cardiac glycoside effective in the treatment of congestive heart failure and rapid atrial arrhythmias. It increases the force of the cardiac contraction through its effects on the sodium-potassium ATPase system. Digoxin significantly increases the stroke volume, thus increasing the cardiac output. It also decreases AV nodal conduction, thus slowing the heart rate. Therapeutic effects begin in about half an hour and peak at 24 hours.

Pharmacokinetics

Onset: 5–30 minutes
Peak Effects: 1–5 hours
Duration: 3–4 days
Half-Life: 34–44 hours

Indications

Digoxin is used in congestive heart failure and supraventricular tachy-dysrhythmias, especially atrial flutter and atrial fibrillation.

Contraindications

Digoxin should not be given to any patient showing any of the signs or symptoms of digitalis toxicity. It also should not be administered to patients in ventricular fibrillation.

Precautions

Patients receiving digoxin should be constantly monitored for signs and symptoms of digitalis toxicity. Extreme care should be used when administering digoxin to patients with myocardial infarction, because they are prone to digitalis toxicity. Digitalis toxicity is potentiated in patients with hypokalemia, hypomagnesemia, and hypercalcemia. Digitalis crosses the placenta and thus can affect the fetal heart in much the same manner as the mother's.

Side Effects

Digoxin can cause numerous side effects. Noncardiac side effects include anorexia, nausea, vomiting, abdominal pain, diarrhea, fatigue, depression, drowsiness, yellow vision, headache, dizziness, hallucinations, sweating, itching, and rash. Cardiac side effects include dysrhythmias, bradycardias, tachycardias, various degrees of heart block, hypotension, and cardiac arrest.

Interactions

Many drugs have potential interaction problems with digoxin. Quinidine and the calcium channel blockers (verapamil, nifedipine, and diltiazem) can increase serum digoxin levels. The administration of digoxin concomitantly with beta-blockers can cause severe bradycardia. Diuretics can cause potassium depletion, which can lead to digitalis toxicity.

Dosage

The dosage is 0.25 to 0.5 mg given by slow IV push. Digoxin is generally given intravenously in the treatment of supraventricular tachydysrhythmias.

ANTICOAGULANTS

Drugs that inhibit blood clot formation (*anticoagulants*) play an important role in emergency medicine. Many significant medical problems result from either embolic or thrombotic events. These include acute coronary syndrome, acute embolic and thrombotic strokes, pulmonary embolism, and deep venous thrombosis. Deep venous thrombosis is a risk factor for the development of pulmonary embolisms and other thrombotic events.

Several drugs are available that inhibit coagulation. The most common of these is warfarin sodium (Coumadin). Warfarin is only available in an oral form and it takes several days to achieve therapeutic blood levels. Thus, its role in emergency medicine is rather limited.

Another common anticoagulant, heparin, can only be administered parenterally. Thus, it is easily administered and rapidly effective. The half-life of heparin is short and any bolus must be followed by a continuous infusion until the condition is resolved or the patient switched to oral warfarin.

Low-molecular-weight heparin (enoxaparin) has become increasingly popular in emergency medicine. Normal heparin has a molecular weight of 5000 to 30 000 Da, whereas low-molecular-weight heparin has a molecular weight of 1000 to 10 000 Da. Because of this, low-molecular-weight heparin has greater bioavailability, is easier to dose, and has fewer effects on platelet function.

For the most part, anticoagulant therapy should be guided by blood coagulation studies [prothrombin time (PT) and partial thromboplastin times (PTT)]. These are unavailable in the prehospital setting. However, in certain cases, the benefits gained from early coagulation may exceed any risks of administering the drugs without baseline coagulation studies.

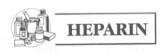 **HEPARIN**

Class: Anticoagulant

Description

Heparin is a rapid-acting anticoagulant prepared from bovine lung tissue or porcine intestinal mucosa.

Mechanism of Action

Heparin enhances the inhibitory actions of antithrombin III–thrombin complex, blocking the conversion of prothrombin to thrombin and preventing the conversion of fibrinogen to fibrin.

Pharmacokinetics

Onset: Immediate
Peak Effects: 2–3 minutes
Duration: 2–6 hours
Half-Life: 90 minutes

Indications

Heparin is used to inhibit clot formation in unstable angina and non-Q-wave myocardial infarction. It is also used to prevent pulmonary embolism and deep venous thrombosis in patients predisposed to such problems.

Contraindications

Heparin is contraindicated in patients with known hypersensitivity to the drug, to pork products, and to beef products.

Precautions

Do not use heparin in patients with active major bleeding or thrombocytopenia. Use with caution in the elderly or any patient with increased risk of bleeding. Heparin should be used with caution in chronic alcoholism, in patients with a history of atrophy or anaphylaxis, and during pregnancy (especially the last trimester).

Side Effects

Reported central nervous system side effects include confusion and dizziness. Cardiovascular side effects include edema, chest pain, and irregular heartbeat. Irritation, pain, erythema, or bruising may occur at the injection site. Other side effects are bleeding complications, angioedema, rash, and urticaria.

Interactions

Interactions with heparin have been reported with nonsteroidal anti-inflammatory drugs, warfarin, and antiplatelet agents. Intravenous nitroglycerin may decrease anticoagulation activities. Protamine antagonizes the effects of heparin.

Dosage

Adult dose. 5000 units IV followed by infusion based on laboratory values.
Pediatric dose. 50 units/kg followed by IV infusion based on laboratory values.

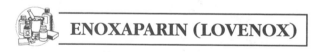

ENOXAPARIN (LOVENOX)

Class: Anticoagulant

Description

Enoxaparin is a low-molecular-weight heparin derivative.

Mechanism of Action

Enoxaparin accelerates the formation of antithrombin III–thrombin complex and deactivates thrombin. It also prevents the conversion of fibrinogen to fibrin.

Pharmacokinetics

Onset: 3–5 hours
Peak Effects: 3–5 hours
Duration: Varies
Half-Life: 4.5 hours

Indications

Enoxaparin is used to inhibit clot formation in unstable angina and non-Q-wave myocardial infarction. It is also used to prevent pulmonary embolism and deep venous thrombosis in patients predisposed to such problems.

Contraindications

Enoxaparin is contraindicated in patients with known hypersensitivity to the drug, to pork products, or to heparin.

Precautions

Do not use enoxaparin in patients with active major bleeding or thrombocytopenia. Use with caution in the elderly or any patient with increased risk of bleeding.

Side Effects

Reported central nervous system side effects include confusion and dizziness. Cardiovascular side effects include edema, chest pain, and irregular heartbeat. Irritation, pain, erythema, or bruising may occur at the injection site. Other side effects are bleeding complications, angioedema, rash, and urticaria.

Interactions

Interactions with enoxaparin have been reported with nonsteroidal anti-inflammatory drugs, warfarin, and antiplatelet agents.

Dosage

Adult dose. 1 mg/kg SQ for unstable angina/MI; 0.5 mg/kg for pulmonary embolism.
Pediatric dose. 1 mg/kg SQ.

FIBRINOLYTICS

A myocardial infarction begins with the formation of a blood clot (thrombus) in a coronary artery. This clot results in complete occlusion of the artery and subsequent interruption of blood flow to the area of the myocardium supplied by that artery. Usually, the coronary artery is already partially obstructed by atherosclerosis. These obstructions are often the narrowest (or tightest) portions of the artery and the site of thrombus formation.

Following arterial occlusion, the portion of the myocardium supplied by the obstructed artery becomes ischemic. At this point the ischemia can be reversed with minimal permanent injury to the muscle if the blood supply can be restored. However, if the occlusion continues, the myocardium will become injured and will eventually die. There is a window of 6 hours after the onset of pain to restore perfusion to the injured myocardium. There are several ways perfusion can be restored, including percutaneous transluminal coronary angioplasty (PTCA), coronary artery bypass grafting (CABG), and fibrinolytic therapy. PTCA requires access to a cardiac catheterization lab and subsequent coronary arteriogram to identify the occlusion. Then, a special balloon catheter is introduced into the diseased artery. The balloon is placed at the site of the occlusion and filled, resulting in dilation of the occlusion. This process is time consuming and not available in every hospital. Likewise, CABG requires an initial arteriogram followed by major surgery to bypass the obstruction. Fibrinolytic therapy, unlike the other procedures, does not require coronary angiography and can be performed in any community hospital and, in some places, in the prehospital setting.

Fibrinolytic therapy is the administration of a drug to dissolve the blood clot in the coronary artery causing an acute myocardial infarction. There are three major types of fibrinolytics available in the United States: streptokinase (Streptase), anistreplase (Eminase, Apsac), and alteplase (tPA, Activase). Aspirin, a platelet aggregation inhibitor, is included in this discussion because it has proved highly effective in reducing mortality following myocardial infarction.

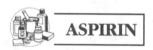 **ASPIRIN**

Class: Platelet aggregator inhibitor and anti-inflammatory agent

Description

Aspirin is an anti-inflammatory agent and an inhibitor of platelet function. This makes it a useful agent in the treatment of various thromboembolic diseases such as acute myocardial infarction.

Mechanism of Action

Aspirin blocks the formation of the substance thromboxane A_2, which causes platelets to aggregate and arteries to constrict. This results in an overall reduction in mortality associated with myocardial infarction. It also appears to reduce the rate of nonfatal reinfarction and nonfatal stroke.

Pharmacokinetics

> **Onset:** 5–30 minutes
> **Peak Effects:** 15–120 minutes
> **Duration:** 1–4 hours
> **Half-Life:** 15–20 minutes

Indications

Aspirin is used for new chest pain suggestive of acute coronary syndrome and signs and symptoms suggestive of recent stroke. Several studies have shown that early aspirin administration (within 3 hours of acute coronary syndrome symptom onset) is associated with a significantly decreased risk of death. However, other studies have shown that aspirin is underused in prehospital care in the treatment of chest pain and acute coronary syndrome.

Contraindications

Aspirin is contraindicated in patients with known hypersensitivity to the drug. It is relatively contraindicated in patients with active ulcer disease and asthma.

Precautions

Aspirin can cause gastrointestinal upset and bleeding. Enteric-coated aspirin, if available, should be used in patients who have a tendency for gastric irritation and bleeding with aspirin. Aspirin should be used with caution in patients who report allergies to the nonsteroidal anti-inflammatory (NSAID) class of drugs. Doses higher than recommended can actually interfere with possible benefits.

Side Effects

Aspirin can cause heartburn, gastrointestinal bleeding, nausea, vomiting, wheezing, and prolonged bleeding.

Interactions

When administered together, aspirin and other anti-inflammatory agents may cause an increased incidence of side effects and increased blood levels of both drugs. Administration of aspirin with antacids may reduce the blood levels of the drug by decreasing absorption.

Dosage

The recommended dosage for aspirin is 160 to 325 mg taken as soon as possible after the onset of chest pain. Low-dose aspirin therapy (80–160 mg) using 1–2 baby asprin (81 mg each) is often preferred because it can be chewed and swallowed and is often a little more palatable; many myocardial infarction patients are nauseated. Aspirin is often given as part of a thrombolytic therapy protocol.

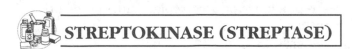 **STREPTOKINASE (STREPTASE)**

Class: Fibrinolytic

Description

Streptokinase is a potent fibrinolytic. It is derived from the bacteria Group C, β-hemolytic streptococci.

Mechanism of Action

Streptokinase acts with plasminogen (present in the blood) to produce a so-called activator complex. This activator complex converts plasminogen to the enzyme plasmin. Plasmin then digests fibrin and fibrinogen, resulting in the dissolution of clots that cause coronary occlusion.

Pharmacokinetics

Onset: <1 hour
Peak Effects: 80 minutes
Duration: 2–36 hours
Half-Life: 83 minutes

Indication

Streptokinase is used for acute coronary syndrome.

Contraindications

Streptokinase is absolutely contraindicated in the following cases:

1. Active internal bleeding
2. Suspected aortic dissection
3. Traumatic CPR (rib fractures, pneumothorax)
4. Severe, persistent hypertension
5. Recent head trauma or known intracranial tumor
6. History of stroke in the past 6 months
7. Pregnancy

It is relatively contraindicated (i.e., the risks must be weighed against the potential benefits) in the following cases:

1. History of trauma or major surgery in the past 2 months
2. Initial blood pressure greater than 180 systolic or 110 diastolic that is controlled by medical treatment
3. Active peptic ulcer or blood in stool
4. History of stroke, tumor, brain surgery, or head injury
5. Known bleeding disorder or current use of warfarin (Coumadin)
6. Significant liver dysfunction or kidney failure
7. Exposure to streptokinase or anistreplase during the preceding 12 months
8. Known cancer or illness with possible thoracic, abdominal, or intracranial abnormalities
9. Prolonged CPR

Precautions

Streptokinase may be ineffective if administered within 12 months of prior streptokinase or anistreplase therapy. Anaphylaxis can occur with streptokinase therapy. Emergency resuscitative drugs and equipment should be immediately available. Reperfusion dysrhythmias are common once the occluded artery opens. Antidysrhythmic medications should be immediately available.

Side Effects

Streptokinase can cause bleeding, allergic reactions, anaphylaxis, fever, nausea, and vomiting.

Interactions

Streptokinase should be used with caution in patients on anticoagulation therapy.

Dosage

Streptokinase should be administered at 1.5 million units over 1 hour. This is typically part of a streptokinase protocol in which aspirin, an antihistamine, and a corticosteroid are administered before administering streptokinase. The antihistamine and corticosteroid are given to prevent a possible allergic reaction to the drug.

Streptokinase must be reconstituted immediately prior to administration. The manufacturer's recommendations for reconstitution, which accompany the drug, should be followed explicitly. Streptokinase should be administered intravenously, preferably through an IV pump.

ANISTREPLASE (EMINASE, APSAC)

Class: Fibrinolytic

Description

Anistreplase is a potent fibrinolytic. It is a derivative of the plasminogen-streptokinase activator complex and is derived from the bacteria Group C, β-hemolytic streptococci.

Mechanism of Action

Anistreplase is an inactive derivative that is activated when administered. Plasmin is produced from plasminogen (present in the blood). Plasmin then digests fibrin and fibrinogen, resulting in the dissolution of clots that cause coronary occlusion.

Pharmacokinetics

Onset: Immediate
Peak Effects: 45 minutes
Duration: 6–48 hours
Half-Life: 105–120 minutes

Indication

Anistreplase is used for acute coronary syndrome.

Contraindications

Anistreplase is absolutely contraindicated in the following cases:

1. Active internal bleeding
2. Suspected aortic dissection
3. Traumatic CPR (rib fractures, pneumothorax)
4. Severe persistent hypertension
5. Recent head trauma or known intracranial tumor
6. History of stroke in the past 6 months
7. Pregnancy

It is relatively contraindicated (i.e., the risks must be weighed against the potential benefits) in the following cases:

1. History of trauma or major surgery in the past 2 months
2. Initial blood pressure greater than 180 systolic or 110 diastolic that is controlled by medical treatment
3. Active peptic ulcer or blood in stool
4. History of stroke, tumor, brain surgery, or head injury
5. Known bleeding disorder or current use of warfarin (Coumadin)
6. Significant liver dysfunction or kidney failure
7. Exposure to streptokinase or anistreplase during the preceding 12 months
8. Known cancer or illness with possible thoracic, abdominal, or intracranial abnormalities
9. Prolonged CPR

Precautions

Anistreplase may be ineffective if administered within 12 months of prior streptokinase or anistreplase therapy. Anaphylaxis can occur with anistreplase therapy. Emergency resuscitative drugs and equipment should be immediately available. Reperfusion dysrhythmias are common once the occluded artery opens. Antidysrhythmic medications should be immediately available.

Side Effects

Anistreplase can cause bleeding, allergic reactions, anaphylaxis, fever, nausea, and vomiting.

Interactions

Anistreplase should be used with caution in patients on anticoagulation therapy.

Dosage

Anistreplase (30 units) should be injected slowly over 4 to 5 minutes in a one-time dose. This is typically part of an Eminase protocol in which aspirin, an antihistamine, and a corticosteroid are administered before administering anistreplase. The antihistamine and corticosteroid are given to prevent a possible allergic reaction to the drug.

Anistreplase must be reconstituted immediately prior to administration and used within 30 minutes of reconstitution. The manufacturer's recommendations for reconstitution, which accompany the drug, should be followed exactly. When mixing the drug, the paramedic must be careful not to shake it. Instead, it should be gently rolled in the vial to mix it.

Anistreplase should be administered by slow intravenous bolus.

ALTEPLASE, TISSUE PLASMINOGEN ACTIVATOR (ACTIVASE)

Class: Fibrinolytic

Description

Alteplase (tPA) is a potent fibrinolytic. It is a tissue plasminogen activator produced through recombinant DNA technology.

Mechanism of Action

Alteplase is an enzyme that converts plasminogen (present in the blood) to the enzyme plasmin. It also produces a limited amount of fibrinogen in the absence of fibrin. When administered, alteplase binds to the fibrin in a thrombus and converts the plasminogen into plasmin. Plasmin then digests fibrin and fibrinogen, causing the dissolution of clots that cause coronary occlusion.

Pharmacokinetics

Onset: 5–10 minutes
Peak Effects: 5–10 minutes
Duration: Varies
Half-Life: 26.5 minutes

Indication

Alteplase is used for acute coronary syndrome.

Contraindications

Alteplase is absolutely contraindicated in the following cases:

1. Active internal bleeding
2. Suspected aortic dissection
3. Traumatic CPR (rib fractures, pneumothorax)
4. Severe, persistent hypertension
5. Recent head trauma or known intracranial tumor
6. History of stroke in the past 6 months
7. Pregnancy

Fibrinolytics

It is relatively contraindicated (i.e., the risks must be weighed against the potential benefits) in the following cases:

1. History of trauma or major surgery in the past 2 months
2. Initial blood pressure greater than 180 systolic or 110 diastolic that is controlled by medical treatment
3. Active peptic ulcer or blood in stool
4. History of stroke, tumor, brain surgery, or head injury
5. Known bleeding disorder or current use of warfarin (Coumadin)
6. Significant liver dysfunction or kidney failure
7. Known cancer or illness with possible thoracic, abdominal, or intracranial abnormalities
8. Prolonged CPR

Precautions

Alteplase does not appear to have the problem with readministration associated with streptokinase or anistreplase. Anaphylaxis can occur with alteplase therapy but is very rare. Emergency resuscitative drugs and equipment should be immediately available. Reperfusion dysrhythmias are common once the occluded artery opens. Antidysrhythmic medications should be immediately available.

Side Effects

Alteplase can cause bleeding, allergic reactions, anaphylaxis, fever, nausea, and vomiting.

Interactions

Alteplase should be used with caution in patients on anticoagulation therapy.

Dosage

The dosage regimen for alteplase is controversial. The manufacturer recommends a total dose of 100 mg; 10 mg is administered as an IV bolus over 1 to 2 minutes, followed by an infusion of 50 mg over the first hour, 20 mg over the second hour, and 20 mg over the third hour. A more popular dosing regimen is the accelerated or front-loaded regimen. In this case, 15 mg of the drug is administered as an IV bolus over 1 to 2 minutes. This is followed by an IV infusion of 50 mg over the first hour and 35 mg over the second hour. Alteplase must be reconstituted immediately prior to administration. The manufacturer's recommendations for reconstitution, which accompany the drug, should be followed exactly. Alteplase should be administered intravenously. An initial bolus should be administered over 1 to 2 minutes followed by an IV infusion, preferably through an IV pump.

RETAPLASE RECOMBINANT (RETAVASE)

Class: Fibrinolytic

Description

Retaplase is a DNA recombinant human tissue-type plasminogen activator (tPA) that acts as a catalyst in the cleavage of plasminogen to plasmin.

Mechanism of Action

Retaplase causes an increase in the formation of plasmin by increasing the conversion of plasminogen to plasmin. It is effective in degrading the fibrin matrix of a clot and is thus an effective fibrinolytic.

Pharmacokinetics

Onset: <5 minutes
Peak Effects: Varies
Duration: Varies
Half-Life: 13–16 minutes

Indications

Retaplase is used for acute coronary syndrome.

Contraindications

Retaplase is absolutely contraindicated in the following cases:

1. Active internal bleeding
2. Suspected aortic dissection
3. Traumatic CPR (rib fractures, pneumothorax)
4. Severe, persistent hypertension
5. Recent head trauma or known intracranial tumor
6. History of stroke in the past 6 months
7. Pregnancy

It is relatively contraindicated (i.e., the risks must be weighed against the potential benefits) in the following cases:

1. History of trauma or major surgery in the last 2 months
2. Initial blood pressure greater than 180 systolic or 110 diastolic that is controlled by medical treatment
3. Active peptic ulcer disease or blood in stool
4. History of stroke, tumor, brain surgery, or head injury
5. Known bleeding disorder or current use of warfarin (Coumadin)
6. Significant liver dysfunction or kidney failure

7. Known cancer or illness with possible thoracic, abdominal, or intracranial abnormalities

8. Prolonged CPR

Precautions

Retaplase does not appear to have the problems with readministration associated with streptokinase or anistreplase. Anaphylaxis can occur with retaplase therapy, but it is very rare. Emergency resuscitative drugs and equipment should be immediately available. Antidysrhythmic medications should be readily available.

Side Effects

Retaplase can cause bleeding, allergic reactions, anaphylaxis, fever, nausea, and vomiting.

Interactions

None in ACLS setting.

Dosage

Adult dose. 10 units IV over 2 minutes. Repeat 10 units IV (over 2 minutes) in 30 minutes (20 units total dose).
Pediatric dose. Not indicated.

ALKALINIZING AGENTS

Alkalinizing drugs, such as sodium bicarbonate, are used to buffer the acids present in the body during and after cardiac arrest and other serious conditions. Normal body pH is 7.4 (7.35 to 7.45). During hypoxia, the serum pH may fall quickly. Sodium bicarbonate will help correct metabolic (usually lactic acid) acidosis until hypoxia is corrected. The following reaction illustrates the role of sodium bicarbonate in acid-base balance:

$$H^+ \quad + \quad HCO_3^- \quad \leftrightarrow \quad H_2CO_2 \quad \leftrightarrow \quad H_2O \quad + \quad CO_2$$

| Acids (strong) | Bicarbonate | Carbonic acid | Water | Carbon dioxide |

Bicarbonate combines with the strong acids, usually lactic acid, and forms a weak, volatile acid (carbonic acid). This acid then is broken down into carbon dioxide and water. The two end products are then removed via the lungs and the kidneys, respectively.

Excessive administration of sodium bicarbonate may cause metabolic alkalosis, which may be worse than the metabolic acidosis being treated. Primary treatment of metabolic acidosis in the setting of hypoxia or cardiac arrest includes adequate oxygenation and blood pressure support.

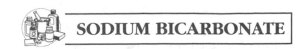

SODIUM BICARBONATE

Class: Alkalinizing agent

Description

Sodium bicarbonate is a salt that provides bicarbonate to buffer metabolic acidosis, which can accompany several disease processes.

Mechanism of Action

For many years sodium bicarbonate was the cornerstone of ACLS care. Controlled studies have shown that sodium bicarbonate was ineffective in the treatment of cardiac arrest. In many instances it has actually been associated with many adverse reactions. Sodium bicarbonate is occasionally used in the treatment of certain types of drug overdose. The most common example is drugs in the tricyclic class of antidepressants. Overdosage of these drugs has serious effects including life-threatening cardiac dysrhythmias. TCA excretion from the body is enhanced by making the urine more alkaline (raising the pH). Sodium bicarbonate is sometimes administered to increase the pH of the urine to speed excretion of the drug from the body.

Pharmacokinetics

Onset: Immediate
Peak Effects: <15 minutes
Duration: 1–2 hours
Half-Life: Not applicable

Indications

Sodium bicarbonate is used late in the management of cardiac arrest, if at all. Hyperventilation, prompt defibrillation, and the administration of epinephrine and lidocaine should always precede use of sodium bicarbonate. Because these therapies take at least 10 minutes to carry out, sodium bicarbonate should rarely be administered in the first 10 minutes of a resuscitation. Sodium bicarbonate is also indicated in TCA overdose, phenobarbital overdose, severe acidosis refractory to hyperventilation, and known hyperkalemia.

Contraindications

When used in the management of the situations described earlier, there are no absolute contraindications.

Precautions

Sodium bicarbonate can cause metabolic alkalosis when administered in large quantities. It is important to calculate the dosage based on patient weight and size.

Side Effects

There are few side effects when sodium bicarbonate is used in the emergency setting.

Interactions

Most catecholamines and vasopressors (e.g., dopamine and epinephrine) can be deactivated by alkaline solutions such as sodium bicarbonate. Sodium bicarbonate should not be administered in conjunction with calcium chloride. A precipitate can form, which may clog the IV line.

Dosage

The usual dose of sodium bicarbonate is 1 mEq/kg body weight initially followed by 0.5 mEq/kg of body weight every 10 minutes. When possible, the dosage of sodium bicarbonate should be based on the results of arterial blood gas studies. Sodium bicarbonate should be administered only as an IV bolus.

CARDIAC PAIN MANAGEMENT (ANALGESICS)

Drugs that have proved to be effective in alleviating pain are referred to as analgesics. Although they may be administered in many different types of emergencies, they are used most often for the treatment of emergencies involving the cardiovascular system, especially myocardial infarction. Analgesics are covered in detail in Chapter 15. This section covers morphine and nitrous oxide.

Morphine is derived from the opium plant. It has impressive analgesic and hemodynamic effects. Nitronox, a 50 percent mixture of oxygen and nitrous oxide that can be easily inhaled by the patient, is entirely different from the other analgesic agents discussed. Its analgesic effects are also very potent yet disappear within a few minutes after the cessation of administration. Thus, Nitronox can be given for many types of pain in the field without fear of impairing subsequent physical examination in the emergency department. In addition to its analgesic effects, Nitronox delivers oxygen to the patient, which makes it useful in cardiac emergencies.

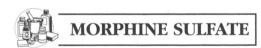 **MORPHINE SULFATE**

Class: Narcotic analgesic

Description

Morphine is a central nervous system depressant and a potent analgesic. Although morphine sulfate is one of the most potent analgesics known to humans, it also has hemodynamic properties that make it extremely useful in emergency medicine.

Mechanism of Action

Morphine sulfate is a central nervous system depressant that acts on opiate receptors in the brain, providing both analgesia and sedation. It increases peripheral venous capacitance and decreases venous return. This effect is sometimes called a chemical phlebotomy. Morphine also decreases myocardial oxygen demand. This action is due to both the decreased systemic vascular resistance and the sedative effects of the drug. Patient apprehension and fear can significantly increase myocardial oxygen demand and in some cases can conceivably increase the size of myocardial infarction. The hemodynamic properties of morphine make it one of the most important drugs used in the treatment of pulmonary edema. Morphine is frequently administered to patients who have signs and symptoms of pulmonary edema but who are not having chest pain.

Pharmacokinetics

Onset: Immediate (IV), 15–30 minutes (IM)
Peak Effects: 20 minutes (IV), 30–60 minutes (IM)
Duration: 2–7 hours
Half-Life: 1–7 hours

Indications

Morphine is used for severe pain associated with myocardial infarction, kidney stones, and so forth and pulmonary edema either with or without associated pain.

Contraindications

Morphine should not be used in patients who are volume depleted or severely hypotensive because of the hemodynamic effects described earlier. Morphine should not be administered to any patient with a history of hypersensitivity to the drug or to patients with undiagnosed head injury or abdominal pain.

Precautions

Morphine is a narcotic derivative of opium. It has a high tendency for addiction and abuse and is thus covered under the Controlled Substances Act of 1970. It is classified as a Schedule II drug. Consequently, there are special considerations involved in the handling of the drug. Many emergency medical services (EMS) have opted to use the synthetic analgesics, including nalbuphine and pentazocine, instead of morphine and meperidine because of these problems. Morphine causes severe respiratory depression in high doses. This is especially true in patients who already have some form of respiratory impairment. The narcotic antagonist naloxone (Narcan) should be readily available whenever morphine is administered.

Side Effects

Morphine can cause nausea, vomiting, abdominal cramps, blurred vision, constricted pupils, altered mental status, headache, and respiratory depression.

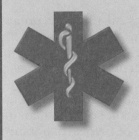

CASE PRESENTATION

At 1300 hours an ALS unit is dispatched to a mobile home park to aid a 61-year-old male complaining of chest pain. The patient is conscious and breathing.

On arrival paramedics are met at the door by the patient's wife. She states that she and her husband had attended church. During the service, he began to feel short of breath. She noticed that he was sweating heavily and appeared pale. She drove him home. The patient took two nitroglycerin sprays (0.4 mg) with no relief. Initially, he would not let her call the ambulance. Finally, he agreed that she could call the ambulance.

As paramedics approach the patient, they see a man sitting in a reclining chair. The patient appears in obvious distress.

On Examination

CNS:	The patient is conscious, alert, and oriented × 4; appears in obvious distress
Resp:	Respirations are 24 and shallow; lung sounds clear bilaterally; trachea is midline; no signs of trauma
CVS:	Carotid and radial pulses are present and weak; skin is pale, cool, and diaphoretic
ABD:	Soft and nontender
Muscl/Skel:	Patient able to move extremities on command; no weaknesses to hand grip

Vital Signs

Pulse:	96/min, regular, weak	
Resp:	24/min, shallow	
BP:	144/94 mmHg	
SpO$_2$:	88 percent	
ECG:	Regular sinus rhythm with ST elevation	
Hx:	**P**	No provoking factors
	Q	Squeezing pain
	R	Radiating to left shoulder and jaw
	S	8/10, worst pain ever
	T	Started suddenly about 2 hours ago
Past Hx:	The patient's wife states that her husband has had several episodes of chest pain in the past month but has not seen his doctor during that time. He was diagnosed with angina 2 years ago. He has nitroglycerin spray, which he has used more often this month than ever in the past. Nitroglycerin is the patient's only prescription home medication. The patient has no recent history of operations, ulcers, or hypertension.	

Treatment

Oxygen was administered by nonrebreather mask at 12 lpm and tolerated by the patient. The patient was hooked up to the ECG monitor, and a regular sinus rhythm with ST elevation was noted. The ST elevation was confirmed in MCL leads 1 and 6. An intravenous line with an 18-gauge catheter was established and run TKO. Paramedics administered nitroglycerin spray (0.4 mg) from their drug kit. The patient stated that the pain was not relieved by the oxygen or the nitroglycerin. The base hospital ordered 2.5 mg of morphine IV. The morphine was given, and transport to the hospital was started. En route the patient stated that the chest pain was 6/10 and a second dose of 2.5 mg of morphine was given, with moderate relief. A second 18-gauge IV was started and run TKO. ASA 325 mg was given by mouth. The patient stated the pain was now 2/10. He was pale, cool, and diaphoretic but appeared less anxious. The base hospital was contacted and advised of the patient findings. The base hospital physician agreed with the findings of the paramedics and prepared to follow through with the fibrinolytic protocol on the patient's arrival at the hospital pending evaluation of a 12-lead ECG.

Interactions

The CNS depression associated with morphine can be enhanced when administered with antihistamines, antiemetics, sedatives, hypnotics, barbiturates, and alcohol.

Dosage

There are many different approaches to the administration of morphine. An initial dose in the range of 2 to 10 mg intravenously is standard. This dose can be augmented with additional doses of 2 mg every few minutes and can be continued until the pain is relieved or until signs of respiratory depression occur.

To attain desired effects, IM injection usually requires 5 to 15 mg based on the patient's weight. However, morphine is routinely given intravenously in emergency medicine and is often administered with an antiemetic agent such as promethazine (Phenergan) to help prevent the nausea and vomiting that often accompany morphine administration. The antiemetics also tend to potentiate morphine's effects. Morphine can also be given intramuscularly and subcutaneously.

NITROUS OXIDE (NITRONOX, ENTONOX)

Class: Analgesic and anesthetic gas

Description

Nitronox is a blended mixture of 50 percent nitrous oxide and 50 percent oxygen that has potent analgesic effects. The Entonox unit consists of one tank that contains both nitrous oxide and oxygen. The Entonox tank must be shaken to mix the gases prior to use.

Mechanism of Action

Nitrous oxide is a CNS depressant with analgesic properties. In the prehospital setting it is delivered in a fixed mixture of 50 percent nitrous oxide and 50 percent oxygen. When inhaled, it has potent analgesic effects. These effects quickly dissipate, however, within 2 to 5 minutes after cessation of administration. The Nitronox unit consists of one oxygen and one nitrous oxide cylinder. The gases are fed into a blender that combines them at the appropriate concentration. The mixture is then delivered to a modified demand valve for administration to the patient. Nitronox must be self-administered. It is effective in treating many varieties of pain encountered in the prehospital setting including pain from many types of trauma. The high concentration of oxygen delivered along with the nitrous oxide will increase the oxygen tension in the blood, thus reducing hypoxia.

Pharmacokinetics

Onset: 2–5 minutes
Peak Effect: 205 minutes
Duration: 2–5 minutes
Half-Life: Unknown

Indications

Nitrous oxide is used for pain of musculoskeletal origin (particularly fractures), burns, suspected ischemic chest pain, and states of severe anxiety including hyperventilation.

Contraindications

Nitronox should not be used with any patient who cannot comprehend verbal instructions or who is intoxicated with alcohol or other drugs. It should not be administered to any patient with a head injury who exhibits an altered mental status. Nitronox should not be administered to any patient with COPD because the high concentration of oxygen (50 percent) might result in respiratory depression. Nitrous oxide tends to diffuse into closed spaces more readily than either carbon dioxide or oxygen. Many COPD patients have air-containing blebs in their lungs, and nitrous oxide can concentrate in these blebs causing them to swell. Swollen blebs may rupture, causing a pneumothorax.

Nitronox should not be administered to patients with a thoracic injury suspicious of pneumothorax, because the gas may accumulate in the pneumothorax, increasing its size. Also, patients with severe abdominal pain and distension, suggestive of bowel obstruction, should not receive Nitronox. Nitrous oxide can concentrate in pockets of an obstructed bowel, possibly leading to rupture.

Precautions

Nitronox should only be used in areas that are well ventilated. When the gas is used in the patient compartment of an ambulance, it is recommended that a scavenging system be in place. Nitrous oxide exists in a liquid state inside the gas cylinder. Heat present in the air, the cylinder wall, or the various regulators and lines causes the liquid to vaporize. This vaporization process makes the cylinder tank and lines cool to touch. Following prolonged use, frost may develop on the cylinder, regulator, or lines. In very cold environments, generally less than 21°F (6°C), the liquid may be slow to vaporize, and administration may be impossible.

Side Effects

The nitrous oxide–oxygen mixture can cause dizziness, light-headedness, altered mental status, hallucinations, nausea, and vomiting.

Interactions

Nitrous oxide can potentiate the effects of other central nervous system depressants such as narcotics, sedatives, hypnotics, and alcohol.

Dosage

Nitronox should only be self-administered. Continuous administration may take place until the pain is significantly relieved or the patient drops the mask. The patient care record should document the duration of drug administration.

DIURETICS

One of the most common cardiovascular emergencies that emergency personnel are called on to treat is congestive heart failure. Congestive heart failure occurs when the heart loses its ability to pump blood effectively. When this occurs, the venous vessels leading to the heart become engorged. Failure of the left side of the heart causes a buildup of blood in the pulmonary circulation. Failure of the right side of the heart results in congestion of the peripheral circulation, which usually manifests as peripheral edema. Common signs of right heart failure include jugular venous distension, ascites, and pedal (ankle or pretibial) edema.

In the treatment of congestive heart failure, the primary objectives are to increase the cardiac output and to reduce pulmonary and peripheral edema. Although the inotropic effects of digitalis preparations will increase cardiac output, the rate of onset is relatively slow, making this drug less than ideal in acute pulmonary edema. In acute heart failure the most effective therapy is to reduce venous filling pressure. Venous filling pressure can be reduced mechanically by applying rotating tourniquets, which are placed on three of the extremities to decrease venous return. Phlebotomy (drawing blood out of the circulatory system) can also be employed. The preferred method, however, is the administration of potent diuretics.

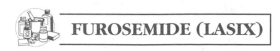 **FUROSEMIDE (LASIX)**

Class: Diuretic

Description

Furosemide is a potent diuretic that inhibits sodium and chloride reabsorption in the kidneys and causes venous dilation.

Mechanism of Action

Furosemide is a loop diuretic that inhibits the reabsorption of both sodium and chloride in the kidneys. It is extremely useful in the treatment of congestive heart failure and pulmonary edema. The effects of furosemide are twofold. First, following administration furosemide causes venous dilation. This effect usually occurs within 5 minutes and causes a reduction in preload, thus decreasing cardiac work. The second effect of furosemide is the diuretic effect, which begins 5 to 15 minutes after administration.

Pharmacokinetics

Onset: 5–10 minutes (vasodilation), 5–30 minutes (diuresis)
Peak Effects: 30 minutes (vasodilation), 20–60 minutes (diuresis)
Duration: 2 hours (vasodilation), 6 hours (diuresis)
Half-Life: 30 minutes

Indications

Furosemide is used in congestive heart failure and pulmonary edema.

Contraindications

Usage in pregnancy should be limited to life-threatening situations in which the benefits of furosemide outweigh the risks. Furosemide has been known to cause fetal abnormalities. It should not be administered to patients with a known allergy to the sulfa class of medications.

Precautions

Dehydration, electrolyte depletion, and hypotension can result from excessive doses of potent diuretics. Thus, blood pressure should be frequently monitored when furosemide is administered. Furosemide should be protected from light.

Side Effects

Furosemide can cause headache, dizziness, hypotension, volume depletion, potassium depletion, dysrhythmias, diarrhea, nausea, and vomiting.

Interactions

Furosemide should not be administered in the same line as amrinone (Inocor) because a chemical reaction can occur between the two, causing the formation of a precipitate in the intravenous line. Administration of furosemide with other diuretics can lead to severe volume depletion and electrolyte imbalance.

Dosage

The standard dosage of furosemide is 40 mg given by slow IV push in patients already on chronic oral furosemide therapy and 20 mg intravenously in patients who are not taking the drug orally on a regular basis. Dosages as high as 80 to 120 mg intravenously may be indicated in severe cases. Furosemide should be given intravenously in emergency situations.

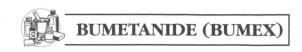

BUMETANIDE (BUMEX)

Class: Diuretic

Description

Bumetanide is a potent diuretic with a rapid rate of onset and a short duration of action.

Mechanism of Action

Like furosemide, bumetanide is a loop diuretic that inhibits the reabsorption of sodium chloride in the kidneys and thus causes a net diuresis; 1 mg of bumetanide has the diuretic potency of 40 mg of furosemide.

Pharmacokinetics

Onset: 1–2 minutes
Peak Effects: 15–30 minutes
Duration: 3.5–4.0 hours
Half-Life: 60–90 minutes

Indications

Bumetanide is used in congestive heart failure and pulmonary edema.

Contraindications

Usage in pregnancy should be limited to life-threatening situations in which the benefits of using bumetanide outweigh the risks.

Precautions

Dehydration and electrolyte depletion can result from excessive doses of potent diuretics. Patients who have experienced allergic reactions to furosemide have not experienced those same reactions when administered bumetanide, which suggests that this drug may be used in patients with furosemide allergy who are in need of rapid diuresis.

Side Effects

Bumetanide can cause muscle cramps, dizziness, hypotension, headache, nausea, and vomiting.

Interactions

Bumetanide can potentiate the effects of the various antihypertensive agents and should be used with caution in patients taking these agents.

Dosage

The usual initial dose of bumetanide is 0.5 to 1.0 mg given during a period of 1 to 2 minutes. A second or third dose can be administered at 2- to 3-hour intervals if required. The total daily dosage should not exceed 10 mg.

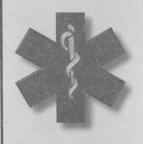

CASE PRESENTATION

Paramedics are called at 0800 hours to a residence to help a woman having difficulty breathing. Dispatch states that the woman is conscious and breathing. On arrival paramedics find a 71-year-old female sitting in a recliner in the living room. She is in severe respiratory distress. Paramedics immediately place the chair into the upright position.

On Examination

CNS:	The patient is conscious, alert, and oriented × 4; appears in obvious respiratory distress and is very restless
Resp:	Respirations are 40 and shallow; lung sounds are diminished bilaterally with loud crackles audible; two- to three-word dyspnea; trachea is midline; no signs of trauma
CVS:	Carotid and radial pulses are weak and regular; skin is pale, lips are blue, and the patient is cool and diaphoretic to touch
ABD:	Soft and nontender
Muscl/Skel:	Patient able to move extremities on command; no weaknesses to hand grip

Vital Signs

Pulse:	120/min, regular, weak
Resp:	40/min, shallow, bilateral loud crackles
BP:	180/108 mmHg
SpO$_2$:	80 percent
ECG:	Sinus tachycardia
Hx:	The patient's husband states that his wife has been complaining of mild SOB for the past 2 days. She has not been able to lie down to sleep because it increases the difficulty of breathing. Therefore she has been sitting in the recliner to sleep. This morning her breathing is worse. She is having difficulty speaking now. He was not sure what to do and finally called the ambulance.
Past Hx:	The patient has a history of congestive heart failure and is currently taking Lasix 20 mg twice per day, Slo-K (potassium), and digoxin.

Treatment

Oxygen was administered by nonrebreather mask at 15 lpm and not well tolerated by the patient. An IV of normal saline was initiated and run TKO. The patient was hooked up to the ECG monitor, and a sinus tachycardia was noted. Nitroglycerin spray was administered, with no relief. Following the nitrospray, paramedics administered 2.5 mg of morphine followed by 80 mg of Lasix (double the patient's home daily dose of Lasix as per their standing orders). Paramedics attempted to assist the patient's respirations with a bag-valve-mask device, but the patient became anxious and combative. The nonrebreather mask was placed back on the patient. The patient did not experience any improvement from the nitroglycerin spray but seemed more relaxed after administration of morphine. En route the patient was treated with two more doses of nitroglycerin spray, 5 minutes apart, and the patient began to experience some relief of her SOB. She was able to speak short sentences and was no longer cyanotic on arrival at the hospital. At the hospital the patient was started on intravenous nitroglycerin and was given another 80 mg of Lasix, with significant improvement.

Bumetanide injection can be given by either the IV or intramuscular route. In the emergency setting, the IV route is preferred.

NATRIURETIC PEPTIDES

Natriuretic peptides are a group of naturally occurring substances that counteract the effects of the renin–angiotensin system. Thus, they cause vasodilation, stimulating the kidneys to increase sodium excretion (natriuresis) and water loss. They appear to be effective in the management of congestive heart failure because they decrease preload and promote sodium and water loss.

Three types of natriuretic peptides have been identified:

- *Atrial natriuretic peptide (ANP)*. ANP is produced in the atria. The identification of ANP was the first indication that the heart also has some endocrine functions.
- *Brain natriuretic peptide (BNP)*. BNP is synthesized in the ventricles but named BNP as is was first identified in the porcine brain.
- *C-type natriuretic peptide (CNP)*. CNP is produced in the brain.

Both ANP and BNP are released in response to atrial and ventricular stretch, respectively. They cause vasorelaxation, inhibition of aldosterone secretion in the adrenal cortex, and inhibition of renin secretion in the kidney. Both ANP and BNP will cause natriuresis and a reduction in intravascular volume. These effects are amplified by antagonism of antidiuretic hormone (ADH). The physiological effects of CNP are different from those of ANP and BNP. CNP has a hypotensive effect, but no significant diuretic or natriuretic actions.

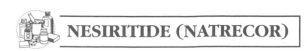

NESIRITIDE (NATRECOR)

Class: Natriuretic peptide

Description

Nesiritide is a genetically engineered form of a naturally occurring substance called B-type (brain) natriuretic peptide (hBPN). It represents a new class of medications.

Mechanism of Action

Nesiritide causes vasodilation through relaxation of vascular smooth muscle. It also causes diuresis and loss of sodium in the kidney (natriuretic effect).

Pharmacokinetics

Onset: 15 minutes
Peak Effects: Varies
Duration: >60 hours (dose related)
Half-Life: 18 minutes

Indications

Nesiritide is used for the treatment of acutely decompensated congestive heart failure (CHF) in patients who have dyspnea at rest or with minimal physical activity.

Contraindications

Nesiritide should not be administered to people with known hypersensitivity to the drug. It should not be used in patients who have a blood pressure of <90 mmHg and cardiogenic shock. It should not be used in patients with CHF secondary to valvular heart disease.

Precautions

Use with caution in patients receiving angiotensin-converting enzyme inhibitors. Safety in pediatrics and pregnancy has not been established. All physiological monitors should be in place prior to administering nesiritide.

Side Effects

Nesiritide has been associated with headaches, back pain, catheter pain, fever, injection site pain, and leg cramps. Hypotension has been reported as well as dysrhythmias.

Interactions

None reported.

Dosage

Adult dose. Initial bolus of 2 mcg/kg over 60 seconds followed by continuous infusion of 0.01 mcg/kg/min. Blood pressure must be constantly monitored.
Pediatric dose. Not indicated.

ANTIANGINAL AGENTS

A common manifestation of advanced cardiovascular disease is angina pectoris, which results from a narrowing of the coronary arteries due to the buildup of atherosclerotic plaques, or coronary artery vasospasm. In exercise and other stressful situations, the amount of blood that can be carried by the coronary arteries may not be sufficient to meet the oxygen demands of the myocardium. This results in myocardial hypoxia, causing the classic pain syndrome called angina pectoris. Sublingual nitroglycerin usually gives immediate relief by dilating the coronary arteries and decreasing cardiac work. In recent years there have been trials in which nitroglycerin has been administered to patients suffering myocardial infarction in the hope of decreasing the extent of myocardial damage. Nitroglycerin is often administered to patients complaining of chest pain to rule out angina as the cause. When cardiac pain is not relieved by nitroglycerin, morphine and other potent analgesics are administered.

Nitroglycerin is usually administered sublingually (SL). Recently, however, it has been given intravenously in certain cases of unstable angina and acute myocardial infarction.

Calcium-ion *antagonists,* such as nifedipine (Procardia), have proved effective in the management of angina, especially when there is coronary artery vasospasm.

 ## NITROGLYCERIN (NITROSTAT)

Class: Nitrate

Description

Nitroglycerin is a potent smooth muscle relaxant used in the treatment of angina pectoris.

Mechanism of Action

Nitroglycerin is a rapid smooth muscle relaxant that reduces cardiac work and, to a lesser degree, dilates the coronary arteries. This results in increased coronary blood flow and improved perfusion of the ischemic myocardium. Relief of ischemia causes reduction and alleviation of chest pain. Pain relief following nitroglycerin administration usually occurs within 1 to 2 minutes, and therapeutic effects can be observed up to 30 minutes later. Nitroglycerin also causes vasodilation, which decreases preload; decreased preload leads to decreased cardiac work. This feature, in conjunction with coronary vasodilation, reverses the effects of angina pectoris.

Pharmacokinetics

Onset: 1–3 minutes (SL)
Peak Effects: 5–10 minutes (SL)
Duration: 20–30 minutes (SL)
Half-Life: 1–4 minutes

Indications

Nitroglycerin is used for chest pain associated with angina pectoris, chest pain associated with acute myocardial infarction, and acute pulmonary edema (unless accompanied by hypotension).

Contraindications

Nitroglycerin is contraindicated in patients who are hypotensive or who may have increased intracranial pressure. It should not be administered to patients in shock.

Precautions

Patients taking nitroglycerin may develop a tolerance for the drug, which necessitates increasing the dose. Headache is a common side effect of nitroglycerin administration and results from vasodilation of cerebral vessels. Nitroglycerin deteriorates quite rapidly once the bottle is opened. When a bottle of nitroglycerin is opened, it should be dated. Nitroglycerin should also be protected from light. Blood pressure and the other vital signs should always be monitored during nitroglycerin administration.

Side Effects

Nitroglycerin can cause headache, dizziness, weakness, tachycardia, hypotension, orthostasis, skin rash, dry mouth, nausea, and vomiting.

Interactions

Nitroglycerin can cause severe hypotension when administered to patients who have recently ingested alcohol. It can cause orthostatic hypotension when used in conjunction with beta-blockers.

Dosage

One tablet (0.4 mg) is administered sublingually for routine angina pectoris. This dose can be repeated in 3 to 5 minutes as required. Usually, more than three tablets should not be administered in the prehospital setting. Nitroglycerin should be administered sublingually. Care should be taken to ensure that it is not swallowed. IV nitroglycerin is used in the emergency department and intensive care units, but the sublingual route is adequate for most prehospital situations. Nitroglycerin is also available in patches and in ointment form for transdermal administration.

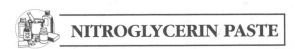 **NITROGLYCERIN PASTE**

Class: Nitrate

Description

Nitroglycerin paste contains a 2 percent solution of nitroglycerin in a special absorbent paste. When placed on the skin, nitroglycerin is absorbed into the systemic circulation. In many cases it may be preferred over nitroglycerin tablets because of its longer duration of action.

Pharmacokinetics

    Onset: 30 minutes (topical)
    Peak-Effects: Varies
    Duration: 3–6 hours (topical)
    Half-Life: 1–4 minutes

Mechanism of Action

Nitroglycerin is a rapid smooth muscle relaxant that reduces cardiac work and, to a lesser degree, dilates the coronary arteries. This results in increased coronary blood flow and improved perfusion of the ischemic myocardium. Relief of ischemia causes reduction and alleviation of chest pain. Pain relief following transcutaneous nitroglycerin administration usually occurs within 5 to 10 minutes, and therapeutic effects can be observed up to 30 minutes later. Nitroglycerin also causes vasodilation, which decreases preload; decreased preload leads to decreased cardiac work. This feature, in conjunction with coronary vasodilation, reverses the effects of angina pectoris.

Indications

Nitroglycerin paste is used for chest pain associated with angina pectoris and chest pain associated with acute myocardial infarction.

Contraindications

Nitroglycerin paste is contraindicated in patients with increased intracranial pressure. It should not be administered to patients who are hypotensive or in shock.

Precautions

Patients taking the drug routinely may develop a tolerance and require an increased dose. Headache is a common side effect of nitroglycerin administration and occurs as a result of vasodilation of the cerebral vessels.

Postural syncope sometimes occurs following the administration of nitroglycerin; it should be anticipated and the patient kept supine when possible. It is important to monitor blood pressure constantly.

Side Effects

Nitroglycerin can cause headache, dizziness, weakness, tachycardia, hypotension, orthostasis, skin rash, dry mouth, nausea, and vomiting.

Interactions

Nitroglycerin can cause severe hypotension when administered to patients who have recently ingested alcohol. It can cause orthostatic hypotension when used in conjunction with beta-blockers.

Dosage

Generally 1/2 to 1 inch (1.25 to 2.50 cm) of the Nitro-Bid Ointment is applied. Measuring applicators are supplied.

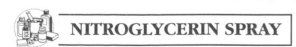

NITROGLYCERIN SPRAY

Class: Nitrate

Description

Nitroglycerin spray is a special preparation of nitroglycerin in an aerosol form that delivers precisely 0.4 mg of nitroglycerin per spray.

Mechanism of Action

Nitroglycerin is a rapid smooth muscle relaxant that reduces cardiac work and, to a lesser degree, dilates the coronary arteries. This results in increased coronary blood flow and improved perfusion of the ischemic myocardium. Relief of ischemia causes reduction and alleviation of chest pain. Pain relief following nitroglycerin administration usually occurs within 1 to 2 minutes, and peak effects occur within 4 minutes. Therapeutic effects can be observed up to 30 minutes later. Nitroglycerin also causes vasodilation, which decreases preload; decreased preload leads to decreased cardiac work. This feature, in conjunction with coronary vasodilation, reverses the effects of angina pectoris.

Pharmacokinetics

Onset: 1–3 minutes (SL)
Peak Effects: 5–10 minutes (SL)
Duration: 20–30 minutes (SL)
Half-Life: 1–4 minutes

Indications

Nitroglycerin spray is used for chest pain associated with angina pectoris and chest pain associated with acute myocardial infarction.

Contraindications

Nitroglycerin is contraindicated in patients who are hypotensive, who are in shock, or who may have increased intracranial pressure.

Precautions

Patients taking nitroglycerin routinely may develop a tolerance for the drug. Headache is a common side effect of nitroglycerin administration and results from dilation of cerebral blood vessels. This effect should be anticipated. The blood pressure should be monitored during nitroglycerin therapy.

Side Effects

Nitroglycerin can cause headache, dizziness, weakness, tachycardia, hypotension, orthostasis, skin rash, dry mouth, nausea, and vomiting.

Interactions

Nitroglycerin can cause severe hypotension when administered to patients who have recently ingested alcohol. It can cause orthostatic hypotension when used in conjunction with beta-blockers.

Dosage

One spray (0.4 mg) should be sprayed under the tongue at the onset of an attack of angina. No more than three sprays are recommended in a 25-minute period. (The spray should not be inhaled.) Nitroglycerin spray should be applied to the sublingual mucous membranes in the manner described earlier for nitroglycerin tablets (Nitrostat).

A dangerously elevated blood pressure is a hypertensive emergency. A hypertensive crisis is defined as a sudden increase in the systolic and diastolic blood pressure, causing a functional disturbance of the central nervous system, the heart, or the kidneys. Hypertensive emergencies call for prompt and efficient care by prehospital providers.

Hypertensive emergencies are often divided into two categories: hypertensive emergencies and hypertensive urgencies. A hypertensive emergency is a situation in which the blood pressure must be lowered within 1 hour. A hypertensive urgency is a situation in which the blood pressure should be lowered within 24 hours. Hypertensive emergencies develop when the blood pressure exceeds 130 mmHg diastolic pressure (with or without symptoms) or any elevated blood pressure associated with end-organ symptoms. End-organ symptoms include chest pain, dyspnea, altered mental status, seizures, stroke, nosebleed, or hypertensive encephalopathy. In many cases the emergency develops not from the absolute blood pressure value but from how rapid the value is achieved. Rapid elevations in blood pressure are poorly tolerated by the body and more apt to cause end-organ symptoms.

Hypertensive encephalopathy is the most devastating complication of hypertension. Signs and symptoms include severe headache, nausea and vomiting, and an altered mental state. The altered mental state can range from lethargy or confusion to coma. Neurological symptoms, including blindness, inability to speak, muscle twitches, weakness, or paralysis, may be present as well. The treatment is to lower blood pressure as rapidly and as safely as possible.

Hypertension is a chronic disease. An elevated blood pressure is not uncommon in the emergency setting. Elevated blood pressure should only be treated if there are significant end-organ changes (i.e., altered mental status). In cases where the blood pressure must be lowered, labetalol or sodium nitroprusside should be used. The drug should be initiated at a low dose and increased until the blood pressure is controlled. Nifedipine (Procardia) was used for many years in the acute treatment of hypertensive emergencies. However, complications (i.e., stroke) were reported and the popular press published several articles on the adverse effects of nifedipine. Because of this, it is no longer used in this setting.

NIFEDIPINE (PROCARDIA, ADALAT)

Class: Calcium channel blocker

Description

Nifedipine is a calcium channel blocker that is used in the treatment of hypertension.

Mechanism of Action

Nifedipine causes relaxation of the smooth muscles that encircle the peripheral blood vessels, principally the arterioles. This relaxation results in peripheral vasodilation, a decrease in peripheral vascular resistance, and a decrease in both the systolic and diastolic blood pressure. Nifedipine is also effective in reducing coronary artery spasm in angina. Nifedipine can be used in hypertension associated with pregnancy if hydralazine is not available.

Pharmacokinetics

Onset: 1–5 minutes (SL), 5–20 minutes [by mouth (PO)]
Peak Effects: 20–30 minutes (SL), 1–2 hours (PO)
Duration: 2–4 hours
Half-Life: 2–5 hours

Indications

Nifedipine is used in hypertension and angina pectoris.

Contraindications

Nifedipine is contraindicated in patients with known hypersensitivity to the drug. It should not be administered to patients who are hypotensive.

Precautions

Nifedipine can cause a significant drop in blood pressure. Thus, blood pressure should be frequently monitored. Nifedipine should be used with caution in patients with heart failure. It should not be administered to patients receiving IV β-blockers.

Side Effects

Nifedepine can cause nausea, vomiting, dizziness, headache, bradycardia, heart block, hypotension, and asystole.

Interactions

Nifedepine should not be administered to patients receiving intravenous β-blockers because of an increased risk of congestive heart failure, bradycardia, and asystole.

Dosage

Several small puncture holes should be placed in one 10 mg capsule before placing it under the tongue, where it can be absorbed. Alternatively, the capsule can be bitten by the patient and swallowed with approximately the same rate of onset. In severe hypertension the medical control physician may order an initial dose of 20 mg. Nifedipine should only be administered orally or sublingually, as described earlier.

SODIUM NITROPRUSSIDE (NITROPRESS, NIPRIDE)

Class: Antihypertensive and vasodilator

Description

Sodium nitroprusside is a potent vasodilating agent used in the management of hypertensive crisis when a prompt reduction in blood pressure is required.

Mechanism of Action

Sodium nitroprusside acts by dilating both peripheral arteries and peripheral veins. This reduction in peripheral vascular resistance results in an immediate reduction in blood pressure, which is generally proportional to the rate of drug administration. Sodium nitroprusside administration is usually accompanied by an increase in heart rate.

Although not approved for this use, sodium nitroprusside is occasionally used in the management of severe congestive heart failure. The dilation of the peripheral veins results in decreased blood return to the heart (preload). In addition, the dilation of the peripheral arteries reduces the pressure against which the heart has to pump (afterload). This results in a net increase in cardiac output in patients with severe congestive heart failure (see Figure 7–10).

Because sodium nitroprusside is such a potent agent, the blood pressure, pulse rate, respiratory status, and EKG should be constantly monitored during drug administration.

Pharmacokinetics

Onset: <1 minute
Peak Effects: 1–5 minutes
Duration: 1–10 minutes
Half-Life: 2.7–7.0 days

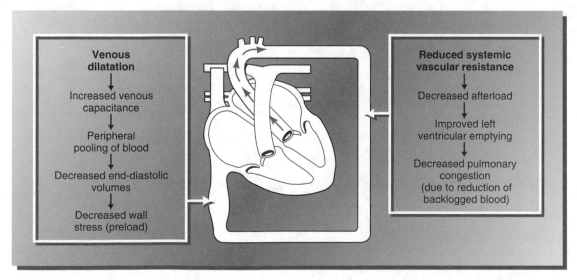

FIGURE 7–10 Actions of sodium nitroprusside.

Indication

Hypertensive crisis in which a prompt reduction in blood pressure is essential.

Contraindications

None when used in the management of life-threatening hypertensive crisis.

Precautions

Once the sodium nitroprusside infusion is prepared, it should be immediately wrapped in an opaque material, usually aluminum foil, to protect it from light. Once exposed to light, the drug is quickly inactivated. Sodium nitroprusside should not be used in children or pregnant women in the prehospital setting. The dosage should be reduced somewhat in elderly patients. The constant monitoring of blood pressure and pulse is essential throughout sodium nitroprusside administration.

Side Effects

Sodium nitroprusside can cause dizziness, headache, hypotension, chest pain, dyspnea, palpitations, nausea, and vomiting.

Interactions

The effects of sodium nitroprusside can be potentiated when administered with other antihypertensive agents.

Dosage

The standard dose is 50 mg of sodium nitroprusside diluted in 500 mL of D_5W. This will give a concentration of 100 μg/mL. The initial dose should be 0.5 μg/kg/min (see Figure 7–11). The typical dosage range is from 0.5 to 8.0 μg/kg/min. Sodium nitroprusside should only be diluted in D_5W or normal saline and administered by slow IV infusion using a minidrip ad-

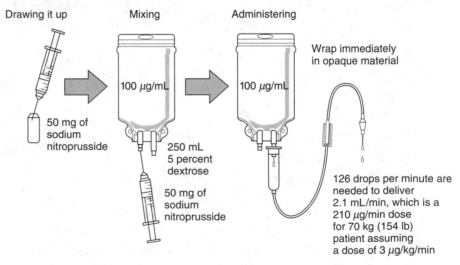

FIGURE 7–11 Preparation of sodium nitroprusside infusion.

ministration set (preferably through an IV pump). *This medication should never be given by IV bolus.*

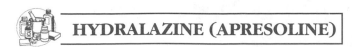

HYDRALAZINE (APRESOLINE)

Class: Antihypertensive and vasodilator

Description

Hydralazine is a potent vasodilating agent used to lower blood pressure in cases of hypertensive crisis.

Mechanism of Action

Hydralazine, like sodium nitroprusside, relaxes vascular smooth muscle, primarily in the arterial system, thus causing decreased arterial pressure (diastolic greater than systolic), decreased peripheral resistance, and increased cardiac output. Hydralazine causes postural hypotension to a lesser degree than does sodium nitroprusside. The effects of hydralazine are usually seen within 5 to 10 minutes after the initiation of therapy.

Pharmacokinetics

Onset: 5–15 minutes (IV), 10–40 minutes (IM)
Peak Effects: <80 minutes
Duration: 2–6 hours
Half-Life: 2–8 hours

Indications

Hydralazine is used in hypertensive crisis in which a prompt reduction in blood pressure is required and hypertension complicating pregnancy (preeclampsia).

Contraindications

Hydralazine should not be administered to patients with a known history of hypersensitivity to the drug, coronary artery disease, or rheumatic heart disease involving the mitral valve.

Precautions

The administration of hydralazine may cause angina pectoris or ECG changes because of the increased cardiac output. This drug should not be used in the prehospital phase of emergency medical care of children because of limited experience with the drug in these cases. The blood pressure, pulse rate, respiratory status, and ECG should be monitored at all times during hydralazine therapy. Headache, nausea, and vomiting have been known to occur following hydralazine therapy and should be expected.

Side Effects

Hydralazine can cause headache, dizziness, altered mental status, tachycardia, dysrhythmias, orthostasis, chest pain, nausea, and vomiting.

Interactions

The effects of hydralazine can be potentiated when administered with other antihypertensive agents.

Dosage

The usual dosage of hydralazine in the management of hypertensive crisis is 20 to 40 mg given by slow IV bolus. This dose can be repeated in 4 to 6 hours if required. If an IV line cannot be established, then the same dosage of the drug can be given by intramuscular injection. The blood pressure and ECG should be continuously monitored. Parenteral hydralazine should be administered by slow IV bolus. When necessary, however, the drug can be administered by intramuscular injection.

OTHER CARDIOVASCULAR DRUGS

The following agent does not readily fit into the classes of drugs discussed thus far.

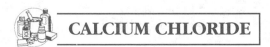

CALCIUM CHLORIDE

Class: Calcium supplement

Description

Calcium chloride provides elemental calcium in the form of the cation (Ca^{2+}). Calcium is required for many physiological activities.

Mechanism of Action

Calcium chloride replaces calcium in cases of hypocalcemia. Calcium chloride causes a significant increase in the myocardial contractile force and appears to increase ventricular automaticity. Although frequently used for many years in the management of cardiac arrest, especially that resulting from asystole and electromechanical dissociation, recent studies have presented data that seriously question the role of calcium chloride, even in these situations. Calcium chloride is an antidote for magnesium sulfate and can minimize some of the side effects of calcium channel blocker usage.

Pharmacokinetics

Onset: Immediate
Peak Effects: Unknown
Duration: Varies
Half-Life: Not applicable

Indications

Calcium chloride is used in acute hyperkalemia (elevated potassium), acute hypocalcemia (decreased calcium), and calcium channel blocker toxicity (nifedipine, verapamil, and diltiazem).

Contraindications

Caution is warranted when calcium chloride is administered to patients receiving digitalis, because it may precipitate digitalis toxicity.

Precautions

It is extremely important to flush the IV line between administrations of calcium chloride and sodium bicarbonate to avoid precipitation. Calcium chloride can cause tissue necrosis at the injection site. It should always be administered through an IV that is patent and running well.

Side Effects

Calcium chloride can cause bradycardia, dysrhythmias, syncope, nausea, vomiting, and cardiac arrest.

Interactions

Calcium chloride will interact with sodium bicarbonate and form a precipitate. In addition, calcium chloride can cause elevated digoxin levels, and possibly digitalis toxicity, when administered to patients receiving digitalis preparations.

Dosage

The standard dose for calcium chloride is 2 to 4 mg/kg intravenously. This dose may be repeated every 10 minutes as required. Calcium chloride should only be given intravenously in the emergency setting.

SUMMARY

All of the medications discussed in this chapter are only of value when used in conjunction with other treatment modalities. Without appropriate cardiopulmonary resuscitation, the medications used in the management of cardiac arrest are not effective. As mentioned, the dosages presented in this chapter are based on nationally accepted regimens. Paramedics should become familiar with the routine dosages and protocols used in their areas.

KEY WORDS

adrenergic receptors. Receptors specific to norepinephrine- and epinephrine-like substances.

adrenergic system. The part of the nervous system that prepares the body to deal with various stresses, whether real or imagined. Also referred to as the sympathetic nervous system.

aerobic metabolism. The process of generating energy with the aid of oxygen.

agonist. A drug or other substance that causes a physiological response.

anaerobic metabolism. The process of generating energy without the aid of oxygen.

antagonist. A drug or other substance that blocks a physiological response or that blocks the action of another drug or substance.

automaticity. The capacity of self-depolarization. Refers to the pacemaker cells of the heart.

catecholamine. A class of hormones that act on the autonomic nervous system. They include epinephrine, norepinephrine, and similar compounds.

cholinergic system. A division of the autonomic nervous system that is responsible for controlling vegetative functions. Also called the parasympathetic nervous system.

chronotrope. A drug or substance that affects the heart rate.

concomitant. Occurring at the same time.

dopaminergic receptor. Receptor in the renal and splanchnic vessels that maintains vasodilation.

dromotrope. A drug or substance that affects the conduction velocity of the heart.

endogenous. Coming from inside the body.

homeostasis. The natural tendency of the body to maintain a relatively constant internal environment.

hypoxic drive. Respiratory control system commonly present in patients with chronic obstructive pulmonary disease whereby respirations are dependent on changes in the concentration of oxygen as opposed to changes in the concentration of carbon dioxide.

inotrope. A drug or substance that affects the contractile force of the heart.

lactic acid. An organic acid normally present in tissue. One form of lactic acid in muscle and blood is a product of the change of the carbohydrates glucose and glycogen to energy during physical exercise.

neurotransmitter. A substance that is released from the axon terminal of a presynaptic neuron on excitation and that travels across the synaptic cleft to either excite or inhibit the target cell. Examples include acetylcholine, norepinephrine, and dopamine.

pheochromocytoma. A tumor of the adrenal gland that causes too much release of two hormones (epinephrine and norepinephrine). Signs include high blood pressure, headache, sweating, high blood sugar level, nausea, vomiting, and fainting spells.

pulse oximetry. An assessment modality that measures the oxygen saturation level of the blood through a noninvasive sensor placed on a finger or earlobe.

retrolental fibroplasia. A disorder caused by giving excess amounts of oxygen to premature infants. A fiber-like tissue forms behind the lens of the eye.

stroke volume. The amount of blood ejected by the heart in one cardiac contraction.

sympathomimetic. A drug or substance that causes effects such as those of the sympathetic nervous system (also called adrenergic).

torsade de pointes. A form of ventricular tachycardia in which the morphology of the QRS appears to change (the axis rotates). It is often drug induced but may be the result of low potassium levels in the blood (hypokalemia) or profound slow heart beat (bradycardia).

Wolff-Parkinson-White syndrome. A disorder of the heart characterized by early contraction of the heart muscle.

8

DRUGS USED IN THE TREATMENT OF RESPIRATORY EMERGENCIES

OBJECTIVES

After completing this chapter, the reader should be able to:

1. Discuss the devices commonly used to administer oxygen in the field.

2. Discuss pulse oximetry and end-tidal carbon dioxide detection and describe the prehospital use of both.

3. Discuss the pathophysiology and prehospital management of asthma and status asthmaticus.

4. Describe and list the indications, contraindications, and dosages for the following beta agonists used in respiratory emergencies: epinephrine 1:1000, albuterol, levalbuterol, racemic epinephrine, terbutaline, isoetharine, metaproterenol, and aminophylline.

5. Describe and list the indications, contraindications, and dosages for the following anticholinergics: atropine and ipratropium.

6. Describe and list the indications, contraindications, and dosages for magnesium sulfate.

7. Describe and list the indications, contraindications, and dosages for the following corticosteroids: methylprednisolone and hydrocortisone.

8. Discuss the indications and considerations in the use of neuromuscular blockers.

9. Describe and list the indications, contraindications, and dosages for the following medications used as neuromuscular-blocking agents: succinylcholine, pancuronium, vecuronium, atricurium, and rocuronium.

10. Discuss the role of induction agents in rapid-sequence induction and detail the pharmacology of diazepam, midazolam, ketamine, and etomidate.

11. List the steps in performing rapid-sequence induction (RSI) intubation.

12. List the steps in performing pharmacologically-assisted intubation (PAI).

INTRODUCTION

Oxygen is the most important drug for use in the management of respiratory emergencies. In addition to oxygen, however, several pharmacological agents have proved quite effective in relieving respiratory distress. In this chapter medications commonly used in the prehospital treatment of respiratory emergencies are discussed. These medications include the following:

Gases

Oxygen

Beta Agonists

Epinephrine 1:1000

Albuterol/salbutamol (Proventil, Ventolin)

Levalbuterol (Xopenex)

Racemic epinephrine (microNefrin, Vaponefron)

Terbutaline (Brethine, Bricanyl)

Isoetharine (Bronkosol)

Metaproterenol (Alupent)

Xanthines

Aminophylline (Somophyllin)

Anticholinergics

Atropine (sulfate)

Ipratropium (Atrovent)

Mineral

Magnesium sulfate

Induction Agents

Diazepam (Valium)

Midazolam (Versed)

Ketamine (Ketalar)

Etomidate (Amidate)

Corticosteroids

Methylprednisolone (Solu-Medrol)

Hydrocortisone (Solu-Cortef)

Neuromuscular Blockers

Succinylcholine (Anectine)

Pancuronium bromide (Pavulon)

Atracurium (Tracrium)

Vecuronium (Norcuron)

Rocuronium bromide (Zemuron)

Sympathomimetics are among the most frequently used agents in the treatment of respiratory emergencies. The principal sympathomimetics include epinephrine, isoetharine, terbutaline, metaproterenol, and albuterol. In treating cardiovascular emergencies it is highly desirable to activate β_1-adrenergic receptors. When treating patients in respiratory distress, however, it is desirable to activate β_2-receptors. Unfortunately, most of the agents that activate β_2-receptors also have some effect on β_1-receptors. When activated, β_1-receptors cause an increase in heart rate and myocardial contractile force, whereas β_2-receptors cause peripheral vasodilation and, most important, bronchodilation. Common side effects of these medications include palpitations, anxiety, and dizziness. Considerable effort has been devoted to isolation of pharmacological agents that act principally on β_2-receptors. Currently, levalbuterol and albuterol are the sympathomimetic agents most frequently used in the prehospital phase of emergency medical care. They are chemically related to epinephrine but tend to be more selective than epinephrine for β_2-receptors.

Another agent used in the management of respiratory emergencies is aminophylline. Aminophylline, chemically unrelated to the catecholamines, belongs to a class of drugs called *xanthines*. A commonly encountered drug within the xanthines class is caffeine. Aminophylline causes relaxation of the bronchiole smooth musculature and bronchodilation.

Although not discussed in detail here, corticosteroids play a major role in the treatment of respiratory diseases. Asthma and many cases of *chronic obstructive pulmonary disease (COPD)* have inflammation as the underlying cause. Although the β-agonists help reverse bronchospasm, they do little for the underlying inflammation. Corticosteroids have a very long rate of onset (1 to 4 hours), and thus their effects are not usually seen in the prehospital setting.

Some systems have added neuromuscular-blocking agents to their paramedic drug lists. These medications are very effective in providing muscle relaxation for endotracheal intubation. However, because they remove a patient's protective reflexes and cause apnea, they should only be used by personnel with experience in their use.

OXYGEN

Oxygen administration is an important aspect of patient care. It is essential in cases that involve suspected *hypoxia* of any cause, chest pain due to myocardial ischemia, asthma, and cardiorespiratory arrest.

Oxygen Administration

Administering oxygen to a hypoxic patient raises his or her oxygen level by increasing the

- Inspired percentage of oxygen
- Oxygen concentration at the alveolar level
- Arterial oxygen levels
- Amount of oxygen delivered to the patient's cells

Oxygen administration decreases hypoxia and reduces the volume of respiration necessary to oxygenate the blood. It also reduces the myocardial work demanded to maintain given arterial oxygen tension.

There are no absolute contraindications to oxygen administration. However, it should be used with caution in premature infants and patients who are prone to carbon dioxide retention (hypoxic drive). It should be administered at lower flow rates with COPD patients (1 to 3 L delivered via nasal cannula). If a patient develops respiratory depression, breathing should be assisted with a bag-valve-mask device. When ventilating via a bag-valve-mask device, 100 percent oxygen is used. When providing oxygen to a premature infant, the mask is held over the face, not directly on it.

Oxygen Devices

Devices commonly used to administer oxygen in the field include the nasal cannula, the simple face mask, the nonrebreather mask, and, to a lesser extent, the Venturi mask.

Nasal Cannula

The *nasal cannula* is a frequently used device that is comfortable and is easily tolerated by the patient. It can deliver oxygen concentrations ranging from 24 to 44 percent. The oxygen flow rates for the nasal cannula vary from 1 to 6 lpm.

Simple Face Mask

The *simple face mask* delivers an oxygen concentration of 40 to 60 percent. Flow rates administered through the simple face mask range from 8 to 12 lpm. No fewer than 6 lpm should be administered through this device, because expired carbon dioxide can accumulate in the mask. Flow rates in excess of 8 lpm are needed to "wash out" any expired carbon dioxide.

The simple face mask provides oxygen to patients who are suffering from moderate hypoxia. Disadvantages include that it may feel confining to the patient, it muffles the patient's speech, and it requires a tight face seal. Because the mask covers the patient's face, it should be used with caution in cases that involve nausea or vomiting. With the pediatric patient, a flow rate of 6 to 8 lpm is generally considered acceptable.

Nonrebreather Mask

When the patient inhales, the 100 percent oxygen contained in the reservoir is drawn into the mask and the patient's respiratory passages. Ambient air is prevented from entering the mask by the rubber flap that closes over the inlet-outlet ports during inspiration. When the patient exhales, the flapper valve is open to allow the expired air an exit. A one-way valve situated between the mask and the reservoir prevents the expired air from entering the reservoir bag.

The *nonrebreather mask* delivers the highest concentration of oxygen. When supplied at a flow rate of 15 lpm, it can deliver an 80 to 100 percent oxygen concentration. No fewer than 8 lpm of oxygen should be administered through this device. Because the nonrebreather mask is a relatively closed system, it restricts the inspiration of ambient air. Therefore, its reservoir bag should not be allowed to deflate totally or be allowed to kink. Otherwise, the patient might suffocate.

The nonrebreather mask is similar to the simple face mask in that it requires a tight seal. A tight seal may be difficult to obtain with some patients because they find the mask confining. This device should be employed with caution in nauseated patients. Its main application lies in the treatment of severely hypoxic patients—those suffering respiratory compromise, shock, acute myocardial infarction, trauma, or carbon monoxide poisoning.

Venturi Mask

With the *Venturi mask,* relatively precise concentrations of oxygen can be provided. This device is not commonly used in prehospital care and is used in the treatment of COPD patients. To control the amount of ambient air taken in by a patient, some Venturi masks are supplied with dial selection, and others come with interchangeable caps. These devices deliver oxygen concentrations of 24, 28, 35, or 40 percent. The liter flow depends on the oxygen concentration desired.

Ventilation

In the field, paramedics are called on in many cases to provide ventilatory support. Situations will range from those that involve apneic patients to less obvious cases in which patients are experiencing depressed respiratory function.

When a patient is unconscious, his or her respiratory center may not function at a satisfactory level. A significant decrease in the patient's rate or depth of breathing will lead to decreased respiratory minute volume, hypercarbia, hypoxia, and a lowered pH. If not corrected, respiratory or cardiac arrest may occur. To achieve effective ventilatory support, an adequate rate and volume of oxygen must be delivered—at least 800 mL of oxygen at a rate of 12 to 20 breaths per minute.

Pulse Oximetry

Pulse oximetry is now widely used in emergency care. The pulse oximeter is a quick and accurate tool that can objectively determine the oxygenation status of the patient. The pulse oximeter provides immediate and continuous evaluation of oxygen delivery to body tissues. It quantifies the effects of interventions including oxygen therapy, medication, suctioning, and ventilatory assistance. In addition, oximetry often detects problems with oxygenation before blood pressure, pulse, and respirations would reveal such a problem. Pulse oximetry, when available, should be used in virtually any patient care situation. In fact, it has been referred to as the fifth vital sign. It should be used during the patient assessment process to determine the patient's baseline value. It should also be used to guide patient care and to monitor the patient's response to paramedic interventions. Normal SpO_2 varies between 95 and 100 percent. Readings between 91 and 94 percent indicate mild hypoxia and warrant further evaluation and supplemental oxygen administration. Readings between 86 and 91 percent indicate moderate hypoxia. These patients should receive 100 percent supplemental oxygen. Readings of 85 percent or lower indicate severe hypoxia and warrant immediate intervention, including the administration of 100 percent oxygen, ventilatory assistance, or both. The goal of therapy is to maintain the SpO_2 in the normal (95 to 99 percent) range.

The incidence of false readings with pulse oximetry is small. When it does occur, the oximeter generates an error signal or a blank screen. Causes of false readings include carbon monoxide poisoning, high-intensity lighting, and certain hemoglobin abnormalities. The absence of a pulse in an extremity will give a false reading. In hypovolemia and in severely anemic patients, the pulse oximetry reading may be misleading. Although the SpO_2 reading may be normal, the total amount of hemoglobin available to carry oxygen may be so markedly decreased that the patient will remain hypoxic at the cellular level.

Pulse oximetry is now an important part of emergency care, including prehospital care. Like the electrocardiogram (ECG) monitor, it provides important information related to the patient. It is important to remember that it is only an additional tool. It does not replace other assessment or monitoring skills. Prehospital care providers cannot depend solely on pulse oximetry reading to guide care; they must always consider and treat the whole patient. The reliability and validity of the pulse oximeter are well documented.

Capnography

Capnography is the measurement of exhaled carbon dioxide concentrations. The devices that make such measurements are called capnometers or end-tidal carbon dioxide ($ETCO_2$) detectors. Their use in prehospital care has increased significantly, most commonly to assess proper placement of an endotracheal tube. The absence of carbon dioxide from the exhaled air strongly indicates that the tube is in the esophagus; its presence indicates proper tracheal placement. Capnography can be used to ensure proper tube placement following insertion and to monitor tube placement during ventilation and cardiopulmonary resuscitation (CPR).

Capnometers are available either as disposable colorimetric devices or as electronic monitors. They are attached either in-line or alongside the endotracheal tube and the ventilation device. A color change in the colorimetric device or a light on the electronic monitor confirms proper tube placement. On the colorimetric device, the low CO_2 content of inspired air makes the device purple, whereas the higher CO_2 content of expired air makes it yellow. Some electronic devices now combine pulse oximetry, $ETCO_2$ detection, blood pressure, pulse rate, respiratory rate, and temperature monitors in one unit.

Although capnography is accurate, the $ETCO_2$ level falls precipitously during cardiac arrest. Therefore, these patients may not cause a color change on the capnometer detector despite proper placement of the endotracheal tube.

Capnography is being used with increasing frequency to monitor nonintubated patients as well. $ETCO_2$ is proportional to pulmonary perfusion and thus, in turn, to systemic perfusion. It can provide important information with regard to patient condition, especially in cases of bronchospastic disease (asthma, COPD) where it can help with early determinations of whether a patient's respiratory status is changing. Likewise, capnography can also monitor perfusion status and provide an early indication of impending shock. As with pulse oximetry, you should use a capnometer only in conjunction with other methods of assessing endotracheal placement. It does not replace actually visualizing the endotracheal tube's passage through the vocal cords.

ASTHMA

Asthma is a common respiratory illness that affects many people. Whereas deaths from other respiratory diseases have been steadily declining, deaths from asthma have significantly increased during the past decade or so. Most of the increased asthma deaths have occurred in patients who are 45 years of age or older. Approximately 50 percent of patients who die from asthma do so before reaching the hospital. Thus, emergency medical service (EMS) personnel are frequently called on to treat patients suffering an asthma attack.

Prompt recognition, followed by appropriate treatment, can significantly improve the patient's condition and enhance chances of survival.

Pathophysiology of Asthma

Asthma is a chronic inflammatory disorder of the airways. In susceptible individuals, this inflammation causes symptoms usually associated with widespread but variable airflow obstruction. The major characteristic of asthma is reversible lower airway obstruction. This obstruction is caused by edema, mucus, and smooth muscle spasm; typically, all three factors are involved. An obstruction narrows the diameter of the smaller, smooth muscle–walled bronchioles. The natural dilation of the airways during inhalation allows air to enter these narrowed airways. However, contraction of the airways on exhalation and the obstruction caused by asthma combine to prevent air from escaping.

Air becomes trapped behind the obstruction, preventing continued ventilation of the alveoli, and oxygen–carbon dioxide exchange may be severely impaired. Hypoxemia and hypercarbia result, with the degree of respiratory distress increasing with the severity of obstruction and number of airways involved.

Asthma may be triggered by one of many different factors. These items, commonly referred to as triggers or inducers, vary from one individual to the next. In allergic individuals, environmental *allergens* are a major cause of inflammation. These allergens may occur both indoors and outdoors. In addition to allergens, asthma may be triggered by cold air, exercise, foods, irritants, and certain medications. Often a specific trigger cannot be identified.

Within minutes of exposure to the offending trigger, a two-phase reaction occurs. The first phase of the reaction is characterized by the release of chemical mediators such as histamine. These mediators cause contraction of the bronchial smooth muscle and leakage of fluid from peribronchial capillaries. This results in both bronchoconstriction and bronchial *edema*. These two factors can significantly decrease expiratory airflow, causing the typical "asthma attack." Often, the asthma attack resolves spontaneously in 1 to 2 hours or may be aborted by the use of inhaled bronchodilator medications such as albuterol. However, within 6 to 8 hours after exposure to the trigger, a second reaction occurs. This late phase is characterized by inflammation of the bronchioles as cells of the immune system (eosinophils, neutrophils, and lymphocytes) invade the mucosa of the respiratory tract. This leads to additional edema and swelling of the bronchioles and a further decrease of expiratory airflow.

The second phase of the reaction does not typically respond to inhaled beta agonist drugs such as epinephrine or albuterol. Instead, anti-inflammatory agents such as corticosteroids are often required. It is important to point out that the severe inflammatory changes seen in an acute asthma attack do not develop over a few hours or even a few days. The inflammation often begins several days or several weeks before the onset of the actual asthma attack.

Status Asthmaticus

Status asthmaticus is defined as a severe, prolonged asthma attack that cannot be broken by repeated doses of epinephrine or albuterol. It is a serious medical emergency that requires prompt recognition, treatment, and transport. The patient suffering from status asthmaticus frequently has a greatly distended chest from continual air trapping. Breath sounds, and often wheezing, may be absent. The patient is usually exhausted, severely acidotic, and dehydrated. Paramedics should recognize that respiratory arrest is imminent and be prepared for endotracheal intubation. Transport should be immediate, with aggressive treatment continued en route.

Management of Asthma

Treatment of asthma is designed to correct hypoxia, reverse any *bronchospasm,* and treat inflammatory changes associated with the disease. Oxygen should be administered at a high concentration (100 percent). Intravenous access should be established, and the patient should be placed on an ECG monitor. Initial treatment should be directed at reversing any bronchospasm present. The most commonly used drugs are inhaled beta agonist preparations such as albuterol (Ventolin, Proventil) (see Table 8–1). These drugs can be easily administered with a small-volume, oxygen-powered nebulizer. The patient's response to these medications should be monitored and documented.

In addition to beta agonists, early administration of corticosteroids should be considered. Although the inhaled beta agonists will help with bronchoconstriction, they will do little for the underlying inflammation,

TABLE 8–1

Drugs Used in the Treatment of Asthma

Mechanism of Action	Medication
Bronchodilators	
Nonspecific agonists	Epinephrine
	Ephedrine
Beta$_2$ specific agonists	
Inhaled (short-acting)	Albuterol (Ventolin, Proventil)
	Levalbuterol (Xopenex)
	Metaproterenol (Alupent)
	Terbutaline (Brethine)
	Bitolterol (Tornalate)
Inhaled (long-acting)	Salmeterol (Serevent)
Methylxanthines	Theophylline (Theo-Dur, Slo-Bid)
	Aminophylline
Anticholinergics	Atropine
	Ipratropium (Atrovent)
Anti-Inflammatory Agents	
Glucocorticoids	
Inhaled	Beclomethasone (Beclovent)
	Flucticasone (Flovent)
	Triamcinolone (Azmacort)
Oral	Prednisone (Deltasone)
Injected	Methyprednisolone (Solu-Medrol)
	Dexamethasone (Decadron)
Leukotriene antagonists	Zafirlukast (Accolate)
	Zileuton (Zyflo)
Mast-Cell Membrane Stabilizer	Cromolyn (Intal)

which is the principal problem. If paramedics anticipate a long transport time, medical control may request the administration of methylprednisolone or similar corticosteroid. However, the beneficial effects of corticosteroid administration will probably not be detected until 6 to 8 hours following administration.

If symptoms are severe and do not improve with administration of the inhaled beta agonists, the intravenous administration of aminophylline may be indicated. If the patient is not currently taking a theophylline preparation, paramedics administer a loading dose of 5 to 6 mg/kg of aminophylline over 20 to 30 minutes. This dose should be followed by a maintenance infusion of 0.8 to 1.0 mg/kg/hr. Both the inhaled beta agonists and aminophylline may increase heart rates and/or cause tremors, nausea, and vomiting.

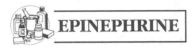 **EPINEPHRINE**

Class: Sympathetic agonist

Description

Epinephrine is a naturally occurring catecholamine. It is a potent α- and β-adrenergic stimulant; however, its effect on β-receptors is more profound.

Mechanism of Action

Epinephrine acts directly on α- and β-adrenergic receptors. Its effect on β-receptors is much more profound than its effect on α-receptors. The effects of epinephrine include increased heart rate, cardiac contractile force, systemic vascular resistance, and increased blood pressure. It also causes bronchodilation due to its effects on β_2-adrenergic receptors. It is occasionally used to treat the bronchoconstriction accompanying asthma and COPD and is also effective in treating bronchoconstriction associated with anaphylaxis.

Epinephrine's effects usually appear within 90 seconds of administration, and they are usually of short duration. Occasionally the drug must be readministered in 15 to 30 minutes if needed. Epinephrine 1:1000 is given subcutaneously to ensure a steady and prolonged action. Inhaled β-agonists are preferred over epinephrine in the treatment of bronchospasm because they have fewer undesirable side effects.

Pharmacokinetics

Onset: 3–10 minutes [subcutaneous (SC)]
Peak Effects: 20 minutes (SC)
Duration: 20–30 minutes (SC)
Half-Life: Not applicable

Indications

Epinephrine is used in bronchial asthma, exacerbation of some forms of COPD, and anaphylaxis.

Contraindications

Because of the cardiac effects seen with the administration of epinephrine, it should not be administered to patients with underlying cardiovascular disease or hypertension. Patients with profound anaphylactic reactions, characterized by hypotension and shock, are usually peripherally vaso-constricted, which will delay absorption of the drug from the subcutaneous site of injection. In these cases, epinephrine 1:10 000 should be administered intravenously.

Precautions

Epinephrine should be protected from light. Also, as with the other cate-cholamines, it tends to be deactivated by alkaline solutions. Any patient receiving epinephrine 1:1000 should be carefully monitored for changes in blood pressure, pulse, and ECG. Palpitations, anxiety, nausea, and headache are fairly common side effects.

Side Effects

Epinephrine can cause palpitations, anxiety, tremulousness, headache, dizziness, nausea, and vomiting. Because of its strong inotropic and chronotropic properties, epinephrine increases myocardial oxygen demand. Even in low doses it can cause myocardial ischemia. These effects should be kept in mind when administering epinephrine in the emergency setting.

Interactions

The effects of epinephrine can be intensified in patients who are taking antidepressants.

Dosage

The standard dose of epinephrine 1:1000 ranges from 0.3 to 0.5 mg administered subcutaneously, depending on the patient's weight and overall medical condition; 0.3 mg is the usual starting dose for adults. The dose for pediatric patients is 0.01 mg/kg administered subcutaneously. In the pre-hospital phase of emergency medical care, epinephrine 1:1000 should only be administered subcutaneously (except in the case of pediatric cardiac arrest).

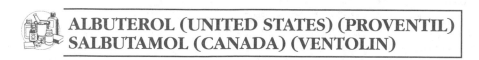

ALBUTEROL (UNITED STATES) (PROVENTIL) SALBUTAMOL (CANADA) (VENTOLIN)

Class: Sympathetic agonist

Description

Albuterol is a sympathomimetic that is selective for β_2-adrenergic receptors.

Mechanism of Action

Albuterol is a selective β_2-agonist with a minimal number of side effects. It causes prompt bronchodilation and has a duration of action of approximately 5 hours.

Pharmacokinetics

Onset: 5–15 minutes (inhaled)
Peak Effects: 1.0–1.5 hours
Duration: 3–6 hours
Half-Life: <3 hours

Indications

Albuterol is used in bronchial asthma and reversible bronchospasm associated with chronic bronchitis and emphysema.

Contraindications

Albuterol should not be administered to any patient with a known history of hypersensitivity to the drug.

Precautions

As with any sympathomimetic, the patient's vital signs must be monitored. Caution should be used when administering albuterol to elderly patients and those with cardiovascular disease or hypertension. Lung sounds should be auscultated before and after each treatment. Ideally, the patient's peak flow rate should be measured both before and after drug administration.

Side Effects

Albuterol can cause palpitations, anxiety, dizziness, headache, nervousness, tremor, hypertension, arrhythmias, chest pain, nausea, and vomiting.

Interactions

The possibility of developing unpleasant side effects increases when albuterol is administered with other sympathetic agonists. β-blockers may blunt the pharmacological effects of albuterol.

Dosage

Albuterol can be administered by metered-dose inhaler or small-volume nebulizer. A common initial dose is two sprays when using a metered-dose inhaler. Each spray delivers 90 μg of albuterol. When using a small-volume nebulizer, the standard adult dose is 2.5 mg (0.5 mL of a 0.5 percent solution diluted in 2.5 mL of normal saline). This amount is typically delivered over 5 to 15 minutes. Albuterol (Ventolin) is also available in the Rotohaler form. A special 200 μg Rotocap is placed in the device and inhaled by the patient. Albuterol should only be administered by inhalation.

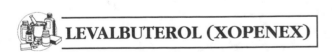 **LEVALBUTEROL (XOPENEX)**

Class: Sympathetic agonist

Description

Levalbuterol is a sympathomimetic that is selective for β₂-adrenergic receptor.

Mechanism of Action

Levalbuterol is a selective β_2-adrenergic agonist that causes relaxation of bronchial smooth muscle, thus decreasing airway resistance and increasing vital capacity. Levalbuterol is a chemical variant of albuterol with greater affinity for the β_2-adrenergic receptors.

Pharmacokinetics

Onset: 5–15 minutes
Peak Effects: 1–1.5 hours
Duration: 3–6 hours
Half-Life: 3.3 hours

Indications

Levalbuterol is used in the treatment of bronchospasm associated with reversible obstructive airway disease (asthma, chronic bronchitis, emphysema).

Contraindications

Levalbuterol is contraindicated in patients with known hypersensitivity to the drug.

Precautions

Levalbuterol should be used with caution in patients with cardiac ischemia. Try one treatment, measuring peak flow before and after treatment. Lung sounds should be auscultated before and after each treatment.

Side Effects

Tremors, anxiety, dizziness, headache, insomnia, nausea, palpitations, tachycardia, and hypertension have been associated with levalbuterol administration.

Interactions

The possibility of developing unpleasant side-effects increase when levalbuterol is administered with other sympathetic agonists. β-blockers may blunt the pharmacologic effects of levalbuterol.

Dosage

Adult dose. A standard nebulizer dose is 0.63 mg in 3.0 mL normal saline every 6 to 8 hours.

Pediatric dose. Children less than 12 years old is 0.31 mg in 3.0 mL normal saline three times a day.

RACEMIC EPINEPHRINE (microNEFRIN, VAPONEFRIN)

Class: Sympathetic agonist

Description

Racemic epinephrine is slightly different chemically from the epinephrine compounds that have been discussed previously. Compounds that differ only in their chemical arrangement are called *isomers*. This particular form is frequently used in children to treat croup.

Mechanism of Action

Racemic epinephrine stimulates both α- and β-adrenergic receptors. However, racemic epinephrine has a slight preference for β_2-adrenergic receptors and causes bronchodilation. It also has some effect in relieving the subglottic edema associated with croup. Racemic epinephrine should only be administered by inhalation.

Pharmacokinetics

> **Onset:** <5 minutes
> **Peak Effects:** 5–15 minutes
> **Duration:** 1–3 hours
> **Half-Life:** Not applicable

Indication

Racemic epinephrine is used to treat croup (laryngotracheobronchitis).

Contraindications

Racemic epinephrine should not be used in the management of epiglottitis.

Precautions

Racemic epinephrine can result in tachycardia and possibly dysrhythmias. Vital signs should be monitored. Many patients develop "rebound worsening" 30 to 60 minutes after the initial treatment and after the effects of racemic epinephrine have worn off. Thus, all children who receive racemic epinephrine should be transported to the hospital. Most hospitals have an institutional policy that requires all children who have received racemic epinephrine to be admitted for at least 24 hours in case rebound worsening occurs.

Dosage

A standard dose is 0.25 to 0.75 mL racemic epinephrine diluted with 2 mL normal saline (2.25 percent) and administered via a standard aerosol nebulizer. It should only be used initially and not repeated. Racemic epinephrine should be given only by inhalation, generally by small-volume nebulizer, diluted with 2 to 3 mL of normal saline.

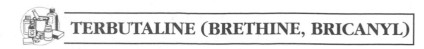

TERBUTALINE (BRETHINE, BRICANYL)

Class: Sympathetic agonist

Description

Terbutaline is a synthetic sympathomimetic that is selective for β_2-adrenergic receptors.

Mechanism of Action

Terbutaline, because of its effects on β_2-adrenergic receptors, causes immediate bronchodilation with minimal cardiac effects. Its onset of action is similar to that of epinephrine. Terbutaline is also used to suppress preterm labor.

Pharmacokinetics

Onset: <5 minutes (SC), 5–30 minutes (inhaled)
Peak Effects: 30–60 minutes (SC), 1–2 hours (inhaled)
Duration: 1.5–4.0 hours (SC), 3–4 hours (inhaled)
Half-Life: 3–4 hours

Indications

Terbutaline is used in bronchial asthma and reversible bronchospasm associated with chronic bronchitis and emphysema.

Contraindications

Terbutaline should not be administered to any patient with a history of hypersensitivity to the drug.

Precautions

As with any sympathomimetic, the patient's vital signs must be monitored. Caution should be used when administering terbutaline to elderly patients and those with cardiovascular disease or hypertension. Lung sounds should be auscultated before and after each treatment. Ideally, the patient's peak flow rate should be measured both before and after drug administration.

Side Effects

Terbutaline can cause palpitations, anxiety, dizziness, headache, nervousness, tremor, hypertension, dysrhythmias, chest pain, nausea, and vomiting.

Interactions

The possibility of developing unpleasant side effects increases when terbutaline is used with other sympathetic agonists. β-blockers may blunt the pharmacological effects of terbutaline.

Dosage

The standard dose is two inhalations, 1 minute apart, from a metered-dose inhaler. Terbutaline can also be administered by subcutaneous injection. The usual dose is 0.25 mg. This dose can be repeated in 15 to 30 minutes if needed. Terbutaline should only be administered by inhalation or by subcutaneous injection as described herein.

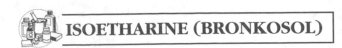
ISOETHARINE (BRONKOSOL)

Class: Sympathetic agonist

Description

Isoetharine is a sympathomimetic similar in chemical structure to epinephrine. It exhibits a slight specificity for β_2-adrenergic receptors, thus reducing the potential for cardiac toxicity.

Mechanism of Action

Isoetharine is a β-agonist with slight selectivity for β_2-adrenergic receptors, causing pulmonary bronchodilation. Its onset of action is similar to that of epinephrine. However, it has a longer duration of effect.

Pharmacokinetics

Onset: Immediate
Peak Effects: 5–15 minutes
Duration: 1–4 hours
Half-Life: Not applicable

Indications

Isoetharine is used in bronchial asthma and reversible bronchospasm associated with chronic bronchitis and emphysema.

Contraindications

Isoetharine should not be administered to any patient with a history of hypersensitivity to any of the ingredients.

Precautions

As with any sympathomimetic, the patient's vital signs must be monitored. Caution should be used when administering isoetharine to elderly patients and those with cardiovascular disease or hypertension. Lung sounds should be auscultated before and after each treatment. Ideally, the patient's peak flow rate should be measured both before and after drug administration.

Side Effects

Isoetharine can cause palpitations, anxiety, dizziness, headache, nervousness, tremor, hypertension, dysrhythmias, chest pain, nausea, and vomiting.

Interactions

The possibility of developing unpleasant side effects increases when isoetharine is administered with other sympathetic agonists. β-blockers may blunt the pharmacological effects of isoetharine.

Dosage

There are three major ways to administer isoetharine, each with different dosages. They are as follows:

Method of Administration	Usual Dose	Dilution
Metered-dose inhaler	2 inhalations	Undiluted
Oxygen aerosolization	0.5 milliliters	1:3 with saline
Intermittent positive-pressure breathing	0.5 milliliters	1:3 with saline

Isoetharine should be administered only by one of the methods listed.

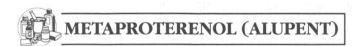

METAPROTERENOL (ALUPENT)

Class: Sympathetic agonist

Description

Metaproterenol is a sympathomimetic that is selective for β_2-adrenergic receptors.

Mechanism of Action

Metaproterenol is a selective β_2-agonist and is an effective bronchodilator. Its duration of effect is up to 4 hours.

Pharmacokinetics

Onset: 1 minute
Peak Effects: 1 hour
Duration: 1–5 hours
Half-Life: Not applicable

Indications

Metaproterenol is used in bronchial asthma and reversible bronchospasm associated with chronic bronchitis and emphysema.

Contraindications

Metaproterenol should not be used in patients with cardiac dysrhythmias or significant tachycardia.

Precautions

As with any sympathomimetic, the patient's vital signs must be monitored. Caution should be used when administering metaproterenol to elderly patients and those with cardiovascular disease or hypertension. Lung sounds should be auscultated before and after each treatment. Ideally, the patient's peak flow rate should be measured both before and after drug administration.

Side Effects

Metaproterenol can cause palpitations, anxiety, dizziness, headache, nervousness, tremor, hypertension, dysrhythmias, chest pain, nausea, and vomiting.

Interactions

The possibility of developing unpleasant side effects increases when metaproterenol is administered with other sympathetic agonists. β-blockers may blunt the pharmacological effects of metaproterenol.

Dosage

Metaproterenol may be administered by metered-dose inhaler. Each spray contains 0.65 mg of metaproterenol. The usual single dose is two to three inhalations, a minute apart, as needed. Metaproterenol may also be administered by small-volume nebulizer. The typical adult dose is 0.2 to 0.3 mL of metaproterenol diluted in 2.5 mL of normal saline. This dose is usually administered over 5 to 15 minutes. Metaproterenol should be administered by inhalation only in the emergency setting.

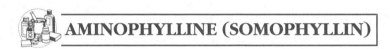

AMINOPHYLLINE (SOMOPHYLLIN)

Class: Xanthine

Description

Aminophylline is a xanthine bronchodilator that sometimes proves effective in cases in which sympathomimetics have not been effective.

Mechanism of Action

Aminophylline achieves its bronchodilation effects via a different mechanism than the sympathomimetics. It relaxes bronchial smooth muscle but does not act on adrenergic receptors. Aminophylline also stimulates the respiratory center in the brain. This effect is particularly useful in the treatment of infants with apnea. In addition to bronchodilation, aminophylline has mild diuretic properties, increases the heart rate and cardiac output, and may precipitate dysrhythmias. Because of its mild diuretic and inotropic effects, aminophylline is also used in the management of congestive heart failure and pulmonary edema. In prehospital emergency care, aminophylline is usually given by slow IV infusion. Some systems also carry aminophylline suppositories for use in special situations.

Pharmacokinetics

Onset: 15 minutes
Peak Effects: 15 minutes
Duration: Varies
Half-Life: 4 hours

Indications

Aminophylline is used in bronchial asthma, reversible bronchospasm associated with chronic bronchitis and emphysema, congestive heart failure, and pulmonary edema.

Contraindications

Aminophylline should not be administered to any patient with a history of hypersensitivity to the drug. It should not be used in patients who have uncontrolled cardiac dysrhythmias.

Precautions

Extreme caution should be used when administering aminophylline to any patient with a history of cardiovascular disease or hypertension. Any patient receiving aminophylline should have a cardiac monitor. One should be alert for any signs of cardiac irritability, especially premature ventricular contractions (PVCs) and tachycardia. Hypotension can occur following rapid administration.

Side Effects

Aminophylline can cause tachycardia, dysrhythmias, palpitations, chest pain, nervousness, headache, seizures, nausea, and vomiting.

Interactions

Aminophylline should not be administered to patients who are on chronic theophylline therapy (Slo-Bid, Theo-Dur, and so on) until the amount of drug in the blood has been obtained (theophylline level). Concomitant use with β-blockers and drugs of the erythromycin class of antibiotics may lead to theophylline toxicity.

Dosage

Two major regimens are used in administering aminophylline. The first is for use in patients in whom fluid overload or edema does not appear to be present (i.e., acute bronchial asthma): Place 250 or 500 mg in 90 or 80 mL of 5 percent dextrose, respectively. This can be done with a 100 mL IV bag or with a Buretrol- or Volutrol-type administration set. This solution is then infused over 20 to 30 minutes. This mechanism of slow infusion tends to reduce the chances of dysrhythmias. In patients with congestive heart failure, or for whom any additional fluid might be dangerous, a more concentrated infusion is prepared: Place 250 or 500 mg (2 to 5 mg/kg) in 20 mL of 5 percent dextrose in water. This solution is then infused over 20 to 30 minutes using a Buretrol- or Volutrol-type administration set. Parenteral aminophylline should only be given by slow intravenous (IV) infusion by one of the regimens discussed earlier.

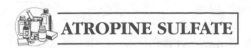

ATROPINE SULFATE

Class: Anticholinergic

Description

Atropine is a parasympatholytic (anticholinergic) that is derived from parts of the *Atropa belladonna* plant.

Mechanism of Action

Atropine sulfate is a potent parasympatholytic. It is used in the treatment of respiratory emergencies, because it causes bronchodilation and drying of respiratory tract secretions. Atropine acts by blocking acetylcholine receptors, thus inhibiting parasympathetic stimulation. With the release of ipratropium, atropine has fallen into relative disuse in the treatment of reactive airway disease.

Pharmacokinetics

Onset: 5–30 minutes (inhaled)
Peak Effects: 1–4 hours (inhaled)
Duration: 2–4 hours (inhaled)
Half-Life: 2–3 hours

Indications

Atropine is used in bronchial asthma and reversible bronchospasm associated with chronic bronchitis and emphysema.

Contraindications

Atropine sulfate should not be used in patients hypersensitive to the drug. It is not indicated for the acute treatment of bronchospasm, for which rapid response is required.

Precautions

The patient's vital signs must be monitored during therapy with atropine. Caution should be used when administering atropine to elderly patients and those with cardiovascular disease or hypertension. Lung sounds should be auscultated before and after each treatment. Ideally, the patient's peak flow rate should be measured both before and after drug administration.

Side Effects

Atropine can cause palpitations, anxiety, dizziness, headache, nervousness, rash, nausea, and vomiting.

Interactions

There are few interactions in the prehospital setting.

Dosage

Atropine is usually administered with a β-agonist. Typically, 0.5 to 1.0 mg of atropine is placed in 2 to 3 mL of normal saline. This dose is administered by small-volume nebulizer with or without a β-agonist.

How Supplied

Atropine is supplied in ampules and vials containing 1.0 mg in 1 mL of solution.

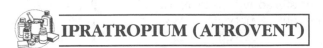 **IPRATROPIUM (ATROVENT)**

Class: Anticholinergic

Description

Ipratropium is an anticholinergic (parasympatholytic) bronchodilator that is chemically related to atropine.

Mechanism of Action

Ipratropium is a parasympatholytic used in the treatment of respiratory emergencies. It causes bronchodilation and dries respiratory tract secretions. Ipratropium acts by blocking acetylcholine receptors, thus inhibiting parasympathetic stimulation.

Pharmacokinetics

> **Onset:** Varies
> **Peak Effects:** 1.5–2.0 hours
> **Duration:** 4–6 hours
> **Half-Life:** 1.5–2.0 hours

Indications

Ipratropium is used in bronchial asthma and reversible bronchospasm associated with chronic bronchitis and emphysema.

Contraindications

Ipratropium should not be used in patients hypersensitive to the drug. It is not indicated for the acute treatment of bronchospasm, for which rapid response is required.

Precautions

The patient's vital signs must be monitored during therapy with ipratropium. Caution should be used when administering it to elderly patients and those with cardiovascular disease or hypertension. Lung sounds should be auscultated before and after each treatment. Ideally, the patient's peak flow rate should be measured both before and after drug administration.

Side Effects

Ipratropium can cause palpitations, anxiety, dizziness, headache, nervousness, rash, nausea, and vomiting.

Interactions

There are few interactions in the prehospital setting.

Dosage

Ipratropium is usually administered with a β-agonist. Typically, 500 μg of Atrovent is placed in a small-volume nebulizer. A β-agonist can be added if desired. This solution is then administered by small-volume nebulizer with or without a β-agonist. Atrovent is also available in a metered-dose inhaler.

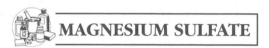 **MAGNESIUM SULFATE**

Class: Mineral

Description

Magnesium sulfate is a salt that dissociates into the magnesium cation (Mg^{2+}) and the sulfate anion when administered. Magnesium is an essential element in numerous biochemical reactions that occur within the body.

Mechanism of Action

Magnesium acts as a physiological calcium channel blocker and blocks neuromuscular transmission. Magnesium sulfate has been used for years in the management of preterm labor and the hypertensive disorders of pregnancy (preeclampsia and eclampsia). Its usage in obstetrics is discussed in Chapter 11.

Pharmacokinetics

    Onset: Immediate (IV), 1 hour (IM)
    Peak Effects: Varies
    Duration: 1 hour
    Half-Life: Not applicable

Indications

Magnesium sulfate is used in severe bronchospasm, in severe refractory ventricular fibrillation or pulseless ventricular tachycardia, after myocardial infarction for prophylaxis of dysrhythmias, and in torsade de pointes (multiaxial ventricular tachycardia).

Contraindications

Magnesium sulfate should not be administered to patients who are in shock, who have persistent, severe hypertension, who have a third-degree atrioventricular (AV) block, who routinely undergo dialysis, or who are known to have a decreased calcium level (hypocalcemia).

Precautions

Magnesium sulfate should be administered slowly to minimize side effects. Any patient receiving intravenous magnesium sulfate should have continuous cardiac monitoring as well as frequent monitoring of vital signs. If possible, the knee and biceps deep tendon reflexes should be checked prior to magnesium therapy. It should be used with caution in patients with known renal insufficiency. Hypermagnesemia (elevated magnesium) can occur following magnesium sulfate administration. Calcium salts (calcium chloride or calcium gluconate) should be available as an antidote for magnesium sulfate in case serious side effects occur.

Side Effects

Magnesium sulfate can cause flushing, sweating, bradycardia, decreased deep tendon reflexes, drowsiness, respiratory depression, dysrhythmias, hypotension, hypothermia, itching, and rash.

Interactions

Magnesium sulfate can cause cardiac conduction abnormalities if administered in conjunction with digitalis.

Dosage

The standard dosage is 2 g over 2 to 5 minutes.

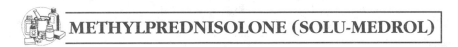

METHYLPREDNISOLONE (SOLU-MEDROL)

Class: Corticosteroid and anti-inflammatory

Description

Methylprednisolone is a synthetic steroid with potent anti-inflammatory properties.

Mechanism of Action

Corticocosteroids have multiple actions in the body. They have potent anti-inflammatory properties and inhibit many of the substances that cause inflammation (cytokines, interleukin, interferon) and also inhibit the synthesis of pro-inflammatory enzymes. The pharmacological actions of the steroids are vast and complex. In general medical practice, steroids have a wide range of uses. Effective as anti-inflammatory agents, they are used in the management of allergic reactions, asthma, and anaphylaxis. Methylprednisolone is considered an intermediate-acting steroid with a plasma half-life of about 3 to 4 hours.

Pharmacokinetics

Onset: Varies
Peak Effects: 4–8 days [intramuscular (IM)]
Duration: 1–5 weeks (IM)
Half-Life: 3.5 hours

Indications

Methylprednisolone is used in severe anaphylaxis, asthma or COPD, and urticaria (hives).

Contraindications

There are no major contraindications to the use of methylprednisolone in the acute management of severe anaphylaxis.

Precautions

A single dose of methylprednisolone is all that should be given in the prehospital phase of care. Long-term steroid therapy can cause gastrointestinal bleeding, prolonged wound healing, and suppression of adrenocortical steroids.

Side Effects

Methylprednisolone can cause fluid retention, congestive heart failure, hypertension, abdominal distension, vertigo, headache, nausea, malaise, and hiccups.

Interactions

There are few interactions in the prehospital setting.

Dosage

The standard dosage of methylprednisolone in the management of severe anaphylaxis is 125 to 250 mg administered intravenously. Methylprednisolone may be administered intravenously or intramuscularly, but the intravenous route is preferred in emergency medicine.

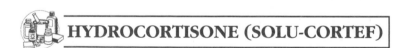 **HYDROCORTISONE (SOLU-CORTEF)**

Class: Corticosteroid and anti-inflammatory

Description

Hydrocortisone is a potent corticosteroid with anti-inflammatory properties.

Mechanism of Action

Corticocosteroids have multiple actions in the body. They have potent anti-inflammatory properties and inhibit many of the substances that cause inflammation (cytokines, interleukin, interferon) and also inhibit the synthesis of pro-inflammatory enzymes. The pharmacological actions of the steroids are vast and complex. Hydrocortisone is considered a short-acting steroid with a plasma half-life of 90 minutes. Like the other adrenocorticosteroids, it is effective as an adjunct in the management of severe anaphylaxis.

Pharmacokinetics

Onset: Immediate
Peak Effects: 4–8 hours
Duration: 1.0–1.5 days
Half-Life: 90 minutes

Indications

Hydrocortisone is used in severe anaphylaxis, asthma or COPD, and urticaria (hives).

Contraindications

There are no major contraindications to the use of hydrocortisone in the acute management of anaphylaxis.

Precautions

A single dose of hydrocortisone is all that should be given in the prehospital phase of care. Long-term steroid therapy can cause gastrointestinal bleeding, prolonged wound healing, and suppression of adrenocortical steroids.

Side Effects

Hydrocortisone can cause fluid retention, congestive heart failure, hypertension, abdominal distension, vertigo, headache, nausea, malaise, and hiccups.

Interactions

There are few interactions in the prehospital setting.

Dosage

The standard dosage of hydrocortisone in the management of severe anaphylaxis is 40 to 250 mg administered intravenously.

Route

The IV route is preferred in emergency medicine. However, hydrocortisone can be administered intramuscularly when an IV cannot be started.

NEUROMUSCULAR BLOCKERS

Establishment and protection of the airway has the highest priority in emergency care. On certain occasions patients who are still responsive may have trouble maintaining their airway and may require endotracheal intubation. This situation most commonly occurs in patients with drug overdoses, in patients with status epilepticus, and in trauma patients with closed-head injuries. Often, however, intubation is difficult because of the presence of gag reflexes, clenched teeth, or general combativeness. In these cases endotracheal intubation can be carried out after administration of a neuromuscular-blocking agent.

Neuromuscular-blocking agents are drugs that cause muscle relaxation, thus facilitating endotracheal intubation (see Table 8–2). All skeletal muscles, including the muscles of respiration, respond to these drugs. Following administration, the patient will become apneic and require mechanical ventilation. Neuromuscular-blocking agents have no effect on the patient's level of consciousness or pain sensation. Neuromuscular-blocking drugs are classified as *depolarizing* and *nondepolarizing* based on their mechanism of action. The most commonly used depolarizing drug is succinylcholine, and vecuronium and pancuronium are the most frequently used nondepolarizing agents.

1. *Succinylcholine (Anectine).* Succinylcholine is a depolarizing neuromuscular blocker commonly used in emergency medicine. It acts in approximately 60 to 90 seconds and lasts approximately 3 to 5 minutes. Succinylcholine causes muscle fasciculations progressing to total paralysis, including paralysis of the diaphragm.

2. *Pancuronium (Pavulon).* Pancuronium is a long-acting, nondepolarizing neuromuscular-blocking agent. It acts in 30 to 45 seconds and lasts 30 to 60 minutes.

3. *Vecuronium (Norcuron).* Vecuronium is a nondepolarizing neuromuscular-blocking agent with a rapid onset and short duration of action. It has fewer cardiovascular side effects than succinylcholine and does not cause fasciculations.

4. *Atracurium (Tracrium).* Atracurium is a nondepolarizing neuromuscular-blocking agent with a rapid onset and short to intermediate duration of action.

5. *Rocuronium (Zemuron).* Rocuronium is a nondepolarizing neuromuscular-blocking agent with a rapid to intermediate onset, depending on dose, and an intermediate duration of action. At equivalent doses, rocuronium has approximately the same clinically effective duration of action as vecuronium.

Depolarizing Blocking Agents

Succinylcholine is the only therapeutic depolarizing blocking agent. Although it is similar to nondepolarizing blockers in its therapeutic effect, its mechanism of action differs. Because succinylcholine is absorbed poorly from the gastrointestinal tract, the preferred administration route is IV. Succincylcholine is metabolized in the liver and excreted via the kidneys.

TABLE 8–2

Common Neuromuscular Blockers Used in Rapid-Sequence Induction (RSI)

Generic	Trade	Class	Adult Dose	Pediatric Dose	Onset	Duration
Succinylcholine	Anectine	Depolarizing	1.0–1.5 mg/kg	1.0–2.0 mg/kg	30–60 seconds (IV) 2–3 minutes (IM)	2–3 minutes (IV) 10–30 minutes (IM)
Pancuronium	Pavulon	Nondepolarizing	0.04–0.1 mg/kg	0.04–0.1 mg/kg	35–45 seconds	30–60 minutes
Vecuronium	Norcuron	Nondepolarizing	0.08–0.10 mg/kg	≥1 year: adult dose	<1 minute	25–40 minutes
Atracurium	Tracrium	Nondepolarizing	0.4–0.5 mg/kg	1 month–2 years: 0.3–0.4 mg/kg	1–2 minutes	60–70 minutes
Rocuronium	Zemuron	Nondepolarizing	0.6 mg/kg	>2 years: adult dose 0.6 mg/kg	30–60 seconds	30–60 minutes

Pharmacodynamics

Succinylcholine has a biphasic effect. In phase I blockade, it acts like acetylcholine and depolarizes the synaptic membrane of the muscle. However, succinylcholine is not inactivated by cholinesterase, so the depolarization persists, resulting in brief periods of excitation, manifested by muscle fasciculations (uncoordinated contractions of muscle fibers), followed by muscle paralysis and flaccidity. Phase II is normally not seen except in high drug concentrations. Succinylcholine is the drug of choice for short-term muscle relaxation, such as during intubation. The primary adverse drug reactions to succinylcholine are the same as those to nondepolarizing blockers: prolonged apnea and cardiovascular alterations. Patients commonly experience muscle pain from the fasciculations that occur in phase I.

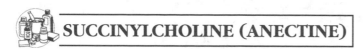 **SUCCINYLCHOLINE (ANECTINE)**

Class: Depolarizing neuromuscular blocker

Description

Succinylcholine is a short-acting, depolarizing skeletal muscle relaxant used to facilitate endotracheal intubation.

Mechanism of Action

Succinylcholine is a short-acting, depolarizing skeletal muscle relaxant. Like acetylcholine, it combines with cholinergic receptors in the motor nerves to cause depolarization. Neuromuscular transmission is thus inhibited, which renders the muscles unable to be stimulated by acetylcholine. Following IV injection, complete paralysis is obtained within 30 to 60 seconds and persists for approximately 2 to 3 minutes. Effects then start to fade, and a return to normal is seen within 6 minutes. Muscle relaxation begins in the eyelids and jaw. It then progresses to the limbs, the abdomen, and finally the diaphragm and intercostals. It has no effect on consciousness.

Pharmacokinetics

> **Onset:** 30–60 seconds (IV), 2–3 minutes (IM)
> **Peak Effects:** 1–3 minutes
> **Duration:** 2–3 minutes (IV), 10–30 minutes (IM)
> **Half-Life:** 5–10 minutes

Indication

Succinylcholine is used to achieve temporary paralysis when endotracheal intubation is indicated and muscle tone or seizure activity prevents it.

Contraindications

Succinylcholine is contraindicated in patients with a history of hypersensitivity to the drug. It should not be used with penetrating eye injuries or in patients with a history of narrow-angle glaucoma. Succinylcholine should not be administered by persons inexperienced with its use.

Precautions

Succinylcholine should not be administered unless personnel skilled in endotracheal intubation are present and ready to perform the procedure. Oxygen therapy equipment should be readily available, as should all emergency resuscitative drugs and equipment. Fractures have been reported in children following the use of depolarizing neuromuscular blockers due to strong and sustained muscle fasciculations. Cardiac arrest and ventricular dysrhythmias have been reported when succinylcholine was administered to patients with severe burns and severe crush injuries.

Side Effects

Succinylcholine can cause wheezing, respiratory depression, apnea, aspiration, dysrhythmias, bradycardia, sinus arrest, hypertension, hypotension, increased intraocular pressure, and increased intracranial pressure.

Interactions

Certain drugs can enhance the neuromuscular-blocking action of succinylcholine: lidocaine, procainamide, β-blockers, magnesium sulfate, and other neuromuscular blockers.

Dosage

The dosage for succinylcholine is 1 to 1.5 mg/kg administered intravenously. The preferred route for succinylcholine administration is intravenously. It can be administered intramuscularly if required, however.

Nondepolarizing Blocking Agents

The nondepolarizing blocking agents, also called competitive or stabilizing agents, are derived curare alkaloids and their synthetic analogues. We discuss four such agents: pancuronium bromide, vecuronium bromide, atracurium, and rocuronium bromide. These drugs produce intermediate to prolonged muscle relaxation, such as that required for intubation and ventilation during surgery. Because nondepolarizing blockers are poorly absorbed from the gastrointestinal tract, they are administered parenterally, with the IV route preferred. A variable but large proportion of the nondepolarizing agents is excreted unchanged in the urine. Some of the newer drugs, such as pancuronium and vecuronium, are metabolized partially in the liver.

Pharmacodynamics

The nondepolarizing blockers compete with acetylcholine at the cholinergic sites of the skeletal muscle membrane. This action blocks acetylcholine's neurotransmitter action, preventing the muscle membrane from depolarizing. The effect can be counteracted clinically by anticholinesterase drugs, such as neostigmine or pyridostigmine, which inhibit the action of acetylcholinesterase, the enzyme that destroys acetylcholine.

The initial muscle weakness produced by the drugs quickly changes to flaccid paralysis that affects the muscles in a specific sequence. The first muscles to exhibit flaccid paralysis are those innervated by the motor portions of the cranial nerves and small, rapidly moving muscles in the eyes, face, and neck. Next, the limb, abdomen, and trunk muscles become flaccid.

Finally, the intercostal muscles and diaphragm are paralyzed. Recovery from the paralysis usually occurs in the reverse order.

Because these drugs do not cross the blood–brain barrier, no alterations in consciousness or pain perception occur. Thus patients are aware of what is happening to them and may experience extreme anxiety and pain, but they cannot communicate their feelings.

Nondepolarizing blockers are used for intermediate or prolonged muscle relaxation. They facilitate endotracheal intubation and are used during surgery to decrease the amount of anesthetic required and to facilitate manipulations. They are also used to paralyze patients who need ventilatory support but who fight the endotracheal tube and ventilator.

Pancuronium selectively blocks the vagus nerve and may result in tachycardia, cardiac arrhythmias, and hypertension.

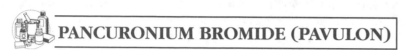

PANCURONIUM BROMIDE (PAVULON)

Class: Nondepolarizing neuromuscular blocker

Description

Pancuronium bromide is a derivative of curare and is used to provide muscle relaxation to facilitate endotracheal intubation.

Mechanism of Action

Pancuronium competes with acetylcholine for cholinergic receptor sites on the postjunctional membrane. This results in paralysis of muscle fibers served by the occupied neuromuscular junction. It does not cause an initial depolarization wave, as does succinylcholine. The onset of action of pancuronium is 30 to 45 seconds, and the effect may persist for up to 60 minutes. Effects may begin to subside after 35 to 45 minutes.

Pharmacokinetics

Onset: 30–45 seconds
Peak Effects: 3–5 minutes
Duration: 30–60 minutes
Half-Life: 2 hours

Indication

Pancuronium is used to achieve temporary paralysis when endotracheal intubation is indicated and muscle tone, seizures, or laryngospasm prevents it.

Contraindications

Pancuronium is contraindicated in patients with a history of hypersensitivity to the drug. It should not be administered by persons inexperienced with its use.

Precautions

Pancuronium should not be administered unless personnel skilled in endotracheal intubation are present and ready to perform the procedure.

Oxygen therapy equipment should be readily available, as should all emergency resuscitative drugs and equipment. Hypotension can occur. Thus, the vital signs must be constantly monitored. Pancuronium can increase intracranial pressure. In patients with head injuries, vecuronium is often preferred.

Side Effects

Pancuronium can cause wheezing, respiratory depression, apnea, aspiration, dysrhythmias, bradycardia, sinus arrest, hypertension, hypotension, increased intraocular pressure, and increased intracranial pressure.

Interactions

Certain drugs can enhance the neuromuscular-blocking action of pancuronium: lidocaine, procainamide, β-blockers, magnesium sulfate, certain antibiotics (aminoglycosides), and other neuromuscular blockers.

Dosage

The adult and pediatric dosage for pancuronium is 0.04 to 0.1 mg/kg administered intravenously. Repeat doses of 0.01 to 0.02 mg/kg administered intravenously may be required every 20 to 40 minutes.

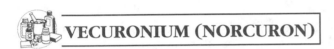

VECURONIUM (NORCURON)

Class: Nondepolarizing neuromuscular blocker

Description

Vecuronium is a derivative of pancuronium and is used to provide muscle relaxation to facilitate endotracheal intubation.

Mechanism of Action

Vecuronium has a similar mechanism of action as pancuronium. However, it is approximately one-third more potent, with a shorter duration of effect. Vecuronium competes with acetylcholine for cholinergic receptor sites on the postjunctional membrane. This competition results in paralysis of muscle fibers served by the occupied neuromuscular junction. It does not cause an initial depolarization wave, as does succinylcholine. The onset of action of vecuronium is <1 minute, with good to excellent intubation conditions within 2.5 to 3 minutes.

Pharmacokinetics

Onset: <1 minute
Peak Effects: 3–5 minutes
Duration: 25–40 minutes
Half-Life: 30–80 minutes

Indication

Vecuronium is used to achieve temporary paralysis when endotracheal intubation is indicated and muscle tone or seizure activity prevents it.

Contraindications

Vecuronium is contraindicated in patients with a history of hypersensitivity to the drug.

Precautions

Vecuronium should not be administered unless personnel skilled in endotracheal intubation are present and ready to perform the procedure. Oxygen therapy equipment should be readily available, as should all emergency resuscitative drugs and equipment.

Side Effects

Vecuronium can cause wheezing, respiratory depression, apnea, aspiration, dysrhythmias, bradycardia, sinus arrest, hypertension, hypotension, increased intraocular pressure, and increased intracranial pressure.

Interactions

Certain drugs can enhance the neuromuscular-blocking action of vecuronium: lidocaine, procainamide, β-blockers, magnesium sulfate, and other neuromuscular blockers.

Dosage

Adult dose. Vecuronium is 0.08 to 0.10 mg/kg administered intravenously. Neuromuscular blockade should last 25 to 30 minutes.

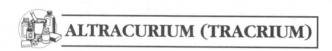

ALTRACURIUM (TRACRIUM)

Class: Nondepolarizing neuromuscular blocker

Description

Atracurium is used to provide muscle relaxation to facilitate endotracheal intubation.

Mechanism of Action

Atracurium has a similar mechanism of action as vecuronium. Atracurium competes with acetylcholine for cholinergic receptor sites on the postjunctional membrane. This competition results in paralysis of muscle fibers served by the occupied neuromuscular junction. It does not cause an initial depolarization wave, as does succinylcholine. The onset of action of atracurium is 2 minutes, with good to excellent intubation conditions within 2.5 to 3 minutes.

Pharmacokinetics

Onset: 2 minutes
Peak Effects: 3–5 minutes
Duration: 60–70 minutes
Half-Life: 20 minutes

Indication

Atracurium is used to achieve temporary paralysis when endotracheal intubation is indicated and muscle tone or seizure activity prevents it.

Contraindications

Atracurium is contraindicated in patients with a history of hypersensitivity to the drug.

Precautions

Atracurium should not be administered unless personnel skilled in endotracheal intubation are present and ready to perform the procedure. Oxygen therapy equipment should be readily available, as should all emergency resuscitative drugs and equipment. Use with caution in asthmatics.

Side Effect

Atracurium can cause wheezing, respiratory depression, apnea, aspiration, dysrhythmias, bradycardia, sinus arrest, hypertension, hypotension, increased intraocular pressure, and increased intracranial pressure.

Interactions

Certain drugs can enhance the neuromuscular-blocking action of atracurium: lidocaine, procainamid, β-blockers, magnesium sulfate, and other neuromuscular blockers.

Dosage

Adult dose. Atracurium is 0.4 to 0.5 mg/kg administered intravenously. Neuromuscular blockade should last 60 to 70 minutes.

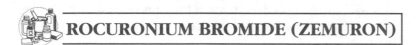

ROCURONIUM BROMIDE (ZEMURON)

Class: Nondepolarizing neuromuscular blocker

Description

Rocuronium is a nondepolarizing neuromuscular-blocking agent with a rapid to intermediate onset, depending on dose, and intermediate duration of action.

Mechanism of Action

Rocuronium acts by binding competitively to cholinergic receptors at the motor end plate to antagonize the action of acetylcholine, an effect that is reversible in the presence of acetylcholinesterase inhibitors, such as neostigmine and edrophonium.

Pharmacokinetics

Onset: 30–60 seconds
Peak Effects: 1–3 minutes
Duration: 30–60 minutes
Half-Life: 14–18 minutes

Indications

Rocuronium is indicated as an adjunct to general anesthesia to facilitate both rapid-sequence (initiated at 60 to 90 seconds postadministration) and routine endotracheal intubation and to provide skeletal muscle relaxation during surgery or mechanical ventilation.

Contraindications

Rocuronium is contraindicated in patients with a history of hypersensitivity to the drug.

Precautions

Rocuronium should be administered in carefully adjusted dosages by or under the supervision of experienced clinicians who are familiar with its actions and the possible complications of its use. Rocuronium is associated with a slight elevation of heart rate and blood pressure; tachycardia may occur in children.

Side Effects

Bronchospasm is a side effect of rocuronium.

Interactions

Intensity and duration of paralysis may be prolonged by pretreatment with succinylcholine, general anesthesia (inhalation), lidocaine, quinidine, procainamide, beta-adrenergic-blocking agents, potassium-losing diuretics, or magnesium.

Dosage

Rapid-sequence tracheal intubation dosage for adults and children is 600 μg (0.6 mg)/kg. Maintenance dose is 100 to 200 μg (0.1 to 0.2 mg)/kg continuous infusion.

INDUCTION AGENTS

Neuromuscular-blocking agents have no effect on consciousness. Thus, when performing rapid-sequence induction (RSI) on all but unconscious patients, it is necessary to first administer a sedative/hypnotic induction agent. Administering a neuromuscular blocker to a conscious patient can be terrifying because they will be unable to move or breathe, yet will remain conscious and alert throughout the procedure.

The classic anesthetic induction agent is the barbiturate thiopental sodium. In emergency medicine and in the prehospital setting, common induction agents used for RSI include the benzodiazepines diazepam (Valium) and midazolam (Versed). These are effective in that they are rapid acting and have significant amnestic properties. In addition, two short-acting induction agents, ketamine (Ketalar) and etomidate (Amidate), are frequently used. Ketamine is a dissociative agent that does not affect breathing or airway reflexes. It is primarily used in children because of its tendency to cause hallucinations in older patients. Etomidate is an ultra-fast-acting nonbarbiturate, nonbenzodiazepine sedative/hypnotic popular in EMS.

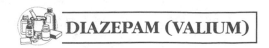 **DIAZEPAM (VALIUM)**

Class: Anticonvulsant and sedative

Description

Diazepam is a benzodiazepine that is frequently used as an anticonvulsant, sedative, and hypnotic.

Mechanism of Action

Benzodiazepines bind to specific sites on gamma-aminobutyric acid (GABA) Type A receptors within the brain. GABA is the major inhibitory neurotransmitter of the central nervous system. Benzodiazepines have no direct effect on the GABA receptors, but do potentiate the effects of GABA within the brain. Increased GABA levels cause sedation. Through this mechanism, the benzodiazepines display their hypnotic, anxiolytic, and anticonvulsant effects. Their usefulness, however, is limited by a broad range of side effects including sedation, ataxia, amnesia, alcohol and barbiturate potentiation, tolerance development, and abuse potential.

In emergency medicine, diazepam is principally used for its anticonvulsant properties. It suppresses the spread of seizure activity through the motor cortex of the brain. It does not appear to abolish the abnormal discharge focus, however. Diazepam, one of the most frequently prescribed medications in the United States, is used in the management of anxiety and stress. It is effective in treating the tremors and anxiety associated with alcohol withdrawal. It is also an effective skeletal muscle relaxant, which makes it an effective adjunct in orthopedic injuries. It is a good premedication for minor operative procedures and cardioversion because it induces amnesia, which dimishes the patient's recall of such procedures.

Pharmacokinetics

> **Onset:** 1–5 minutes (IV), 15–30 minutes (IM)
> **Peak Effects:** 15 minutes (IV), 30–45 minutes (IM)
> **Duration:** 15–60 minutes
> **Half-Life:** 20–50 hours

Indications

Diazepam is used in major motor seizures, status epilepticus, premedication before cardioversion, skeletal muscle relaxant, and acute anxiety states.

Contraindications

Diazepam should not be administered to any patient with a history of hypersensitivity to the drug.

Precautions

Because diazepam is a relatively short-acting drug, seizure activity may recur. In such cases, an additional dose may be required. Flumazenil (Romazicon), a benzodiazepine antagonist, should be available to use as an antidote if required. Injectable diazepam can cause local venous irritation.

To minimize irritation, it should only be injected into relatively large veins and should not be given faster than 1 mL/min.

Side Effects

Diazepam can cause hypotension, drowsiness, headache, amnesia, respiratory depression, blurred vision, nausea, and vomiting.

Interactions

Diazepam is incompatible with many medications. Whenever diazepam is given intravenously in conjunction with other drugs, the IV line should be adequately flushed. The effects of diazepam can be additive when used in conjunction with other CNS depressants and alcohol.

Dosage

In the management of seizures, the usual dose of diazepam is 5 to 10 mg IV. In many instances it may be necessary to give diazepam directly into the vein, because the seizure activity will prevent the insertion of an indwelling catheter. When given directly into a vein, it is essential that a large vein, preferably in the antecubital fossa, be used. In acute anxiety reactions, the standard dosage is 2 to 5 mg administered intramuscularly.

To induce amnesia prior to cardioversion, a dosage of 5 to 15 mg of diazepam is given intravenously. Peak effects are seen in 5 to 10 minutes. Diazepam should be given intravenously by slow IV push. It can be injected intramuscularly, but absorption via this route is variable. When an IV line cannot be started, parenteral diazepam can be administered rectally with a similar onset of action.

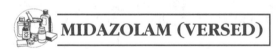 **MIDAZOLAM (VERSED)**

Class: Sedative and hypnotic

Description

Midazolam is a benzodiazepine with strong hypnotic and amnestic properties.

Mechanism of Action

Benzodiazepines bind to specific sites on GABA Type A receptors within the brain. GABA is the major inhibitory neurotransmitter of the central nervous system. Benzodiazepines have no direct effect on the GABA receptors, but do potentiate the effects of GABA within the brain. Increased GABA levels cause sedation. Through this mechanism, the benzodiazepines display their hypnotic, anxiolytic, and anticonvulsant effects. Their usefulness, however, is limited by a broad range of side effects including sedation, ataxia, amnesia, alcohol and barbiturate potentiation, tolerance development, and abuse potential.

Midazolam is a potent but short-acting benzodiazepine used widely in medicine as a sedative and hypnotic. It is three to four times more potent than diazepam. Its onset of action is approximately 1.5 minutes when administered intravenously and 15 minutes when administered intramuscularly. Midazolam has impressive amnestic properties. Like the other benzodiazepines, it has no effect on pain.

Pharmacokinetics

Onset: 1.5 minutes (IV), 15 minutes (IM)
Peak Effects: 20–60 minutes
Duration: <2 hours (IV), 1–6 hours (IM)
Half-Life: 1–4 hours

Indication

Midazolam is used as a premedication before cardioversion and other painful procedures.

Contraindications

Midazolam should not be administered to any patient with a history of hypersensitivity to the drug. It should not be used in patients who have narrow-angle glaucoma, Midazolam should not be administered to patients in shock with depressed vital signs, or who are in alcoholic coma.

Precautions

Emergency resuscitative equipment must be available prior to the administration of midazolam. Vital signs must be continuously monitored during and after drug administration. Midazolam has more potential than the other benzodiazepines to cause respiratory depression and respiratory arrest. Flumazenil (Romazicon), a benzodiazepine antagonist, should be available to use as an antidote if required.

Side Effects

Midazolam can cause laryngospasm, bronchospasm, dyspnea, respiratory depression and arrest, drowsiness, amnesia, altered mental status, bradycardia, tachycardia, premature ventricular contractions, and retching.

Interactions

The effects of midazolam can be accentuated by CNS depressants such as narcotics and alcohol.

Dosage

When used for sedation, midazolam must be administered cautiously, because the amount of medication required to achieve sedation varies from individual to individual. Typically, 1 to 2.5 mg are administered by slow IV injection. Usually, it is best to dilute midazolam with normal saline or D_5W prior to IV administration. Midazolam can be administered intramuscularly at a dose of 0.07 to 0.08 mg/kg (average adult dose of 5 mg). Recently, many centers have been administering midazolam intranasally or by mouth to sedate children prior to suturing of lacerations.

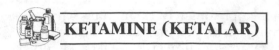
KETAMINE (KETALAR)

Class: Anesthetic agents and analgesic agent

Description

Ketamine is a phencyclidine derivative that is unique among sedative, hypnotic, and analgesic agents. It is used as an induction agent for rapid-sequence induction/intubation and for sedation. Ketamine has strong amnestic properties.

Mechanism of Action

Ketamine is thought to cause a dissociation between the cortical and limbic system, resulting in a seemingly awake patient who is dissociated from the environment. It has powerful analgesic and sedative properties.

Pharmacokinetics

Onset: <1 minute (IV), <5 minutes (IM)
Peak Effects: Varies
Duration: 10–15 minutes (IV), 20–30 minutes (IM)
Half-Life: 1–2 hours

Indication

Ketamine is used as a sedative and induction agent for RSI (particularly in children).

Contraindications

Ketamine is contraindicated in those with a significant elevation in blood pressure and in those who have a hypersensitivity to the drug.

Precautions

Ketamine can cause hallucinations following waking (emergence hallucinations) that can be quite severe. The incidence of hallucinations is higher in adults than in children. Much of this can be avoided by keeping the environment quiet when the patient emerges from anesthesia. Ketamaine is usually used with a low dose of a benzodiazipine such as lorazepam, diazepam, or midazolam. Resuscitation equipment must be immediately available. All monitors (ECG, SpO_2, $ETCO_2$) must be in place prior to administration. Monitor vital signs closely.

Side Effects

Side effects associated with ketamine include increased hallucinations, increased skeletal muscle tone, nausea, and vomiting. Protective airway reflexes may actually be enhanced with ketamine.

Interactions

Recovery time may be prolonged if narcotics and barbiturates are also used.

Dosage

The usual dose is 0.5 to 1.0 mg/kg IV given over 30 to 60 seconds. For the IM route, 2 to 4 mg/kg may be used.

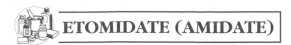

ETOMIDATE (AMIDATE)

Class: Sedative and hypnotic

Description

Etomidate is an ultra-short-acting, nonbarbiturate, nonbenzodiazepine hypnotic. It does not have any analgesic properties. It is used as an induction agent for RSI.

Mechanism of Action

Etomidate produces a rapid induction of anesthesia with minimal respiratory and cardiovascular effects. Unlike other types of sedative/hypnotics, etomidate does not cause histamine release.

Pharmacokinetics

Onset: 10–20 seconds
Peak Effects: <1 minute
Duration: 3–5 minutes
Half-Life: 30–70 minutes

Indication

Etomidate is used as an induction agent for rapid-sequence induction/intubation.

Contraindication

Etomidate is contraindicated in patients with a hypersensitivity to the drug.

Precautions

Etomidate should be used with caution in patients with marked hypotension, severe asthma, or severe cardiovascular disease.

Side Effects

Side effects associated with etomidate include myoclonic skeletal muscle movement, apnea, hyperventilation or hypoventilation, laryngospasm, hypertension or hypotension, tachycardia or bradycardia, nausea, and vomiting.

Interaction

Verapamil may cause prolonged respiratory depression and apnea.

Dosage

Give 0.1 to 0.3 mg/kg IV over 15 to 30 seconds.

Precautions

Before administering any neuromuscular-blocking agent, it is essential that paramedics have equipment ready for airway management as soon as the patient becomes apneic. In addition, because a neuromuscular-blocking agent has no effect on pain sensation and mental status, it should not be administered to alert patients without first administering a sedative or analgesic. Most emergency patients have eaten or drunk something in the hours prior to the onset of the emergency. Thus, virtually every emergency patient is considered to have a full stomach.

Neuromuscular blockade and endotracheal intubation may cause vomiting, which increases the risk of aspiration. Consequently, special precautions must be taken to gain rapid control of the airway as soon as the drug is administered. As a result, this procedure is often referred to as RSI.

RAPID-SEQUENCE INDUCTION

The procedure for RSI is as follows: Place the patient in a supine position. Preoxygenate with 100 percent oxygen for 5 minutes (spontaneous respirations) or ventilate with a bag-valve-mask device and 100 percent oxygen for at least five tidal volumes prior to intubation to facilitate nitrogen washout (allows 3 to 5 minutes of apnea without serious hypoxemia).

1. Establish IV normal saline with large-bore catheter (two IVs if time and personnel permit).
2. Monitor ECG, SpO_2, waveform capnography, and vital signs as closely as possible throughout procedure.
3. Perform a thorough neurological exam.
4. Prepare for rapid administration of fentanyl, midazolam, lidocaine, atropine, and succinylcholine.
5. Assemble and prepare equipment (suction, endotracheal tube, endotracheal tube stylet, syringe, lubricant, and cricothyrotomy and PTTV kits).
6. Administer lidocaine 1.5 mg/kg IV push if head is injured or increased intracranial pressure is suspected.
7. Administer atropine 1.0 mg IV push if
   - Bradycardia is present (fentanyl may induce bradydysrhythmias)
   - Cervical-spine injury
   - Patients under age 16 (pediatric dose 0.02 mg/kg IV push)
8. Prepare paralytic agents.
9. Administer fentanyl 1.0 to 3.0 µg/kg slow IV push.
10. Administer midazolam 0.05 to 0.1 mg/kg slow IV push or for the adult patient, 2.5 to 5.0 mg if the blood pressure is over 100 systolic.
11. As patient becomes relaxed, approximately 1 to 2 minutes after administration of midazolam, apply cricoid pressure (Sellick's maneuver) to occlude the esophagus and maintain

pressure until the endotracheal tube is in place and the cuff is inflated.

12. Check adequacy of sedation and administer 1.5 mg/kg succinylcholine or 0.01 mg/kg vecuronium IV push and stop ventilating if doing so.

13. Apnea and jaw relaxation are indications that the patient is sufficiently relaxed to proceed with endotracheal intubation. If patient is not adequately relaxed, then administer atropine and a second dose of succinylcholine 1.5 mg/kg.

14. Position head, visualize larynx, and intubate.

15. Observe lung inflations, check endotracheal tube for fogging, and auscultate the chest for adequate ventilation. Ventilate with 100 percent oxygen at 16 to 20 per minute. (Use $ETCO_2$ to determine effective ventilatory rate.)

16. Inflate cuff on endotracheal tube.

17. Release cricoid pressure.

18. Reassess patient's vital signs.

19. The effects of the succinylcholine will wear off in 3 to 5 minutes (vecuronium will wear off in 25 to 30 minutes).

20. Medical control or standing orders may request the administration of pancuronium or vecuronium if continued paralysis is warranted.

21. The maintenance dose of pancuronium is 0.01 mg/kg; the maintenance dose of vecuronium is 0.01 mg/kg.

22. Assess patient for adequacy of sedation. It may be necessary to administer more fentanyl or midazolam for long transports; the effects of both generally last approximately 30 minutes.

PHARMACOLOGICALLY-ASSISTED INTUBATION

An alternative to rapid-sequence induction is the use of many of the same medications, without the use of paralytics. This procedure is referred to as pharmacologically-assisted intubation (PAI). The advantage to this procedure is that paralytics are not used, and a reversal of some of the respiratory depressant effects (from the narcotic fentanyl) is possible with the administration of Narcan. A disadvantage to this procedure occurs in the patient with trismus or a clenched jaw. In spite of the administration of the PAI medications, it may be impossible to pass the endotracheal tube. In this case a surgical airway may be warranted.

The procedure for PAI is as follows: Place the patient in a supine position. Preoxygenate with 100 percent oxygen for 5 minutes (spontaneous respirations) or ventilate with a bag-valve-mask device and 100 percent oxygen for at least five tidal volumes prior to intubation to facilitate nitrogen washout (allows 3 to 5 minutes of apnea without serious hypoxemia).

1. Establish IV normal saline with large-bore catheter. Monitor ECG SpO_2, and vital signs as closely as possible throughout procedure.

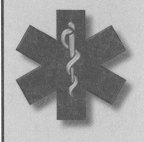

CASE PRESENTATION

EMS is called to a residence to help a female patient complaining of shortness of breath. The patient is conscious and breathing. En route dispatch informs the paramedics that the patient has a history of COPD and uses an inhaler. On arrival paramedics are met by the patient's son, who takes them to the bedroom where the patient is sitting up in bed. The patient, an 88-year-old woman, is in obvious respiratory distress. She is leaning forward and struggling to breathe.

On Examination

CNS:	The patient is conscious, alert, and oriented × 4; she is able to answer questions with short answers only (less than 4 words); patient is clearly frightened
Resp:	Respirations are 42 and shallow; patient is wheezing; wheezes are heard throughout all lung fields on expiration; trachea is midline; no signs of trauma
CVS:	Carotid and radial pulses are present and weak; skin is warm and dry
ABD:	Soft and nontender
Muscl/Skel:	Patient able to move extremities on command; no weaknesses to hand grip

Vital Signs

Pulse:	120/min, irregular, weak
Resp:	42/min, shallow
BP:	152/110 mmHg
SpO$_2$:	88 percent
ECG:	Sinus rhythm with unifocal PVCs at 4 to 6 per minute

Hx: Patient has emphysema and was recently hospitalized for it and then discharged 2 days ago. She has had a cold for the past 2 weeks and states that changes in weather cause her "lungs to act up." She has been getting progressively worse, and her son states that the inhaler that she uses ran out this afternoon. She has no chest pain and denies any recent trauma.

PHx: She has had emphysema, which seems to get worse during the winter months, for 20 years. She has been hospitalized numerous times for "breathing problems." The patient had a "heart attack" 2 years ago. Medications include Ventolin and Becloforte inhalers, synthroid, and verapamil; she has no allergies.

Treatment

Oxygen was administered by nasal cannula at 6 lpm, and 5 mg of salbutamol (Ventolin) was administered by an oxygen-powered nebulizer. With coaching, the patient relaxed and her breathing improved slightly. The patient was hooked up to the ECG monitor and a sinus tachycardia was noted. En route to the hospital, a second dose of 5 mg of salbutamol and 500 mg of ipratropium bromide (Atrovent) were administered via a nebulizer. On arrival at the hospital, the patient was able to speak normally and the wheezing had diminished significantly. The SpO$_2$ had increased to 96 percent. Her prescription for the inhalers was refilled, and after an overnight stay in the hospital she was released.

2. Prepare for rapid administration of fentanyl, midazolam, lidocaine, and atropine. Assemble and prepare equipment (suction, endotracheal tube, endotracheal tube stylet, syringe, lubricant, and cricothyrotomy and PTTV kits).

3. Administer lidocaine 1.5 mg/kg IV push.

4. Administer atropine 1.0 mg IV push if
   - Bradycardia is present (fentanyl may induce bradydys-rhythmias)
   - Cervical-spine injury
   - Patients under age 16 (pediatric dose 0.02 mg/kg IV push)

5. Administer fentanyl 1.0 µg/kg IV push or for the adult patient 100 µg initially, redosing with 50 µg or 0.5 µg/kg increments as necessary to a maximum of 4 µg/kg.

6. Administer midazolam 0.09 to 0.3 mg/kg slow IV push or for the adult patient 2.5 to 5.0 mg if the patient is responsive to voice or pain and blood pressure is over 100 systolic. Redose with up to three 1 mg boluses if necessary, the blood pressure is over 100 systolic, and the patient becomes responsive to voice or pain.

7. As patient becomes relaxed, approximately 1 to 2 minutes after administration of midazolam, apply cricoid pressure.

8. Check adequacy of sedation and administer additional fentanyl and midazolam if required.

9. Position head, visualize larynx, apply lidocaine spray, and intubate. Observe lung inflations, check endotracheal tube for fogging, and auscultate the chest for adequate ventilation. Ventilate with 100 percent oxygen at 16 to 20 per minute. Monitor ECG, vital signs, and SpO$_2$ every 3 to 5 minutes.

Maintenance of Sedation

Fentanyl may be repeated 0.5 µg/kg or 50 µg for the adult patient every 20 to 30 minutes, as needed. Midazolam may be repeated 0.05 mg/kg or 2.5 mg for the adult patient every 20 to 30 minutes, as needed. Lorazepam 0.05 to 0.1 mg/kg (<2 mg/min) or 2.0 to 4.0 mg, may be given for the adult patient every 4 to 8 hours to a maximum of 8 mg.

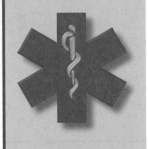

CASE PRESENTATION

At 1830 hours paramedics are called to a rural residence 45 minutes from the hospital to aid a 45-year-old woman complaining of shortness of breath. She is conscious and breathing. On arrival paramedics are met by the patient's husband, who leads them to the living room. There, paramedics find a patient leaning forward in a chair. The patient is using home oxygen by nasal cannula and an oxygen-powered nebulizer. The patient appears very anxious and in severe respiratory distress.

On Examination

CNS: The patient is conscious, alert, and oriented × 4; in extreme respiratory distress

Resp: Respirations are 36 and shallow; wheezes are heard unaided by stethoscope; there are tight, barely audible wheezes in the apices bilaterally and no sounds heard in the bases; trachea is midline; no signs of trauma

CVS: Carotid and radial pulses are present and weak; skin is pale and cool

ABD: Soft and nontender

Muscl/Skel: Patient able to move extremities on command; no weaknesses to hand grip

Vital Signs

Pulse: 140/min, regular, weak

Resp: 36/min, shallow

BP: 144/94 mmHg

SpO$_2$:   82 percent

ECG: Sinus tachycardia

Hx: Patient has a 20-year history of asthma and was taking Ventolin by inhaler twice a day, Becloforte twice a day, and home oxygen by nasal cannula at 4 lpm as needed and during sleep. The patient was talking to her granddaughter on the phone. She became very upset during the telephone call and then became short of breath. The patient put on her oxygen (which provided no relief) and also took one dose (2.5 mg) of albuterol with an oxygen-powered nebulizer (which also provided no relief).

Treatment

Paramedics administered 5 mg of Ventolin and 500 µg of Atrovent by nebulizer mask as per standing orders, and the patient was coached to take a breath and hold it. The patient was very agitated, and the coaching had little effect. An IV was initiated and run TKO. The patient was hooked up to the ECG monitor and a sinus tachycardia was noted. The base hospital was contacted, and the paramedics were directed to administer 125 mg of Solu-Medrol IV push and to continue administering Ventolin. The patient's condition deteriorated en route to the hospital. Although the patient was conscious, she was fatigued and unable to follow verbal commands. The base hospital was contacted, and the paramedics were directed to sedate and intubate the patient. The procedure was explained to the patient; 100 µg of fentanyl (Sublimaze) and 2.5 mg of midazolam (Versed) were administered IV. Sellick's maneuver was applied to occlude the esophagus, at which point 1.5 mg/kg of succinylcholine (Anectine) was given IV. Once the jaw relaxed, the patient was intubated and bilateral breath sounds were confirmed. The patient was admitted to the intensive care unit on arrival at the hospital.

Notes

A Glasgow Coma Scale score of 9 or less indicates the need for intubation unless the decreased loss of consciousness can be readily reversed (e.g., hypoglycemia or narcotic overdose).

The sedative effect of midazolam diminishes after approximately 2 hours. The duration of action of fentanyl may be as short as 30 minutes (and reversible with naloxone).

Lorazepam may be used for patients with seizure disorder.

The dosage of benzodiazepines should be reduced in patients over 50 years of age or if hypotension is present.

SUMMARY

Respiratory emergencies are a serious and potentially fatal condition if not treated immediately. Prompt recognition of the signs and symptoms of respiratory distress is essential. Oxygen is the primary drug for treating any respiratory problem. Many types of medical problems, especially asthma and anaphylaxis, respond only to the medications discussed in this chapter.

KEY WORDS

allergens. A foreign substance that can cause an allergic response in the body but is only harmful to some people.

bronchospasm. An abnormal contraction of the bronchi, resulting in narrowing and blockage of the airway. A cough with wheezing is the usual symptom. Bronchospasm is the main feature of asthma and bronchitis.

capnography. A system for measuring the concentration of exhaled carbon dioxide.

chronic obstructive pulmonary disease (COPD). A pulmonary disease characterized by a decreased ability of the lungs to perform the function of ventilation.

edema. An abnormal pooling of fluid in the tissues.

hypoxia. A state in which insufficient oxygen is available to meet the oxygen requirements of the cells.

pH. A scientific method of expressing the acidity or alkalinity of a solution. It is the logarithm of the hydrogen ion concentration divided by 1. The higher the pH, the more alkaline the solution. The lower the pH, the more acidic the solution.

pulse oximetry. An assessment modality that measures the oxygen saturation level of the blood through a noninvasive sensor placed on a finger or earlobe.

DRUGS USED IN THE TREATMENT OF METABOLIC-ENDOCRINE EMERGENCIES

9

OBJECTIVES

After completing this chapter, the reader should be able to:

1. Define the term *hormone.*
2. Discuss the function and location of the pancreas.
3. List two functions of the pancreas.
4. Discuss the function of glucagon.
5. Define *diabetes mellitus.*
6. Discuss the function of insulin and its relation to glucose metabolism.
7. Compare and contrast type I (insulin-dependent) and type II (non-insulin-dependent) diabetes mellitus.
8. Compare and contrast diabetic ketoacidosis and hypoglycemia.
9. Describe and list the indications, contraindications, and dosages for insulin, glucagon, $D_{50}W$, and thiamine.

INTRODUCTION

Glands that secrete *hormones* directly into the blood, without the aid of ducts, are called *endocrine glands.* A hormone is a chemical substance produced by an organ or specialized cells that regulates or controls the activities of another organ. Hormones are typically released directly into the bloodstream where they are transported to the target issues. With the exception of the pancreas, they rarely cause emergency disorders. Occasionally the thyroid, the endocrine gland that controls metabolic rate, begins secreting excess thyroid hormones. This disorder, called hyperthyroidism, is characterized by increased heart rate, loss of body weight, insomnia, dry skin, hair loss, and nervousness. A rare but severe form of thyroid dysfunction is called *thyroid storm.* Thyroid storm causes fever, tachycardia, dehydration, and a change in mental status. Although this chapter is devoted to metabolic-endocrine emergencies, we primarily discuss the pancreatic disorder *diabetes mellitus.*

DIABETES MELLITUS

The pancreas is located in the retroperitoneal space, within the folds of the small intestine. Within the pancreas is an area called the *islets of Langerhans.* The islets of Langerhans have three types of cells that secrete three different hormones. The α cells secrete the hormone *glucagon.* The β cells secrete *insulin.* A third hormone, called *somatostatin,* is secreted from the delta cells. Insulin is required for the passage of glucose into the cells. Without insulin the blood glucose level rises. Glucagon causes stored carbohydrates, especially glycogen, to be broken down to glucose. When the blood sugar level falls, glucagon is released, which then causes a release of stored carbohydrates. Somatostatin inhibits the secretion of both insulin and glucagon. Functionally, it is similar to growth hormone.

Diabetes mellitus is caused when β cells of the pancreas reduce the amount of insulin secreted. In addition, the relative number of insulin receptors decreases. These two factors contribute to an increasing level of glucose in the blood, which results in increased thirst (polydipsia), increased hunger (polyphagia), and increased urination (polyuria). The hunger results because the various body cells are glucose depleted. The thirst is due to a relative dehydration that occurs when glucose spills over into the urine. Glucose spillage into the urine takes water with it, which results in the polyuria and polydipsia characteristic of hyperglycemia. If allowed to progress untreated, the patient will eventually lapse into diabetic coma. Patients in diabetic coma have warm, dry skin. Clinically they are dehydrated. They may exhibit rapid, deep respirations (*Kussmaul respirations*), which are part of the body's attempt to rid itself of accumulated acids. Because the signs and symptoms occur early, most patients seek medical care before coma ensues. Once diagnosed, the patient will most likely be placed on hypoglycemic agents. If an excessive amount of insulin is taken, or if the patient fails to eat properly, then *hypoglycemia* can develop (see Table 9–1).

TYPES OF DIABETES

Generally, diabetes mellitus can be divided into two different categories. Type I diabetes, or insulin-dependent diabetes, usually begins in the early years. Patients who have type I diabetes must take insulin. Type II diabetes, or non-insulin-dependent diabetes, usually begins later in life and tends to be associated with obesity. Type II diabetes can often be controlled without using insulin. It is important for paramedics to understand the difference between these two forms of diabetes.

Type I Diabetes Mellitus

Type I diabetes mellitus is a serious disease characterized by inadequate production of insulin by the endocrine pancreas. The cause of type I diabetes is not well understood. One theory is that a viral infection attacks the pancreatic β cells, thus slowing or stopping insulin production. Another theory proposes that the body's immune system mistakenly targets the pancreatic β

TABLE 9–1

Typical Findings in Diabetic-Induced Altered Mental Status

Hypoglycemia

Scene Size-up	Initial Assessment	Signs and Symptoms	Vitals/Physical	History	Causes	Management
Presence of syringes, insulin, glucometers, lower extremity prosthetic devices	Chief complaint may reveal patient or family awareness of diabetic condition; may complain of confusion, restlessness, weakness	Weakness/ uncoordination	**Vitals**	History of diabetes, cardiac, renal, or vascular disease	Patient has taken too much insulin	Check blood sugar level
		Lethargy/confusion	Weak or full, rapid pulses			
		Headache	Cold clammy skin	Obesity, endocrine problems; exertion, infection	Patient has overexerted, thus reducing glucose levels	Administer dextrose as per protocol/ standing order
		Irritable, nervous behavior	Diaphoresis			
		Hunger, thirst, polyuria	Pupils normal to dilated			
	Acute onset	Chest pain		Slow healing wounds, poor peripheral perfusion, scarring of fingers; provisional amputations		
		Shortness of breath				
		Nausea, vomiting, diarrhea				
	Airway compromise (vomitus, tongue)	Malaise				
		Abdominal pain				
		May appear intoxicated				
		Coma (severe cases)				

Diabetic Ketoacidosis (DKA/Hyperglycemia)

Scene Size-up	Initial Assessment	Signs and Symptoms	Vitals/Physical	History	Causes	Management
Presence of syringes, insulin, glucometers, lower extremity prosthetic devices	Chief complaint may reveal patient or family awareness of diabetic condition; may complain of confusion, restlessness, weakness	Polyuria, polydypsia, polyphagia	**Vitals**	History of diabetes, cardiac disease, renal disease, vascular disease, endocrine problems	Patient has not taken insulin	Check blood sugar level
		Nausea, vomiting	Weak, rapid pulses			
		Tachycardia	Kussmaul respirations	Family history of diabetes	Patient has overeaten, flooding the body with carbohydrates	Fluids
		Deep, rapid respirations	Low blood pressure in later stages			Insulin
		Warm, dry skin				
	Gradual onset	Fruity odor on breath	Poor skin turgor, pallor, delayed capillary refill related to dehydration		Patient has infection that disrupts glucose/insulin balance	
		Abdominal pain	**Physical**			
	"Fruity" smell of ketones on patient's breath	Falling blood pressure	Injection sites; medical alert jewelry			
		Fever (occasionally)				
	Airway compromise	Decreased level of consciousness	Slow healing wounds, poor peripheral perfusion			
			Scarring of fingers; Provisional amputations			

267

cells as foreign and attacks them. In either case, heredity appears to be a factor in increasing a person's chances of contracting the disease.

With type I diabetes mellitus, the patient must take daily doses of insulin. In the normal state, the intake of glucose, such as in a meal, results in the release of insulin. Insulin promotes the uptake of glucose by the cells. Type I diabetes generally begins with decreased insulin secretion, subsequently leading to elevated blood glucose levels. However, because insulin is required for glucose to enter into the various body cells, they become glucose depleted despite increased blood glucose levels.

In diabetes, a drop in insulin levels is accompanied by a steady accumulation of glucose in the blood. As the cells become glucose depleted, they begin to use other sources of energy. Therefore, various harmful by-products, such as *ketones* and *organic acids*, are produced. When these by-products start to accumulate, several of the classic findings of diabetic ketoacidosis appear. If the various acids and ketones continue to collect in the blood, severe metabolic acidosis occurs and coma ensues. Severe acidosis can result in serious brain damage or death.

As the concentration of glucose in the blood continues to rise, the kidneys begin excreting glucose in the urine. When glucose is spilled into the urine, it takes water with it, resulting in osmotic diuresis, which dehydrates the patient.

Type II Diabetes Mellitus

Type II diabetes mellitus occurs more commonly than type I does. Like type I, it is characterized by decreased insulin production by the endocrine pancreas. As mentioned previously, type II diabetes usually begins later in life. It is often associated with obesity but can occur in nonobese patients. Increased body weight causes a relative decrease in the number of available insulin receptors. In addition, the insulin receptors become defective and less responsive to insulin. The pancreas also becomes less responsive to stimulation from increased blood glucose levels. Thus, insulin is not secreted as needed, increasing blood glucose levels even further.

The first approach in treating type II diabetes is to encourage the patient to lose weight by reducing the intake of carbohydrates. Physicians may also prescribe oral hypoglycemic agents. These medications tend to stimulate increased insulin secretion from the pancreas and to promote an increase in the number of insulin receptors on the cells. Both actions tend to lower blood glucose levels. If diet and oral agents fail, insulin may be required.

Type II diabetes does not usually result in diabetic ketoacidosis. In type II diabetes, the patient makes enough insulin to maintain pH homeostasis but not enough to supply all of the body's needs. It can, however, develop into a life-threatening emergency termed *nonketotic hyperosmolar coma.* In type II diabetes, when blood glucose levels exceed 600 mg/dL (33.3 mmol/L), the high osmolality of the blood causes an osmotic diuresis and dehydration of body cells. It is difficult to distinguish diabetic ketoacidosis from nonketotic hyperosmolar coma in the field. Therefore, the prehospital treatment of both emergencies is identical.

DIABETIC KETOACIDOSIS (DIABETIC COMA)

Diabetic *ketoacidosis* is a serious complication of diabetes mellitus. It occurs when insulin levels become inadequate to meet the metabolic demands of the body.

Pathophysiology

Diabetic ketoacidosis develops as blood glucose levels increase and individual cells become glucose depleted. The body begins spilling sugar into the urine, which causes a significant osmotic diuresis and serious dehydration, evidenced by dry, warm skin and mucous membranes. As cellular glucose depletion continues, ketones and acids are produced. Subsequently, the blood becomes acidotic. Deep respiration begins as the body tries to compensate for the metabolic acidosis. If ketoacidosis is uncorrected, coma will follow.

Clinical Presentation

The onset of diabetic ketoacidosis is slow, lasting from 12 to 24 hours. In its early stages, the signs and symptoms include increased thirst, excessive hunger, excessive urination, and malaise. Increased urination results from osmotic diuresis accompanying glucose spillage into the urine. Intensified thirst is caused by the body's attempt to replace fluids lost by increased urination. Diabetic ketoacidosis is characterized by nausea, vomiting, marked dehydration, tachycardia, and weakness. The skin is usually warm and dry. Coma is not uncommon. The breath may have a sweet or acetone-like character because of the increased ketones in the blood. Very deep, rapid respirations, called *Kussmaul respirations*, also occur. Kussmaul respirations represent the body's attempt to compensate for the metabolic acidosis produced by ketones and organic acids present in the blood.

Diabetic ketoacidosis is often associated with infection or decreased insulin intake. It may be complicated by several electrolyte imbalances. The most significant is decreased potassium. Initially, potassium levels will be high, but will rapidly fall as the glucose level falls and potassium is driven intracellularly. Overall, levels of potassium will be low. Decreased potassium (hypokalemia) can lead to serious dysrhythmias or even death.

Ketoacidosis can occur in patients who fail to take their insulin or who take an inadequate amount over an extended period. Persons not previously diagnosed as diabetic occasionally present in ketoacidosis.

HYPOGLYCEMIA (INSULIN SHOCK)

Hypoglycemia occurs when insulin levels are excessive. Hypoglycemia is an urgent medical emergency because a prolonged hypoglycemic episode can result in serious brain injury.

Pathophysiology

Hypoglycemia, sometimes called insulin shock, lies at the other end of the spectrum from diabetic ketoacidosis. Hypoglycemia can occur if a patient accidentally or intentionally takes too much insulin or eats an inadequate amount of food after taking insulin. If the patient is untreated, the insulin will cause the blood glucose level to drop to a very low level. *Hypoglycemia is a true medical emergency.* If the patient is not treated quickly, he or she can sustain serious injury to the brain because it receives most of its energy from glucose metabolism.

TABLE 9–2			
Route	Onset	Peak	Duration
SC (rapid acting)	30 min to 1 hr	2 to 10 hr	5 to 16 hr
SC (intermediate acting)	1 to 2 hr	4 to 15 hr	22 to 28 hr
SC (long acting)	4 to 8 hr	10 to 30 hr	36 hr

Clinical Presentation

The clinical signs and symptoms of hypoglycemia are many and varied. An abnormal mental status is the most important. In the earliest stages of hypoglycemia, the patient may appear restless or impatient or complain of hunger. As the blood sugar level falls lower, he or she may display inappropriate anger (even rage) or a variety of bizarre behaviors. Sometimes the patient may be placed in police custody for such behaviors or be involved in an automobile accident.

Physical signs may include diaphoresis and tachycardia. If the blood sugar level falls to a critically low level, the patient may sustain a *hypoglycemic seizure* or become comatose.

In contrast to diabetic ketoacidosis, hypoglycemia can develop quickly. A change in mental status can occur without warning. When encountering a patient behaving bizarrely, paramedics should always consider the possibility of hypoglycemia.

In this chapter we discuss *insulin, glucagon, 50 percent dextrose in water ($D_{50}W$),* and *thiamine.* All of these agents, except thiamine, are primarily used in the management of the diabetic patient. Thiamine may be administered before $D_{50}W$ to patients with coma of an unknown origin and in whom alcoholism is suspected.

There are three major classifications of injectable insulin. *Regular insulin* is classified as rapid acting. *Lente* or *NPH insulin* is classified as intermediate acting. Long-lasting insulin is called *ultralente.* Table 9–2 helps illustrate the relationship among the three classes.

INSULIN

Patients with type I diabetes mellitus require insulin to control their blood glucose level. Insulin may also be given to type II diabetics. Four sources of insulin are available:

- Beef insulin: from bovine pancreas
- Pork insulin: from porcine pancreas
- Human insulin: from recombinant deoxyribonucleic acid (DNA)
- Human insulin: from an enzymatic conversion of pork insulin through which the pork insulin molecule becomes identical to the insulin produced by the human pancreas

Insulin is available in three concentrations:

- U 40, or 40 units of insulin per milliliter
- U 100, or 100 units of insulin per milliliter
- U 500, or 500 units of insulin per milliliter

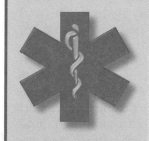

CASE PRESENTATION

At 2130 hours on a Saturday evening, paramedics are called to respond to a residence to aid a patient who is unconscious and unresponsive. Dispatch reports that the caller is unable to "wake up" his wife. The husband meets the paramedics as they arrive. He says that his wife is a diabetic and that the ambulance has been called several times before. Paramedics find the patient lying in bed in the master bedroom. The man says that his wife has been sick for a couple of days now and has been in bed for most of that time. Paramedics try to awaken the patient by gently shaking her, but there is no response. There is no evidence of trauma or of a fall. The patient is a 40-year-old woman who is unconscious and unresponsive. She is breathing adequately and has both a radial and a carotid pulse. Both, however, are weak.

On Examination

CNS: The patient is unconscious and unresponsive

Resp: Respirations are 24 per minute and shallow; lungs are clear bilaterally, with equal air entry; trachea is midline; no signs of trauma

CVS: The radial and carotid pulses are present but weak; skin is pale and quite diaphoretic

ABD: Soft and nontender in all four quadrants; no sign of vomiting

Muscl/Skel: No apparent injuries; no pitting edema

Vital Signs

Pulse: 112/minute

Resp: 24/minute, shallow

BP: 118/78 mmHg

SpO$_2$: 92 percent

ECG: Sinus tachycardia

Past Hx: The patient's husband states that the patient has been a diabetic for most of her life. He also shows paramedics the insulin vials in the refrigerator (Humulin N and Humulin R). The patient has had a low-grade fever for 2 days and has not been eating because of nausea. She is also alcoholic.

Treatment

To confirm your diagnosis of hypoglycemia, paramedics decide to take a blood glucose reading. While one paramedic prepares to check the level, another administers oxygen by nonrebreather mask at 15 lpm. An IV is initiated with an 18-gauge catheter and, prior to connecting the IV tubing, paramedics draw a red-top blood tube for analysis. They also use the hub of the needle to obtain a blood sample for glucose testing. An IV of normal saline is initiated and run at a TKO rate. The blood glucose reading is 40 mg/dL (2.2 mmol/L). At this time paramedics administer 100 mg of thiamine IV because of the history of alcoholism and 50 mL (25 g) of $D_{50}W$. Following administration of the $D_{50}W$, a fluid bolus of 20 mL of normal saline is administered to flush the IV line. Almost immediately following the $D_{50}W$ administration, the patient begins to make sounds and move about. The patient awakens and is surprised to see the paramedics. After a few minutes she is alert and oriented, although still a little lethargic. Paramedics decide to transport her to the hospital for assessment and monitor both vital signs and blood glucose levels en route. During the transport she tells paramedics that although she has not been eating normally, she was taking her regular amount of insulin.

Insulin is not effective when taken orally because the gastrointestinal (GI) tract breaks down the protein molecule before it reaches the bloodstream. All insulin, however, may be given by subcutaneous (SC) injection. Absorption of SC insulin varies according to the injection site and the vascular supply and degree of tissue hypertrophy at the injection site. Regular (unmodified) insulin may be given intravenously (IV) or intramuscularly (IM) as well.

After absorption into the bloodstream, insulin is distributed throughout the body. Insulin-response tissues are located in the liver, adipose tissue, and muscle. Insulin is metabolized primarily in the liver and to a lesser extent in the muscle tissue; it is excreted in the feces and urine.

The exact times for onset, peak, and duration are not absolute. They may vary not only from patient to patient but from injection to injection in the same patient. If insulin absorption is altered, the onset of action, peak concentration level, and duration of action are also altered. If insulin absorption occurs more rapidly, the onset of action and peak concentration times occur more rapidly. Conversely, if insulin absorption is prolonged, onset of action and peak concentration are delayed, and duration of action is prolonged.

Insulin is an anabolic, or building, hormone. It promotes the storage of glucose as glycogen, increases protein and fat synthesis, and inhibits the breakdown of glycogen, protein, and fat.

Insulin is indicated for type I diabetes mellitus. It may also be required for patients with type II diabetes mellitus when other methods of maintaining normal blood glucose level are ineffective. Patients with type II diabetes mellitus may find the usual methods of maintaining a normal blood glucose level ineffective during times of emotional or physical stress (such as surgery and infection) or contraindicated because of pregnancy or hypersensitivity. These patients may need insulin to control blood glucose levels more stringently. Insulin is also indicated for two of the comas that are complications of diabetes: diabetic ketoacidosis (more common with type I diabetes mellitus) and hyperosmolar hyperglycemic nonketotic syndrome (more common with type II diabetes mellitus).

Sometimes insulin is prescribed for patients who do not have diabetes mellitus. Because insulin stimulates cellular uptake of potassium, it may be administered with hypertonic glucose to patients with severe hyperkalemia. This insulin and glucose mixture produces a shift of serum potassium into cells and lowers the serum potassium level for a short time.

All insulin has the same effect in the body. The advantages or disadvantages of a particular kind of insulin reflect the differences in onset of action, peak concentration, and duration of action, as well as concentration, source, and purity. Many different insulin preparations are available; several are available in more than one concentration.

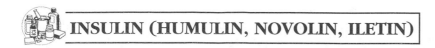

INSULIN (HUMULIN, NOVOLIN, ILETIN)

Class: Hormone and antihyperglycemic

Description

Insulin is a protein secreted by the β cells of the islets of Langerhans. It is responsible for promoting the uptake of glucose by the cells. In diabetics, in whom insulin secretion has diminished, supplemental insulin must be obtained by injection. Older forms of insulin are derived from animals (bovine and porcine). However, animal insulin is not identical to human insulin. Consequently, many patients develop antibodies to animal insulin, rendering it less effective. Human insulin can be manufactured through genetic engineering (recombinant DNA technology). Genetically engineered insulin (Humulin, Novolin) is chemically identical to the insulin hormone secreted by the pancreas. Patients do not develop antibodies to human insulin as they do to animal insulin.

Mechanism of Action

Insulin, when administered, is distributed throughout the body. It combines with insulin receptors present on the cell membranes, which promotes glucose entry into the cell and lowers the blood glucose level.

Pharmacokinetics

Onset: 0.5–1.0 hour
Peak Effects: 2–3 hours
Duration: 5–7 hours
Half-Life: 13 hours

Indications

Insulin is used in diabetic ketoacidosis, *hyperglycemia*, and hyperkalemia.

Contraindications

Insulin should be administered only when hyperglycemia or ketoacidosis has been confirmed. A blood glucose approximation should be obtained in all diabetic emergencies. Every emergency medical service (EMS) unit carrying insulin and 50 percent dextrose should also carry Dextrostix reagent strips or an electronic glucose determination device for approximating blood glucose levels. Based on the results of the blood glucose test, and in conjunction with the physical examination, the differential field diagnosis between hypoglycemia and ketoacidosis can usually be made. If there is any doubt about the etiology of diabetic coma, glucose should be administered. Insulin is almost always administered in the emergency department and not during the prehospital phase of emergency medical care.

Precautions

Repeated measurements of the blood glucose level, including possible administration of glucose, are necessary.

Side Effects

Insulin may cause hypoglycemia. Itching, swelling, redness, and frank allergic reactions may occur following administration of animal-derived insulins.

Interactions

Certain drugs, such as the corticosteroids, can increase the blood glucose level. Patients receiving these drugs may require a higher dose of insulin. The signs and symptoms of hypoglycemia may be masked in patients receiving β-blockers. Paramedics must always determine the blood glucose level.

Dosage

A standard dose for diabetic coma is 5 to 10 units of regular insulin IV followed by an infusion at 0.1 unit per kilogram per hour; 5 to 20 units of regular insulin can be administered subcutaneously or intramuscularly if there is not an immediate need for intravenous insulin. In an emergency setting insulin should be given intravenously, intramuscularly, or subcutaneously.

GLUCAGON

Unlike insulin and the oral antidiabetic agents, which decrease the blood glucose level, glucagon increases it. This hyperglycemic agent is a hormone normally produced by the α cells of the islets of Langerhans in the pancreas. After SC, IM, or IV injection, glucagon is absorbed rapidly (Table 9–3). It cannot be taken orally because it is a protein, and it would be destroyed in the GI tract. Glucagon is distributed throughout the body, although its effect occurs primarily in the liver. The exact metabolic fate of glucagon is unknown, although it is degraded extensively in the liver. Glucagon is removed from the body by the liver and the kidneys.

Glucagon regulates the rate of glucose production through glycogenolysis, gluconeogenesis, and lipolysis. A glucagon deficiency results in hypoglycemia. Although glucagon stimulates insulin secretion, insulin antagonizes glucagon's action through a negative feedback system.

Glucagon is used for emergency treatment of severe hypoglycemia. It is also used as an antidote for β-blocker overdose. Glucagon is ineffective in poorly nourished or starving patients.

TABLE 9–3			
Absorption Rate of Glucagon			
Route	Onset	Peak	Duration
SC, IM, IV	5 to 20 min	30 min	1 to 2 hr

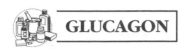 **GLUCAGON**

Class: Hormone and antihypoglycemic

Description

Glucagon is a protein secreted by the α cells of the pancreas. Glucagon for parenteral administration is extracted from beef and pork pancreas. It is used to increase the blood glucose level in cases of hypoglycemia in which an IV cannot be immediately placed.

Mechanism of Action

Glucagon is a hormone secreted by the pancreas. When released it causes a breakdown of stored glycogen to glucose. It also inhibits the synthesis of glycogen from glucose. Both actions tend to cause an increase in circulating blood glucose. In hypoglycemia the administration of glucagon increases blood glucose levels. The drug of choice in the management of insulin-induced hypoglycemia is still $D_{50}W$. A return to consciousness is seen almost immediately following the administration of glucose. A return to consciousness following the administration of glucagon usually takes from 5 to 20 minutes. Glucagon is only effective if there are sufficient stores of glycogen in the liver. Glucagon exerts a positive inotropic action on the heart and decreases renal vascular resistance.

Indications

Glucagon is used in hypoglycemia and β-blocker overdose.

Contraindications

Because glucagon is a protein, hypersensitivity may occur. Glucagon should not be administered to patients with a known hypersensitivity to the drug.

Precautions

Glucagon is only effective if there are sufficient stores of glycogen within the liver. In an emergency situation intravenous glucose is the agent of choice. Glucagon should be administered with caution to patients with a history of cardiovascular or renal disease.

Side Effects

Although side effects are rare, glucagon can cause hypotension, dizziness, headache, nausea, and vomiting.

Interactions

Few interactions with glucagon are reported in the emergency setting.

Dosage

A standard initial dose is 0.25 to 0.5 units administered intravenously. If an IV cannot be obtained, 1 mg of glucagon can be administered intramuscularly.

Route

Glucagon can be administered intravenously, intramuscularly, or subcutaneously.

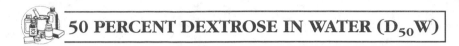

50 PERCENT DEXTROSE IN WATER (D$_{50}$W)

Class: Carbohydrate

Description

Dextrose is used to describe the six-carbon sugar *d-glucose*, which is the principal form of carbohydrate used by the body.

Mechanism of Action

Dextrose supplies supplemental glucose in cases of hypoglycemia. Serious brain injury can occur if hypoglycemia is prolonged. Thus, in hypoglycemia the rapid administration of glucose is essential. When the hypoglycemic patient is comatose, glucose cannot be given by mouth and should be given as an IV D$_{50}$W solution.

Pharmacokinetics

Onset: <1 minute
Peak Effects: Varies
Duration: Varies
Half-Life: Not applicable

Indication

Dextrose is used in hypoglycemia and coma of unknown origin.

Contraindications

There are no major contraindications to the IV administration of D$_{50}$W to a patient with suspected hypoglycemia. Even if a patient were suffering from ketoacidosis, the amount of glucose present in 50 mL of 50 percent dextrose would not adversely affect the clinical outcome; 50 percent dextrose should be used with caution in patients with increased intracranial pressure because the dextrose load may worsen cerebral edema.

Precautions

It is important to use a Dextrostix or obtain a Glucometer reading and draw a sample of blood before initiating an IV infusion and giving 50 percent dextrose. Localized venous irritation may occur when smaller veins are used. Infiltration of 50 percent dextrose may result in tissue necrosis. Fifty percent dextrose should never be administered as part of a "coma cocktail." "Coma cocktails" involve the empiric administration of 50 percent dextrose, thiamine, and naloxone (and in some cases, flumazenil) to unresponsive patients in an attempt to correct the cause of their unresponsiveness and awaken them. "Coma cocktails" are a poor prehospital practice. Therapy should always be guided by objective data such as patient assessment findings and blood glucose determination.

Side Effects

Side effects can include tissue necrosis and phlebitis at the injection site.

Interactions

There are no interactions in the emergency setting.

Dosage

The standard dosage of 50 percent dextrose in hypoglycemia is 25 g (50 mL of a 50 percent solution) administered intravenously. If an initial dose is ineffective, a second dose of 25 g may also be given; 50 percent dextrose should be diluted 1:1 with sterile water for pediatric administration (thus forming $D_{25}W$). The pediatric dose is 0.5 to 1.0 g/kg of body weight by slow, intravenous bolus.

Route

Dextrose is only given intravenously. Concentrated glucose solutions can cause venous irritation if administered for an extended period.

THIAMINE

Thiamine is used primarily to prevent and treat thiamine deficiency syndromes such as beriberi, Wernicke's encephalopathy, and peripheral neuritis associated with pellagra. Thiamine malabsorption may occur in patients with alcoholism, cirrhosis, or GI disease, requiring supplements. In most cases thiamine administration does not result in adverse reactions or toxicity. Various nonspecific reactions that have been reported include nausea, anxiety, sweating, and sensations of warmth. Allergic reactions, ranging from itching and uticaria to cardiovascular failure and death, have occurred with parenteral administration.

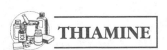 **THIAMINE**

Class: Vitamin

Description

Thiamine is an important vitamin commonly referred to as vitamin B_1. It is required for the conversion of pyruvic acid to acetyl coenzyme A.

Mechanism of Action

A vitamin is a substance that the body cannot manufacture but that is required for metabolism. Most of the vitamins required by the body are obtained through the diet. Thiamine is required for the conversion of pyruvic acid to acetyl coenzyme A. Without this step, a significant amount of the energy available in glucose cannot be obtained. The brain is extremely sensitive to thiamine deficiency. Chronic alcohol intake interferes with the absorption, intake, and use of thiamine. A significant percentage of alcoholics have thiamine deficiency. During extended periods of fasting, neurological symptoms owing to thiamine deficiency may occur. These symptoms include Wernicke's encephalopathy and Korsakoff's psychosis. Wernicke's encephalopathy is an

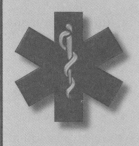

CASE PRESENTATION

At 1630 hours on a Thursday afternoon, paramedics are called to respond to a suburban residence to aid a patient who is unresponsive. The emergency medical dispatcher reports that the caller is a 9-year-old girl who just came home from school and cannot wake up her mother.

Paramedics are met by the young girl as they arrive at the small frame residence. Tearfully she tells them that her mother is a diabetic and that the ambulance has been called several times before. As paramedics enter the residence, they notice that someone had been preparing a meal. They find the mother lying on the floor in the living room. The girl tells them that her mother's name is Tanya. Paramedics call to Tanya and gently shake her shoulder, but there is no response. There is no evidence of trauma or of a fall. The patient is a 30-year-old woman who is unconscious and unresponsive. She is breathing adequately and has both a radial and a carotid pulse. Both, however, are weak.

On Examination

CNS: The patient is unconscious and unresponsive

Resp: Respirations are 30 per minute and shallow; lungs are clear bilaterally, with equal air entry; trachea is midline; no signs of trauma

CVS: Radial and carotid pulses present but weak; skin is pale and quite diaphoretic

ABD: Soft and nontender in all four quadrants; no sign of vomiting

Muscl/Skel: No apparent injuries; no pitting edema

Vital Signs

Pulse: 112/min

Resp: 30/min, shallow

BP: 118/78 mmHg

SpO$_2$: 92 percent

ECG: Sinus tachycardia

Past Hx: Her daughter states that the patient has been a diabetic for as long as she can remember. She also shows you insulin vials in the refrigerator (Humulin N and Humulin R). The daughter does not know when her mother last ate. However, they usually eat at 5 P.M.

Treatment

Based on physical findings, the patient history obtained from the daughter, and the presence of insulin in the refrigerator, paramedics suspect that the patient is hypoglycemic. To confirm, they decide to determine the blood glucose level. While one paramedic prepares to do this, another administers oxygen by nonrebreather mask at 15 lpm. By medical control protocol, they are able to begin definitive advanced life support procedures. Paramedics perform venipuncture with an

18-gauge catheter and, prior to connecting the IV tubing, draw a red-top blood tube for analysis. They also use the hub of the needle to obtain a blood sample for glucose testing. An IV of D_5W (normal saline is also acceptable) is initiated and run at a TKO rate. The blood glucose reading is 40 mg/dL (2.2 mmol/L). At this time 50 mL (25 g) of $D_{50}W$ is administered. Following administration of the $D_{50}W$, a fluid bolus of 25 mL of D_5W is administered to flush the IV line.

Almost immediately following the $D_{50}W$ administration, the patient begins to make sounds and move about. The patient awakens and is surprised to see the paramedics. She is very apologetic and somewhat embarrassed. She insists that she is fine now and refuses transport to the hospital. After paramedics are sure that the patient is conscious, alert, and in no further danger, they inform her of the risks of refusing transport. She acknowledges the risks and signs the release form. Paramedics aseptically discontinue the IV, apply an adhesive strip, and leave the scene.

acute and reversible encephalopathy characterized by an unsteady gait, eye muscle weakness, and mental derangement. Korsakoff's psychosis is a significant memory disorder and may be irreversible. Any comatose patients, especially those who are suspected to be alcoholic, should receive IV thiamine in addition to the administration of 50 percent dextrose or naloxone.

Pharmacokinetics

Onset: Rapid
Peak Effects: Varies
Duration: Varies
Half-Life: Not applicable

Indication

Thiamine is used for coma of unknown origin, especially if alcohol may be involved, and delirium tremens.

Contraindications

There are no contraindications to the administration of thiamine in the emergency setting.

Precautions

A few cases of hypersensitivity to thiamine have been reported. Thiamine should never be administered as part of a "coma cocktail." "Coma cocktails" involve the empiric administration of 50 percent dextrose, thiamine, and naloxone (and in some cases, flumazenil) to unresponsive patients in an attempt to correct the cause of their unresponsiveness and awaken them. "Coma cocktails" are a poor prehospital practice. Therapy should always be guided by objective data such as patient assessment findings and blood glucose determination.

Side Effects

Few side effects are reported with thiamine usage. However, hypotension, dyspnea, and respiratory failure have been reported with its use.

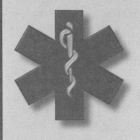

CASE PRESENTATION

Late in the afternoon on a warm September day, paramedics are dispatched to a residence to help a patient "not feeling well." The emergency medical dispatcher reports that the patient is a 60-year-old man who is reportedly conscious and alert. On arrival paramedics are directed into the patient's bedroom by his wife. The patient is lying in bed, propped up by two pillows. The patient says he has been feeling ill for over 48 hours. He also reports that he has had rather severe abdominal pain accompanied by nausea and vomiting. However, he has been able to tolerate some clear liquids. He has not been able to keep down any food. He denies any diarrhea or any other problems and is sure that this is the flu.

On Examination

CNS:	The patient is conscious, alert, and oriented × 4
Resp:	Respirations are 32/minute, deep and labored; lungs are clear bilaterally, with equal air entry; trachea is midline; no signs of trauma
CVS:	Both radial and carotid pulses are present but weak; skin is slightly pale and dry
ABD:	Soft and nontender in all four quadrants
Muscl/Skel:	No apparent injuries; no pitting edema

Vital Signs

Pulse:	140/min
Resp:	32/min, shallow, labored
BP:	92/54 mmHg
SpO$_2$:	94 percent
ECG:	Sinus tachycardia
Past Hx:	Past medical history includes insulin-dependent diabetes mellitus (type I). His wife states that the patient has not taken insulin since he has been sick.

Treatment

Oxygen is administered by nonrebreather mask at 12 lpm. The rapid, deep respirations are consistent with Kussmaul respirations. One paramedic prepares an IV of normal saline while another performs venipuncture with a 16-gauge catheter. Blood is drawn for a red-top tube and the hub of the needle is used to obtain a blood sample for glucose testing. The IV of normal saline is connected to the catheter and run at 150 mL/hr. The blood glucose reading exceeds 400 mg/dL (22.22 mmol/L). Paramedics suspect the patient is in early diabetic ketoacidosis. Care provided during transport to the hospital is primarily supportive and includes monitoring of vital signs and fluid replacement.

At the emergency department the patient's blood glucose reading is 880 mg/dL (48.88 mmol/L). His serum ketones are positive at 1:16 dilution. An arterial blood gas reveals a pH of 7.16, pCO_2 of 30 Torr, and pO_2 of 190 Torr (on 40 percent mask), which is generally consistent with a partially compensated metabolic acidosis. He is started on an insulin drip and admitted to the hospital. A chest X ray reveals a right lower lobe pneumonia, which the emergency department physician feels contributed to the development of diabetic ketoacidosis. Following a 3-day course of antibiotics and aggressive fluid therapy, the patient is discharged.

Interactions

There are no interactions in the emergency setting.

Dosage

The emergency dose of thiamine is 100 mg administered intravenously or intramuscularly.

Route

Thiamine can be given either intravenously or intramuscularly. The intravenous route is preferred in emergency medicine.

SUMMARY

Diabetes mellitus is probably the most common metabolic-endocrine emergency seen in the prehospital phase of emergency medical care. Hypoglycemia, if not immediately treated, can result in serious and permanent brain damage. It is important to remember that acute metabolic-endocrine disorders can cause a wide range of signs and symptoms, from bizarre behavior to coma.

Prehospital drug administration should be guided by available data. Paramedics should always determine the blood glucose level. If it is low, 50 percent dextrose is administered. If alcoholism is suspected, administration of thiamine should be considered. If narcotic abuse is possible, administration of naloxone is considered. The "coma cocktail" is a thing of the past. Prehospital care should be based on physical exam findings and the patient's medical history.

KEY WORDS

diabetes mellitus. An endocrine disorder characterized by inadequate insulin production by the β cells of the islets of Langerhans in the pancreas.

endocrine glands. Glands that secrete hormones directly into the blood.

hormones. Chemical substances released by a gland that control or affect other glands or body systems.

hyperglycemia. A complication of diabetes characterized by excessive levels of blood glucose.

hypoglycemia. A complication of diabetes characterized by low levels of blood glucose. It often occurs from too high a dose of insulin or from inadequate food intake following a normal insulin dose. Sometimes called *insulin shock*, hypoglycemia is a true medical emergency.

ketoacidosis. A complication of diabetes due to decreased insulin secretion or intake. It is characterized by high levels of glucose in the blood, metabolic acidosis, and, in advanced stages, coma. Ketoacidosis is often called *diabetic coma*.

Kussmaul respirations. A very deep, gasping respiratory pattern found in diabetic coma.

DRUGS USED IN THE TREATMENT OF NEUROLOGICAL EMERGENCIES 10

OBJECTIVES

After completing this chapter, the reader should be able to:

1. Describe the treatment for a patient with a blunt or penetrating head injury.

2. Describe and list the indications, contraindications, and dosages for dexamethasone, mannitol, and methylprednisolone.

3. List three acute, nontraumatic neurological disorders.

4. Describe and list the indications, contraindications, and dosages for the following drugs used in the treatment of seizures: diazepam, lorazepam, midazolam, phenytoin, fosphenytoin, and phenobarbital.

INTRODUCTION

Emergencies involving the nervous system can be devastating. In addition, they are also notoriously difficult to manage. Signs and symptoms of neurological disorders can range from slight headache to coma. They may be temporary or permanent. Prompt recognition and treatment are essential.

NEUROLOGICAL TRAUMA

Head injuries are an all-too-common result of automobile and motorcycle collisions. Although encased within the protective skull, the brain is quite susceptible to injury. Following craniocerebral trauma, cerebral edema occurs within 24 hours.

The primary treatment of patients with blunt or penetrating head injury is supportive. Airway management is of paramount importance, and continuous monitoring of blood pressure to detect occult blood loss in major trauma is mandatory. Pharmacological agents that have been used in the management of neurological emergencies include *dexamethasone,* which is thought to be of use in reducing brain edema, and *mannitol,* an osmotic diuretic that is also useful in reducing brain edema and is faster acting than dexamethasone.

High-dose methylprednisolone (Solu-Medrol) was recommended as an emergency treatment for acute spinal cord injury. This recommendation was a result of three studies called the National Acute Spinal Cord Injury Studies (NASCIS 1, NASCIS 2, and NASCIS 3). However, scrutiny of these studies revealed numerous flaws, and subsequent studies failed to reproduce the results seen in the NASCIS trials. Furthermore, several studies found that the side effects associated with such massive doses of steroids were harmful and that, in most cases, any possible benefits were not worth the associated risks. EMS personnel should refer to local protocols and practices with regard to the use of high-dose steroids for acute spinal cord injury.

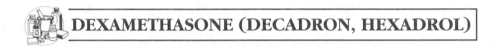

DEXAMETHASONE (DECADRON, HEXADROL)

Class: Corticosteroid

Description

Dexamethasone is a synthetic steroid chemically related to the natural hormones secreted by the adrenal cortex.

Mechanism of Action

Corticocosteroids have multiple actions in the body. They have potent anti-inflammatory properties and inhibit many of the substances that cause inflammation (cytokines, interleukin, interferon) and also inhibit the synthesis of pro-inflammatory enzymes. Dexamethasone is a long-acting steroid with a plasma half-life of 3 to 4 hours. In general medical practice, steroids have a wide range of uses. Effective as anti-inflammatory agents, they are used in the management of allergic reactions and occasionally as an adjunctive agent in the management of shock. The role of steroids in the management of cerebral edema remains controversial. The mechanism by which and extent to which dexamethasone decreases cerebral edema, if indeed it does, are unclear.

Pharmacokinetics

> **Onset:** <1 hour
> **Peak Effects:** <1 hour
> **Duration:** Varies [intravenous (IV)], 6 days [intramuscular (IM)]
> **Half-Life:** 3–4 hours

Indications

Dexamethasone is used in cerebral edema, anaphylaxis, asthma, and exacerbation of chronic obstructive pulmonary disease (COPD).

Contraindications

There are no major contraindications to the use of dexamethasone in the emergency setting.

Precautions

A single dose of dexamethasone is all that should be given in the prehospital phase of care. Long-term steroid therapy can cause gastrointestinal bleeding, prolonged wound healing, and suppression of adrenocortical steroids.

Side Effects

Dexamethasone can cause fluid retention, congestive heart failure, hypertension, abdominal distention, vertigo, headache, nausea, malaise, and hiccups.

Interactions

There are few interactions in the prehospital setting.

Dosage

The dose of dexamethasone varies considerably from physician to physician. The usual range is 4 to 24 mg; 12 mg administered intravenously (IV) is a commonly used dose. High-dose dexamethasone therapy, however, with up to 100 mg of the drug, is sometimes given.

Route

Dexamethasone is administered intravenously or intramuscularly; the intravenous route is preferred in the emergency setting.

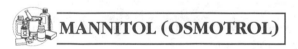

MANNITOL (OSMOTROL)

Class: Osmotic diuretic

Description

Mannitol is a six-carbon sugar compound that has osmotic diuretic properties.

Mechanism of Action

Mannitol is an osmotic diuretic that inhibits sodium and water absorption in the kidneys. It promotes movement of fluid from the intracellular into the extracellular space. Because it dehydrates brain tissue, mannitol has proved effective in the management of cerebral edema and reduces intracranial pressure.

Pharmacokinetics

Onset: 15 minutes
Peak Effects: 3–8 hours
Duration: Varies
Half-Life: 100 minutes

Indications

Mannitol is used for acute cerebral edema and blood transfusion reactions.

Contraindications

Mannitol should not be used in any patient with acute pulmonary edema or severe pulmonary congestion. It should not be used in any patient who is profoundly hypovolemic.

Precautions

Rapid administration of mannitol can cause a transitory increase in intravascular volume and can result in congestive heart failure. The diuresis that accompanies mannitol therapy can cause sodium depletion.

One problem in the use of mannitol in the prehospital phase of emergency medical care is crystallization of the drug. The more concentrated the solution, the more tendency it has to crystallize at low temperatures. Crystallization begins as temperatures approach 45°F. Anytime a concentrated solution of mannitol is used, usually 15 percent or greater, an in-line filter should be present. It is important to remember that microscopic crystals appear long before those that can be seen by the naked eye. If mannitol solution crystallizes, it should be warmed slowly in boiling water until the crystals disappear. It should be removed from emergency medical service (EMS) vehicles that are not parked in heated areas during colder weather.

Side Effects

Mannitol can cause chills, headache, dizziness, lethargy, mental status change, chest pain, nausea, and vomiting.

Interactions

Mannitol should not be administered with whole blood or packed red blood cells because it can damage the red blood cells.

Dosage

The typical adult dose of mannitol is 1.5 to 2.0 g/kg of body weight administered intravenously. This dose can be given as a slow IV bolus or IV infusion. The slower rate of infusion helps eliminate the chances of inducing circulatory overload and congestive heart failure.

Route

Mannitol should be given intravenously.

METHYLPREDNISOLONE (SOLU-MEDROL)

Class: Corticosteroid and anti-inflammatory

Description

Methylprednisolone is an intermediate-acting corticosteroid related to the natural hormones secreted by the adrenal cortex.

Mechanism of Action

Corticocosteroids have multiple actions in the body. They have potent anti-inflammatory properties and inhibit many of the substances that cause inflammation (cytokines, interleukin, interferon) and also inhibit the synthesis of pro-inflammatory enzymes. Methylprednisolone is an intermediate-acting synthetic steroid. In general medical practice, steroids have a wide range of uses. Effective as anti-inflammatory agents, they are used in the management of allergic reactions and occasionally as an adjunctive agent in the management of shock. The role of steroids in the management of neurological emergencies remains controversial. It is generally agreed that a large single dose of steroids has little harmful effect. Consequently, it is used in patients with spinal cord injury both in the emergency department and in the prehospital setting.

Pharmacokinetics

Onset: Varies
Peak Effects: 4–8 days (IM)
Duration: 1–5 weeks (IM)
Half-Life: 3.5 hours

Indications

Methylprednisolone may be used as a treatment option in spinal cord injury, anaphylaxis, asthma, and exacerbation of COPD.

Contraindications

There are no major contraindications to the use of methylprednisolone in the emergency setting.

Precautions

A single dose of methylprednisolone is all that should be given in the prehospital phase of care. Long-term steroid therapy can cause gastrointestinal bleeding, prolonged wound healing, and suppression of adrenocortical steroids.

Side Effects

Methylprednisolone can cause fluid retention, congestive heart failure, hypertension, abdominal distension, vertigo, headache, nausea, malaise, and hiccups.

Interactions

There are few interactions in the prehospital setting.

Dosage

Spinal cord injury. High-dose methylprednisolone is used as a treatment option for spinal cord injuries. An initial bolus of 30 mg/kg is administered intravenously over a 15-minute period. This dose is followed 45 minutes later by a maintenance infusion of 5.4 mg/kg/hr for 24 to 48 hours.

Asthma, COPD, or allergic reactions. For other emergencies, 80 to 125 mg is usually administered intravenously or intramuscularly.

NONTRAUMATIC NEUROLOGICAL EMERGENCIES

There are many acute nontraumatic neurological disorders. Drugs, poisonings, and metabolic derangements can precipitate neurological emergencies. Little can be done for stroke and brain tumors in the prehospital phase of emergency medical care. Seizures attributable to epilepsy and other disorders can be managed in the field, however.

Seizures are one of the most frequently encountered neurological emergencies. One seizure followed by another seizure, without an intervening period of consciousness, is called *status epilepticus* and constitutes a serious threat to life. Status epilepticus should be terminated as quickly as possible.

The most common drug used to terminate seizure activity is IV diazepam (Valium). Phenytoin (Dilantin) and phenobarbital are also effective, however. We discuss these three drugs and their roles in prehospital care next.

Benzodiazepines

Benzodiazepines produce many effects, including daytime and preanesthetic sedation, sleep inducement, relief of anxiety and tension, skeletal muscle relaxation, and anticonvulsant activity. In the prehospital setting, benzodiazepines are primarily used as skeletal muscle relaxants, for preprocedure sedation (such as cardioversion), and for anticonvulsant activity.

Benzodiazepines are absorbed well from the gastrointestinal (GI) tract and distributed widely in the body. In the prehospital setting, benzodiazepines are almost always given parenterally. All benzodiazepines are metabolized in the liver and excreted primarily in the urine. Onset of action when administered IV is 1 to 5 minutes, with peak immediate and duration of 15 minutes to 1 hour.

The principal sites of action for benzodiazepines are the cerebral cortex and the limbic, thalamic, and hypothalamic levels of the *central nervous system* (CNS).

In most cases benzodiazepines are preferred over barbiturates because of their effectiveness and safety. Benzodiazepines offer many advantages, including fewer adverse reactions, decreased potential for abuse, fewer drug interactions, a wide margin of safety between therapeutic and toxic dosages that makes overdoses less likely, and a reduced risk of physical and psychological dependence with therapeutic dosages.

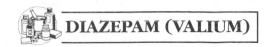

DIAZEPAM (VALIUM)

Class: Anticonvulsant and sedative

Description

Diazepam is a benzodiazepine that is frequently used as an anticonvulsant, sedative, and hypnotic.

Mechanism of Action

Benzodiazepines bind to specific sites on gamma-aminobutyric acid (GABA) Type A receptors within the brain. GABA is the major inhibitory neurotransmitter of the central nervous system. Benzodiazepines have no direct effect on the GABA receptors, but do potentiate the effects of GABA within the brain. Increased GABA levels cause sedation. Through this mechanism, the benzodiazepines display their hypnotic, anxiolytic, and anticonvulsant effects. Their usefulness, however, is limited by a broad range of side effects including compromised sedation, ataxia, amnesia, alcohol and barbiturate potentiation, tolerance development, and abuse potential.

In emergency medicine, diazepam is principally used for its anticonvulsant properties. It suppresses the spread of seizure activity through the motor cortex of the brain. It does not appear to abolish the abnormal discharge focus, however. Diazepam, one of the most frequently prescribed medications in the United States, is used in the management of anxiety and stress. It is effective in treating the tremors and anxiety associated with alcohol withdrawal. It is also an effective skeletal muscle relaxant, which makes it an effective adjunct in orthopedic injuries. It is a good premedication for minor operative procedures and cardioversion because it induces amnesia, which diminishes the patient's recall of such procedures.

Pharmacokinetics

Onset: 1–5 minutes (IV), 15–30 minutes (IM)
Peak Effects: 15 minutes (IV), 30–45 minutes (IM)
Duration: 15–60 minutes
Half-Life: 20–50 hours

Indications

Diazepam is used in major motor seizures, status epilepticus, premedication before cardioversion, skeletal muscle relaxant, and acute anxiety states.

Contraindications

Diazepam should not be administered to any patient with a history of hypersensitivity to the drug.

Precautions

Because diazepam is a relatively short-acting drug, seizure activity may recur. In such cases, an additional dose may be required. Flumazenil

(Romazicon), a benzodiazepine antagonist, should be available to use as antidote if required. Injectable diazepam can cause local venous irritation. To minimize irritation, it should only be injected into relatively large veins and should not be given faster than 1 mL/min.

Side Effects

Diazepam can cause hypotension, drowsiness, headache, amnesia, respiratory depression, blurred vision, nausea, and vomiting.

Interactions

Diazepam is incompatible with many medications. Whenever diazepam is given intravenously in conjunction with other drugs, the IV line should be adequately flushed. The effects of diazepam can be additive when used in conjunction with other CNS depressants and alcohol.

Dosage

In the management of seizures, the usual dose of diazepam is 5 to 10 mg IV. In many instances it may be necessary to give diazepam directly into the vein, because the seizure activity will prevent the insertion of an indwelling catheter. When given directly into a vein, it is essential that a large vein, preferably in the antecubital fossa, be used. In acute anxiety reactions, the standard dosage is 2 to 5 mg administered intramuscularly.

To induce amnesia prior to cardioversion, a dosage of 5 to 15 mg of diazepam is given intravenously. Peak effects are seen in 5 to 10 minutes. Diazepam should be given intravenously by slow IV push. It can be injected intramuscularly, but absorption via this route is variable. When an IV line cannot be started, parenteral diazepam can be administered rectally with a similar onset of action.

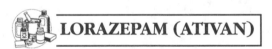

LORAZEPAM (ATIVAN)

Class: Anticonvulsant and sedative

Description

Lorazepam is a benzodiazepine that is used as an anticonvulsant, sedative, and hypnotic.

Mechanism of Action

Benzodiazepines bind to specific sites on GABA, Type A receptors within the brain. GABA is the major inhibitory neurotransmitter of the central nervous system. Benzodiazepines have no direct effect on the GABA receptors, but do potentiate the effects of GABA within the brain. Increased GABA levels cause sedation. Through this mechanism, the benzodiazepines display their hypnotic, anxiolytic, and anticonvulsant effects. Their usefulness, however, is limited by a broad range of side effects including compromised sedation, ataxia, amnesia, alcohol and barbiturate potentiation, tolerance development, and abuse potential.

Lorazepam is a benzodiazepine with a shorter half-life than that of diazepam. Its onset of action is approximately the same. It is used in the management of anxiety and stress. It is a good premedication for minor operative procedures and cardioversion because it induces *amnesia,* which diminishes the patient's recall of such procedures. Lorazepam is often used in pediatrics as an anticonvulsant because of its shorter half-life. Like diazepam, lorazepam suppresses the spread of seizure activity through the motor cortex of the brain. It does not appear to abolish the abnormal discharge focus.

Pharmacokinetics

Onset: 1–5 minutes (IV), 15–30 minutes (IM)
Peak Effects: 15–20 minutes (IV), 2 hours (IM)
Duration: 6–8 hours
Half-Life: 10–20 hours

Indications

Lorazepam is used in major motor seizures, in status epilepticus, as premedication before cardioversion, and for acute anxiety states.

Contraindications

Lorazepam should not be administered to any patient with a history of hypersensitivity to the drug.

Precautions

Lorazepam should be diluted with normal saline or D_5W prior to intravenous administration. Because lorazepam is a relatively short-acting drug, seizure activity may recur. In such cases, an additional dose may be required. Flumazenil (Romazicon), a benzodiazepine antagonist, should be available to use as an antidote if required.

Side Effects

Lorazepam can cause hypotension, drowsiness, headache, amnesia, respiratory depression, blurred vision, nausea, and vomiting.

Interactions

The effects of lorazepam can be additive when used in conjunction with other CNS depressants and alcohol.

Dosage

The usual dose of lorazepam is 0.5 to 2.0 mg when given intravenously. The dose can be increased to 1.0 to 4.0 mg when given intramuscularly. It can be given rectally when an IV cannot be placed. The medication should be drawn up into a syringe. A small, red, rubber pediatric feeding tube can be attached to the syringe. The feeding tube should be inserted 2 to 4 cm into the rectum and the drug administered. Often it is necessary to hold the buttocks together to help the patient retain the drug.

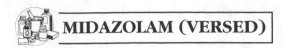

MIDAZOLAM (VERSED)

Class: Sedative, anticonvulsant, and hypnotic

Description

Midazolam is a benzodiazepine with strong hypnotic and amnestic properties.

Mechanism of Action

Benzodiazepines bind to specific sites on GABA, Type A receptors within the brain. GABA is the major inhibitory neurotransmitter of the central nervous system. Benzodiazepines have no direct effect on the GABA receptors, but do potentiate the effects of GABA within the brain. Increased GABA levels cause sedation. Through this mechanism, the benzodiazepines display their hypnotic, anxiolytic, and anticonvulsant effects. Their usefulness, however, is limited by a broad range of side effects including compromised sedation, ataxia, amnesia, alcohol and barbiturate potentiation, tolerance development, and abuse potential.

Midazolam is a potent but short-acting benzodiazepine used widely in medicine as a sedative, anticonvulsant, and hypnotic. It is three to four times more potent than diazepam. Its onset of action is approximately 3–5 minutes when administered intravenously and 15 minutes when administered intramuscularly. Midazolam has impressive amnestic properties. Like the other benzodiazepines, it has no effect on pain.

Pharmacokinetics

Onset: 3–5 minutes (IV), 15 minutes (IM)
Peak Effects: 20–60 minutes
Duration: <2 hours (IV), 1–6 hours (IM)
Half-Life: 1–4 hours

Indications

Midazolam is used as a premedication before cardioversion and other painful procedures. It is also an effective anticonvulsant.

Contraindications

Midazolam should not be administered to any patient with a history of hypersensitivity to the drug. It should not be used in patients who have narrow-angle glaucoma. Midazolam should not be administered to patients in shock, with depressed vital signs, or who are in alcoholic coma.

Precautions

Emergency resuscitative equipment must be available prior to the administration of midazolam. Vital signs must be continuously monitored during and after drug administration. Midazolam has more potential than the other benzodiazepines to cause respiratory depression and respiratory arrest. Flumazenil (Romazicon), a benzodiazepine antagonist, should be available to use as an antidote if required.

Side Effects

Midazolam can cause laryngospasm, bronchospasm, dyspnea, respiratory depression and arrest, drowsiness, amnesia, altered mental status, bradycardia, tachycardia, premature ventricular contractions, and retching.

Interactions

The effects of midazolam can be accentuated by CNS depressants such as narcotics and alcohol.

Dosage

When used for sedation, midazolam must be administered cautiously, because the amount of medication required to achieve sedation varies from individual to individual. Typically, 1 to 2.5 mg are administered by slow IV injection. Higher doses may be required when used as an anticonvulsant. Usually, it is best to dilute midazolam with normal saline or D_5W prior to IV administration. Midazolam can be administered intramuscularly at a dose of 0.07 to 0.08 mg/kg (average adult dose of 5 mg). Recently, many centers have been administering midazolam intranasally or by mouth to sedate children prior to suturing of lacerations.

Hydantoins

Phenytoin and phenytoin sodium are the most commonly prescribed anticonvulsant agents. In the prehospital setting, phenytoin may be used as a second-line drug for the treatment of seizures and as a second-line antidysrhythmic.

Hydantoin anticonvulsants are usually absorbed slowly, rapidly distributed, and extensively protein bound. They are metabolized in the liver and excreted in the urine.

In most cases, the hydantoin anticonvulsants can stabilize nerve cells against hyperexcitability. Phenytoin's primary site of action appears to be the motor cortex, where the drug inhibits the spread of seizure activity. Phenytoin also exhibits antidysrhythmic properties similar to those of quinidine or procainamide. Because of its clinical efficacy and relatively low toxicity, phenytoin is the most commonly prescribed anticonvulsant.

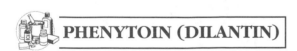 **PHENYTOIN (DILANTIN)**

Class: Anticonvulsant and antidysrhythmic

Description

Phenytoin is a long-acting anticonvulsant. It is also used as an antidysrhythmic because it depresses spontaneous ventricular depolarization.

Mechanism of Action

Phenytoin produces a voltage- and frequency-dependent blockade of sodium channels in rapidly discharging nerve cells. Thus, it stops sustained repetitive firing such as that occurring during a seizure. Because of this it prevents the spread of seizure discharge.

Phenytoin is an effective anticonvulsant. Its onset of action, however, is longer than that of diazepam. In most emergency situations the seizure should first be controlled with Valium. If seizure activity recurs, phenytoin can be administered. Phenytoin also is used to treat dysrhythmias caused by digitalis toxicity. This use of the drug is discussed in Chapter 7.

Pharmacokinetics

Onset: 3–5 minutes
Peak Effects: 1–2 hours
Duration: Varies
Half-Life: 22 hours

Indications

Phenytoin is used in major motor seizures, status epilepticus, and dysrhythmias caused by digitalis toxicity.

Contraindications

Phenytoin should not be given to any patient with a history of hypersensitivity to the drug. It is contraindicated in cases of bradycardia and high-grade heart block. It should not be administered to patients who take the drug chronically for seizures until the blood level has been determined.

Precautions

Intravenous administration of phenytoin should not exceed 50 mg/min. Signs of central nervous system depression or hypotension may occur. Elderly patients are at increased risk of developing side effects from phenytoin administration. Extravasation should be avoided. Any patient receiving intravenous phenytoin should have continuous cardiac monitoring as well as frequent monitoring of vital signs.

Side Effects

Phenytoin can cause drowsiness, dizziness, headache, hypotension, dysrhythmias, itching, rash, nausea, and vomiting.

Interactions

Phenytoin must never be diluted in dextrose-containing solutions such as D_5W. It should be diluted in normal saline or other non-glucose-containing crystalloids.

Dosage

The loading dose of phenytoin is typically 10 to 15 mg/kg. This dose should be administered no faster than 50 mg/min. Phenytoin should be diluted with normal saline, because dilution with 5 percent dextrose may result in precipitation of the drug. In emergency medicine phenytoin should be administered intravenously only.

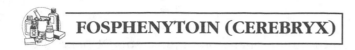

FOSPHENYTOIN (CEREBRYX)

Class: Anticonvulsant

Description

Fosphenytoin is a prodrug of phenytoin. It is converted to phenytoin after parenteral administration. Unlike phenytoin, fosphenytoin can be given by intramuscular injection when IV access is unavailable.

Mechanism of Action

Fosphenytoin is an effective anticonvulsant with properties similar to those of phenytoin. Like phenytoin, it suppresses seizure activity in the brain.

Pharmacokinetics

Onset: <15 minutes (IM)
Peak Effects: 30 minutes (IM)
Duration: Varies
Half-Life: 15 minutes to convert to phenytoin (phenytoin half-life: 22 hours)

Indications

Fosphenytoin is used in major motor seizures. Like phenytoin, it has unlabeled use as an antidysrhythmic, particularly for digitalis-induced dysrhythmias.

Contraindications

Hypersensitivity to the phenytoin (hydantoin) class of medications. Fosphenytoin should not be used in seizures caused by hypoglycemia, bradycardia, or complete or partial heart block.

Precautions

Use with caution in patients with impaired kidney function, alcoholism, hypotension, heart block, bradycardia, respiratory depression, or severe heart disease. An ECG monitor and a pulse oximeter should be used whenever administering fosphenytoin. Vital signs should be checked regularly during administration.

Side Effects

Side effects associated with fosphenytoin include dizziness, somnolence, drowsiness, bradycardia, heart block, blurred vision, and hypotension. These are reduced with slower administration.

Interactions

Alcohol decreases the effects of fosphenytoin.

Dosage

The IV loading dose is 15 to 20 mg phenytoin-equivalent (PE) per kilogram administered at 100 to 150 mg/minute. IV maintenance dose is 4 to 6 mg PE/kg per day. IM administration is possible if IV access cannot be attained.

Barbiturates

The long-acting barbiturate phenobarbital is also one of the most widely employed anticonvulsants. Phenobarbitol is used in the long-term treatment of *epilepsy* and is prescribed selectively for acute treatment of status epilepticus.

The barbiturate anticonvulsants are metabolized in the liver, and metabolites and unchanged drugs are excreted in the urine. Phenobarbitol provides an onset of action within 30 minutes after oral administration. Peak anticonvulsant effect occurs in 8 to 12 hours. The onset after IV administration occurs within 5 to 15 minutes, with peak anticonvulsant effect within 30 minutes. Phenobarbitol has an extremely long half-life of 2 to 6 days.

 PHENOBARBITAL (LUMINAL)

Class: Anticonvulsant and barbiturate

Description

Phenobarbital belongs to a class of drugs called *barbiturates*. It is used as a sedative and an anticonvulsant.

Mechanism of Action

Phenobarbital increases the action of the inhibitory neurotransmitter of GABA in the brain. It also appears to inhibit the release of glutamate (an excitatory neurotransmitter) from nerve endings. It is through these actions that phenobarbital exerts its sedative and anticonvulsant properties.

Barbiturates have many uses in medicine. They are central nervous system depressants and are used as anticonvulsants and in the management of insomnia and anxiety. Phenobarbital is an effective anticonvulsant of relatively low toxicity. It depresses the sensory cortex, decreases motor activity, alters cerebellar function, and causes drowsiness, sedation, and hypnosis.

Pharmacokinetics

Onset: 5–15 minutes (IV)
Peak Effects: 30 minutes (IV)
Duration: 4–6 hours (IV)
Half-Life: 2–6 days

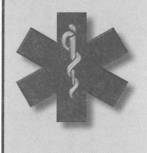

CASE PRESENTATION

At 2:30 P.M. paramedics are called with fire department first responders to a motorcycle collision. On arrival they find an 18-year-old male, unhelmeted rider. Bystanders state that he lost control of the motorcycle on a corner and slid head first into the cement retaining wall.

The patient is unconscious and unresponsive to deep pain. He is lying on his left side. His head is being supported by a bystander, who states that the patient has been unconscious and unresponsive since he arrived.

On Examination

CNS: The patient is unconscious and unresponsive; pupils are bilaterally constricted; abnormal flexion (decorticate posture) bilaterally

Resp: Respirations are 30 per minute and deep; lungs are clear bilaterally with equal air entry; trachea is midline; no signs of trauma to the neck or chest

CVS: Both radial and carotid pulses are present and weak; skin is pale and diaphoretic

ABD: Soft and nontender in all four quadrants

Muscl/Skel: No other injuries noted

Vital Signs

Pulse: 50/min

Resp: 30/min, deep

BP: 160 by palpation

SpO$_2$: 87 percent

ECG: Sinus bradycardia

Past Hx: The patient's history is unknown.

Treatment

Fire department first responders assist with spinal immobilization while a paramedic inserts an oropharyngeal airway and begins to ventilate the patient with a bag-valve-mask device and 100 percent oxygen. The patient is moved to an ALS ambulance following rapid immobilization and stabilization on a long spine board. During transport the patient's condition remains largely unchanged except as follows: (1) Respiration rate increases to 36 per minute, (2) blood pressure increases to 210/120 mmHg, (3) oxygen saturation (as measured by pulse oximetry) increases to 91 percent, and (4) pupils become uneven (right > left). Because of the critical nature of this patient's injuries, the following procedures were completed: endotracheal intubation with in-line c-spine stabilization, IV line × 2, 14-gauge catheter (per trauma protocol), normal saline TKO, and mannitol 1.5 g/kg. Total scene time was 10 minutes, and transport time to the hospital was 8 minutes. There were no changes in patient condition en route. On arrival at the hospital the patient was immediately taken to CT, where an epidural hematoma was visualized. The patient was taken emergently to surgery, where the epidural hematoma was decompressed. The patient was transferred to the neurology ICU, where he remains.

Indications

Phenobarbital is used in major motor seizures, status epilepticus, and acute anxiety states.

Contraindications

Phenobarbital should not be administered to any patient with a history of hypersensitivity to barbiturates.

Precautions

Respiratory depression and hypotension can occur following IV administration of phenobarbital. Constant monitoring of respiratory pattern and blood pressure is essential. Administration of phenobarbital to children may result in hyperactive behavior.

Side Effects

Phenobarbital can cause drowsiness, altered mental status, agitation, hypoventilation, apnea, bradycardia, hypotension, syncope, headache, nausea, and vomiting.

Interactions

Phenobarbital may enhance the sedative effects of other sedatives including alcohol, narcotics, antihistamines, and antidepressants.

Dosage

The standard dosage of phenobarbital in the management of status epilepticus is 100 to 250 mg given slowly by IV.

SUMMARY

In the management of acute head injury, mannitol has proved effective in reducing cerebral edema. Airway management and ventilation are important aspects of acute head injury management. It is important to remember that stabilization of the cervical spine, maintenance of the airway, and supplemental delivery of oxygen are of primary importance.

In a general motor seizure, as occasionally occurs, the primary treatment is that of protecting the patient from injury. It is important to remember that most epileptic patients are already taking orally one or two anticonvulsant medications. The judicious use of the parenteral agents

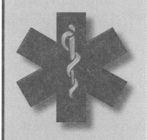

CASE PRESENTATION

At 0900 hours paramedics are called to the local high school to help a 16-year-old boy with reported seizures. Dispatch reports that the boy has had one seizure in the last 10 minutes and is now into his second seizure. The boy has a history of epilepsy and takes medication for it. He is unconscious and unresponsive. Three minutes later paramedics arrive at the school and are met by a very frantic teacher, who leads them to a classroom. There they find the patient lying on the floor. The desks have been moved away from the patient, and the patient has been placed in the recovery position. The patient appears to be postictal now.

On Examination

CNS: The patient is unconscious and unresponsive

Resp: Respirations are 32 per minute and shallow; trachea is midline; no external signs of trauma

CVS: Both the radial and carotid pulses are present but are rapid and weak; skin is pale and diaphoretic

ABD: Soft and nontender in all four quadrants; no signs of vomiting; patient has been incontinent of urine

Muscl/Skel: No injuries detected

Vital Signs

Pulse: 120/min

Resp: 36/min, shallow

BP: 124/82 mmHg

SpO$_2$: 90 percent

ECG: Sinus tachycardia

Past Hx: The teacher states that the patient has epilepsy. She shows paramedics a prescription bottle of Dilantin from the patient's coat pocket. The patient had the first seizure at 0850, and the second started at 0900. She does not know if he has been sick or experienced any recent trauma.

Treatment

One paramedic performs oropharyngeal suction to remove some frothy sputum from the patient's mouth and then ventilates the patient with a bag-valve-mask unit with 100 percent oxygen. Following contact with the base hospital, another paramedic is preparing to give lorazepam (Ativan) IV push. An 18-gauge IV is initiated in the right antecubital fossa and secured in place with tape and Kling in case the patient has another seizure. The patient's blood glucose level is checked from the blood in the IV hub, and it is 100 mg/dL (5.6 mmol/L). He then begins to seize, and paramedics administer lorazepam 2–4 mg IV push. If that does not terminate the seizure, a repeat dose of 2-4 mg may be given. Paramedics administer the first dose of lorazepam, and the seizure subsides in 1 minute. Within 5 minutes the patient is in the postictal stage. He is transported to the hospital without incident and without further seizure. At the hospital the patient's Dilantin level is checked to see if it was too low. The Dilantin level obtained from the blood is 3.4 mg/L (therapeutic level is 10 to 20 mg/L). IV Dilantin is administered, and the patient admitted to the intensive care unit. He does well, with no additional seizures, and is released with an increased daily dosage of Dilantin.

discussed in this chapter is therefore indicated. It is helpful to the emergency physician to obtain blood samples from seizure patients prior to the administration of an anticonvulsant. Some authorities believe that a significant percentage of patients who have general motor seizures do so because they fail to follow instructions on ordered medications. Blood studies taken before the administration of anticonvulsants will aid the physician in making a diagnosis.

KEY WORDS

amnesia. A loss of memory.

benzodiazepine. A class of drugs frequently used to relieve anxiety and insomnia and to induce sedation.

central nervous system. The central portion of the nervous system, namely the brain and spinal cord.

epilepsy. A group of nervous system disorders characterized by the presence of seizures.

seizures. A sudden change in nervous function. The symptoms can range from a slight alteration in mental status to violent, generalized, uncontrollable contraction of muscles.

status epilepticus. A state of repeated seizures without an intervening period of consciousness.

DRUGS USED IN THE TREATMENT OF OBSTETRICAL AND GYNECOLOGICAL EMERGENCIES

11

OBJECTIVES

After completing this chapter, the reader should be able to:

1. List three obstetrical and gynecological emergencies that require intervention with pharmacological agents.

2. Describe and list the indications, contraindications, and dosages for oxytocin.

3. List the signs and symptoms of hypertensive disorders of pregnancy.

4. Distinguish among gestational hypertension, preeclampsia, and eclampsia.

5. Describe and list the indications, contraindications, and dosages for magnesium sulfate.

6. Describe the management of a patient in preterm labor.

7. Describe and list the indications, contraindications, and dosages for terbutaline.

8. Define the following terms: *abruptio placenta, eclampsia, ectopic pregnancy, placenta previa, postpartum hemorrhage, preeclampsia,* and *spontaneous abortion.*

INTRODUCTION

Prehospital care for most obstetrical and gynecological emergencies is supportive. There are three complications, however, that necessitate intervention with pharmacological agents. These are the hypertensive disorders of pregnancy, severe vaginal bleeding, and preterm labor. *Magnesium sulfate* has proved effective in controlling the convulsions associated with eclampsia. *Pitocin,* a drug chemically identical to the hormone oxytocin, is effective in causing uterine contraction and will control many cases of postpartum vaginal bleeding. *Terbutaline*, a β_2-agonist, is effective in the suppression of preterm labor.

SEVERE VAGINAL BLEEDING

Vaginal bleeding that occurs during the first trimester of pregnancy is usually due to *spontaneous abortion* or *ectopic pregnancy*. During the third trimester of pregnancy, vaginal bleeding is most frequently caused by either *abruptio placenta* or *placenta previa*.

Bleeding following childbirth is common. Hypovolemic shock can develop when blood loss is in excess of 500 mL. Severe vaginal bleeding can be a life-threatening emergency, necessitating immediate therapy. The management of severe vaginal bleeding is similar to that employed with any other type of severe hemorrhage. Initial treatment should include airway maintenance, administration of supplemental oxygen, and infusion of intravenous volume expanders. In addition, the intravenous (IV) administration of Pitocin in postpartum hemorrhage can be effective in controlling severe vaginal bleeding.

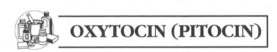

OXYTOCIN (PITOCIN)

Class: Hormone and uterine stimulant

Description

Oxytocin is a naturally occurring hormone that is secreted by the posterior pituitary.

Mechanism of Action

Oxytocin causes contraction of uterine smooth muscle and lactation. Oxytocin is used to induce labor in selected cases and is also effective in inducing uterine contractions following delivery, thereby controlling *postpartum hemorrhage.* When a baby is placed on the breast, the sucking action causes the posterior pituitary to release oxytocin. It is important to remember this inherent mechanism whenever confronted by a patient suffering moderate to severe postpartum bleeding.

Pharmacokinetics

Onset: Immediate (IV), 3–7 minutes (IM)
Peak Effects: Varies
Duration: 1 hour (IV), 2–3 hours (IM)
Half-Life: 3–5 minutes

Indication

Oxytocin is used for postpartum hemorrhage.

Contraindications

In the prehospital setting, oxytocin should be administered only to patients suffering severe postpartum bleeding. Before administration it is essential to verify that the baby *and the placenta* have been delivered and that there is not an additional fetus in the uterus.

Precautions

Excess oxytocin can cause overstimulation of the uterus and possible uterine rupture. Hypertension, cardiac dysrhythmias, and anaphylaxis have been reported in conjunction with the administration of oxytocin. Vital signs and uterine tone should be monitored.

Side Effects

Oxytocin can cause hypotension, dysrhythmias, tachycardia, seizures, coma, nausea, and vomiting in the mother. When administered prior to delivery, oxytocin can cause fetal hypoxia, fetal asphyxia, fetal arrhythmias, and possibly fetal intracranial bleeding.

Both oxytocin and antidiuretic hormone (ALH) are secreted from the posterior pituitary and are similar in chemical structure. Because of this, oxytocin may have some ADH effects—especially in higher doses. These include water restriction and, to a lesser degree, vasoconstriction.

Interactions

Oxytocin can cause hypertension when administered in conjunction with vasoconstrictors such as norepinephrine.

Dosage

Following are two regimens for the administration of oxytocin in the management of patients with postpartum hemorrhage: (1) 3 to 10 units can be administered intramuscularly following delivery of the placenta or (2) 10 to 20 units can be placed in either 500 or 1000 mL of D_5W, 0.9 percent normal saline, or lactated Ringer's solution. This should be titrated according to the severity of the bleeding and the uterine response. Oxytocin should only be administered intramuscularly or by slow IV infusion.

HYPERTENSIVE DISORDERS OF PREGNANCY

In addition to vaginal bleeding, paramedics should be aware of several pregnancy-associated problems known collectively as *hypertensive disorders of pregnancy* (formerly called *toxemia of pregnancy*). These disorders are characterized by hypertension, weight gain, edema, protein in the urine, and, in late stages, seizures. Hypertensive disorders of pregnancy occur in approximately 5 percent of pregnancies. They are thought to be caused by abnormal vasospasm in the mother, which results in increased blood pressure and other associated symptoms. The hypertensive disorders of pregnancy generally include the following:

Gestational hypertension (GH).   GH is characterized by a blood pressure of 140/90 level or greater in pregnancy in a patient who was previously normotensive. GH is the early stage of the disease process. It is important to remember that blood pressure usually drops in pregnancy, and a blood pressure reading of 130/80 may be elevated.

Preeclampsia.   Preeclamptic patients are those who have hypertension, abnormal weight gain, edema, headache, protein in the urine, epigastric pain, and, occasionally, visual disturbances. If untreated, preeclampsia may progress to the next stage, eclampsia.

Eclampsia. Eclampsia is the most serious manifestation of the hypertensive disorders of pregnancy. It is characterized by grand mal seizure activity. Eclampsia is often preceded by visual disturbances, such as flashing lights or spots before the eyes. Also, the development of epigastric pain or pain in the right upper abdominal quadrant often indicates impending seizure. Eclampsia can be distinguished from epilepsy by the history and physical appearance of the patient. Patients who become eclamptic are usually edematous and have markedly elevated blood pressure, whereas epileptics usually have a prior history of seizures and are taking anticonvulsant medications.

The hypertensive disorders of pregnancy tend to occur most often with a woman's first pregnancy. They also appear to occur more frequently in patients with preexisting hypertension. Diabetes mellitus is also associated with an increased incidence of this disease process.

Patients who develop GH and preeclampsia are at increased risk for cerebral hemorrhage, the development of renal failure, and pulmonary edema. Patients who are preeclamptic have intravascular volume depletion, because a great deal of their body fluid is in the third space. If eclampsia develops, death of the mother and fetus frequently results. Eclampsia must be treated aggressively. *Magnesium sulfate* is the drug of choice for controlling the convulsions associated with eclampsia. In addition, it may be necessary to administer an antihypertensive agent, such as those discussed in Chapter 7, to prevent the complications of hypertensive crisis. The decision to administer an antihypertensive in the prehospital phase of emergency medical care rests with the base station physician. Each case should be treated individually.

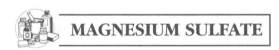

MAGNESIUM SULFATE

Class: Electrolyte

Description

Magnesium sulfate is a salt that dissociates into the magnesium cation (Mg^{2+}) and the sulfate anion when administered. Magnesium is an essential element in numerous biochemical reactions that occur within the body.

Mechanism of Action

Magnesium sulfate is a central nervous system depressant effective in the management of seizures associated with eclampsia. It is used for the initial therapy of convulsions associated with pregnancy. After cessation of seizure activity, other anticonvulsant agents may be administered.

Pharmacokinetics

Onset: Immediate (IV), 1 hour (IM)
Peak Effects: Varies
Duration: 1 hour
Half-Life: Not applicable

Indications

Magnesium sulfate is used in eclampsia (seizures accompanying pregnancy) and preterm labor.

Contraindications

Magnesium sulfate should not be administered to any patient with heart block. It should not be administered to patients who are in shock; who have persistent, severe hypertension; who routinely undergo dialysis; or who are known to have a decreased calcium level (hypocalcemia).

Precautions

Magnesium sulfate, like other central nervous system depressants, can cause hypotension, circulatory collapse, and depression of cardiac and respiratory function. The most immediate danger is respiratory depression. Calcium chloride should be readily available for IV administration as an antidote in case respiratory depression occurs. Magnesium sulfate should be administered slowly to minimize side effects. Any patient receiving intravenous magnesium sulfate should have continuous cardiac monitoring as well as frequent monitoring of vital signs. If possible, the knee and biceps deep tendon reflexes should be checked prior to and during magnesium therapy.

Side Effects

Magnesium sulfate can cause flushing, sweating, bradycardia, decreased deep tendon reflexes, drowsiness, respiratory depression, dysrhythmias, hypotension, hypothermia, itching, and rash.

Interactions

Magnesium sulfate can cause cardiac conduction abnormalities if administered in conjunction with digitalis.

Dosage

The standard dosage for the management of convulsions associated with eclampsia is 2 to 4 g slow IV over 25 min. If an IV cannot be started, magnesium sulfate can be administered intramuscularly. Because of the volume of the drug (5 to 10 mL), the dose should be divided in half and each half administered intramuscularly at a separate site (usually each gluteus).

PRETERM LABOR

Preterm labor is labor that begins before the age of fetal maturity, usually before 36 weeks. If labor begins early, obstetricians often try to suppress it to allow more time for intrauterine fetal development.

There are three approaches to suppressing preterm labor. The first approach is to sedate the mother. Often, labor begins in response to maternal stress or exhaustion. In these cases, a sedative such as Seconal is given. Alternatively, morphine sulfate can be administered (intramuscularly) for sedation.

The second approach to suppressing preterm labor is administration of a fluid bolus. The hormone oxytocin is manufactured and released from the posterior pituitary. Antidiuretic hormone (ADH) is also manufactured and released from the posterior pituitary. ADH causes the kidneys to retain water. In cases of preterm labor, a fluid bolus (1 to 2 L of lactated Ringer's solution or normal saline) is administered. ADH production and release are inhibited through feedback systems. Because ADH and oxytocin come from the same area of the posterior pituitary, suppression of ADH release also suppresses oxytocin release and thus can help suppress preterm labor.

Finally, labor can be suppressed by the use of tocolytics. Although many tocolytics are available, β_2-agonists are frequently used. Stimulation of uterine β_2-receptors causes uterine relaxation and suppression of preterm labor. Common β_2-agonists include terbutaline and ritodrine (Yutopar). Terbutaline is used more frequently in the emergency setting. Magnesium sulfate, previously discussed, is also effective in suppressing preterm labor.

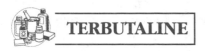 **TERBUTALINE**

Class: Sympathetic agonist and tocolytic

Description

Terbutaline is a synthetic sympathomimetic that is selective for β_2-adrenergic receptors.

Mechanism of Action

Terbutaline, because of its effects on β_2-adrenergic receptors, causes immediate bronchodilation with minimal cardiac effects. It is also used to suppress preterm labor. Stimulation of β_2-adrenergic receptors in the uterus causes uterine relaxation and can suppress labor.

Pharmacokinetics

> **Onset:** <15 minutes [subcutaneous (SC)]
> **Peak Effects:** 30–60 minutes (SC)
> **Duration:** 1.5–4.0 hours (SC)
> **Half-Life:** 3–4 hours

Indication

Terbutaline is used for preterm labor.

Contraindications

Terbutaline should not be administered to any patient with a history of hypersensitivity to the drug.

Precautions

As with any sympathomimetic, the patient's vital signs must be monitored. Caution should be used when administering terbutaline to elderly patients and those with cardiovascular disease or hypertension.

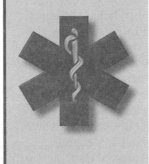

CASE PRESENTATION

An ALS ambulance is called to a rural hospital to transport a maternity patient to a larger city hospital 1 hour away. Paramedics are asked to bring the monitor in with the stretcher. On arrival at the hospital the nurse attending the patient gives the following information: The patient is an 18-year-old female, gravida 1, para 0, in her third trimester of pregnancy. She came to the hospital by private car after suffering a grand mal seizure at home. She had no prior history of seizures, and her pregnancy had been uneventful to date. She evidently was not in labor prior to the seizure. At present the patient is lying on a hospital bed and is not having contractions, as based on the external fetal monitor. The fetal heart rate is stable. The hospital diagnosis is eclampsia.

On Examination

CNS:	The patient is conscious but lethargic
Resp:	Respirations are 24 per minute and shallow; symmetrical chest wall movement with clear bilateral breath sounds
CVS:	Both carotid and radial pulses are present and strong; a systolic flow murmur can be heard; minimal blood loss is noted from the vagina; neck veins are not distended; skin color is normal, warm, and diaphoretic to touch; patient is very edematous
ABD:	Obviously pregnant with no contractions noted
Muscl/Skel:	No apparent injuries
Extremities:	Pedal and finger edema noted

Vital Signs

Pulse:	100/min, regular
Resp:	24/min
BP:	166/112 mmHg
SpO$_2$:	95 percent
ECG:	Normal sinus rhythm

Hospital Treatment

The patient is receiving high-flow, high-concentration oxygen. A large-bore IV was started in the left forearm. Magnesium sulfate is being infused at a rate of 1 g/hr. The receiving hospital was notified and is expecting the patient.

Treatment

The patient is moved to the ambulance stretcher and then to the ambulance. Oxygen is administered at 15 lpm by nonrebreather mask. The pulse oximeter is applied and shows an SpO$_2$ of 96 percent. The cardiac monitor shows a regular sinus rhythm and is checked frequently by the paramedics who are watching for any ECG changes. The IV of magnesium sulfate initiated in the hospital is continued at 1 g/hr. The interior ambulance lights are dimmed to help prevent additional seizure activity. A prefilled syringe of Valium is removed from the lock box in case the patient suffers another seizure.

During transport the patient is continually assessed, with special attention to the IV of magnesium sulfate. Deep tendon reflexes are periodically checked to ensure the magnesium effect is not excessive. The trip to the hospital is uneventful. On arrival at the receiving facility, an emergency sonogram is obtained. It shows a fetal age of 37 weeks (±2 weeks). Labor is induced, and the patient delivers a healthy female infant 18 hours later.

Side Effects

Terbutaline can cause palpitations, anxiety, dizziness, headache, nervousness, tremor, hypertension, dysrhythmias, chest pain, nausea, and vomiting.

Interactions

The possibility of developing unpleasant side effects increases when terbutaline is used with other sympathetic agonists. β-blockers may blunt the pharmacological effects of terbutaline.

Dosage

Terbutaline should be administered initially by subcutaneous injection. The initial dose should be 0.25 mg administered subcutaneously. This dose can be repeated in 30 minutes to 1 hour as required. A terbutaline drip can be used to provide ongoing suppression of labor. It can be prepared by placing 5 mg of terbutaline in 500 mL of lactated Ringer's solution or normal saline. The drip should be started at 30 mL/hr (5 μg/min). This can be slowly increased to a maximum dose of 80 μg/min as required.

SUMMARY

Most obstetrical and gynecological emergencies are not managed in the field. Prehospital treatment should include stabilization of the airway, administration of supplemental oxygen, and replacement of intravascular volume. In severe postpartum bleeding, the administration of Pitocin is often effective. In the hypertensive disorders of pregnancy, magnesium sulfate may be used during the prehospital phase of emergency medical care to control convulsions. The definitive treatment of preeclampsia and eclampsia is delivery of the fetus.

KEY WORDS

abruptio placenta. A premature separation of the placenta from the uterus before birth. Because it often results in severe bleeding, it is considered to be a serious condition.

eclampsia. The most serious manifestation of the hypertensive disorders of pregnancy. It is characterized by grand mal seizure activity. Eclampsia is often preceded by visual disturbances, such as flashing lights or spots before the eyes. Also, the development of epigastric pain or pain in the right upper abdominal quadrant often indicates impending seizure. Patients who become eclamptic are usually edematous and have markedly elevated blood pressure.

ectopic pregnancy. The implantation of a developing fetus outside the uterus, often in the fallopian tube.

placenta previa. A condition in which the placenta partly or completely covers the opening of the cervix. It is the most common cause of painless bleeding in the third trimester.

postpartum hemorrhage. The loss of 500 mL or more blood in the first 24 hours following delivery.

preeclampsia. A manifestation of the hypertensive disorders of pregnancy characterized by hypertension, abnormal weight gain, edema, headache, protein in the urine, epigastric pain, and, occasionally, visual disturbances. If untreated, preeclampsia may progress to the next stage, eclampsia.

spontaneous abortion. A fetal loss, also called a miscarriage, that occurs of its own accord. Most spontaneous abortions occur before the 12th week of pregnancy. Many occur 2 weeks after conception and are mistaken for menstrual periods.

12

TOXICOLOGICAL EMERGENCIES IN PREHOSPITAL CARE

OBJECTIVES

After completing this chapter, the reader should be able to:

1. Discuss the importance of toxicological emergencies in prehospital care.

2. Discuss the role of regional poison centers in the management of the poisoned patient.

3. Describe the key historical information required in the management of a toxicological emergency.

4. Describe the various routes of exposure to toxic substances.

5. Describe the general management of the patient exposed to a toxin, including decontamination and elimination.

6. Define the term *toxidrome* and describe the common toxidromes encountered in prehospital care.

7. Describe the signs, symptoms, and management (including antidotes where appropriate) of the following toxic exposures and overdoses: acetaminophen, anticholinergics, neuroleptics, beta-blockers, calcium channel blockers, carbon monoxide, cyanide, cyclic antidepressants, digoxin/digitalis, ethylene glycol, iron, isopropyl alcohol, lithium, methanol, narcotics and narcotic antagonists, organophosphates and carbamates, salicylates, and selective serotonin reuptake inhibitors (SSRIs).

INTRODUCTION

Toxicology is a rapidly evolving science that can provide the prehospital care provider with a fascinating window into the field of pharmacology and pharmacokinetics. The management of toxin exposure and overdoses represents a constantly expanding aspect of prehospital care. Maintaining clinical competence in managing these patients reflects a significant challenge because new medications and chemicals, each with its own unique toxicological potential, are continuously being introduced. The approach to the poisoned or overdosed patient can be likened to a form of detective work. The clinical clues required to manage these patients are often subtle, and providers must be aware that virtually any patient presentation may be directly or indirectly related to a toxicological problem. Without suspicion, even the most obvious clinical clues can go unnoticed.

In this chapter, the discussion focuses not only on prescription drugs but also on nonprescription toxins that may be encountered in prehospital care. There are similarities between many of the agents presented here and those used by terrorists as weapons of mass destruction. The attacks on the United States on September 11, 2001, significantly changed the way prehospital care is practiced in the world. Terrorism has brought once obscure chemical and biological agents to the forefront of medical care. As a result, antidotes and palliative drugs are now routinely stocked on ambulances and rescue vehicles. The modern emergency medical service (EMS) provider must be familiar with common antidotes and treatments for many of the chemical and biological weapons available throughout the world. These agents will be addressed in more detail in Chapter 16, *Weapons of Mass Destruction.*

REGIONAL POISON CENTERS

Once the possibility of a poisoning or overdose has been identified, several resources are available to assist in patient management. Traditionally, a hospital-based medical director has provided guidance and direction for the management of toxicological emergencies. In recent years the emergence of toxicology as a distinct discipline has led to the development of regional poison centers whose role is to provide information and advice to caregivers encountering poisoned patients. Poison information specialists are typically nurses and pharmacists with specialized training in toxicology. They are generally available 24 hours per day to provide telephone advice to prehospital care providers, laypeople, and hospital medical staff. They can serve as an extremely valuable resource to care providers, particularly in rural settings where the decision to transfer a patient to a larger center can be a difficult one. The prehospital care provider should not overlook the potential benefit of consultation with a regional poison center.

PATIENT HISTORY

The history constitutes an essential part of the initial approach to the toxicology patient. Like all detective work, suspicion is the foundation for discovering the truth; the truth in this case is the identity, quantity, and time of exposure to the toxic substance. Despite its importance, the history is frequently confusing and inconsistent in this patient population. The problem is related to factors such as illicit drug use, associated psychiatric illnesses, and in some cases a lack of awareness on the part of both the patient and the care provider that an exposure has actually occurred.

A thorough history includes *what* agent the patient was exposed to, *how much* of the agent, *when* the exposure occurred (time), *how* the exposure occurred (*route of exposure*), *where* (location) the exposure occurred, and any *treatment* the patient may have received prior to the arrival of the prehospital care provider.

The importance of identifying the agent in question is obvious. Knowing which agent is involved can allow the care provider to plan decontamination, provide initial treatment, and anticipate problems before they actually occur. With some toxic agents, immediate management is required in the field, whereas others can have therapy initiated in the emergency department. In the latter cases, it is extremely useful to provide hospital staff with all available information so that they can prepare for the patient's arrival. Some agents have antidotes that can be lifesaving if used appropriately. In circumstances in which the toxic agent cannot be identified or an antidote is not available, management may be limited to supportive care. Searching the scene for pill bottles, poisons, evidence of drug abuse, venomous plants, and animals is paramount. Whenever possible, toxicological evidence, especially pill bottles and medication dispensers, should be transported to the hospital for review by a physician.

The dose or amount of toxin can be very helpful in predicting the occurrence or severity of clinical symptoms. It may also help to determine the need for decontamination procedures and antidote treatment. Making note of the date on prescription medication containers and the number of pills still present can assist in quantifying the dosage.

The time of exposure is important for several reasons. First, it allows an estimation of the degree of toxicity (however, many toxins have delayed symptom onset). Second, it allows some planning for decontamination and management. Finally, some agents (salicylates and acetaminophen) require blood levels to determine the need for treatment. Interpretation of these blood levels often requires knowledge of the time of ingestion. Reviewing the patient's recent activities and time of symptom onset with family members or friends can be very helpful.

Potential routes of exposure include *oral ingestion, inhalation, dermal exposure, injection* (*intra-* or *extravascular*), and *mucosal absorption*. The route of exposure guides treatment (e.g., gastric decontamination would not be indicated in a patient who has had dermal exposure).

The location of the exposure can be helpful in identifying the agent (e.g., an agricultural worker who develops symptoms shortly after spraying organophosphate pesticides on a wheat field). The route of exposure can be crucial in ensuring the safety of the care provider because some toxins can be airborne (e.g., carbon monoxide) or spread through patient contact (e.g., organophosphate pesticides).

Identifying any treatment provided prior to medical attention is also important. The occurrence of vomiting is relevant because it suggests some emptying of residual gastric toxins has already occurred. Although no longer widely used and potentially dangerous, syrup of ipecac is still available and may be administered by laypeople. If administered, the prehospital care provider must anticipate vomiting and take steps to prevent aspiration of gastric contents.

GENERAL APPROACH TO THE POISONED PATIENT

As emphasized earlier, the foundation of managing the poisoned patient is a clinical suspicion supplemented by clues present at the scene and in the presentation of the patient. The initial approach to the poisoned patient includes early attention to *airway, breathing,* and *circulation.* Airway control should occur early where indicated, followed by establishment of vascular access. Because vomiting is a frequent occurrence in the poisoned patient, aspiration is a significant risk and should be anticipated and prevented wherever possible. *Vital signs* must be recorded early because they can provide clues to both the type of toxin and the severity of the overdose. *Cardiac monitoring* is crucial because many toxic exposures are associated with serious dysrhythmias. In the setting of tricyclic antidepressant overdose, the presence of a wide QRS complex may guide treatment, as discussed in greater detail later in the chapter. *Blood glucose level* should be measured in all patients with altered level of consciousness because hypoglycemia can often be misinterpreted as an intoxicated state. As discussed previously, both the patient and care providers must be protected from further exposure to the toxin. Discussion of physical exam findings is deferred to the later review of specific toxidromes.

Decontamination and enhancing *elimination* of toxins in the poisoned patient may have a role in prehospital care. Traditional approaches include *syrup of ipecac, gastric lavage*, and *activated charcoal* with or without a cathartic agent (an agent that enhances bowel motility and speeds transit through the gut). Syrup of ipecac acts by inducing vomiting and thereby decreasing further absorption of remaining toxins from the gastrointestinal tract. Its usage has largely fallen out of favor recently due to a lack of evidence for improved patient outcome as well as significant concerns regarding its safety. The largest safety concern relates to the fact that altered level of consciousness is relatively common in toxic ingestions, and combining reduced consciousness with induced emesis creates considerable risk of airway compromise and aspiration. Gastric lavage remains a relatively commonly utilized method of in-hospital gastric decontamination. Although its efficacy remains somewhat unproven, it is occasionally utilized in cases of recent ingestion or in agents known to slow gastric emptying. Gastric lavage is impractical for most prehospital settings because it requires multiple personnel and may be associated with significant complications such as aspiration and esophageal rupture. Activated charcoal has been shown to be effective in decreasing the toxicity in certain oral ingestions and in agents with enterohepatic circulation. Charcoal is by no means effective for all orally ingested toxins. Its use is relatively safe; the largest risk is aspiration in the event that vomiting ensues and the patient is unable to protect his or her airway. It is sometimes combined with a cathartic agent such as sorbitol or magnesium citrate to help speed passage of toxins through the small and large bowel and thereby limit absorption. Although cathartic agents may improve elimination somewhat, the resultant frequent and voluminous bowel movements can create a suboptimal patient care environment in the back of an ambulance. To summarize, activated charcoal likely represents the only truly safe and efficacious method of enhancing toxin elimination in the prehospital setting.

TOXIDROMES

A *toxidrome* is a set of clinical signs that are considered diagnostic of certain toxins or classes of toxins. Although not all toxins have their own unique toxidrome, an ability to recognize the common toxidromes can greatly enhance toxin identification and thereby aid patient care in certain circumstances. The clinical reliability of toxidromes is limited in cases of mixed overdoses, for which physical findings can be contradictory.

Perhaps the most common toxidrome encountered in prehospital care is that of the narcotized patient (*narcotic* or *opiate toxidrome*). Whether self-induced or iatrogenic, the classic triad of decreased level of consciousness, respiratory depression, and constricted pupils (miosis) is seen with frequency and, when present, can guide therapy. Although this triad generally holds for the common narcotics, including morphine, heroin, and codeine, it is important to remember that not all narcotics cause pupillary constriction. Meperidine (Demerol), propoxyphene (Darvon), pentazocine (Talwin), and others may not demonstrate miosis.

Another relatively common toxidrome is that of *anticholinergic* toxicity, as commonly seen with dimenhydrinate and tricyclic antidepressant overdoses. These patients commonly display both central signs and peripheral antimuscarinic signs. Peripheral signs are typically more common and include dry skin and mucous membranes, thirst, dysphagia, blurred vision, fixed dilated pupils, tachycardia, fine red (scarlatiniform) rash, hyperthermia, abdominal distension with decreased or absent bowel sounds, and urinary urgency or retention. Central signs include lethargy, confusion, restlessness, delirium, hallucinations, ataxia, seizures, and in severe cases cardiopulmonary collapse. Agents that can cause this toxidrome include dimenhydrinate and cyclic antidepressants. A common mnemonic for remembering the clinical signs of anticholinergic syndrome is "*hot* as a Hades, *blind* as a bat, *dry* as a bone, *red* as a beet, *mad* as a Hatter."

The *cholinergic toxidrome*, as is classically seen with organophosphate pesticide poisoning, can present with a complex cascade of signs that include muscarinic, nicotinic, and central nervous system (CNS) signs and symptoms. Once again, the multiple clinical signs can be simplified through the use of a mnemonic. The muscarinic symptoms are described by the mnemonic *DUMBELS*, in which the signs include defecation, urination, miosis, bronchorrhea, excitation (muscular), lacrimation, and salivation or seizures. The nicotinic symptoms can be summarized by a mnemonic based on the days of the week, *MTWtHF*, which stands for muscle weakness and paralysis, tachycardia, weakness, hypertension, and fasiculations.

The *sympathomimetic syndrome* can present with various symptoms depending on which class of agents is involved. Alpha-adrenergic agents include phenylephrine, methoxamine, and phenylpropanolamine and typically present with hypertension (HTN) and reflex bradycardia secondary to vasoconstriction of resistance vessels. Beta-adrenergic agents include theophylline, caffeine, and metoproterenol and typically present with tachycardia with or without hypotension (secondary to excessive stimulation of the sinus node or vascular smooth muscle dilatation).

SPECIFIC TOXIC AGENTS ENCOUNTERED IN PREHOSPITAL CARE

The following sections summarize some of the commonly encountered toxins in prehospital care. The list of agents discussed is by no means comprehensive but emphasizes those that may require specific treatment.

Acetaminophen

Acetaminophen is found in many over-the-counter medications and, as such, is a commonly encountered overdose. The primary concern in this overdose is the potential for irreversible hepatic injury. Therapy is aimed at preventing hepatotoxicity. A specific antidote, *N*-acetylcysteine, is available but is generally reserved for use in the hospital.

Route of Exposure	Oral.
Mechanism of Toxicity	Metabolism is primarily hepatic; the production of toxic metabolites results in direct hepatic toxicity. Ninety percent is conjugated with glucuronic or sulfuric acid in the liver to form nontoxic compounds that are excreted in the urine. An additional 2 percent is excreted unchanged in the urine. A toxic byproduct formed by this process is normally conjugated with hepatic glutathione and subsequently excreted in the urine. When glutathione stores are depleted, as in a massive overdose, hepatotoxicity occurs.
Toxic Dose	*Acute ingestion:* Doses greater than 7.5 g or 140 mg/kg are predictive of hepatotoxicity in an adult. Hepatotoxicity is rare in children. Certain drugs such as cimetidine and ethanol are protective in acute overdose because they compete with acetaminophen.
	Chronic ingestion: Variable toxicity can occur at low doses, especially in chronic alcoholics who have higher levels of acetaminophen and thus develop toxic metabolites more readily.
	Toxicity can be accurately predicted using serum (assuming the time of ingestion is known).
Signs and Symptoms	Signs and symptoms are classified into stages (see Table 12–1).
Prehospital Management	Supportive care should be provided, including airway support as indicated and activated charcoal where permitted by medical direction guidelines.
In-Hospital Management	Treatment with *N*-acetylcysteine (NAC) either orally or intravenously is the mainstay of therapy in cases of confirmed toxicity. Lavage

TABLE 12–1

Stage	Time Postingestion	Characteristics
I	1/2 to 24 hours[a]	Anorexia, nausea, vomiting, malaise, pallor, and diaphoresis
II	24 to 48 hours	Abdominal pain, liver tenderness, elevated liver enzymes, and oliguria
III	72 to 96 hours	Peak liver enzyme abnormalities, jaundice, hypoglycemia, coagulopathies, and encephalopathy
IV	4 days to 2 weeks	Resolution of hepatotoxicity or progressive hepatic failure

[a]Some patients may be completely asymptomatic during stage I.

is sometimes used if the patient presents within 2 hours of ingestion. Toxicity and the need for NAC therapy are determined by measurement of serum levels. These serum levels are most useful if measured 4 hours postingestion but can be used up to 25 hours postingestion. The level is plotted on the Rumack-Matthew nomogram for acetaminophen poisoning. Hepatotoxicity can be prevented with NAC therapy but once present is generally irreversible. NAC therapy is most effective if initiated within 8 hours of ingestion but in some circumstances is used even later. Liver transplant has been performed as a lifesaving measure in rare cases.

Anticholinergics

Anticholinergic properties can be found in many agents including both prescription drugs and drugs of abuse. Drugs with anticholinergic properties include tricyclic antidepressants, antihistamines, phenothiazines, and antiparkinsonian drugs. Dimenhydrinate, an antiemetic, is a drug with anticholinergic properties that is commonly used recreationally, especially among adolescents. Some plants and mushrooms (including the hallucinogenic varieties that are used recreationally) also have anticholinergic properties.

Route of Exposure	Oral, intravenous (IV), or dermal.
Mechanism of Toxicity	As described previously, cholinergic blockade occurs both centrally and peripherally and involves both muscarinic and nicotinic receptors. Different agents have different degrees of effect on the two receptor types and, as such, can have slightly different presentations.
Toxic Dose	Variable.
Signs and Symptoms	See earlier description of anticholinergic toxidrome. (*Remember:* Hot as Hades, blind as a bat, dry as a bone, red as a beet, mad as a Hatter.)
Prehospital Management	Conservative supportive care is the mainstay of therapy. Monitoring of airway, breathing, and circulation supplemented with IV access and cardiac monitoring is indicated in all but the most minor overdoses. Activated charcoal may be useful.
In-Hospital Management	Supportive care should be provided as in prehospital management. Lavage may be indicated even late in overdose because of the effects that anticholinergics have on delaying gastric emptying. Seizures and agitation are treated with benzodiazepines. Dysrhythmias can be treated with conventional therapy with the exception that Class Ia drugs (quinidine,

disopyramide, and procainamide) should be avoided because of the quinidine-like effects of some anticholinergics. The use of physostigmine, a reversible acetylcholinesterase inhibitor, remains controversial. It may aggravate dysrhythmias and seizures, and as such its use is limited to severe toxicity unresponsive to conventional therapy. Indications may include uncontrollable agitation, hemodynamically unstable dysrhythmias, and coma with respiratory depression, malignant hypertension, or refractory hypotension. Physostigmine can potentiate toxicity in tricyclic antidepressant overdose and should be avoided. Toxic symptoms of anticholinergics are generally evident within 4 to 6 hours of ingestion, and patients asymptomatic at that point can generally be safely discharged.

Neuroleptics

Neuroleptics are a broad class of agents which include the antipsychotics and some tranquilizers. The two most commonly encountered neuroleptic classes are the butyrophenones (such as haloperidol and droperidol) and the phenothiazines (such as chlorpromazine). These agents are typically prescribed to patients with significant psychiatric illness and, as such, are frequently seen in overdose settings. Significant adverse reactions can occur to these agents even when taken at normally prescribed dosages.

Route of Exposure	Oral, IV, or intramuscular (IM).
Mechanism of Toxicity	Act by blocking neurotransmission involving dopaminergic, adrenergic, muscarinic, and histaminic receptors. Therapeutic and toxicologic effects vary from agent to agent depending on the degree of blockage of each receptor subtype.
Toxic Dose	Variable.
Signs and Symptoms	Adverse reactions are common and may occur even in the setting of normal therapeutic dosages. These reactions include the following: Dystonic reaction which features involuntary muscle spasm including torticollis, facial grimacing, opisthotonos (flexion adduction of the arms), oculogyric crisis, and laryngeal spasm. Treatment is diphenhydramine or benztropine. Akathisia which features restlessness, jittery feeling, and insomnia. May be treated with benztropine, amantidine, or propranolol. Parkinsonism featuring resting tremor, rigidity, and masked facies. May be treated with benztropine or amantidine. Tardive dyskinesia which features lip smacking, tongue protrusion, grimacing, and chewing motion.

Neuroleptic malignant syndrome (NMS) which is a life-threatening condition (10% mortality rate) featuring hyperthermia, rigidity, altered mental status, and autonomic instability.

Symptoms of acute overdose are highly variable and can include any of the previously described conditions as well as CNS depression (ranging from sedation to coma), respiratory depression, hypo or hyperthermia, pinpoint pupils (especially phenothiazines), anticholinergic symptoms, hypotension with reflex tachycardia, cardiac dysrhythmias, and prolongation of the PR and QT intervals (with resultant ventricular dysrhythmias such as torsade de pointes).

Prehospital Management ABCs, cardiac monitoring, nalaxone, and chemstrip if altered LOC. Treat hypotension with crystalloid (normal saline) and norepinephrine or phenylephrine as needed. Ventricular dysrhythmias should be treated initially with bicarbonate (1–2 mEq/kg IV bolus) followed by lidocaine or phenytoin. Torsade de pointes should be treated initially with magnesium, followed by isoproterenol or overdrive pacing as needed. Seizures should be treated using standard methods including benzodiazapines, phenytoin, or phenobarbital.

In-Hospital Management Consists of supportive care including all the aforementioned methods. Gastrointestinal decontamination should be performed using activated charcoal and gastric lavage if the patient is intubated and a short interval has elapsed since the time of ingestion. Class 1A antidysrhythmics such as quinidine and procainamide should be avoided because they may exacerbate the cardiac toxicity. Cooling or warming techniques may be needed to control extremes of temperature. Management of NMS includes muscle relaxation using benzodiazepines and, if necessary, neuromuscular blockade. Dantrolene and bromocriptine, a dopamine agonist, have been used with mixed results in the treatment of NMS.

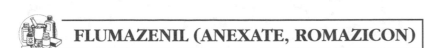

FLUMAZENIL (ANEXATE, ROMAZICON)

Class: Benzodiazepine antagonist

Description

Flumazenil is a benzodiazepine antagonist. It is used to reverse the sedative effects of benzodiazepines, especially respiratory depression.

Mechanism of Action

Flumazenil antagonizes the actions of the benzodiazepines in the central nervous system. Particularly, it inhibits their actions on the gamma-aminobutyric acid–benzodiazepine complex. It is used to reverse the sedative effects of the benzodiazepines.

Pharmacokinetics

Onset: 1–5 minutes
Peak Effects: 6–10 minutes
Duration: 2–4 hours
Half-Life: 54 minutes

Indications

Fumazenil is used for complete and partial reversal of CNS and respiratory depression caused by benzodiazepines including the following agents: Valium, Versed, Ativan, Halcion, Restoril, Dalmane, Tranxene, Serax, Klonopin, Ambien, Doral, ProSom, Centrax, and Xanax. Flumazenil should *not* be used as a diagnostic agent for benzodiazepine overdose in the manner naloxone is used for narcotic overdose. The potential of inducing a life-threatening benzodiazepine withdrawal reaction in patients addicted to benzodiazepines with flumazenil is not worth the perceived benefits.

Contraindications

Flumazenil is contraindicated in patients with a known hypersensitivity to the drug or to benzodiazepines. It should not be administered to patients who have received benzodiazepines to control life-threatening conditions such as status epilepticus. It should not be used in patients with tricyclic antidepressant overdoses.

Precautions

Flumazenil should be administered with caution to patients dependent on benzodiazepines. Benzodiazepine withdrawal can be life threatening. Signs and symptoms of benzodiazepine withdrawal include tachycardia, hypertension, anxiousness, confusion, and seizures. The effects of flumazenil can wear off, resulting in the return of sedation. Following administration, patients should be monitored for signs of resedation and respiratory depression. Flumazenil should never be administered as part of a "coma cocktail." "Coma cocktails" involve the empiric administration of 50 percent dextrose, thiamine, and naloxone (and in some cases, flumazenil) to unresponsive patients in an attempt to correct the cause of their unresponsiveness and awaken them. "Coma cocktails" are a poor prehospital practice. Therapy should always be guided by objective data such as patient assessment findings and blood glucose determination.

Side Effects

Flumazenil can cause fatigue, headache, agitation, nervousness, dizziness, flushing, confusion, convulsions, dysrhythmias, nausea, and vomiting.

Interactions

There are few interactions in the emergency setting.

Dosage

The standard dose of flumazenil is 0.2 mg intravenously administered over 30 seconds. This dose can be repeated, as required, up to a maximum dose of 1.0 mg. Flumazenil should only be given intravenously in the emergency setting.

Beta-Blockers

Although intentional overdose on beta-blockers is relatively rare, toxic symptoms occur frequently. True overdoses are often life threatening and difficult to manage because of the profound hemodynamic effects. Glucagon is the primary antidote and is often the only useful treatment modality.

Route of Exposure	Generally oral; occasionally ocular.
Mechanism of Toxicity	Beta-blockers cause blockade of both β_1- and β_2-receptors in the adrenergic nervous system. This blockade can affect several organ systems, most notably the cardiovascular (bradycardia, atrioventricular [AV] block, or vasodilation) and respiratory (bronchospasm or congestive heart failure).
Toxic Dose	The toxic dose is highly variable. Toxicity is more likely in the setting of underlying heart disease.
Signs and Symptoms	Bradycardia, AV blockade, and hypotension are common. Tachycardia has been reported with some β-blockers such as practolol, pindolol, and sotalol. Hypotension is a result of negative chronotropy (bradycardia) and negative inotropy (decreased cardiac contractility). Changes in mental status, ranging from confusion to seizures or coma, have been described. Bronchospasm and congestive heart failure can occur. Beta-blockers can mask the normal adrenergic signs and symptoms of hypoglycemia. In addition, they can impair recovery from hypoglycemia.
Prehospital Management	Supportive care, including airway management, is provided where indicated. Activated charcoal may be indicated. Symptomatic patients with abnormal vital signs may respond to atropine or catecholamines (epinephrine) but more frequently require glucagon therapy. Glucagon acts by augmenting heart rate, AV conduction, and myocardial contractility. The required dose for glucagon therapy in this setting is typically 3 to 10 mg given as a bolus. This dosage is frequently problematic in that few EMS vehicles carry these quantities of glucagon in the field. Cases unresponsive to these pharmacological interventions

may be supported with fluid therapy and/or transcutaneous pacing. Seizures can be treated with benzodiazepines (diazepam or lorazepam) or in refractory cases phenytoin or phenobarbital. Bronchospasm can be treated with β_2-agonists and in severe cases amino-phylline.

In-Hospital Management	Supportive care should be provided as in prehospital management. Patients often require intensive care unit (ICU) support including continuous glucagon infusion with or without pressor therapy (dopamine or epinephrine).

Calcium Channel Blockers

The clinical presentation of calcium channel blocker overdose can be extremely variable depending on the agent involved but is often clinically similar to beta-blocker toxicity. Although calcium therapy can be useful, major overdoses are often dependent on inotrope therapy (epinephrine or dopamine) and occasionally glucagon.

Route of Exposure	Oral, sublingual, or intravenous.
Mechanism of Toxicity	Virtually any cell utilizing calcium can be affected, most notably myocardium, the sino-atrial (SA) and AV nodes, and the AV nodal conduction pathway. Metabolism occurs in the liver.
Toxic Dose	The toxic dose is variable. The effects are generally more severe in the presence of underlying cardiovascular disease.
Signs and Symptoms	Hypotension, bradycardia, and AV conduction blocks are common. The extent of these effects is dependent on the specific agent ingested. Nonspecific features include lethargy, slurred speech, nausea, vomiting, coma, and respiratory depression.
Prehospital Management	Supportive care is provided as required. Activated charcoal may be indicated. In cases of severe toxicity, calcium chloride or calcium gluconate may be given intravenously in a dosage of 10 cc of a 10 percent solution. Calcium therapy is occasionally but not universally effective. Other therapeutic options for cardiac toxicity include atropine, isoproterenol, and transcutaneous pacing. Intravenous glucagon therapy has also been tried with some success in cases unresponsive to calcium and pressors. Hypotension may be partially responsive to IV fluids and inotropes (dopamine and norepinephrine).

In-Hospital Management	Supportive care should be provided as in pre-hospital management. Decontamination may include gastric lavage as well as the use of activated charcoal. Prolonged toxicity is common, and observation for extended periods is often required. Severe cases may require ICU admission with assisted ventilation and inotropic therapy.

Carbon Monoxide

Carbon monoxide (CO) exposure, both intentional and accidental, is a common toxicological problem. Death is not infrequent, and long-term neurological sequelae are also common. Oxygen is the mainstay of therapy, and hyperbaric oxygen therapy may be indicated in severe cases.

Route of Exposure	Inhalation is the most common route of exposure and is caused by blocked ventilation of furnace, chimney, or automobile exhaust systems. Carbon monoxide exposure is also common in smoke inhalation and can be seen with ingestion or inhalation of paint thinners (containing methylene chloride, which can be metabolized to CO).
Mechanism of Toxicity	CO binds hemoglobin to form carboxyhemoglobin, thereby reducing the availability of hemoglobin to carry oxygen and thus inducing hypoxemia. It may also impair cellular oxygenation by competing with oxygen for binding sites of enzymes on the cytochrome chain. The affinity of hemoglobin for CO is 250× that of O_2. CO also binds directly to both cardiac and skeletal myoglobin, thereby decreasing contractility. In the CNS, CO can induce cerebral edema and necrosis of white matter.
Toxic Dose	Variable.
Signs and Symptoms	Signs and symptoms depend on levels:

<10 percent:	Generally asymptomatic; smokers often run levels up to 10 percent
10–20 percent:	Headache and dyspnea
20–30 percent:	Headache, fatigue, and visual disturbance
40–50 percent:	Tachycardia and altered level of consciousness; may precipitate angina
>60 percent:	Coma, seizures, and cherry red skin

Levels can only be measured via blood testing in the hospital. At levels greater than 40 percent, virtually any organ system can be affected. Pulmonary effects include noncardiogenic pulmonary edema, congestive heart failure, and aspiration. CNS effects include ataxia, nystagmus, hearing loss, tinnitus, papilledema, retinal hemorrhages, coma, and seizures. Cardiovascular system (CVS) effects include dysrhythmias, ST and T wave changes on electrocardiogram (ECG), and occasionally ischemia or infarction. Renal effects include rhabdomyolysis or myoglobinuria and acute renal failure. Although the occurrence of cherry red skin is commonly described in the presence of CO poisoning, it is actually a rare finding and its absence does not rule out CO poisoning. Pallor or cyanosis is seen relatively frequently in CO poisoning.

Prehospital Management Supportive care supplemented by O_2 (via 100 percent nonrebreather mask) and airway management should be provided as required. Oxygen acts to decrease the half-life of CO:

$t_{1/2}$ room air = 320 minutes

$t_{1/2}$ 100 percent O_2 = 60–80 minutes

$t_{1/2}$ hyperbaric O_2 = 20–30 minutes

The measured O_2 saturation is unreliable in the setting of CO poisoning because the unit cannot differentiate between carboxyhemoglobin and oxyhemoglobin. As such it gives a falsely high saturation reading. The difference between an accurately measured O_2 saturation and the falsely elevated oximetry measurement is known as the saturation gap and is characteristic of CO poisoning. Unfortunately, accurate measurement of the O_2 saturation requires the use of arterial blood gases and therefore is generally not possible in a prehospital care setting.

In-Hospital Management Supportive care should be provided as in prehospital management. Use of hyperbaric oxygen therapy remains controversial but may offer benefit in patients with severe symptoms and neurological deficits. Indications for hyperbaric O_2 therapy include patients with significant neurological abnormalities, patients with cardiovascular abnormalities, or symptomatic pregnant patients. Some studies suggest symptomatic patients with levels >20 to 25 percent warrant hyperbaric O_2 therapy. Long-term neurological sequelae occur, and some centers routinely use psychometric testing to monitor neurological function.

Cyanide

Cyanide is a substance with a somewhat notorious history commonly found in many industrial products, medications, and plants. It is found in many manufacturing plants and laboratories and is produced in the burning of some plastics, wool, silk, and furniture. It is found in plant material, including apricot, peach, and cherry pits, and in some poisons. It is an uncommon but potentially deadly toxin; patients who have been exposed to it can be treated using a specific antidote kit that may be life saving if used early.

Route of Exposure	Inhalation, ingestion, intravenous, or dermal contact.
Mechanism of Toxicity	Cyanide binds a key cellular enzyme, cytochrome oxidase, causing cellular asphyxia and thus affecting virtually all organ systems.
Toxic Dose	Highly variable.
Signs and Symptoms	Most commonly present very quickly postexposure as unconscious, noncyanosed patients with hypotension and bradycardia; death occurs in seconds to minutes. In less severe cases or very early postexposure, the patient may have headache, dyspnea, confusion, or seizures with hypotension. Permanent neurological sequelae can occur in survivors. A bitter almond odor may be detected by care providers.
Prehospital Management	Recognition of cyanide exposure is the key to management because the window for implementing therapy is extremely short. As always, initial supportive care, including airway, breathing and circulation, is paramount. A specific antidote, known as the Pasadena Cyanide Antidote Kit, is available and is often kept on site at industrial sites using cyanide products. Some EMS systems, particularly in rural settings, carry the antidote kit. The kit contains three different products: amyl nitrite pearls for inhalation, sodium nitrite solution for intravenous use, and sodium thiosulfate for intravenous use. The amyl nitrite pearls are meant to be broken and inhaled by the victim immediately, and the sodium nitrite is meant to be given immediately on establishment of IV access. Both nitrite products work by inducing methemoglobinemia—a form of hemoglobin that scavenges cyanide. Sodium thiosulfate works by converting cyanide to thiocyanate, a much less toxic compound that is gradually excreted in the urine. If the symptoms are relatively mild, sodium thiosulfate should be used alone, because methemoglobinemia can itself be dangerous and is only valuable in truly life-threatening cases of cyanide poison-

ing. Base physician contact or poison center consultation should come early in the course of managing cyanide poisoning.

In-Hospital Management Supportive care should be provided as in prehospital management. Inhalational exposures related to closed-space combustion can often present with concurrent cyanide and carbon monoxide toxicity, and both must be treated aggressively. In cases requiring nitrite therapy, methemoglobin levels must be closely monitored. Intravenous hydroxycobalamin (vitamin B_{12}) can be a useful adjunct because it combines with cyanide to form a nontoxic cyanocobalamin that is excreted renally. Hyperbaric oxygen has no proven role in cyanide poisoning, although it may be indicated in cases of concurrent CO poisoning. For oral cyanide ingestion, charcoal may be beneficial.

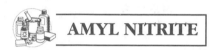

AMYL NITRITE

Class: Vasodilator/cyanide antidote

Description

Amyl nitrite is a potent vasodilator and an antidote for cyanide poisoning.

Mechanism of Action

Amyl nitrite, which is chemically related to nitroglycerin, has been used for many years in the treatment and symptomatic relief of angina. It is also effective in the emergency management of cyanide poisoning. It is supplied in a glass inhalant that can be broken and inhaled immediately. Amyl nitrite causes the oxidation of hemoglobin to a compound called *methemoglobin.* Methemoglobin reacts with the toxic cyanide ion to form *cyanomethemoglobin,* which can be enzymatically degraded. This serves to remove cyanide from the blood.

Pharmacokinetics

Onset: 10–30 seconds
Peak Effects: 30 seconds
Duration: 3–5 minutes
Half-Life: Not applicable

Indication

Cyanide poisoning.

Contraindications

There are no contraindications to the use of amyl nitrite in the management of cyanide poisoning.

Precautions

Headache and hypotension have been known to occur following the inhalation of amyl nitrite. Amyl nitrite is a drug of abuse and should be kept in a secure place with the narcotics. It has a horrible odor resembling dirty sweat socks.

Side Effects

Amyl nitrite can cause severe headache, weakness, dizziness, flushing, cold sweats, tachycardia, syncope, orthostatic hypotension, nausea, and vomiting.

Interactions

The hypotensive effects of amyl nitrite can be potentiated by antihypertensive agents, β-blockers, and certain antiemetics (phenothiazines).

Dosage

One to two inhalants of amyl nitrite should be crushed and inhaled. This should be maintained until the patient has reached an emergency department. Therapeutic effects diminish after approximately 20 minutes. Amyl nitrite should be administered by inhalation only.

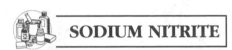 **SODIUM NITRITE**

Class: Nitrate/cyanide antidote

Description

Sodium nitrite is a nitrate salt and a part of the Pasadena Cyanide Antidote Kit (Figure 12–1). It is seldom used alone in the treatment of cyanide poisoning; instead, it is usually used with sodium thiosulfate and amyl nitrite. When used together, these compounds are more effective than when used alone.

Mechanism of Action

Sodium nitrite converts hemoglobin to methemoglobin. Methemoglobin has a high affinity for cyanide and can actually draw cyanide from the cells. The methemoglobin–cyanide complex is still toxic (but less so than cyanide bound to cytochrome a_3) and must be detoxified by sodium thiosulfate. The mechanism of action of sodium nitrite is not fully understood.

Pharmacokinetics

> **Onset:** 2–5 minutes
> **Peak Effects:** 30–70 minutes
> **Duration:** Varies
> **Half-Life:** Not applicable

Indications

Cyanide poisoning as a part of the Pasadena Cyanide Antidote Kit.

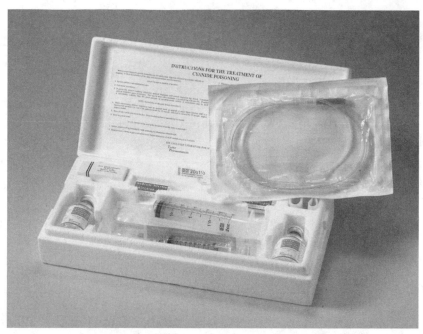

FIGURE 12–1   Cyanide antidote kit.

Contraindications

Sodium nitrite should not be administered to asymptomatic patients following exposure to cyanide. It should not be administered to patients with smoke inhalation and combined carbon monoxide and cyanide poisoning unless hyperbaric oxygen therapy is available and such therapy has already been initiated.

Precautions

Excessive methemoglobinemia may occur, especially when doses larger than those recommended are administered to children. Hypotension is common following rapid administration of sodium nitrite due to its vasodilating properties and can be minimized by slow IV administration. Blood pressure should be monitored carefully during sodium nitrite administration, and the infusion rate slowed if hypotension occurs.

Patients with smoke inhalation and combined carbon monoxide and cyanide poisoning with elevated carboxyhemoglobin levels should not be given sodium nitrite unless treatment in a hyperbaric oxygen chamber is available and such treatment has been initiated.

Side Effects

Excessive methemoglobinemia may occur, especially with doses exceeding those recommended. Hypotension may occur with rapid intravenous infusion.

Interactions

None when used in the setting of cyanide poisoning.

Dosage

Adult dose: Give amyl nitrite until IV access available, then administer 300 mg (10 mL of 3 percent solution) sodium nitrite IV. Subsequent doses of 150 mg can be administered in 30 minutes as needed or if there is no response to the first dose.

Pediatric dose: 10 mg/kg IV. Fifty percent of the original dose can be administered in 30 minutes as needed.

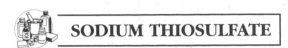

SODIUM THIOSULFATE

Class: Cyanide antidote

Description

Sodium thiosulfate is a part of the Pasadena Cyanide Antidote Kit. It is seldom used alone in the treatment of cyanide poisoning; instead, it is usually used with sodium nitrite and amyl nitrite. When used together, these compounds are more effective than when used alone.

Mechanism of Action

The major route of detoxification of cyanide in the body is conversion to thiocyanate. The thiocyanate is then removed by the kidneys.

Pharmacokinetics

Onset: 2–5 minutes
Peak Effects: Varies
Duration: Varies
Half-Life: Not applicable

Indications

Cyanide poisoning as a part of the Pasadena Cyanide Antidote Kit.

Contraindications

None when used in the treatment of cyanide poisoning.

Precautions

Sodium thiosulfate is most effective as a cyanide antidote when used in conjunction with nitrites.

Side Effects

Nausea, vomiting, and joint aches are common. Psychosis reported with higher doses. Side effects are mild and of minor importance compared to the risks associated with cyanide poisoning.

Interactions

None when used in the setting of cyanide poisoning.

Dosage

Adult dose: Administer following sodium nitrite and/or amyl nitrite. The initial dose is 12.5 (50 mL of 25 percent solution) IV over 10 minutes. Repeat half original dose if signs recur.

Pediatric dose: The initial dose in children is 400 (300 to 500) mg/kg body weight given intravenously as indicated above.

Cyclic Antidepressants (Tricyclics)

Despite the introduction of various new classes of antidepressant agents in recent years, tricyclics continue to be widely prescribed. Unfortunately, the clinical benefit of these agents is often offset by their lethal potential in the setting of overdose. Cardiac toxicity, predominantly in the form of lethal dysrhythmias, is the clinical hallmark, and intravenous bicarbonate therapy continues to be an essential part of management. Examples of agents in this class include amitriptyline and nortriptyline.

Route of Exposure	Oral.
Mechanism of Toxicity	Multiple physiological effects lead to clinical toxicity. Blockage of norepinephrine, dopamine, and serotonin reuptake at the presynaptic receptor leads to eventual norepinephrine depletion. Tricyclics also possess some anticholinergic activity, calcium channel blocking activity, and alpha-blocking activity. Cardiac toxicity is related to antagonism of cardiac fast sodium channels (quinidine-like effects), resulting in prolonged QRS complexes, as well as blockade of potassium efflux, resulting in QT interval prolongation. Metabolism is almost entirely hepatic, with a half-life of approximately 24 hours at therapeutic doses. In the setting of overdose, the half-life can be as much as 72 hours.
Toxic Dose	Highly variable.
Signs and Symptoms	Symptoms include dizziness, confusion, blurred vision, and dry mouth. Signs can be classified into three categories: cardiovascular, CNS, and anticholinergic. Cardiovascular signs include conduction blocks, hypotension, dysrhythmias, and cardiac arrest. CNS signs include delirium, agitation, extrapyramidal signs, myoclonus, seizures, and coma. Anticholinergic signs occur as described previously and include tachycardia, mydriasis, decreased bowel sounds, urinary retention, and hyper- or hypothermia. The earliest and most sensitive sign of cyclic antidepressant overdose is tachycardia. Life-threatening dysrhythmias are generally preceded by prolongation of the QRS complex.

Prehospital Management	Supportive care, including airway support, should be provided as indicated. Multidose activated charcoal is indicated. Intravenous access and fluid therapy are indicated if hypotension is present. Sodium bicarbonate remains a mainstay of therapy and has the following specific indications: hypotension, ventricular dysrhythmias, seizure activity (bicarbonate is not therapeutic for the seizure itself, but seizure activity is considered predictive of impending cardiac dysrhythmias, which may be averted with bicarbonate therapy), and wide QRS complexes on cardiac monitor. (The QRS interval requiring bicarbonate therapy remains somewhat controversial—some authors advocate 0.10 seconds, whereas others advocate that it be reserved for complexes >0.16 seconds; base physician contact is generally indicated where possible.)
	Several mechanisms have been postulated for the therapeutic effects of bicarbonate, including increased protein binding of tricyclic antidepressant (TCA) in an alkaline environment (thus there is less free TCA to induce cardiac toxicity), alkalinization increasing the amount of unionized TCA, which appears to be less able to bind the sodium channel, and alkalinization causing free TCA to be pulled out of cardiac tissue. Additionally, some evidence suggests that the sodium in sodium bicarbonate helps to overcome the sodium channel blockade.
	Hypotension unresponsive to bicarbonate and IV fluid may require inotrope therapy. Seizure activity unresponsive to bicarbonate therapy may be treated with benzodiazepines such as diazepam or lorazepam. Mechanical hyperventilation may be of some value in reducing cardiac and CNS toxicity.
In-Hospital Management	Supportive care should be provided as in prehospital management. Gastric lavage may be indicated if less than 2 hours postingestion. Cases of suspected toxicity require an observation period of at least 6 hours to rule out serious sequelae.

Digoxin and Digitalis

Although not as widely used as it once was, digoxin remains a relatively common drug that can cause severe illness and death in the setting of overdose. A specific antidote, digitalis-specific Fab fragments, is available but is not commonly used in the prehospital setting. Digoxin has a relatively narrow therapeutic window, and EMS providers should maintain a high index of suspicion for toxicity in cases in which a patient is known to be taking the drug. It is found in several sources, including prescription medications, plants (most notably foxglove), and certain toad venom.

Route of Exposure	Generally oral; can be related to plant exposure (digitalis is derived from plants, most notably the foxglove plant).
Mechanism of Toxicity	Digoxin and digitalis inhibit the sodium-potassium ATPase, causing potassium efflux and sodium and calcium influx into cells. Toxicity is enhanced in hypokalemia, hypomagnesemia, hypercalcemia, and alkalosis.
Toxic Dose	The toxic dose is highly variable. Patients with underlying heart disease, renal failure, hypothyroidism, and hypoxemia and those using nonsteroidal anti-inflammatory drugs (NSAIDs) are more prone to toxicity.
Signs and Symptoms	Symptoms are nonspecific and include fatigue, anorexia, disorientation, confusion, delerium, hallucinations, gastrointestinal upset, visual halos (green or yellow), slowed conduction in SA and AV nodes, increased PR interval, shortened QT intervals, AV block, asystole, ST-T wave scooping, junctional rhythms, and hemodynamic instability. Virtually any cardiac dysrhythmia can be seen.
Prehospital Management	Supportive care, including fluids and pressor agents for the treatment of hypotension, should be provided. Multidose activated charcoal may be useful. Calcium, which will worsen digoxin toxicity, should *not* be given.
In-Hospital Management	Supportive care should be provided as in prehospital management. Electrolyte abnormalities, including hyperkalemia, should be corrected. Calcium should *not* be given. Magnesium therapy may lessen cardiac toxicity. Phenytoin or dilantin may be helpful for ventricular dysrhythmias. Atropine and pacing may be required for symptomatic bradycardias. Procainamide and quinidine are contraindicated because they may worsen conduction and contractility problems. Digibind (digoxin Fab fragments) can be lifesaving in severe overdose. It acts by directly binding and inactivating digoxin, thereby allowing for rapid excretion by the kidneys. Digibind is indicated in ingestions that are potentially lethal based on the amount of ingested drug (generally 10 mg in an adult), high serum levels (>12.8 to 19.2 mmol/L), marked hyperkalemia, malignant dysrhythmias, resistant bradycardias, and hypotension. Clinical response to Digibind can occur as early as 20 to 30 minutes after administration.

Ethylene Glycol

The toxic alcohols include ethylene glycol, methanol, and isopropyl alcohol. In the case of ethylene glycol, which is most commonly found in antifreeze, ingestion is often accidental and may not be recognized until severe toxicity has occurred. Ethylene glycol poisoning is frequently misdiagnosed as ethanol intoxication, often resulting in suboptimal outcomes. Ethanol therapy helps to avert toxicity, but in severe cases dialysis may be required.

Route of Exposure	Generally oral.
Mechanism of Toxicity	Toxic metabolites are formed, causing acidosis and renal damage. Ethylene glycol is metabolized by alcohol dehydrogenase into several toxic metabolites including glycoaldehyde, glycolic acid, glyoxylic acid, and oxalate. These products take some time to accumulate, and thus signs and symptoms may not appear until 6 to 12 hours after the ingestion. This delay is even more pronounced if ethanol is also ingested because ethanol competes for alcohol dehydrogenase and thereby slows the development of toxic metabolites.
Toxic Dose	The minimal toxic dose is 1 to 2 mL/kg.
Signs and Symptoms	Toxicity is sometimes divided into three phases.
	Phase I is from 1 to 12 hours postingestion and typically presents with signs of intoxication without the smell of ethanol (which prehospital care providers should be able to recognize). CNS symptoms may include ataxia, seizures, and nystagmus. Nausea and vomiting are common in phase I.
	Phase II occurs from 12 to 36 hours postingestion and consists of cardiopulmonary toxicity including hypertension, tachycardia, and tachypnea. In severe poisoning pulmonary edema, congestive heart failure, and shock may develop.
	Phase III occurs from 24 to 72 hours postingestion and is associated with acute renal toxicity consisting of flank pain, costovertebral angle tenderness, decreased urine output, and acute renal failure.
	Not all patients go through these phases; some can present critically ill early postingestion (i.e., within 12 hours). The fluorescent additive in antifreeze can sometimes be seen excreted in the urine.
Prehospital Management	Supportive care, including airway management, should be provided as required. Intravenous fluid therapy is indicated because

dehydration is common and renal perfusion may be compromised. Ethanol therapy is indicated as a means of preventing metabolism to toxic metabolites. Although not widely used in a prehospital care setting, some circumstances (such as long transport times) may warrant the use of oral or IV ethanol therapy. Patients who have been coingesting ethanol have the benefit of having initiated their own therapy.

In-Hospital Management Supportive care should be provided as in prehospital management. Metabolism to toxic metabolites is limited by administering ethanol as a competitive inhibitor of alcohol dehydrogenase. In this way ethanol allows for excretion of unchanged ethylene glycol without metabolism. The half-life of ethylene glycol is 5 hours, whereas with therapeutic ethanol levels it is increased to approximately 17 hours. Serum ethanol levels are used to determine the need for ethanol therapy, which is usually given intravenously but can be given orally in unusual circumstances. Hemodialysis is indicated in cases of renal failure, in severe metabolic acidosis, or as determined by blood levels. Hypocalcemia can occur and, when present, requires treatment. Magnesium is a cofactor in the conversion to nontoxic metabolites, and magnesium supplementation is sometimes required. Bicarbonate is used in cases of profound acidosis. Pyridoxine is used to help promote conversion of glyoxylic acid to its nontoxic metabolite, glycine.

Iron

Iron overdose is relatively common and tends to be seen most frequently in the pediatric population. Symptoms are highly variable, depending on the time since ingestion. A specific antidote, deferoxamine, is available but is generally reserved for use in the hospital.

Route of Exposure Oral.

Mechanism of Toxicity Iron has a direct corrosive effect on gastric and intestinal mucosa that can lead to hemorrhage or perforation. Fluid loss from the gastrointestinal (GI) tract and vasodilation can cause hypotension. Iron is also an intracellular toxin that causes uncoupling of oxidative phosphorylation, leading to impaired generation of ATP and cellular death.

Toxic Dose The toxic dose is somewhat dependent on the form of iron ingested because it is the elemental amount of iron present that is relevant.

Ferrous sulfate tablets contain only 20 percent elemental iron per weight, whereas ferrous fumarate contains 33 percent iron by weight. Taking this into account, 20 to 60 mg/kg of elemental iron has moderate risk of toxicity, whereas >60 mg/kg has high risk for toxicity.

Signs and Symptoms

Some authors describe four distinct stages of iron toxicity, and others describe five. The classification based on four stages is presented here.

Stage 1 (1/2 to 2 hours postingestion): Severe vomiting and diarrhea (often with blood), lethargy, coma, pallor, tachycardia, hypotension, acidosis, hyperglycemia, hypovolemia, shock, renal failure, and death.

Stage 2 (2 to 12 hours postingestion): Relatively asymptomatic period.

Stage 3 (12 to 48 hours postingestion): Recurrence of GI symptoms including bloody emesis and diarrhea, GI perforation, coma, seizures, shock, hepatorenal failure, coagulation defects, hypoglycemia, and severe metabolic acidosis.

Stage 4 (beyond 48 hours postingestion): Pyloric (gastric outlet) strictures. In this stage either death or recovery occurs.

Prehospital Management

Treatment is limited to supportive care including airway support and fluid resuscitation in cases of volume depletion.

In-Hospital Management

Supportive care should be provided as in prehospital management. Iron levels are helpful but do not completely rule out iron toxicity, particularly in the later stages. Levels generally peak 3 to 5 hours postingestion, and levels drawn outside this window may be misleading. Iron tablets can often be seen on X-ray, and, as such, abdominal X-rays may be helpful. Charcoal does not bind iron and is therefore not indicated. Gastric lavage is of limited value because iron can form concretions or bezoars, which are too large to fit in lavage tubing. Whole-bowel irrigation is the decontamination method of choice. Patients with toxic levels or clinical signs and symptoms are treated with deferoxamine, which works by binding with iron to form a water-soluble compound, ferrioxamine, which is renally excreted. A deferoxamine challenge test is sometimes used in which deferoxamine is administered and a change in urine color (vin-rose) is considered diagnostic of a toxic iron ingestion. Charcoal hemoperfusion and exchange transfusions have been used occasionally with some success. Symptomatology always takes precedence over laboratory values in managing cases of suspected iron overdose.

Isopropyl Alcohol

Isopropyl alcohol, commonly known as rubbing alcohol, is a commonly abused toxic alcohol. Although it is far less toxic than methanol or ethylene glycol, in high doses it can induce hypotension unresponsive to conventional therapy and cardiac ischemia.

Route of Exposure	Oral, skin contact, or inhalation.
Mechanism of Toxicity	Isopropyl alcohol is a CNS depressant and vasodilator. In the liver it is metabolized to acetone, which is subsequently excreted by the kidneys.
Toxic Dose	Toxic dose is 0.5 to 1 mL/kg of 70 percent isopropanol (typical concentration).
Signs and Symptoms	Signs of intoxication and CNS depression may appear. It is twice as potent a CNS depressant as ethanol. In severe overdose, hypotension secondary to vasodilation that is largely unresponsive to fluids and pressor therapy can occur. Cardiac ischemia or infarction can occur.
Prehospital Management	Supportive care, including airway management, assisted ventilation, and fluid therapy, should be provided as needed. Gastric lavage and activated charcoal may be indicated for recent ingestions. Ethanol therapy is not indicated.
In-Hospital Management	Supportive care should be provided as in prehospital management. Vasopressor therapy, though of limited value, may be tried. Dialysis is rarely required but may be indicated in cases involving severe, unresponsive hypotension.

Lithium

Lithium is a relatively common medication used in the treatment of certain psychiatric disorders such as bipolar (manic-depressive) disorder. Although overdose is not common, it can be serious. No specific antidote is available, and therapy is generally aimed at enhancing elimination and providing supportive care.

Route of Exposure	Oral.
Mechanism of Toxicity	Lithium replaces sodium, thereby altering cellular processes, membrane structures, response to hormones, and utilization of energy at a cellular level. In the CNS these effects can result in permanent neurological damage. Lithium is excreted almost entirely by the kidneys. Because it decreases renal function, lithium tends to decrease its own clearance and can in fact enhance its own reabsorption by the kidney.
Toxic Dose	The toxic dose is highly variable depending on whether it is an acute or chronic ingestion. Overdose in the setting of chronic ingestion

	tends to be more severe because serum lithium levels are already high, allowing lithium to enter cells (predominantly CNS) more readily. Toxicity is generally more severe in the setting of poor underlying renal function, diuretic use, and dehydration.
Signs and Symptoms	Signs and symptoms are variable depending on levels.
	Low (serum levels less than 1.5 mEq/L): GI symptoms including nausea, vomiting, and diarrhea.
	Moderate (serum levels 1.5 to 3.0 mEq/L): Polyuria followed by urinary and fecal incontinence, muscle weakness (which can progress to myoclonic twitches and muscle rigidity with choreoathetoid movements), and neurological symptoms (which can include restlessness, vertigo, slurred speech, blurred vision, and coma).
	Severe (serum levels >3.0 mEq/L): Seizures, coma, cardiac dysrhythmias, hypotension with peripheral vascular collapse, muscle twitching, and spasticity.
Prehospital Management	Supportive care should be provided as indicated. Virtually all patients with lithium overdoses are volume depleted, and aggressive fluid resuscitation using normal saline is indicated. It remains unclear whether the administration of sodium chloride aids elimination.
In-Hospital Management	Lavage may be helpful if less than 1 hour has elapsed from the time of ingestion. Whole-bowel irrigation has also been shown to be beneficial. Correction of volume depletion is essential and can take several hours. Hemodialysis is indicated in cases of renal failure, of severe cardiovascular or neurological abnormalities, or with high serum levels.

Methanol

Methanol is found in many solutions including wood alcohol, window washer fluid, paint solvent, and industrial solvents. Ingestion is generally accidental, and small doses can be fatal. Although virtually any organ system can be involved, visual disturbances including blindness remain the clinical hallmark. Toxicity is dependent on the formation of toxic metabolites, and thus toxicity is generally delayed for several hours.

Route of Exposure	Generally oral but can be dermal or by inhalation.
Mechanism of Toxicity	Toxic metabolites, predominantly formaldehyde and formic acid, are formed through the metabolism of methanol by alcohol dehydrogenase. These toxic metabolites have direct

toxic effects at a cellular level and result in a profound acidosis that can further accelerate toxicity. Methanol is metabolized by alcohol dehydrogenase to form formaldehyde, which in turn is converted to fomic acid by aldehyde dehydrogenase. Up to 5 percent of ingested methanol may be excreted unchanged by the kidneys and via respiration.

Toxic Dose

Death has been reported with as small a dose as 15 to 30 mL (1 to 2 tablespoons).

Signs and Symptoms

An initial latent period ranging from 6 to 30 hours consists of signs of intoxication and gastrointestinal irritation. Some patients may have a prolonged asymptomatic period, particularly if ethanol has been coingested. Caution must be used, because a lack of symptoms early on does not preclude toxicity.

As toxic metabolites are formed, nausea, vomiting, abdominal pain, and CNS symptoms (ranging from headache and confusion to coma) occur. Ocular toxicity is the hallmark of methanol overdose and can manifest as decreased visual acuity (haziness or "snowfield blindness").

Death is generally related to profound acidosis and severe CNS effects including cerebral edema. Gastrointestinal bleeding secondary to gastritis can occur.

Prehospital Management

Supportive care, including airway management, should be provided as indicated. As with ethylene glycol, oral or IV ethanol therapy has been utilized in some prehospital care settings. Gastric lavage is sometimes used in recent ingestions. Charcoal is not helpful.

In-Hospital Management

Diagnosis can be difficult because blood levels are not always available or reliable at the time of presentation. Laboratory investigation generally reveals an anion gap metabolic acidosis, as well as an osmolar gap. Supportive care augmented by intravenous ethanol therapy is the mainstay of therapy. Hemodialysis is indicated in the presence of visual symptoms, severe acidosis, high serum levels, or an ingestion of greater than 30 mL. Bicarbonate is reserved for cases of profound acidosis. Folate is a cofactor for the conversion of formate to nontoxic by-products and has a role in therapy.

Narcotics and Opioids

Narcotics and opioids are widely used for both medicinal and therapeutic purposes. Overdoses are common, especially in large urban centers. Recognition of these overdoses is important, because a specific antidote (naloxone) is available in most prehospital settings. In hospital settings, Revex, a long-acting opioid antagonist, may be given.

Route of Exposure	Oral, intravenous, intramuscular, or dermal.
Mechanism of Toxicity	Narcotics and opioids act directly on opiate receptors within the CNS, causing CNS depression. Some opioids have mixed agonist and antagonist properties.
Signs and Symptoms	The classic triad of opioid overdose consists of miosis, respiratory depression, and decreased level of consciousness. Certain types of opioids (e.g., meperidine, morphine, propoxyphene, and pentazocine) can present with mydriasis rather than miosis. Occasionally seizures, hypotension, and ventricular dysrhythmias can be seen.
Prehospital Management	Supportive care, including airway management, takes priority over naloxone therapy. Track marks (IV) are helpful diagnostically when present and should always be examined. Following assessment and initial stabilization, early use of naloxone (Narcan) may avert the need for invasive airway control. Patients with opioid overdose can rapidly become combative and violent when given naloxone, and precautions need to be taken to ensure that both the patient and care providers are adequately protected from injury. This may include prophylactic use of restraints. Response to naloxone is often effective for diagnosis as well as treatment.
In-Hospital Management	Supportive care and naloxone therapy are provided as described earlier. Long periods of observation are often required to ensure that sedation does not recur. The duration of action of intravenous naloxone is typically 20 to 120 minutes, which is considerably shorter than the duration of action of most opioids (typically 3 to 6 hours). In cases of severe, prolonged opioid toxicity, continuous naloxone infusion may be indicated.

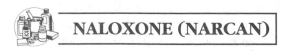

NALOXONE (NARCAN)

Class: Narcotic antagonist

Description

Naloxone is an effective narcotic antagonist. It has proved effective in the management and reversal of overdoses caused by narcotics or synthetic narcotic agents.

Mechanism of Action

Naloxone is chemically similar to the narcotics. However, it has only antagonistic properties. Naloxone competes for opiate receptors in the brain. It also displaces narcotic molecules from opiate receptors. It can reverse respiratory depression associated with narcotic overdose.

Pharmacokinetics

Onset: <2 minutes (IV), 2–10 minutes [IM, endotracheally (ET)]
Peak Effects: <2 minutes (IV), 2–10 minutes (IM, ET)
Duration: 20–120 minutes
Half-Life: 60–90 minutes

Indications

Naloxone is used for the complete or partial reversal of depression caused by narcotics including the following agents: morphine, Demerol, heroin, paregoric, Dilaudid, codeine, Percodan, fentanyl, and methadone. It is also used for the complete or partial reversal of depression caused by synthetic narcotic analgesic agents including the following drugs: Nubain, Talwin, Stadol, and Darvon. Naloxone may be used in the treatment of coma of unknown origin.

Contraindications

Naloxone should not be administered to a patient with a history of hypersensitivity to the drug.

Precautions

Naloxone should be administered cautiously to patients who are known or suspected to be physically dependent on narcotics. Abrupt and complete reversal by naloxone can cause withdrawal-type effects. This includes newborn infants of mothers with known or suspected narcotic dependence.

Naloxone should never be administered as part of a "coma cocktail." "Coma cocktails" involve the empiric administration of 50 percent dextrose, thiamine, and naloxone (and in some cases, flumazenil) to unresponsive patients in an attempt to correct the cause of their unresponsiveness and awaken them. "Coma cocktails" are a poor prehospital practice. Therapy should always be guided by objective data such as patient assessment findings and blood glucose determination.

Side Effects

Side effects associated with naloxone are rare. However, hypotension, hypertension, ventricular dysrhythmias, nausea, and vomiting have been reported.

Interactions

Naloxone may cause narcotic withdrawal in the narcotic-dependent patient. In cases of suspected narcotic dependence, only enough of the drug to reverse respiratory depression should be administered.

Dosage

The standard dosage for suspected or confirmed narcotic or synthetic narcotic overdoses is 1 to 2 mg administered IV. If unsuccessful, then a second dose may be administered 5 minutes later. Failure to obtain reversal after two to three doses indicates another disease process or overdosage on non-opioid drugs. Larger than average doses (2 to 5 mg) have been used in the management of Darvon overdoses and alcoholic coma. An intravenous infusion can be prepared by placing 2 mg of naloxone in 500 mL of D_5W. This gives a concentration of 4 µg/mL; 100 mL/hr should be infused, thus delivering 0.4 mg/hr. In the emergency setting, naloxone should be administered intravenously only. When an IV line cannot be established, intramuscular or subcutaneous (SC) administration can be performed. Naloxone can be administered endotracheally. The dose should be increased to 2.0 to 2.5 times the intravenous dose. Furthermore, naloxone should be diluted in enough normal saline to provide a total of 10 mL of fluid.

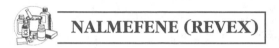 **NALMEFENE (REVEX)**

Class: Opioid antagonist

Description

Nalmefene is an opioid antagonist used for the reversal (partial or complete) of opioid effects, including respiratory and CNS depression.

Mechanism of Action

Nalmefene completely blocks the effects of opioids, including CNS and respiratory depression, without producing any agonist (opioid-like) effects.

Pharmacokinetics

> **Onset:** 2–5 minutes (IV), 15 minutes (IM/SC)
> **Peak Effects:** 5 minutes (IV), 2 hours (IM/SC)
> **Duration:** 4–8 hours
> **Half-Life:** 8.5–10.8 hours

Indications

Nalmefene is used for reversal of opioid effects and management of known or suspected opioid overdose.

Contraindications

Nalmefene should be avoided in patients with known hypersensitivity.

Precautions

Overdose of long-acting opioids may require repeat dosing. Revex should be used with caution in pregnant patients and patients known to be dependent on opioid agents.

Side Effects

Side effects include dysphoria, headache, hypertension, hypotension, tachycardia, vasodilation, abdominal cramps, nausea, joint pain, myalgia, chills, fever, and postoperative pain.

Interactions

No significant interactions have been noted.

Dosage

Adults are administered 0.5 mg/70 kg IV followed by incremental doses of 1.0 mg/70 kg every 2 to 5 minutes (up to a total dose of 1.5 mg/kg).

Organophosphates and Carbamates

Organophosphates and carbamates are commonly found in commercial insecticides. Although rare, toxic exposure to these agents is generally serious and often fatal. Diagnosis is frequently difficult because of the subtle nature of many exposures and generalized symptoms. A contaminated piece of clothing may prolong exposure over several days, further confusing the diagnosis. Atropine is widely used and can be highly effective for treatment of poisoning secondary to these agents.

Route of Exposure	Dermal, oral, ocular, or by inhalation.
Mechanism of Toxicity	Organophosphates and carbamides inhibit acetylcholinesterase activity, leading to increased acetylcholine at nerve synapses and an initial overstimulation followed by disruption of transmission in the CNS, parasympathetic nerve endings and some sympathetic nerve endings, somatic nerve endings, and autonomic ganglia.
Toxic Dose	Highly variable; toxicity can occur with minimal exposure. Recurrent exposure secondary to contaminated clothing is common.
Signs and Symptoms	The CNS symptoms include agitation, drowsiness, seizures, cardiorespiratory depression, coma, and death. The mnemonic DUMBELS can be used to describe the muscarinic signs and symptoms of cholinergic excess, and the mnemonic MTWtHF is used to describe the nicotinic features (see description under "Toxidromes" earlier in this chapter). Miosis is typically present, but in 10 percent of cases mydriasis is present. The history is not always clear in identifying an exposure. A garlic odor may be present.
Prehospital Management	As with all toxicological emergencies, supportive care must be provided immediately. Atropine in doses of 0.5 to 1 mg every 2 to 5 minutes (maximum of 100 mg) reverses the cholinergic symptoms. End points for atropine therapy include drying of secretions, reversal of bradycardia, and pupillary mydriasis. It is important to monitor ventilation closely because diaphragmatic weakness is not treated by atropine. Extreme care must be taken to avoid contamination of care providers by removal of

contaminated clothing and use of gloves and gowns (where available). Contaminated clothing should be removed as soon as practically possible.

In-Hospital Management Supportive care should be provided as in prehospital management. Additional therapies include the use of pralidoxime (2-PAM), which acts to regenerate acetylcholinesterase. Charcoal and lavage may be indicated for oral ingestions.

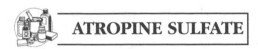

ATROPINE SULFATE

Class: Parasympatholytic

Description

Atropine sulfate is a potent parasympatholytic (anticholinergic). It blocks acetylcholine receptors, thus aiding the management of organophosphate poisonings. Organophosphate poisonings inhibit the enzyme cholinesterase, causing an increase and accumulation of the neurotransmitter acetylcholine. Often, large doses are required to achieve atropinization. Severe poisonings, especially those characterized by paralysis and muscle twitching, require pralidoxime (2-PAM), in addition to atropine.

Mechanism of Action

Atropine sulfate is a potent parasympatholytic and is used to increase the heart rate in hemodynamically significant bradycardias. Hemodynamically significant bradycardias are those slow heart rates accompanied by hypotension, shortness of breath, chest pain, altered mental status, congestive heart failure, and shock. Atropine acts by blocking acetylcholine receptors, thus inhibiting parasympathetic stimulation. Although it has positive chronotropic properties, it has little or no inotropic effect. It plays an important role as an antidote in organophosphate poisonings. Atropine has been shown to be of some use in asystole, presumably because some cases of asystole may be caused by a sudden and tremendous increase in parasympathetic tone. The mechanism by which atropine is effective in asystole is not clear. However, despite no definite proof of its value in asystole, there is little evidence that its use is harmful in this setting.

Pharmacokinetics

Onset: Immediate
Peak Effects: 2–4 minutes
Duration: 4 hours
Half-Life: 2–3 hours

Indications

Organophosphate poisoning, bradycardias that are hemodynamically significant, and asystole.

Contraindications

There are no contraindications to atropine when used in the management of severe organophosphate poisoning.

Precautions

It is important to remove all clothing from a patient who has suffered organophosphate poisoning. The patient must then be completely bathed to remove all residual organophosphate present on the skin. Always be sure to protect the rescuer. Atropine may actually worsen the bradycardia associated with second-degree Mobitz II and third-degree AV blocks. In these cases, go straight to transcutaneous pacing instead of trying atropine.

Side Effects

Atropine sulfate can cause blurred vision, dilated pupils, dry mouth, tachycardia, drowsiness, and confusion.

Interactions

Few in the prehospital setting.

Dosage

One milligram of atropine should be administered initially to determine whether or not the patient is tolerant to atropine. If the patient responds to the diagnostic dose, then most likely he or she is not severely poisoned or is not tolerant to atropine. If there is no improvement, a second dose of 2 to 5 mg may be indicated for an adult (0.05 mg/kg for a child). Doses exceeding 100 mg are sometimes required to treat severe organophosphate poisoning. Following the prehospital initial administration of atropine, prompt transportation to an emergency department is indicated. In severe organophosphate poisoning, atropine sulfate is administered intravenously.

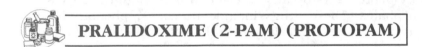

PRALIDOXIME (2-PAM) (PROTOPAM)

Class: Cholinesterase reactivator

Description

Pralidoxime is a cholinesterase reactivator.

Mechanism of Action

Pralidoxime is an antidote for severe organophosphate poisonings. It chemically removes the phosphate group from cholinesterase that was transferred from an organophosphate poison. Once cholinesterase is reactivated, it can deactivate acetylcholine. Pralidoxime also detoxifies some organophosphates by direct chemical reaction. It reverses respiratory depression and skeletal muscle paralysis resulting from organophosphate poisoning.

Pralidoxime should be reserved for severe organophosphate poisonings characterized by muscle twitching and paralysis. It should follow atropinization.

Pharmacokinetics

Onset: Varies
Peak Effects: 5–15 minutes (IV), 10–20 minutes (IM)
Duration: Varies
Half-Life: 0.8–2.7 hours

Indication

Severe organophosphate poisoning.

Contraindications

Pralidoxime should not be used in cases of poisoning resulting from inorganic phosphates or the carbamate class of insecticides.

Precautions

Always protect yourself and other rescuers when caring for the victim of organophosphate poisoning.

Intravenous administration should be carried out slowly because tachycardia, laryngospasm, and muscle rigidity have been seen with rapid administration. When used in conjunction with atropine, the effects of atropinization may be seen much earlier than expected. This is especially true if the atropine dose has been large. Excitement and manic behavior have been known to occur immediately following recovery from unconsciousness in a few cases.

Side Effects

Pralidoxime can cause tachycardia, increased salivation, headache, altered mental status, dizziness, blurred vision, nausea, and vomiting.

Interactions

Patients who have sustained organophosphate poisonings should not receive respiratory depressants because these can potentiate the effects of the organophosphates. These drugs include narcotics, phenothiazines (antiemetics), antihistamines, and alcohol. Pralidoxime should not be used with theophylline preparations (including aminophylline).

Dosage

One to 2 g of pralidoxime should be placed in 250 to 500 mL of normal saline and infused over 30 minutes. Pralidoxime should be administered by IV infusion or slow IV bolus only.

Salicylates

Salicylate (ASA) overdose is commonly encountered and can be fatal if not treated appropriately. These agents are found in a variety of over-the-counter medications and are frequently confused with other analgesics such as ibuprofen and acetaminophen. The clinical presentation is variable depending on the time since ingestion. Although a specific antidote is not available, therapy is aimed at enhancing elimination and thereby preventing long-term sequelae.

Route of Exposure	Oral; occasionally dermal.
Mechanism of Toxicity	Salicylates cause cellular toxicity through the uncoupling of oxidative phosphorylation and induce anion gap metabolic acidosis.
Metabolism	Salicylates are extensively metabolized by the liver; inactive metabolites are excreted by the kidneys.
Toxic Dose	*Acute:* 150 to 300 mg/kg = mild to moderate toxicity; >300 mg/kg = moderate to severe toxicity
	Chronic: Variable
Signs and Symptoms	*Mild to moderate:* Tachypnea, vomiting, diaphoresis, tinnitus, and acid–base disturbances. The tachypnea is typically early in the course of overdose and can result in an early respiratory alkalosis.
	Severe: CNS abnormalities ranging from confusion and delirium to coma secondary to cerebral edema, hypoglycemia (rare), pulmonary edema, coagulopathies and platelet dysfunction, and occasionally hyperthermia. An anion gap metabolic acidosis is the classic acid–base disturbance in the later stages of toxicity. Renal failure is possible.
Prehospital Management	Supportive care, including airway management, should be provided as required. Activated charcoal may be used. Hypoglycemia should be ruled out (especially in children).
In-Hospital Management	Toxicity is determined both by clinical criteria and by plotting blood levels taken at least 6 hours postingestion on the Done nomogram. The nomogram is a guideline only and is not useful for chronic toxicity. A single serum salicylate value is not always conclusive, and repeat levels aimed at determining half-lives are sometimes required. When toxicity is suspected by history and physical exam, therapy is initiated regardless of availability of serum levels. Gastric lavage is utilized in early presentations. Multidose activated charcoal has been shown to decrease absorbtion and toxicity. Renal excretion of salicylate is enhanced by inducing an alkaline diuresis. This is typically accomplished using an IV solution consisting of sodium bicarbonate mixed in D_5W. Potassium supplementation is often required. Hemodialysis is indicated in severe toxicity associated with renal failure, severe CNS or cardiac dysfunction, or severe acidosis not responsive to the alkaline diuresis.

SSRIs

Selective serotonin reuptake inhibitors (SSRIs) are the newest generation of antidepressant agents and are currently prescribed more frequently than more traditional antidepressants such as tricyclics. The popularity of these agents is largely attributable to their improved safety profile, particularly in the setting of overdose. Prototypical agents include fluoxetine (Prozac), trazadone, sertraline, and paroxetine.

Route of Exposure	Oral.
Mechanism of Toxicity	SSRIs block reuptake of serotonin at the presynaptic junction.
Toxic Dose	The toxic dose is variable, but the SSRIs are generally well tolerated even in large overdoses. If used in combination with a monoamine oxidase inhibitor (MAOI), the serotonin syndrome, which is potentially fatal, can occur.
Signs and Symptoms	Overdose with SSRIs is often asymptomatic. Symptoms and signs include agitation, insomnia, CNS excitation, tachycardia, hypertension, and ST depression. Serotonin syndrome can occur when the drug is used in combination with MAOIs. Serotonin syndrome can include hyperthermia, shivering, tremor, myoclonus, seizures, delirium, agitation, rigidity or hypertonia, autonomic instability, coma, and death.
Prehospital Treatment	Only supportive care is provided; no specific treatment is available.
In-Hospital Treatment	Supportive care is supplemented by activated charcoal and lavage (if less than 1 hour postingestion).
	Serotonin syndrome may require aggressive airway management, assisted ventilation, and pharmacological therapy including IV Dantrolene or oral cyproheptadine. Seizures are treated with benzodiazepines, and hypertension can be treated with calcium channel blockers such as nifedipine.

SUMMARY

Paramedics must be diligent in the assessment and treatment of suspected overdose. Without a high index of suspicion, even the most obvious clues can go unnoticed. By reviewing the general principles of toxicology, the paramedic will be better prepared to treat these emergencies.

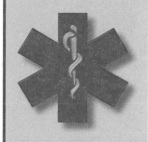

CASE PRESENTATION

Paramedics are dispatched at 14:30 hours on a weekday to a residence in an older neighborhood. Enroute the call taker provides further information. The patient is a 4-year-old female who is unconscious. On arrival a woman in her late 60s runs out of the house carrying a flaccid, unresponsive 4-year-old child.

On Examination

CNS: The child is unresponsive. Her pupils are dilated and unresponsive to light. She is unresponsive to voice and pain.

Resp: Respirations are agonal at 4 per minute and shallow. Her lungs are clear bilaterally with equal air entry. The trachea is midline and there are no signs of trauma.

CVS: The carotid pulse is present, but weak. The radial pulse is absent. Her skin is pale, with cyanotic/gray color to face. Skin is cool and dry.

ABD: Soft and nontender in all four quadrants. There are no signs of vomiting or diarrhea.

Muscl/Skel: No injuries are noted.

Vital Signs:

Pulse: 40 per minute

Resp: 4 per minute and shallow

B/P: 30/?? mmHg

SpO$_2$: error

ECG: 3rd-degree block

Past Hx: The grandmother states that she put her granddaughter down for a nap around 14:00 hours. At about 14:30 she checked on her granddaughter and found her on the floor of the grandmother's bedroom. The girl was unconscious and unresponsive with an open bottle of heart pills beside her. The grandmother called 911. The prescription is for Isoptin (verapamil) 120 mg. There are 10 to 12 pills on the floor. The bottle of 60 is empty.

The granddaughter has no previous illnesses and is in good health. She is not taking any medications, nor does she have any allergies.

Treatment

An OPA is inserted and the patient's respirations are assisted by a bag-valve-mask device with 100% oxygen via a reservoir bag. The patient is placed on a cardiac monitor, which shows a third-degree block. A weak pulse is still present. An intravenous line is initiated with a 20-gauge catheter in the antecubital fossa.

At the earliest moment, paramedics contact the poison control center for advice.

The patient is given fluid bolus of 20 mL/kg. The patient is approximately 25 kg so a bolus of 500 mL is administered. If perfusion does not improve with the bolus, the paramedics will, in consultation with poison control, administer calcium chloride 10 percent at 10 to 25 mg/kg diluted to 50 mL and given over 5 minutes. If calcium is not available, paramedics will consider epinephrine 0.01 mg/kg administered slow IV push.

The patient is prepared for transcutaneous pacing. Because this patient weighs more than 15 kg, the adult pads should work. Although this is unusual in children, the paramedics feel it is indicated because of the profound symptoms and may be required if the patient does not respond to medications. The paramedics realize that atropine does not work on third-degree heart blocks.

Outcome

The patient responded to medications and her heart rate increased to 100 with a junctional rhythm. She was transferred to ICU where she battled an aspiration pneumonia and liver failure (secondary to verapamil). She was eventually discharged from hospital with no complications.

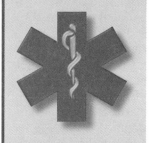

CASE PRESENTATION

Early one evening Waterville EMS is called to a residence in an upscale area of the city. Dispatch reports that they are responding to a "man down," unconscious, unresponsive, and not breathing. On arrival a woman in her 20s meets the paramedics and states that her boyfriend is not breathing. Paramedics are led to the living room, where they find a male in his mid-20s lying supine on the floor. There is emesis near the patient.

On Examination

CNS: The patient is unresponsive; Glasgow Coma Scale score is 3; both pupils are pinpoint yet equal

Resp: Respirations are 6 per minute and very shallow; the airway has residue from vomiting

CVS: The carotid pulse is slow and weak; the radial pulse is absent; skin is pale; lips are blue

ABD: Soft and nontender in all four quadrants; the patient has vomited

Muscl/Skel: No apparent injuries; no pitting edema

Vital Signs

Pulse: 56/min

Resp: 6/min

B/P: 70/52 mmHg

SpO$_2$: 72 percent

ECG: Sinus bradycardia

Past Hx: Initially the patient's girlfriend states that she does not know what happened. She states that her boyfriend is very healthy, has no medical problems, and does not take any medication. Paramedics specifically ask about alcohol or recreational drugs. The girlfriend emphatically states, "No."

Treatment

Police backup is requested. The initial treatment begins with the ABCs. The airway is suctioned, and an oropharyngeal airway is placed. Ventilation by bag-valve-mask device and 100 percent oxygen by reservoir bag is initiated at 24 breaths per minute. Airway compliance is good. An IV of normal saline is prepared and paramedics perform venipuncture with a 16-gauge catheter. Blood is drawn for a red-top tube, and the hub of the needle is used to obtain a blood sample for glucose testing. The IV of normal saline is connected to the catheter, and the fluid is administered at 100 mL/hr.

As one paramedic starts the IV, she looks for previous needle marks and does not find any. The absence of needle marks does not change the paramedic's assessment. Based on the age of the patient (a male in his mid-20s does not just stop breathing), the slow respirations, and the pinpoint pupils, the paramedic is fairly certain that the patient has taken a narcotic or some designer drug.

The patient's girlfriend is questioned once again as to whether her boyfriend uses any drugs. The paramedic tells her that her boyfriend's condition is very serious and that she must be absolutely honest. Finally the girlfriend states that her boyfriend uses heroin. She found him on the floor when she came home and then called for the ambulance after she hid the drugs and syringes.

At this point the police arrive and assist the paramedics. The patient is moved to the stretcher and restrained. The paramedics are concerned for their safety because the patient may be aggressive or violent as he comes out of the coma. His airway is still patent, and intubation is not required at this time. Narcan is administered intravenously in 1.0 mg dosages. The paramedics carefully titrate the dose to increase the respiratory rate. The stretcher and patient are moved to the ambulance, and a police officer agrees to accompany the paramedics to the hospital. The patient is not fighting against the bag-valve-mask device or straining against the restraints. The patient's girlfriend gives the paramedics the rest of the drugs and the syringe.

En route to the hospital a paramedic monitors the patient's vital signs closely. Respirations increase to 20 per minute, and the patient is placed on oxygen by nonrebreather mask at 15 lpm. The pulse rate increases to 112 per minute, and blood pressure increases to 124/82 mmHg. The blood glucose reading is 125 mg/dL (7.0 mmol/L). The half-life of Narcan is likely to be less than that of the narcotic. Thus, the patient's level of consciousness may decrease. On arrival at the hospital, the patient is conscious and verbally abusive and has stable vital signs. While awaiting the results of laboratory tests, the patient gets up, sneaks out the back door, and leaves the emergency department unseen.

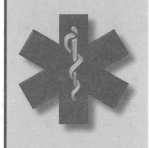

CASE PRESENTATION

Paramedics are called to meet the police at a local motel, where they have found an unconscious person in one of the motel suites. On arrival, several police officers escort paramedics to the room, where they find a 42-year-old male lying supine on the bed. He appears to have been alone in the room, and there is an empty bottle of whiskey lying on the floor next to the bed.

On Examination

CNS: The patient is unresponsive; his pupils are pinpoint and unresponsive to light

Resp: Respirations are 4 per minute and shallow; lungs are clear bilaterally, with equal air entry; trachea is midline; no signs of trauma

CVS: The carotid pulse is present but weak; the radial pulse is absent; skin is pale, cool, and dry, with dry mucous membranes

ABD: Soft and nontender in all four quadrants; no signs of vomiting or diarrhea

Muscl/Skel: No injuries are noted

Vital Signs

Pulse: 124/min

Resp: 4/min and shallow

BP: 70/40 mmHg

SpO$_2$: 80 percent

ECG: Sinus tachycardia

Past Hx: The police state that the patient had called his wife earlier in the evening and had threatened to kill himself. His wife then called the police, who managed to track the patient down to this motel. The patient's wife told the police that the patient had been suffering from depression for the past couple of months and had recently begun to drink heavily. The police found two empty pill bottles in the bathroom. One bottle contained amitriptyline (Elavil), and the other contained meperidine (Demerol). Both prescriptions had been filled recently.

Treatment

An OPA is inserted, and the patient's respirations are assisted by a bag-valve-mask device with 100 percent oxygen via a reservoir bag. The patient is placed on a cardiac monitor, which shows a sinus tachycardia with widened QRS complexes at 0.16 mm width. An intravenous line is initiated with a 16-gauge catheter, and a solution of normal saline is run wide open (20 mL/kg fluid bolus); 100 mEq sodium bicarbonate is administered along with 2 mg naloxone. The patient is prepared for transport to the hospital with the assistance of the police. Following the administration of the sodium bicarbonate, the QRS complexes eventually narrow to 0.12 mm. However, the patient's level of consciousness does not change. Once in the ambulance, the patient is intubated. The patient's condition remains unchanged during transport to the hospital. On arrival at the hospital, the patient is treated with gastric lavage and activated charcoal and then admitted to the ICU.

DRUGS USED IN THE TREATMENT OF BEHAVIORAL EMERGENCIES 13

OBJECTIVES

After completing this chapter, the reader should be able to:

1. Define the term *behavioral emergency.*
2. List the intrapsychic causes of altered behavior.
3. Explain interpersonal and environmental causes of behavioral emergencies.
4. Explain organic causes of behavioral emergencies.
5. Describe and list the indications, contraindications, and dosages for the following drugs used in behavioral emergencies: haloperidol, droperidol, chlorpromazine, ziprasidone, olanzapine, diazepam, lorazepam, midazolam, and hydroxyzine.

INTRODUCTION

Behavioral emergencies rarely require pharmacological intervention during the prehospital phase of emergency medical care. There are situations, however, in which emergency personnel may be called on to administer a sedative or similar agent. Among these are acute anxiety reactions and paranoid psychoses. Occasionally, it may be necessary to administer a sedative to friends or family of a patient who has been severely injured or who has recently died.

UNDERSTANDING BEHAVIORAL EMERGENCIES

A *behavioral emergency* is an intrapsychic, environmental, situational, or organic alteration that results in behavior that cannot be tolerated by the patient or other members of society. It usually requires immediate attention.

Intrapsychic Causes

Intrapsychic causes of altered behavior arise from problems within the person. Such behavior usually results from an acute stage of an underlying psychiatric condition. A wide range of behaviors can be manifested, including depression, withdrawal, catatonia, violence, suicidal acts, homicidal acts, paranoid reactions, phobias, hysterical conversion, disorientation, and disorganization. In the field, behavioral emergencies resulting from intrapsychic causes are less common than those resulting from other causes, such as alcohol or drug abuse.

Interpersonal and Environmental Causes

Interpersonal and *environmental causes* of behavioral emergencies result from reactions to stimuli outside the person. They often result from overwhelming and stressful incidents, such as the death of a loved one, rape, or a disaster. The change in behavior can frequently be linked to a specific incident or series of incidents. The range of behavior manifested is broad, and a patient's specific symptoms often relate to the type of incident that precipitated them.

Organic Causes

An *organic cause* of altered behavior results from a disturbance in the patient's physical or biochemical state. Such disturbances include drug or substance abuse, alcohol abuse, trauma, medical illness, and dementia. The area of the brain affected by the disturbance determines the type of behavior change.

It is important to consider the possibility of organic disease in *all* behavioral emergencies. As a result, physical assessment of patients with aberrant behavior is extremely important. It may uncover unsuspected causes of the altered behavior, such as drug or alcohol abuse, hypoxia, hypoglycemia, head injury, or meningitis. Common agents used in the acute treatment of behavioral emergencies include haloperidol (Haldol), droperidol (Inapsine), chlorpromazine (Thorazine, Largactil), ziprasidone (Geodon), olanzapine (Zyprexa, Zyprexa Zydis), diazepam (Valium), lorazepam (Ativan), midazolam (Versed), and hydroxyzine (Vistaril, Atarax).

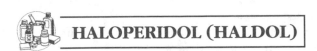

HALOPERIDOL (HALDOL)

Class: Antipsychotic and neuroleptic

Description

Haloperidol is a frequently used major tranquilizer.

Mechanism of Action

Haloperidol is a major tranquilizer of the butyrophenone class that has proved effective in the management of acute psychotic episodes. It has pharmacological properties similar to those of the phenothiazine class of drugs (e.g., Thorazine). Haloperidol appears to block dopamine receptors in the brain associated with mood and behavior. However, its precise mechanism of action is not clearly understood. Haloperidol has weak anticholinergic properties.

Pharmacokinetics

Onset: 30–45 minutes
Peak Effects: 10–20 minutes
Duration: Varies
Half-Life: 3–35 hours

Indication

Haloperidol is used in acute psychotic episodes.

Contraindications

Haloperidol should not be administered in cases in which other drugs, especially sedatives, may be present. It should not be used in the management of dysphoria caused by Talwin because it may promote sedation and anesthesia.

Precautions

Haloperidol may impair mental and physical abilities. Occasionally, orthostatic hypotension may be seen in conjunction with haloperidol use. Caution should be used when administering haloperidol to patients taking anticoagulants. Extrapyramidal or dystonic reactions have been known to occur following the administration of haloperidol, especially in children. Diphenhydramine (Benadryl) should be readily available.

Although haloperidol has not received a "black box" warning from the FDA, paramedics should know that there have been reported adverse cardiovascular efforts, most notably several cases of prolonged QT/QTc and some cases of torsade de pointes. Most, but not all complications, were associated with much higher doses than those used in prehospital care.

Side Effects

Haloperidol can cause extrapyramidal symptoms (EPS), insomnia, restlessness, drowsiness, seizures, respiratory depression, dry mouth, constipation, hypotension, and tachycardia.

Interactions

Antihypertensive medications may increase the likelihood of a patient developing hypotension with haloperidol administration. Haloperidol should be used with caution in patients taking lithium, because irreversible brain damage (encephalopathic syndrome) has been reported when these two drugs are used together.

Dosage

Doses of 2 to 5 mg administered intramuscularly are fairly standard in the management of an acute psychotic episode with severe symptoms. Haloperidol should be given intramuscularly only.

DROPERIDOL (INAPSINE)

Class: Antiemetic and antipsychotic

Description

Droperidol is a butyrophenone derivative that is structurally and pharmacologically related to haloperidol.

Mechanism of Action

Droperidol antagonizes the emetic effects of morphine-like analgesics and other drugs that act on the chemoreceptor trigger zone (CTZ). Its mild alpha-adrenergic blocking properties and direct vasodilation effects may cause hypotension. It acts at the subcortical level to produce sedation and reduce anxiety and minor activities without necessarily inducing sleep.

Pharmacokinetics

Onset: 3–10 minutes
Peak Effects: 30 minutes
Duration: 2–4 hours
Half-Life: 2 hours

Indications

Droperidol is indicated in the treatment of nausea and vomiting in patients refractory to first-line antiemetics. It can be used to produce a tranquilizing effect and as an antipsychotic.

Contraindications

Droperidol is contraindicated in patients with a known hypersensitivity to the drug. Safe usage during pregnancy and in children less than 2 years of age has not been established.

Precautions

Droperidol has received a "black box" warning from the FDA because of reported adverse cardiovascular effects. Most notably, several cases of prolonged QT/QTc intervals and some cases of torsade de pointes have been associated with droperidol administration. Most, but not all complications, were associated with much higher doses than those used in prehospital care.

Droperidol should be used with caution in elderly, debilitated, and other poor-risk patients, including those with Parkinson's disease, hypotension, liver disease, kidney disease, and cardiac disease (including dysrhythmias).

The dosage of droperidol should be decreased in patients who have received other central nervous system (CNS) depressants. Monitor the vital signs and ECG closely. Be aware of possible postural hypotension.

Side Effects

CNS side effects include drowsiness, extrapyramidal symptoms, dystonia, dizziness, restlessness, anxiety, hallucinations, and depression. Cardiovascular side effects reported include hypotension and tachycardia. Other reported side effects include chills, shivering, laryngospasm, and bronchospasm.

Interactions

None reported.

Dosage

Usual dose is 2.5 to 10.0 mg intravenously (IV) or intramuscular (IM).

 ## CHLORPROMAZINE (THORAZINE, LARGACTIL)

Class: Antipsychotic and neuroleptic

Description

Chlorpromazine is an antipsychotic of the phenothiazine type and neuroleptic used in the management of severe psychotic episodes.

Mechanism of Action

Chlorpromazine is a member of the phenothiazine class of drugs. Phenothiazine drugs are thought to block dopamine receptors in the brain that are associated with behavior and mood. Chlorpromazine is also effective in the management of mild alcohol withdrawal and intractable hiccoughs. It is also effective in treating nausea and vomiting, although more appropriate agents are available.

Pharmacokinetics

Onset: 3–5 minutes
Peak Effects: 30–60 minutes
Duration: 4–6 hours
Half-Life: 6 hours

Indications

Chlorpromazine is used in acute psychotic episodes, mild alcohol withdrawal, intractable hiccoughs, and nausea and vomiting.

Contraindications

Chlorpromazine should not be administered to patients in comatose states or who have recently taken a large amount of sedatives. Chlorpromazine should not be administered to patients who may have recently taken hallucinogens because it tends to promote seizures.

Precautions

Chlorpromazine may impair mental and physical abilities. Occasionally, orthostatic hypotension may be seen in conjunction with chlorpromazine use. Extrapyramidal or dystonic reactions have been known to occur following the administration of chlorpromazine, especially in children. Diphenhydramine should be readily available.

Side Effects

Chlorpromazine can cause dry mouth, constipation, blurred vision, dry eyes, sedation, headache, drowsiness, hypotension, and tachycardia.

Interactions

Antihypertensive medications may increase the likelihood of a patient developing hypotension with chlorpromazine administration.

Dosage

The standard dose of chlorpromazine in the management of an acute psychotic episode is 25 to 50 mg administered intramuscularly. Intractable hiccoughs will usually respond to a 25 mg dose of chlorpromazine. Chlorpromazine should only be administered intramuscularly by paramedics.

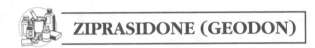

ZIPRASIDONE (GEODON)

Class: Antipsychotic

Description

Ziprasidone is an antipsychotic unrelated to the phenothiazines or butyrophenone classes of antipsychotics. It is known to bind to serotonin, dopamine, histamine, and α_1-adrenergic receptors.

Mechanism of Action

Ziprasidone's mechanism of action is unknown, but is probably related to inhibition of synaptic uptake of serotonin and norepinephrine.

Pharmacokinetics

> **Onset:** Not yet determined for IM route
> **Peak Effects:** Not yet determined for IM route
> **Duration:** Not yet determined for IM route
> **Half-Life:** 7 hours

Indications

Acute psychosis and Tourette's syndrome.

Contraindications

Ziprasidone should not be used in patients with hypersensitivity to the drug. Ziprasidone does not appear to prolong the QT/QTc interval as seen in the butyrophenones. However, it should not be used in patients with a prolonged QT/QTc or history of long QT syndrome.

Precautions

Use with caution in patients with history of seizures, stroke, Alzheimer's disease, or with known cardiovascular disease.

Side Effects

Side effects associated with ziprasidone include myalgias, somnolence, dizziness, tremor, dyskinesia, extrapyramidal effects (dystonia), tachycardia, postural hypotension, nausea, and dry mouth.

Interactions

Carbazepine (Tegretol) may decrease ziprasidone levels. Interactions may occur with antidysrhythmics, antidepressants, and ethanol.

Dosage

Ten to 20 mg IM up to a maximum dose of 40 mg.

OLANZAPINE (ZYPREXA, ZYPREXA ZYDIS)

Class: Antipsychotic

Description

Olanzapine is a rapidly acting oral antipsychotic agent chemically related to clozapine. Zyprexa Zydis is a rapidly dissolving wafer that can be administered orally or placed in a drink.

Mechanism of Action

Olanzapine inhibits synaptic uptake of serotonin and norepinephrine, producing antipsychotic and anticholinergic effects.

Pharmacokinetics

Onset: <30 minutes
Peak Effects: 6 hours
Duration: Varies
Half-Life: 21–54 hours

Indications

Acute psychosis and Alzheimer's disease.

Contraindications

Olanzapine should not be used in patients with hypersensitivity to the drug.

Precautions

Use with caution in patients with a history of cardiovascular disease or conditions that may predispose a patient to hypotension. Do not push orally disintegrating tablet through the blister-pack foil. Peel the foil back and remove the tablet.

Side Effects

Side effects associated with olanzapine include myalgias, somnolence, dizziness, tremor, tachycardia, postural hypotension, nausea, and dry mouth.

Interactions

Olanzapine may enhance the hypotensive effects of antihypertensives.

Dosage

Five to 15 mg PO (via rapidly dissolving tablet). May be placed in a drink. *Never place the tablet in the patient's mouth. Allow them to place it.*

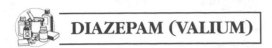

DIAZEPAM (VALIUM)

Class: Sedative, anticonvulsant, and antianxiety agent

Description

Diazepam is a benzodiazepine that is frequently used as a sedative, hypnotic, and anticonvulsant.

Mechanism of Action

Benzodiazepines bind to specific sites on gamma-aminobutyric acid (GABA) Type A receptors within the brain. GABA is the major inhibitory neurotransmitter of the central nervous system. Benzodiazepines have no direct effect on the GABA receptors, but do potentiate the effects of GABA within the brain. Increased GABA levels cause sedation. Through this mechanism, the benzodiazepines display their hypnotic, anxiolytic, and anticonvulsant effects. Their usefulness, however, is limited by a broad range of side effects including compromised sedation, ataxia, amnesia, alcohol and barbiturate potentiation, tolerance development, and abuse potential.

Diazepam, one of the most frequently prescribed medications in the United States, is used in the management of anxiety and stress. It is effective in treating the tremors and anxiety associated with alcohol withdrawal. It is also an effective skeletal muscle relaxant, which makes it an effective adjunct in orthopedic injuries. It is a good premedication for minor operative procedures and cardioversion because it induces amnesia, which diminishes the patient's recall of such procedures. In emergency medicine, diazepam is principally used for its anticonvulsant properties. It suppresses the spread of seizure activity through the motor cortex of the brain. It does not appear to abolish the abnormal discharge focus, however.

Pharmacokinetics

Onset: 1–5 minutes (IV), 15–30 minutes (IM)
Peak Effects: 10 minutes (IV), 30–45 minutes (IM)
Duration: 15–60 minutes
Half-Life: 20–50 hours

Indications

Diazepam is used in acute anxiety states, as a premedication before cardioversion, as a skeletal muscle relaxant, in major motor seizures, and in status epilepticus.

Contraindications

Diazepam should not be administered to any patient with a history of hypersensitivity to the drug.

Precautions

Because diazepam is a relatively short-acting drug, seizure activity may recur. In such cases, an additional dose may be required. Flumazenil (Romazicon), a benzodiazepine antagonist, should be available to use as an antidote if required. Injectable diazepam can cause local venous irritation. To minimize irritation, it should only be injected into relatively large veins and should not be given faster than 1 mL/min.

Side Effects

Diazepam can cause hypotension, tachycardia, drowsiness, headache, amnesia, hallucinations, respiratory depression, blurred vision, nausea, and vomiting.

Interactions

Diazepam is incompatible with many medications. Whenever diazepam is given intravenously in conjunction with other drugs, the IV line should be adequately flushed. The effects of diazepam can be additive when used in conjunction with other CNS depressants and alcohol.

Dosage

In acute anxiety reactions, the standard dosage is 2 to 5 mg administered intramuscularly or intravenously. To induce amnesia prior to cardioversion, a dosage of 5 to 15 mg of diazepam is given intravenously. Peak effects are seen in 5 to 10 minutes. Diazepam should be given intravenously by slow IV push. It can be injected intramuscularly, but absorption via this route is variable. When an IV line cannot be started, parenteral diazepam can be administered rectally with a similar onset of action. In the management of seizures, the usual dose of diazepam is 5 to 10 mg administered IV. In many instances it may be necessary to give diazepam directly into the vein, because the seizure activity will prevent the insertion of an indwelling catheter. When given directly into a vein, it is essential that a large vein, preferably in the antecubital fossa, be used.

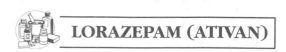

LORAZEPAM (ATIVAN)

Class: Anticonvulsant, sedative, and hypnotic

Description

Lorazepam is a benzodiazepine that is used as an anticonvulsant, sedative, and hypnotic.

Mechanism of Action

Benzodiazepines bind to specific sites on GABA Type A receptors within the brain. GABA is the major inhibitory neurotransmitter of the central nervous system. Benzodiazepines have no direct effect on the GABA receptors, but do potentiate the effects of GABA within the brain. Increased GABA levels cause sedation. Through this mechanism, the benzodiazepines display their hypnotic, anxiolytic, and anticonvulsant effects. Their usefulness, however, is limited by a broad range of side effects including compromised sedation, ataxia, amnesia, alcohol and barbiturate potentiation, tolerance development, and abuse potential.

Lorazepam is a benzodiazepine with a shorter half-life than that of diazepam. Its onset of action is approximately the same. It is used in the management of anxiety and stress. It is a good premedication for minor operative procedures and cardioversion because it induces amnesia, which diminishes the patient's recall of such procedures. Lorazepam is often used in pediatrics as an anticonvulsant because of its shorter half-life. Like diazepam, lorazepam suppresses the spread of seizure activity through the motor cortex of the brain. It does not appear to abolish the abnormal discharge focus.

Pharmacokinetics

Onset: 1–5 minutes (IV), 15–30 minutes (IM)
Peak Effects: 15–20 minutes (IV), 2 hours (IM)
Duration: 6–8 hours
Half-Life: 10–20 hours

Indications

Lorazepam is used in major motor seizures, in status epilepticus, as a premedication before cardioversion, and for acute anxiety states.

Contraindications

Lorazepam should not be administered to any patient with a history of hypersensitivity to the drug.

Precautions

Lorazepam should be diluted with normal saline or D$_5$W prior to intravenous administration. Because lorazepam is a relatively short-acting drug, seizure activity may recur. In such cases, an additional dose may be required. Flumazenil (Romazicon), a benzodiazepine antagonist, should be available to use as antidote if required.

Side Effects

Lorazepam can cause hypotension, drowsiness, headache, amnesia, respiratory depression, blurred vision, nausea, and vomiting.

Interactions

The effects of lorazepam can be additive when used in conjunction with other CNS depressants and alcohol.

Dosage

The usual dose of lorazepam is 0.5 to 2.0 mg when given intravenously. The dose can be increased to 1.0 to 4.0 mg when given intramuscularly.

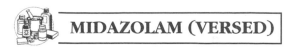

MIDAZOLAM (VERSED)

Class: Sedative and hypnotic

Description

Midazolam is a benzodiazepine with strong hypnotic and amnestic properties.

Mechanism of Action

Benzodiazepines bind to specific sites on GABA Type A receptors within the brain. GABA is the major inhibitory neurotransmitter of the central nervous system. Benzodiazepines have no direct effect on the GABA receptors, but do potentiate the effects of GABA within the brain. Increased GABA levels cause sedation. Through this mechanism, the benzodiazepines display their hypnotic, anxiolytic, and anticonvulsant effects. Their usefulness, however, is limited by a broad range of side effects including compromised sedation, ataxia, amnesia, alcohol and barbiturate potentiation, tolerance development, and abuse potential.

Midazolam is a potent but short-acting benzodiazepine used widely in medicine as a sedative and hypnotic. It is three to four times more potent than diazepam. Its onset of action is approximately 3–5 minutes when administered intravenously and 15 minutes when administered intramuscularly. Midazolam has impressive amnestic properties. Like other benzodiazepines, it has no effect on pain.

Pharmacokinetics

Onset: 3–5 minutes (IV), 15 minutes (IM)
Peak Effects: 20–60 minutes
Duration: <2 hours (IV), 1–6 hours (IM)
Half-Life: 1–4 hours

Indication

Midazolam is used as a premedication before cardioversion and other painful procedures. It is also an effective anticonvulsant.

Contraindications

Midazolam should not be administered to any patient with a history of hypersensitivity to the drug. It should not be used in patients who have narrow-angle glaucoma. Midazolam should not be administered to patients in shock, with depressed vital signs, or who are in alcoholic coma.

Precautions

Emergency resuscitative equipment must be available prior to the administration of midazolam. Vital signs must be continuously monitored during and after drug administration. Midazolam has more potential than the other benzodiazepines to cause respiratory depression and respiratory arrest. Flumazenil (Romazicon), a benzodiazepine antagonist, should be available to use as antidote if required.

Side Effects

Midazolam can cause laryngospasm, bronchospasm, dyspnea, respiratory depression and arrest, drowsiness, amnesia, altered mental status, bradycardia, tachycardia, premature ventricular contractions, and retching.

Interactions

The effects of midazolam can be accentuated by CNS depressants such as narcotics and alcohol.

Dosage

When used for sedation, midazolam must be administered cautiously, because the amount of medication required to achieve sedation varies from individual to individual. Typically, 1 to 2.5 mg are administered by slow IV injection. Usually, it is best to dilute midazolam with normal saline or D_5W prior to IV administration. Midazolam can be administered intramuscularly at a dose of 0.07 to 0.08 mg/kg (average adult dose of 5 mg). Recently, many centers have been administering midazolam intranasally or by mouth to sedate children prior to suturing of lacerations.

 ## HYDROXYZINE (VISTARIL, ATARAX)

Class: Antianxiety agent and sedative

Description

Hydroxyzine is an antianxiety and sedative agent with sedative properties. It is a versatile drug used frequently in emergency medicine.

Mechanism of Action

Hydroxyzine is chemically unrelated to the phenothiazines. Because of its antihistamine properties, hydroxyzine has been shown to exert a calming effect during acute psychotic states. It is an effective antiemetic and muscle relaxant. When administered concurrently with many analgesics, it tends to potentiate their effects.

Pharmacokinetics

Onset: 15–30 minutes
Peak Effects: 1–2 hours
Duration: 4–6 hours
Half-Life: 20 hours

Indications

Hydroxyzine is used to potentiate the effects of narcotics and synthetic narcotics, for nausea and vomiting, and for anxiety reactions.

Contraindications

Hydroxyzine should not be administered to any patient with a history of hypersensitivity to the drug.

Precautions

Hydroxyzine is given by intramuscular injection only. When administered concomitantly with analgesics, the potentiating effects of hydroxyzine should be kept in mind, and the total analgesic dose should be adjusted accordingly.

Side Effects

Hydroxyzine can cause sedation, dizziness, headache, dry mouth, and seizures.

Interactions

The sedative effects of hydroxyzine can be potentiated by CNS depressants such as narcotics, other antihistamines, sedatives, hypnotics, and alcohol.

Dosage

The standard dosage of hydroxyzine in the management of an acute anxiety reaction is 50 to 100 mg administered intramuscularly. The standard antiemetic dose is 25 to 50 mg. Hydroxyzine should be administered by intramuscular injection. Localized burning is a common complaint following an injection of hydroxyzine.

SUMMARY

It is important to consider and rule out physical causes for bizarre behavior before determining that a patient's disorder is of psychiatric origin. Diabetes, head injury, and alcohol intoxication can cause bizarre behavior easily mistaken for psychosis. The psychotic patient is best handled in an emergency department by personnel skilled in psychiatric intervention. However, some patients may require pharmacological intervention before transport is possible.

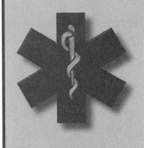

CASE PRESENTATION

Early on a Saturday morning paramedics are dispatched to a local residence to aid a 40-year-old male patient who is acting violently toward his family members. On arrival paramedics are met by the patient's wife and son, who state they were having breakfast when the patient suddenly "snapped." They state that he keeps talking about how everyone is out to get him and that he seems to think that everyone is part of a conspiracy to "frame" him. His wife and son have tried unsuccessfully to calm him down, but he is getting more aggressive toward them with each attempt to talk to him. Just prior to the arrival of the ambulance, he punched his son and told him "they" would have to kill him before he would leave his house. The police are on the way to back the paramedics up. When the police arrive a few minutes later, paramedics approach the patient. He is standing in the kitchen yelling at everyone to get out before he "kills" them.

On Examination

Paramedics are unable to physically assess the patient at this time. A visual survey reveals the following:

CNS: The patient is conscious, able to speak, and appears in good physical health

Resp: His respirations are 28 per minute; no obvious signs of trauma

CVS: His skin is flushed in color

ABD: Unable to assess

Muscl/Skel: No injuries noticed

Vitals Signs

Paramedics are unable to assess the man's vital signs.

Past Hx: Over the past couple of weeks, the patient has had several episodes in which he would start raving about being persecuted by everyone around him. Usually they would only last for several minutes and then he would return to normal without any memory of what had just occurred. This time it has been over 30 minutes. This is the worst episode yet and is the first time he has been physically violent toward his family.

Treatment

The paramedics realize that there are several factors to recognize here. First, the patient is 40 years old and appears to be in good physical health. An attempt to physically restrain him could be dangerous for both the patient and the ambulance crew. Second, there is a history of violence, although paramedics are unsure of the extent of that violence. Medical direction was contacted and gave an order for 5 mg of droperidol (Inapsine) and 2 mg of lorazepam (Ativan) mixed together in the same syringe and then given IM. Advice from the medical director was for the paramedics and police to restrain the patient long enough to give the Inapsine-Ativan mixture and then release the patient and give the medication time to work. The patient was then to be brought to the hospital, with vital signs monitored en route.

A paramedic explained the situation to the police officers, and with a coordinated effort they were able to restrain the patient and give the medications. Ten minutes later the patient had calmed down significantly and was placed on the stretcher and restrained with straps as a precaution. An uneventful trip to the hospital followed. At the hospital he was admitted to the psychiatric service, where he was treated and then released several days later on medications to help prevent further outbursts.

DRUGS USED IN THE TREATMENT OF GASTROINTESTINAL EMERGENCIES

14

After completing this chapter, the reader should be able to:

1. Define the term *antiemetic.*

2. Describe and list the indications, contraindications, and dosages for promethazine, dimenhydrinate, prochlorperazine, metoclopramide, droperidol, and trimethobenzamide.

GASTROINTESTINAL MEDICATIONS

Although many medications are available for use in the treatment of gastrointestinal problems, few are used in prehospital care. The majority of gastrointestinal drugs used in prehospital care are *antiemetics.* These drugs are effective in treating nausea and vomiting. Many of these medications are used concomitantly with narcotics, both to potentiate their effects and to reduce the likelihood of the side effects commonly associated with narcotic usage. Antiemetics commonly used in emergency medicine include promethazine (Phenergan), dimenhydrinate (Gravol, Dramamine), prochlorperazine (Compazine), metoclopramide (Reglan), droperidol (Inapsine), and trimethobenzamide (Tigan).

The major antiemetics include antihistamines, phenothiazines, and serotonin receptor agonists. Antihistamine antiemetics are absorbed well from the gastrointestinal (GI) tract when administered orally.

PROMETHAZINE (PHENERGAN)

Class: Antihistamine and antiemetic

Description

Promethazine is a phenothiazine derivative with potent antihistamine properties and anticholinergic properties.

Mechanism of Action

Promethazine possesses sedative, antihistamine, antiemetic, and anticholinergic properties. It competitively blocks histamine receptors. The duration of action of promethazine is 4 to 6 hours. It is an effective and frequently used antiemetic. Promethazine, unlike hydroxyzine, can be given intravenously. It is often administered with analgesics, particularly narcotics, to potentiate their effect.

Pharmacokinetics

Onset: 5 minutes [intravenously (IV), 20 minutes intramuscularly (IM)]
Peak Effects: Varies
Duration: 4–6 hours
Half-Life: 10–14 hours

Indications

Promethazine is used for nausea and vomiting, motion sickness, and sedation and to potentiate the effects of analgesics.

Contraindications

Promethazine is contraindicated in patients in comatose states and in those who have received a large amount of depressants. Also, it should not be administered to any patient with a history of hypersensitivity to the drug.

Precautions

Promethazine may impair mental and physical abilities. Care must be taken to avoid accidental intra-arterial injection. It should never be administered subcutaneously. Extrapyramidal symptoms (EPS) have been reported following promethazine use. Diphenhydramine (Benadryl) should be available.

Side Effects

Promethazine can cause drowsiness, sedation, blurred vision, tachycardia, bradycardia, and dizziness.

Interactions

The depressant effect on the central nervous system (CNS) of narcotics, sedatives or hypnotics, and alcohol is potentiated by promethazine. An increased incidence of EPS has been reported when promethazine is administered to patients taking monamine oxidase inhibitors (MAOIs).

Dosage

The standard dosage of promethazine in the management of nausea and vomiting is 12.5 to 25 mg administered either intravenously (IV) or intramuscularly (IM). The standard dosage in adjunctive use with analgesics is 25 mg. Promethazine should be given by IV or deep IM injection only. Care must be taken to avoid accidental intra-arterial injection.

 DIMENHYDRINATE (GRAVOL, DRAMAMINE)

Class: Antiemetic

Description

Dimenhydrinate belongs to the antihistamine class of drugs, although it is not commonly used for this action. Its site and action are not precisely known.

Mechanism of Action

The mechanism of action of dimenhydrinate is not precisely known. There is evidence that it acts to depress hyperstimulated labyrinthine functions or associated neural pathways. It is an effective and frequently used antiemetic in Canada. It is often used with analgesics, particularly narcotics.

Pharmacokinetics

Onset: Immediate (IV), 20–30 minutes (IM)
Peak Effects: Varies
Duration: 3–6 hours
Half-Life: Unknown

Indications

Dimenhydrinate is used for the prevention or relief of nausea and vomiting, motion sickness, and drug-induced nausea and vomiting (particularly narcotics).

Contraindications

There are no significant contraindications in the emergency setting.

Precautions

Dimenhydrinate should be used with caution in patients with seizure disorders and asthma. Those who are administered the drug should be cautioned against operating motor vehicles or dangerous machinery because of drowsiness associated with the drug.

Side Effects

Dimenhydrinate can cause drowsiness, dizziness, blurred vision, dry mouth, dry nose and bronchi, and tinnitus.

Interactions

The CNS-depressant effect of narcotics, sedatives or hypnotics, and alcohol is potentiated by dimenhydrinate.

Dosage

The standard dose of dimenhydrinate in the management of nausea and vomiting is 12.5 to 25 mg (diluted) slow IV or 50 to 100 mg IM or by mouth. This dose can be repeated every 4 hours as needed.

 ## PROCHLORPERAZINE (COMPAZINE)

Class: Antiemetic

Description

Prochlorperazine is a phenothiazine derivative. It is highly effective in the treatment of severe nausea and vomiting.

Mechanism of Action

Prochlorperazine is an effective and frequently used antiemetic. It does not prevent vertigo and motion sickness, as do many of the other phenothiazines. Prochlorperazine blocks dopaminergic receptors in the brain. It also has weak anticholinergic properties.

Pharmacokinetics

Onset: 10–20 minutes
Peak Effects: Varies
Duration: 4–12 hours
Half-Life: 24–48 hours

Indications

Prochlorperazine is used in severe nausea and vomiting and acute psychosis.

Contraindications

Prochlorperazine should not be used in patients with a history of hypersensitivity to the drug or the phenothiazine class of medications. It should not be administered to comatose patients or those who have received large amounts of CNS depressants.

Precautions

Prochlorperazine may impair mental and physical abilities. It should never be administered subcutaneously because of local tissue irritation. The incidence of EPS appears to be higher with prochlorperazine than with many of the other phenothiazines. Diphenhydramine (Benadryl) should be available.

Side Effects

Prochlorperazine can cause drowsiness, sedation, blurred vision, tachycardia, bradycardia, dizziness, and hypotension.

Interactions

The CNS-depressant effect of narcotics, sedatives or hypnotics, and alcohol is potentiated by prochlorperazine.

Dosage

The standard dose of prochlorperazine is 5 to 10 mg administered intramuscularly or intravenously. The intravenous route is preferred with severe nausea and vomiting because the onset of action is much more rapid. Often, 10 mg of prochlorperazine is placed into 1 L of normal saline or lactated Ringer's solution and administered.

 METOCLOPRAMIDE (REGLAN)

Class: Antiemetic

Description

Metoclopramide is a medication used in the treatment of gastroesophageal reflux and nausea and vomiting.

Mechanism of Action

Metoclopramide is an effective antiemetic. It stimulates motility of the upper gastrointestinal tract and promotes emptying of the stomach. It increases the tone of the valve between the esophagus and the stomach (lower esophageal sphincter), which reduces reflux of stomach contents into the distal esophagus. Metoclopramide's antiemetic effects appear to result from its blockade of central and peripheral dopamine receptors.

Pharmacokinetics

Onset: 1–3 minutes (IV), 10–15 minutes (IM)
Peak Effects: 1–2 hours
Duration: 1–3 hours
Half-Life: 2.5–6.0 hours

Indications

Metoclopramide is used in severe nausea and vomiting and gastroesophageal reflux.

Contraindications

Metoclopramide should not be used in patients with possible gastrointestinal hemorrhage, bowel obstruction, or perforation. It is also contraindicated in patients with a history of hypersensitivity to the drug.

Precautions

Metoclopramide may impair mental and physical abilities. Mental depression has occurred in patients with and without a prior history of depression following metoclopramide therapy. EPS can occur following metoclopramide administration. Diphenhydramine (Benadryl) should be available.

Side Effects

Metoclopramide can cause drowsiness, fatigue, sedation, dizziness, mental depression, hypertension, hypotension, tachycardia, bradycardia, and diarrhea.

Interactions

The effects of metoclopramide on gastric motility can be antagonized by anticholinergic drugs such as atropine. The CNS-depressant effect of narcotics, sedatives or hypnotics, and alcohol can be potentiated by metoclopramide. Hypertension can result when metoclopramide is administered to patients receiving MAOIs.

Dosage

The standard dose of metoclopramide is 10 to 20 mg administered intramuscularly. Metoclopramide can be administered intravenously for severe or intractable nausea and vomiting. The standard intravenous dose is 10 mg administered by slow IV push over 1 to 2 minutes. Alternatively, 10 mg of metoclopramide can be diluted in 50 mL of normal saline and administered over 15 minutes. The intravenous route is preferred in severe nausea and vomiting because the onset of action is much more rapid.

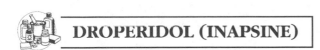

DROPERIDOL (INAPSINE)

Class: Antiemetic and antipsychotic

Description

Droperidol is a butyrophenone derivative that is structurally and pharmacologically related to haloperidol.

Mechanism of Action

Droperidol antagonizes the emetic effects of morphine-like analgesics and other drugs that act on the chemoreceptor trigger zone. Its mild alpha-adrenergic blocking properties and direct vasodilation effects may cause hypotension. It acts at the subcortical level to produce sedation and reduce anxiety and motor activities without necessarily inducing sleep.

Pharmacokinetics

Onset: 3–10 minutes
Peak Effects: 30 minutes
Duration: 2–4 hours
Half-Life: 2 hours

Indications

Droperidol is indicated in the treatment of nausea and vomiting in patients refractory to first-line antiemetics. It can be used to produce a tranquilizing effect and as an antipsychotic.

Contraindications

Droperidol is contraindicated in patients with a known hypersensitivity to the drug. Safe usage during pregnancy and in children less than 2 years of age has not been established.

Precautions

Droperidol has received a "black box" warning from the FDA because of reported adverse cardiovascular effects. Most notably, several cases of prolonged QT/QTc intervals and some cases of torsade de pointes have been associated with droperidol administration. Most, but not all complications, were associated with much higher doses than those used in prehospital care.

    Droperidol should be used with caution in elderly, debilitated, and other poor-risk patients, including those with Parkinson's disease, hypotension, liver disease, kidney disease, and cardiac disease (including dysrhythmias).

    The dosage of droperidol should be decreased in patients who have received other CNS depressants. Monitor the vital signs and ECG closely. Be aware of possible postural hypotension.

Side Effects

CNS side effects include drowsiness, EPS, dystonia, dizziness, restlessness, anxiety, hallucinations, and depression. Cardiovascular side effects reported include hypotension and tachycardia. Other reported side effects include chills, shivering, laryngospasm, and bronchospasm.

Interactions

None reported.

Dosage

Adult dose: 2.5 to 10.0 mg IV or IM.
Pediatric dose: 0.088 to 0.165 mg/kg IV.

 TRIMETHOBENZAMIDE (TIGAN)

Class: Antiemetic

Description

Trimethobenzamide is an antiemetic that does not have the sedative effects of other commonly used antiemetic drugs.

Mechanism of Action

The mechanism of action of trimethobenzamide is unclear. It appears to work on the chemoreceptor trigger zone in the medulla oblongata.

Pharmacokinetics

Onset: 5 minutes (IM)
Peak Effects: 30 minutes (IM)
Duration: 2–3 hours (IM)
Half-Life: 7–9 hours

Indication

Trimethobenzamide is used for severe nausea and vomiting.

Contraindications

The injectable form of trimethobenzamide should not be used in children. Trimethobenzamide should not be administered to patients with a history of hypersensitivity to the drug.

Precautions

The antiemetic effects of trimethobenzamide may render diagnosis more difficult in conditions such as appendicitis. EPS have been reported following administration of trimethobenzamide; however, their incidence appears to be much less than with other antiemetics. Diphenhydramine (Benadryl) should be available. Trimethobenzamide should not be administered intravenously.

Side Effects

Trimethobenzamide can cause blurred vision, diarrhea, dizziness, headache, muscle cramps, and allergic symptoms.

Interactions

The CNS-depressant effects of alcohol may be potentiated by trimethobenzamide.

Dosage

The standard dose of trimethobenzamide is 200 mg administered intramuscularly. Trimethobenzamide should not be administered intravenously.

SUMMARY

Medications are rarely required in the prehospital management of gastrointestinal emergencies. However, many emergency medical services (EMS) systems utilize antiemetics for severe or intractable nausea and vomiting. Prehospital administration of antiemetics decreases the potential for dehydration, improves patient comfort, and reduces exposure of EMS personnel to body fluids. The antiemetics are often used to potentiate the effects of the narcotics. Paramedics are encouraged to be familiar with the antiemetics used in their system.

15

DRUGS USED IN PAIN MANAGEMENT

OBJECTIVES

After completing this chapter, the reader should be able to:

1. Discuss the history of pain management in prehospital care.
2. Explain the characteristics of the ideal analgesic agent for prehospital care.
3. Define the terms *analgesic* and *narcotic.*
4. Describe the analgesics available for use in prehospital care.
5. Describe and list the indications, contraindications, and dosages for the following medications used in pain management: morphine sulfate, meperidine, fentanyl citrate, nitrous oxide, nalbuphine, butorphanol tartrate, and ketorolac.

INTRODUCTION

Emergency medical services (EMS) and the prehospital care of patients have made significant advances during the past decade. The focus of these efforts has been primarily the overall reduction of death and disability in the critically ill or injured patient. However, controversy continues around the extent of prehospital intervention and the influence these efforts have on the outcome of patients. Through these advances, very little attention has been given to the relief of pain and anxiety.

In the early 1970s the focus of prehospital care in the United States and Canada was on the treatment of cardiac arrest and myocardial infarction. Because of the importance of pain relief in the treatment of acute myocardial infarction, a *narcotic* (usually morphine) was included in the treatment protocol for prehospital advanced life support. However, the use of analgesics for pain relief has not been universally accepted beyond their use in myocardial infarction.

Meanwhile, British clinicians took a different view. Baskett introduced the use of a fixed-ratio mixture (50:50) of nitrous oxide and oxygen to the ambulance service in 1969. During the next decade, use of the gas mixture became widespread for both basic and advanced life support systems in Australia, Canada, and the United States.

However, during the past decade there has been a lack of interest in providing adequate pain relief for patients in the prehospital care setting. "In every medical study of analgesia in hospital settings, pain relief in patients was found to be inconsistent, inadequate, and revealing of serious misconceptions or frank ignorance on the part of the physician or nursing staff. Add to this the fact that the uncontrolled prehospital environment argued against the safe administration of any medication, and there is little wonder that relief of pain in patients got a short shrift." And despite the advances made in prehospital care and medical control over the past decade, very little progress has been made in the area of pain relief. "There has been the suggestion (albeit an old chestnut, seemingly resuscitated) that field analgesics will complicate in-hospital management and confuse diagnosis. This attitude, a variation on the old dictum with origins in the 19th and early 20th centuries, appears to have a new lease on life when applied to the prehospital setting. The availability of newer agents given in appropriate doses by appropriate routes should relegate this formerly sound medical truism to the scrap heap of medical myths."[1]

Is the relief of pain in the prehospital setting important? This question can be put to rest by patients who have suffered in agony while trapped in a motor vehicle or by patients with compound fractures who have been bounced around while being moved out of ditches and transported across rural or urban roads. What about the pain experienced by patients with extensive body surface burns? It is not only humanitarian to provide pain relief in prehospital care, but the relief of pain can be of physiological benefit to seriously ill and injured patients.

Perhaps it is time we paid more attention to managing the most common complaint faced in prehospital care today—pain. The ideal analgesic agent for prehospital care has characteristics that are not easily met by one agent. First, the safety of the analgesic must be of prime concern. Second, it must be rapid in onset and short in duration. Rapidity of onset is the function of the route of administration, and that implies the intravenous route. Third, the ease with which an agent is stored and administered is important in prehospital care. For example, the relative bulk and weight of double- or single-tank nitrous oxide–oxygen mixtures have inhibited their frequent use in the prehospital setting. Perhaps, then, the ideal agent has yet to be discovered.

Still, much can be done in the prehospital care setting to relieve pain and anxiety. Basic measures should consist of gentle handling, splinting, and compassionate caring rapport with the patient. Other factors, such as exposure to the cold, may occur during extrication or other prehospital procedures. Exposure may cause shivering and movement of fractures or other painful parts, increasing the patient's discomfort and negating the effect of almost any analgesic agent.

The good news is that pain relief is being reexamined as an important element of prehospital care. This interest is focused not only on agents previously used but also on new drugs and routes of administration. This chapter will prepare paramedics to provide prehospital patients with relief from pain and freedom from fear and anxiety. Many agents appropriate for prehospital care are discussed on the following pages.

---

[1]R. D. Stewart, "Analgesia in the Field," *Prehospital and Disaster Medicine* 4, no. 1 (1989).

Drugs that have proved to be effective in alleviating pain are referred to as *analgesics.* Although they may be administered in many different types of emergencies, they are usually reserved for the treatment of emergencies involving the cardiovascular system, especially myocardial infarction.

As a rule, undiagnosed pain is usually not treated. Early administration of analgesics to these patients may alter physical findings and impair subsequent evaluation by the emergency physician. Some types of pain may be easy to distinguish and are sometimes treated in the prehospital setting. These include chest pain associated with acute myocardial infarction, pain from severe burns, and pain associated with kidney stones.

Analgesics used in prehospital care include the following:

- Morphine sulfate
- Meperidine (Demerol)
- Fentanyl citrate (Sublimaze)
- Nitrous oxide (Nitronox, Entonox)
- Nalbuphine (Nubain)
- Butorphanol tartrate (Stadol)
- Ketorolac (Toradol)

Morphine is derived from the opium plant. It has impressive analgesic and hemodynamic effects. Meperidine, although similar to morphine in its analgesic effects, is considerably different chemically and is synthetically derived. Nalbuphine (Nubain) is also a potent synthetic analgesic. It does not have the hemodynamic effects that morphine does, yet it is often used in emergency medicine because it does not cause respiratory depression and has a low tendency for abuse. Stadol, another of the new breed of synthetic analgesics, is similar to Nubain but is rarely used in treating cardiovascular emergencies. Nitronox, a 50 percent mixture of oxygen and nitrous oxide that can be easily inhaled by the patient, is entirely different from the other analgesic agents discussed. Its analgesic effects are also very potent yet disappear within a few minutes after the cessation of administration. Thus, Nitronox can be given for many types of pain in the field without fear of impairing subsequent physical examination in the emergency department. In addition to its analgesic effects, Nitronox delivers oxygen to the patient, which makes it useful in cardiac emergencies. Ketorolac (Toradol) is the first injectable nonsteroidal anti-inflammatory agent. It is often used in emergency medicine as an analgesic because it does not affect the patient's mental status.

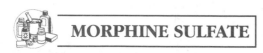 **MORPHINE SULFATE**

Class: Narcotic analgesic

Description

Morphine is a central nervous system (CNS) depressant and a potent analgesic. Although morphine sulfate is one of the most potent analgesics known to humans, it also has hemodynamic properties that make it extremely useful in emergency medicine.

Mechanism of Action

Morphine sulfate is a CNS depressant that acts on opiate receptors in the brain, providing both analgesia and sedation. It increases peripheral venous capacitance and decreases venous return. This effect is sometimes called a chemical phlebotomy. Morphine also decreases myocardial oxygen demand. This action is due to both the decreased systemic vascular resistance and the sedative effects of the drug. Patient apprehension and fear can significantly increase myocardial oxygen demand and in some cases can conceivably increase the size of myocardial infarction. The hemodynamic properties of morphine make it one of the most important drugs used in the treatment of pulmonary edema. Morphine is frequently administered to patients with signs and symptoms of pulmonary edema who are not having chest pain.

Pharmacokinetics

> **Onset:** Immediate [intravenous (IV)], 15–30 minutes [intramuscular (IM)]
> **Peak Effects:** 20 minutes (IV), 30–60 minutes (IM)
> **Duration:** 2–7 hours
> **Half-Life:** 1–7 hours

Indications

Morphine sulfate is used for severe pain associated with myocardial infarction, kidney stones, and so forth and pulmonary edema either with or without associated pain.

Contraindications

Because of the hemodynamic effects described earlier, morphine should not be used in patients who are volume depleted or severely hypotensive. Morphine should not be administered to any patient with a history of hypersensitivity to the drug or to patients with undiagnosed head injury or abdominal pain.

Precautions

Morphine is a narcotic derivative of opium. It has a high tendency for addiction and abuse and is thus covered under the Controlled Substances Act of 1970. It is classified as a Schedule II drug. Consequently, special considerations are involved in the handling of the drug. Many EMS systems have opted to use the synthetic analgesics, such as nalbuphine and pentazocine, instead of morphine and meperidine because of these problems. Morphine causes severe respiratory depression in higher doses. This is especially true in patients who already have some form of respiratory impairment. The narcotic antagonist naloxone (Narcan) should be readily available whenever the drug is administered.

Side Effects

Morphine can cause nausea, vomiting, abdominal cramps, blurred vision, constricted pupils, altered mental status, headache, and respiratory depression.

Interactions

The CNS depression associated with morphine can be enhanced when administered with antihistamines, antiemetics, sedatives, hypnotics, barbiturates, and alcohol.

Dosage

There are many different approaches to the administration of morphine. An initial dose in the range of 2 to 10 mg administered intravenously is standard. This dose can be augmented with additional doses of 2 mg every few minutes and can be continued until the pain is relieved or until signs of respiratory depression occur.

Intramuscular injection usually requires 5 to 15 mg, based on the patient's weight, to attain desired effects. However, morphine is routinely given intravenously in emergency medicine and is often administered with an antiemetic agent such as promethazine (Phenergan). These agents help prevent the nausea and vomiting that often accompany morphine administration. The antiemetics also tend to potentiate morphine's effects. Morphine can also be given intramuscularly and subcutaneously.

MEPERIDINE (DEMEROL)

Class: Narcotic analgesic

Description

Meperidine is a CNS depressant and a potent analgesic. It is used extensively in medicine in the treatment of moderate to severe pain. It is less potent than morphine sulfate; 60 to 80 mg of meperidine are roughly equivalent in action to 10 mg of morphine.

Mechanism of Action

Meperidine is a CNS depressant that acts on opiate receptors in the brain, providing both analgesia and sedation. It does not have the same hemodynamic properties as morphine but has the same tendency for physical dependence and abuse. Because it causes respiratory depression, naloxone should be available whenever meperidine is administered. The rate of onset is slightly faster than morphine, yet its effects are much shorter in duration. Like morphine, meperidine is a Schedule II drug regulated under the Controlled Substances Act of 1970.

Pharmacokinetics

Onset: 5 minutes (IV), 10 minutes (IM)
Peak Effects: 1 hour
Duration: 2 hours (IV), 2–4 hours (IM)
Half-Life: 3–5 hours

Indication

Meperidine is used for moderate to severe pain.

Contraindications

Meperidine should not be administered to patients with known hypersensitivity to the drug. In addition, it should not be administered to patients with undiagnosed abdominal pain or head injury, or to patients who are receiving, or who have recently received, monoamine oxidase inhibitors (e.g., Nardil, Parnate, and Eutron). Therapeutic doses of meperidine have occasionally caused severe, and sometimes fatal, reactions in patients receiving these agents.

Precautions

Meperidine can cause respiratory depression. Naloxone (Narcan) should always be available to reverse the effects of the drug if respiratory depression ensues. Like morphine, meperidine should be kept in a secure, locked box.

Side Effects

Meperidine can cause nausea, vomiting, abdominal cramps, blurred vision, constricted pupils, altered mental status, hallucinations, headache, and respiratory depression.

Interactions

Meperidine should not be administered to patients who are receiving, or who have recently received, monoamine oxidase inhibitors (e.g., Nardil, Parnate, and Eutron). These agents are used for certain types of depression and behavioral disorders. Therapeutic doses of meperidine have occasionally caused severe, and sometimes fatal, reactions in patients receiving these agents.

Dosage

The usual dose used in the treatment of severe pain is 25 to 50 mg administered intravenously. When administered intramuscularly, 50 to 100 mg is a standard dose. Meperidine is often administered with an antiemetic agent such as promethazine (Phenergan). These agents help prevent the nausea and vomiting that often accompany meperidine administration. Meperidine can be administered either intravenously or intramuscularly.

FENTANYL CITRATE (SUBLIMAZE)

Class: Narcotic analgesic

Description

Fentanyl, although chemically unrelated to morphine, produces pharmacological effects and a degree of analgesia similar to those of morphine. On a weight basis, however, fentanyl is 50 to 100 times more potent than morphine, but its duration of action is shorter than that of meperidine or morphine. A parenteral dose of 100 μg of fentanyl is approximately equivalent in analgesic activity to 10 mg of morphine or 75 mg of meperidine.

Mechanism of Action

The principal actions of therapeutic value are analgesic and sedative. Fentanyl is a narcotic analgesic with a rapid onset and a short duration of action. Alterations in respiratory rate and alveolar ventilation, associated with narcotic analgesics, may last longer than the analgesic effect. Large doses may produce apnea. Fentanyl appears to have less emetic activity than other narcotic analgesics.

Pharmacokinetics

Onset: Immediate
Peak Effects: 3–5 minutes (IV)
Duration: 30–60 minutes
Half-Life: 6–8 hours

Indications

Fentanyl is used for maintenance of analgesia, as an adjunct in rapid-sequence induction intubation, and for severe pain.

Contraindications

Contraindications include severe hemorrhage, shock, and known hypersensitivity.

Precautions

Vital signs should be monitored routinely. Fentanyl may produce bradycardia, which may be treated with atropine. However, fentanyl should be used with caution in patients with cardiac bradydysrhythmias.

Fentanyl should be administered with caution to patients with liver and kidney dysfunction because of the importance of these organs in the metabolism and excretion of drugs. As with other CNS depressants, patients who have received fentanyl should have appropriate surveillance. Resuscitation equipment and a narcotic agonist such as naloxone should be readily available to manage apnea.

Side Effects

As with other narcotic analgesics, the most common serious reactions reported to occur with fentanyl are respiratory depression, apnea, muscle rigidity, and bradycardia. If these side effects remain untreated, respiratory arrest, circulatory depression, or cardiac arrest could occur.

Interactions

Other drugs with a depressant effect on the CNS (e.g., barbiturates, tranquilizers, narcotics, and general anesthetics) have an additive or potentiating effect with fentanyl. When patients have received such drugs, the dose of fentanyl required is less than usual. Likewise, following the administration of fentanyl, the dose of other CNS-depressant drugs should be reduced. Severe and unpredictable potentiation by monoamine oxidase inhibitors (MAOIs) has been reported with narcotic analgesics. Because the safety of fentanyl in this regard has not been established, its use in patients who have received MAOIs within 14 days is not recommended.

Dosage

Adult dosages are IV, 25 to 100 μg (0.025 to 0.1 mg); direct IV, slowly over at least 1 minute, preferably over 2 to 3 minutes (not necessary to dilute—may be diluted to facilitate administration); and 100 μg/2 mL diluted in 3 mL of normal saline for a concentration of 20 μg/mL.

Pediatric dosages are 1.7 to 3.3 μg/kg for children 2 to 12 years of age; the dosage should be reduced in very young, elderly, and poor-risk patients.

NITROUS OXIDE (NITRONOX, ENTONOX)

Class: Analgesic and anesthetic gas

Description

Nitronox is a blended mixture of 50 percent nitrous and 50 percent oxygen that has potent analgesic effects.

Mechanism of Action

Nitrous oxide is a CNS depressant with analgesic properties. In the prehospital setting it is delivered in a fixed mixture of 50 percent nitrous oxide and 50 percent oxygen. When inhaled, it has potent analgesic effects. These quickly dissipate, however, within 2 to 5 minutes after cessation of administration. The Nitronox unit consists of one oxygen and one nitrous oxide cylinder. The gases are fed into a blender that combines them at the appropriate concentration. The mixture is then delivered to a modified demand valve for administration to the patient. Nitronox must be self-administered. It is effective in treating many varieties of pain encountered in the prehospital setting, including pain from many types of trauma. The high concentration of oxygen delivered along with the nitrous oxide will increase the oxygen tension in the blood, thus reducing hypoxia.

Pharmacokinetics

Onset: 2–5 minutes
Peak Effects: 2–5 minutes
Duration: 2–5 minutes
Half-Life: Unknown

Indications

Nitrous oxide is used for pain of musculoskeletal origin, particularly fractures; burns; suspected ischemic chest pain; and states of severe anxiety, including hyperventilation.

Contraindications

Nitronox should not be used in any patient who cannot comprehend verbal instructions or who is intoxicated with alcohol or other drugs. It should not be administered to any patient with a head injury who exhibits an altered mental status. Nitronox should not be administered to any patient with chronic obstructive pulmonary disease (COPD) because the high concentration of oxygen (50 percent) might result in respiratory depression. Nitrous oxide tends to diffuse into closed spaces more readily than either carbon dioxide or oxygen. Many COPD patients have air-containing blebs in their lungs, and nitrous oxide can concentrate in these blebs, causing them to swell. Swollen blebs may rupture, causing a pneumothorax. Nitronox should not be administered to patients with a thoracic injury suspicious of pneumothorax, because the gas may accumulate in the pneumothorax, increasing its size. Also, patients with severe abdominal pain and distension suggestive of bowel obstruction should not receive Nitronox. Nitrous oxide can concentrate in pockets of an obstructed bowel, possibly leading to rupture.

Precautions

Nitronox should only be used in areas that are well ventilated. When the gas is used in the patient compartment of an ambulance, a scavenging system should be in place. Nitrous oxide exists in a liquid state inside the gas cylinder. Heat present in the air, in the cylinder wall, or in the various regulators and lines causes the liquid to vaporize. This vaporization process makes the cylinder tank and lines cool to touch. Following prolonged use, frost may develop on the cylinder, regulator, or lines. In very cold environments, generally less than 21°F (6°C), the liquid may be slow to vaporize, and administration may be impossible.

Side Effects

A nitrous oxide–oxygen mixture can cause dizziness, light-headedness, altered mental status, hallucinations, nausea, and vomiting.

Interactions

Nitrous oxide can potentiate the effects of other CNS depressants such as narcotics, sedatives, hypnotics, and alcohol.

Dosage

Nitronox should only be self-administered. Continuous administration may take place until the pain is significantly relieved or until the patient drops the mask. The patient care record should document the duration of drug administration.

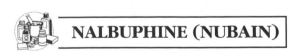

NALBUPHINE (NUBAIN)

Class: Synthetic analgesic

Description

Nalbuphine is a synthetic analgesic agent with a potency equivalent to morphine on a milligram-to-milligram basis.

Mechanism of Action

Like the narcotics, nalbuphine is a centrally acting analgesic that binds to the opiate receptors in the central nervous system. Its onset of action is considerably faster than that of morphine, occurring within 2 to 3 minutes after intravenous administration. Its duration of effect is reported to be 3 to 6 hours. Although nalbuphine causes some respiratory depression in doses up to 10 mg, these effects do not seem to get worse in doses that exceed 10 mg. Naloxone (Narcan) is an effective antagonist and should be available when nalbuphine is administered.

In addition to its effects on opiate receptors, nalbuphine has antagonistic effects similar to those of naloxone. This feature minimizes the abuse potential of the drug and appears to lessen the chances of significant respiratory depression. At this time, nalbuphine is not regulated under the Controlled Substances Act of 1970. Current studies show that it has a minimal tendency for physical dependence and abuse. This property has made nalbuphine increasingly popular in prehospital care. However, recent studies have shown nalbuphine to be somewhat unpredictable in terms of analgesia with many authorities discouraging its use in the prehospital setting.

Pharmacokinetics

Onset: 2–3 minutes (IV), 15 minutes (IM)
Peak Effects: 30 minutes
Duration: 3–6 hours
Half-Life: 5 hours

Indication

Nalbuphine is used for moderate to severe pain.

Contraindications

Nalbuphine should not be administered to patients with head injury or undiagnosed abdominal pain.

Precautions

The primary precaution in using nalbuphine is in patients with impaired respiratory function. Small doses of nalbuphine may cause significant respiratory depression. Naloxone should be readily available. Nalbuphine also has narcotic antagonistic properties. Thus, it should be administered with caution to patients dependent on narcotics, because it may cause withdrawal effects. The dosage of nalbuphine should be reduced in older patients because the effects are less predictable in this age group. Small repeated boluses are often safer than a single large dose.

Side Effects

Nalbuphine can cause headache, altered mental status, hypotension, bradycardia, blurred vision, rash, respiratory depression, nausea, and vomiting.

Interactions

Nalbuphine can potentiate the CNS depression associated with narcotics, sedatives, hypnotics, and alcohol. Because of its antagonistic properties, nalbuphine can cause withdrawal symptoms in patients addicted to narcotics. Nalbuphine can interfere with certain types of anesthesia (nitrous and narcotic techniques) because of its antagonistic properties.

Dosage

The general regimen for nalbuphine administration is 5 mg intravenously initially. This dose may be augmented with additional 2 mg doses if necessary. Nalbuphine is often administered with an antiemetic agent such as promethazine (Phenergan). These agents help prevent the nausea and vomiting that often accompany nalbuphine administration. Nalbuphine can be administered intravenously or intramuscularly.

BUTORPHANOL TARTRATE (STADOL)

Class: Synthetic analgesic

Description

Butorphanol is a synthetic analgesic used frequently in emergency medicine. It is quite potent; the analgesic effects of 2 mg of butorphanol are roughly equivalent to 10 mg of morphine.

Mechanism of Action

Butorphanol is a centrally acting analgesic that binds to the opiate receptors in the central nervous system, causing CNS depression and analgesia. Like nalbuphine, it has some antagonistic (naloxone-like) properties. Although butorphanol can cause respiratory depression, this effect usually plateaus following administration of approximately 4 mg. Currently, butorphanol is not restricted under the 1970 act. Thus it is quite attractive for use in the prehospital phase of emergency medical care.

Pharmacokinetics

Onset: 10–15 minutes (IM), 2–3 minutes (IV)
Peak Effects: 0.5–1.0 hour (IM), 4–5 minutes (IV)
Duration: 3–4 hours
Half-Life: 3–4 hours

Indication

Butorphanol is used for moderate to severe pain.

Contraindications

Butorphanol should not be administered to any patient with a history of hypersensitivity to the drug. Also, it should not be given to patients dependent on narcotics because it may cause some reversal of the narcotic effects. It should not be administered to patients with head injury or undiagnosed abdominal pain.

Precautions

If butorphanol causes marked respiratory depression, then Narcan can be administered to reverse its effects. When administering any potent analgesic, it is possible to mask other signs and symptoms. All analgesics should be administered only after a thorough physical examination. Butorphanol should not be administered to any patient with head injury because it may cause an increase in cerebrospinal pressure. The dosage of nalbuphine should be reduced in older patients because the effects are less predictable in this age group. Small repeated boluses are often safer than a single large dose.

Side Effects

Butorphanol can cause headache, altered mental status, hypotension, bradycardia, blurred vision, rash, respiratory depression, nausea, and vomiting.

Interactions

Like nalbuphine, butorphanol has some narcotic antagonistic properties. Caution should be used when administering butorphanol to patients already dependent on narcotics because it may precipitate withdrawal.

Dosage

The standard dose of butorphanol is 1 mg administered intravenously every 3 to 4 hours. When given intramuscularly, the standard dose is 2 mg. Butorphanol should only be administered intravenously or intramuscularly.

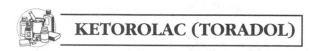

KETOROLAC (TORADOL)

Class: Nonsteroidal anti-inflammatory agent

Description

Ketorolac is the first injectable nonsteroidal anti-inflammatory drug to become available in the United States. It is useful in treating mild to moderate pain.

Mechanism of Action

Ketorolac is a nonsteroidal anti-inflammatory drug (NSAID). It has analgesic, anti-inflammatory, and antipyretic effects. Unlike narcotics, which act on the central nervous system, ketorolac is considered a peripherally acting analgesic. Consequently, it does not have the sedative properties of the narcotics. Ketorolac has been used concomitantly with morphine and meperidine without adverse effects. In dental studies, ketorolac was found to be quite effective as an analgesic.

Pharmacokinetics

> **Onset:**   30 minutes
> **Peak Effects:**   45–60 minutes
> **Duration:**   Varies
> **Half-Life:**   4–6 hours

Indication

Ketorolac is used for mild to moderate pain.

Contraindications

Ketorolac should not be used in patients with a known hypersensitivity to the drug. It should not be administered to patients who report allergies to aspirin or NSAIDs, or to patients currently taking aspirin or NSAIDs.

Precautions

Gastrointestinal (GI) irritation and hemorrhage can result from therapy with NSAIDs. Long-term usage increases the incidence of serious GI side effects. Ketorolac is cleared through the kidneys. Long-term usage can result in renal impairment.

Side Effects

Ketorolac can cause edema, hypertension, rash, itching, nausea, heartburn, constipation, diarrhea, drowsiness, and dizziness.

Interactions

Ketorolac, when administered with other NSAIDs (including aspirin), can worsen the side effects associated with the use of drugs in this class. Intramuscular ketorolac has been found to reduce the diuretic response to furosemide (Lasix).

Dosage

The typical dose of ketorolac is 30 to 60 mg administered intramuscularly. Half the original dose can be repeated every 6 hours. Ketorolac is approved for IV use by the U.S. Food and Drug Administration (FDA); many emergency departments use ketorolac intravenously to obtain more prompt analgesia. The typical intravenous dose is 30 mg. Some practitioners use 60 mg intravenously. Few adverse reactions have been reported with intravenous ketorolac.

SUMMARY

Paramedics can reliably manage most patients who complain of pain. With their expanded understanding of pain medications, oversight by medical direction, and use of critical thinking skills, paramedics are ready to relieve the pain many patients suffer.

KEY WORDS

analgesic. A drug used in the relief of pain.

narcotic. A substance that works on the central nervous system to decrease or relieve the sensation of pain. Narcotic pain killers (analgesics) are made from opium or made artificially.

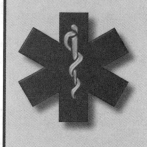

CASE PRESENTATION

At 1430 hours paramedics are called to a football field to help a 16-year-old male who has injured his leg playing football. En route the dispatcher tells the paramedics that the 16-year-old male is conscious and breathing and has a possible fracture of his left leg. On arrival paramedics are directed to the center of the field, where a group of players and coaches are standing. They find their patient lying on the ground with an obviously deformed left ankle. He is wearing football equipment, and first-aid providers have already removed the patient's shoes, socks, and helmet. The patient states that he was running with the ball when he stepped in a small hole in the field. He felt a "pop" in his ankle and then extreme pain. He states he attempted to get up but was unable to because of the pain.

On Examination

CNS:	The patient is conscious, alert, and oriented × 4; in extreme pain
Resp:	Respirations are 24; trachea is midline; no signs of trauma; lung sounds are clear bilaterally
CVS:	Carotid and radial pulses are present and strong; skin is pink and warm
ABD:	Soft and nontender
Extremities:	Arms and right leg intact with good pulses, sensation, and strength; left leg is deformed at the ankle, with the left foot rotated externally; distal pulse is palpable in left foot, although it is cooler to touch than the right foot

Vital Signs

Pulse:	96/min, regular, strong
Resp:	24/min, shallow
BP:	122/80 mmHg
SpO$_2$:	99 percent
ECG:	Regular sinus rhythm
Hx:	The patient is not taking any medications, has no known allergies, and states he is a healthy person.

Treatment

Paramedics examine the patient thoroughly and determine that because of the mechanism of the injury the patient does not need to be spinal immobilized. His left ankle is severely angulated, with obvious external rotation. His left foot is cool to touch but has a strong pulse and is pink in color. During attempts to splint the ankle the patient screams in pain, and therefore paramedics decide to give an analgesic prior to completion of the splinting to make it more bearable for the patient. An IV is initiated using an 18-gauge catheter in the right forearm. The IV of normal saline is run TKVO. Paramedics give the patient 5 mg of morphine IV over 2 minutes as per standing order. The paramedics immobilize the ankle in a pillow splint. The patient is moved to the ambulance. The patient is still in considerable pain, and another 5.0 mg of morphine is administered. The patient's vital signs, especially respirations and blood pressure, are closely monitored. En route to the hospital the patient starts to complain about feeling nauseated and is therefore given 25 mg of dimenhydrinate (Gravol) IV. The rest of the trip to the hospital is uneventful. On arrival at the hospital, the patient is assessed and treated for a severe dislocation fracture of his left ankle.

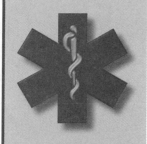

CASE PRESENTATION

At 1900 hours on a fall evening, paramedics are called to the high school football stadium to aid a football player who has injured his shoulder. On arrival they are directed to the sidelines, where the coaches are attending to a player. The player is not wearing shoulder pads and is slouched to his right side.

On Examination

CNS:	The patient is conscious, alert, and oriented × 4; in moderate pain
Resp:	Respirations are 24; trachea is midline
CVS:	Carotid and radial pulses are present; skin is warm and dry
ABD:	Soft and nontender
Extremities:	Dislocation of right shoulder

Vital Signs

Pulse:	88/min, regular
Resp:	18/min, shallow
BP:	118/72 mmHg
SpO$_2$:	96 percent

Hx: The patient is not taking any medications, has no known allergies, and states he is a healthy person. The coaches tell the paramedics that the football player is the team quarterback. He was sacked on a play and landed heavily on his shoulder.

Treatment

On assessment paramedics find that the shoulder is dislocated anteriorly. They give the patient nitrous oxide to self-administer. After several minutes of breathing the nitrous oxide, the patient states that the pain is not as intense. Paramedics sling and swathe the arm and shoulder and move the patient to the ambulance. Once in the unit, they administer 75 mg of meperidine IM in the left deltoid. The combination of nitrous oxide and meperidine give the patient almost total pain relief. The transport to the hospital is uneventful.

16

WEAPONS OF MASS DESTRUCTION

OBJECTIVES

After completing this chapter, the reader should be able to:

1. Define the terms *weapons of mass destruction* and *NBC agent*.
2. Understand the importance of using personal protective equipment during WMD incidents.
3. Describe the common NBC agents and their prehospital treatments: blistering agents, irritant gases, nerve agents, cyanide, viruses, toxins, bacteria, and nuclear agents.

INTRODUCTION

Our world changed on September 11, 2001. The reality of the terrorist attacks against the United States on that day was graphically brought into our living rooms through our television sets. Many witnessed the attacks first hand. These attacks involved careful planning and were specifically designed to target civilians—something that, until that date, had never been witnessed in U.S. history.

Terrorists have clearly indicated their ability and desire to utilize nontraditional weapons in their attacks. They have even embraced a heretofore rare form of terrorism called *homicide bombing.* In homicide bombings, terrorists hide high-power explosives on their bodies or in their cars and detonate these when they are most apt to injure a large number of people—usually civilians. As terrorists resort to nontraditional weapons, the task of protecting a nation and a people becomes more and more difficult.

Emergency medical services (EMS) personnel, by the nature of the work, are on the front line of defense and will play a major role in any future terrorist attacks. Because of this, EMS personnel must be familiar with what has come to be known as *weapons of mass destruction (WMD).* These include *nuclear, biological, and chemical (NBC) agents* that can be introduced through various mechanisms. NBC agents, depending on the particular agent involved, can enter the body through the skin or be ingested, inhaled, or introduced via a vector or weapon. As a general rule, *personal protective equipment (PPE)* can be used to prevent entry of these agents. Many of these agents are known and antidotes and treatment are available.

In this chapter, we address the issue of WMD from a prehospital pharmacological standpoint. The field of WMD is diverse and complicated and it is not possible to discuss it comprehensively within the scope of this book. Instead, we concentrate on common pharmacological agents EMS personnel may be called on to administer (or take) in the event of a terrorist attack.

PERSONAL PROTECTION

Your personal safety and that of your team should always be your main priority when responding to a possible WMD incident. Because of the nature of NBC agents, it is essential that EMS personnel use personal protective equipment (PPE) to minimize the risk of exposure and subsequent illness or death. PPE may involve specialized suits, gloves, boots, and breathing apparatus. It is essential that you understand the suspected WMD agent you are dealing with in order to take the necessary precautions. Always refer to local guidelines and recommendations regarding the use and level of PPE. It is paramount that all personnel who might be called on to respond to a WMD incident be trained in the appropriate protective measures and response. Remember, you cannot help others if you become a victim!

NBC AGENTS OVERVIEW

Many types of NBC agents are available. Many are similar in their effects and actions. In this section, we detail common NBC agents and address emergent prehospital treatment.

Chemical Agents

Chemical agents used in WMD affect people in different ways. The blistering agents cause damage to the skin, eyes, and mucous membranes. The irritants cause pulmonary destruction, ultimately leading to pulmonary edema, hypoxia, and death. The nerve agents affect the autonomic and voluntary nervous systems, causing increased parasympathetic symptoms and ultimately flaccid paralysis. Cyanide profoundly and adversely affects the cellular use of oxygen, resulting in cellular hypoxia and rapid death. These agents are all easily delivered through both conventional and nonconventional weapons.

Blistering Agents

Blistering agents, also called *vesicants,* have been the mainstays of chemical warfare until international treaties banned their use. They are still used by certain rogue nations and pose a threat as WMDs. It is essential that responding personnel wear appropriate respiratory protection when irritant gases are suspected. The three common blistering agents are discussed next.

Mustard

There are no immediate signs of mustard exposure. However, some 4 to 8 hours later, redness of the skin may appear. In addition there may be reddening of the conjunctiva of the eye and associated eye itching and pain. The eyes will often feel gritty. The patient may also exhibit upper respiratory symptoms such as sinus pain, cough, and scratchy throat. Eventually, small fluid-filled blisters (vesicles) will appear. However, no mustard is actually in the blister fluid. Mustard eventually causes cell death.

There is no specific antidote for mustard poisoning. The only initial action is to decontaminate the victim as soon as possible. Decontamination of the mustard gas victim after 5 minutes will not prevent the development of toxic effects, but will protect others from cross-contamination.

Lewisite

The lewisite vapor causes immediate burning and pain in the eyes and exposed mucous membranes. The skin will exhibit a grayish color reflective of tissue destruction within minutes after contact with lewisite. Later, severe damage of the skin, eyes, and airway may appear. Lewisite causes leakage from systemic capillaries resulting in hypovolemia and, ultimately, hypotension.

EMS personnel must be ready to provide airway assistance. Decontamination should be performed as soon as possible. There is an antidote for lewisite called British Anti-lewisite (BAL). If administered early in care, it may decrease some of the internal damage, but will not help skin, airway, or eye damage. Skin lesions from irritant agents should be treated as you would treat a thermal burn with Silvadene or Neosporin. Artificial tears and topical ophthalmic antibiotics may help with eye involvement. Airway involvement may lead to laryngeal edema. EMS personnel should have a low threshold for intubating the patient and providing mechanical ventilation.

Phosgene Oxime

Phosgene oxime and lewisite are similar in their effects. Like lewisite, phosgene causes immediate effects. The vapor causes immediate burning and pain in the eyes and exposed mucous membranes. The skin will exhibit a grayish color reflective of tissue destruction within minutes after contact with phosgene. Later, severe damage of the skin, eyes, and airway may appear.

Decontamination should be performed as soon as possible. There is no antidote for phosgene. Calamine lotion may be applied to the skin. Artificial tears and topical ophthalmic antibiotics may help with eye involvement. Airway involvement may lead to laryngeal edema. EMS personnel should have a low threshold for intubating the patient and providing mechanical ventilation.

Irritant Gases

Irritant gases primarily affect the respiratory system. They include ammonia, chlorine, and phosgene (a different agent than phosgene oxime). There is usually associated eye irritation. Ammonia and chlorine can cause pulmonary edema with high-level exposures—usually taking 2 to 24 hours to develop. These agents physically damage the membranes of the lung, causing fluid to enter the interstitial space and ultimately leading to pulmonary edema. The patient eventually becomes hypoxic. The first symptom is usually shortness of breath which becomes progressively worse.

It is important to remove the victim from the source and administer high-flow, high-concentration oxygen. Mechanical ventilation should be provided as needed. There are no specific antidotes. It is important to remember that pulmonary edema caused by these agents is noncardiac in origin and diuretics may be of limited use. Supplemental oxygen and inhaled bronchodilators are useful. Riot control agents can cause many of the same effects as irritant gases and sometimes it is hard to distinguish between the two.

Nerve Agents

Nerve agents are potent chemicals that profoundly affect the nervous system. They include tabun, sarin, soman, and the organophosphate pesticides. Sarin was used as a WMD in an attack on the subways of Tokyo. Rogue nations have been reportedly stockpiling these agents. Nerve agents are much stronger than—but similar to—many commercial insecticides used in agriculture.

The effects of nerve agents appear almost immediately. Nerve agents, present as both a vapor and a liquid, are capable of being absorbed through the skin or inhaled and absorbed through the respiratory tract. Exposure leads to a series of signs and symptoms. The mnemonic *SLUDGE* can be used to remember these: *S*alivation, *L*acrimation, *U*rination, *D*efecation, and *G*astric *E*mptying. People will begin to exhibit pupillary constriction (miosis). Many will have a runny nose (rhinorrhea) and most will complain of some shortness of breath.

These agents block the activity of the enzyme acetylcholinesterase. Acetylcholinesterase is responsible for breaking down the neurotransmitter acetylcholine in the autonomic nervous system and in the neuromuscular junction. Thus, you have unopposed acetylcholine effects. This causes the patient to exhibit symptoms of parasympathetic stimulation. These result from the direct effects on the parasympathetic nervous system (miosis, increased intestinal contractions) and from stimulation of glands innervated by the parasympathetic nervous system (increased salivation, increased acid secretion in the stomach, runny nose, tearing, and sweating). Likewise, the skeletal muscles will be affected. Initially, there will be some twitching, which will lead to muscle fasciculations. This may lead to seizures or complete motor paralysis. The amount and route of exposure can cause varying symptoms:

- *Mild symptoms* of nerve agent poisoning include miosis, rhinorrhea, shortness of breath, chest tightness, sweating, and muscle fasciculations.

- *Moderate symptoms* include wheezing, profuse airway secretions, respiratory distress, muscle weakness, vomiting, and diarrhea.

- *Severe symptoms* include unconsciousness, seizures, flaccid paralysis, cyanosis, and apnea.

The sooner the onset of symptoms, the more severe the exposure. It is important to remember that, with exposure to liquid nerve agents, the onset of symptoms may be delayed for up to 18 hours. Delay of symptoms is also seen with ingestion of these agents such as might occur when insecticides are used during a suicide attempt.

Treatment of nerve agent poisoning involves the administration of specific antidotes. The antidotes are atropine sulfate and pralidoxime (2-PAM). These are often supplied in a kit referred to as a Mark I kit (Figure 16–1). The Mark I kit contains 2 mg of atropine and 600 mg of 2-PAM in spring-driven

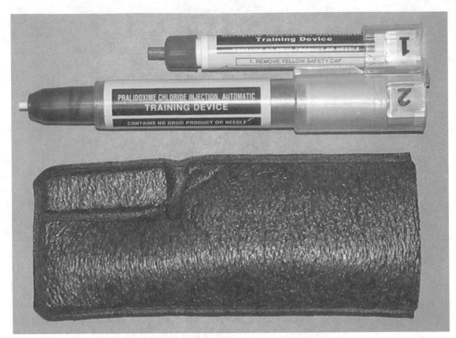

FIGURE 16–1   Mark I Autoinjector.

autoinjectors. Atropine helps to block the effects of acetylcholine at the neuromuscular junction and in the synapses of the autonomic nervous system by binding to acetylcholine receptors. This is a temporary benefit. It is important to remember that larger than usual doses of atropine are usually required for nerve agent poisoning. 2-PAM serves to reactivate the acetylcholinesterase by competitively binding with the nerve agent and releasing the nerve agent from the acetylcholinesterase molecule, thus allowing acetylcholinesterase to again function. If the patient is symptomatic with moderate symptoms, they should be administered one or two Mark I kits and receive additional doses every 5 minutes until ventilatory status improves. For severe exposures, start with two to three Mark I kits and consider the addition of diazepam for seizure prophylaxis. Pediatric patients will require less medication because of their size. Atropine should be dosed at 0.5 mg intramuscularly (IM) for children younger than 2 years of age. Children 2 to 10 years of age should receive 1 mg IM, and children older than 10 years of age should receive 2 mg IM. 2-PAM is given at 15 mg/kg intravenously (IV) to children weighing less than 20 kg. Those weighing more than 20 kg can receive the 600 mg IM adult dose.

Cyanide

Cyanide is a product of many chemical processes and occurs naturally in some foods. It is also produced by combustion when certain items are burned. The two general forms of cyanide are hydrogen cyanide and cyanogen chloride.

Cyanide can enter the body through the respiratory tract, by ingestion, or through the skin. It is rapidly distributed by the blood. Once in the body, the toxin directly poisons the respiratory mechanism of the cells. This leads to cellular hypoxia and, ultimately, death.

Cyanide inactivates an enzyme called *cytochrome* a_3. This enzyme is an important part of cellular respiration and deactivation of the enzyme

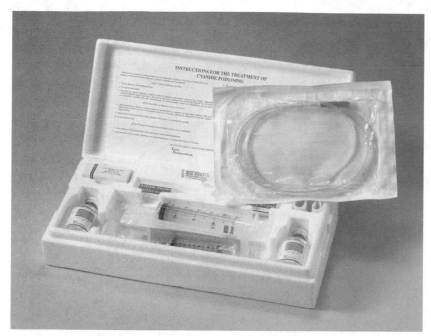

FIGURE 16–2 Cyanide antidote kit.

leads to cellular hypoxia. The administration of supplemental oxygen cannot overcome this problem.

Following exposure, the victim will begin to demonstrate symptoms in 15 to 30 seconds. Initially, the respiratory rate will increase. Later, dizziness, weakness, anxiety, and nausea will occur. Ultimately, the patient will lose consciousness and stop breathing. This progression of events is quite rapid. In fact, many victims of cyanide poisoning die before help reaches them. Occasionally, rescuers have reported the smell of bitter almonds in cyanide victims.

Treatment includes maintenance of the airway and respirations and administration of an antidote. All cyanide exposure victims should receive high-flow, high-concentration oxygen and mechanical ventilation, if required. Antidotal therapy should be provided as soon as possible and involves the administration of a nitrite and a thiosulfate. The nitrite causes the iron in hemoglobin to change to a form called methemoglobin. Methemoglobin has a high affinity for cyanide and can actually remove cyanide off the *cytochrome a₃* enzyme and out of the cells. Once removed, it must be detoxified with sodium thiosulfate where it is excreted by the kidneys. Methemoglobin will gradually return to normal hemoglobin through natural biochemical processes.

The antidotes for cyanide are typically supplied in what is called the Pasadena Cyanide Antidote kit (Figure 16–2). It contains amyl nitrite, sodium nitrite, and sodium thiosulfate. Amyl nitrite is supplied in ampules for inhalation. It can be immediately administered by inhalation or with a bag-valve-mask unit while IV access is obtained. Once IV access is obtained, sodium nitrite can be administered intravenously. Half the original dose can be repeated in 30 minutes as needed. Finally, following nitrite therapy, sodium thiosulfate can be administered intravenously to detoxify and remove the cyanide. The key to successful treatment is early recognition and prompt treatment with the antidotes. The antidotes are much less effective when given individually as compared to giving them in the sequence described.

Biological Agents

Biological agents include those derived from viruses, bacteria, fungi, and other species. In some cases, the biological agent itself is responsible for infection. In others, toxins produced by the bacteria are responsible. The following are common biological agents that can be used as WMD agents.

Viruses

Smallpox

Smallpox is caused by the variola virus. It was declared eradicated from the earth by the World Health Organization in 1980. Two research labs were allowed to keep strains of the variola virus: the Centers for Disease Control and Prevention in Atlanta, Georgia, and the Vector Center in Koltsovo, Russia. Following the fall of the Soviet Union it became uncertain whether all vials of the bacteria at Vector were accounted for. In addition, concerns have been raised that clandestine stockpiles of the virus might remain even though all stocks were supposed to have been destroyed by 1999. Its lethality and ease of transmission make smallpox an attractive WMD agent.

A vaccine for smallpox is available and vaccination against smallpox was routine. However, once the disease was eradicated, vaccine administration stopped. The incubation period for smallpox is approximately 12 days. The signs and symptoms of infection include malaise, fever, chills (rigors), vomiting, headache, and backache. Some patients will develop a delirium. Approximately 2 to 3 days after the onset of symptoms, a rash develops on the face, hands, and forearms, and then spreads to the trunk. The lesions then form red spots and ultimately pustules. The pustules will later scab over.

Prevention of smallpox is by a vaccine, which is administered by forming a scar that lasts 3 to 10 years. Booster doses are administered as needed. Specific therapy for those infected is vaccinia immune globulin, which is most effective when administered within 24 hours of exposure.

Ebola

Ebola virus is one of the deadliest viruses known and causes hemorrhagic fever. It causes death in 50 to 90 percent of all infected patients. It is transmitted through direct contact with the blood, urine, stool, semen, or organs of infected persons. Inhalation transmission has been reported. The incubation period is 2 to 21 days. Hemorrhagic fever usually begins with a sudden onset of fever, weakness, muscle pain, headache, and sore throat. Later, the patient will develop nausea, vomiting, diarrhea, and rash. Organ failure (renal and hepatic) usually begins secondary to internal and external bleeding. The hemorrhagic symptoms usually begin on the fifth day. Ebola is a prime candidate for an agent in a WMD. No vaccines are available, nor is antiviral therapy available. Treatment consists of isolation and supportive care.

Marburg

The Marburg virus is closely related to the ebola virus. It was first identified following an outbreak of hemorrhagic fever in Germany after importation of African green monkeys. The symptoms are similar to ebola. The mortality rate is approximately 25 percent. Marburg can be aerosolized, thus making it an attractive weapon. No vaccine or treatment is available.

Toxins

Botulism

Botulinum toxin, one of the most lethal compounds known to man, is produced by the bacteria *Clostridium botulinum*. Members of the *Clostridium* species are spore formers. Spores are special reproductive cells produced by certain bacteria. In daily medical practice, botulism most commonly results from improperly canned or undercooked foods that contain the bacteria. The bacteria themselves are harmless. But the toxin they produce, although not contagious, is extremely toxic. Without prophylaxis or treatment, victims stand little chance of survival.

There are seven or more types of botulinum toxin. The toxin affects the neuromuscular junction much like a neuromuscular blocker. The first symptoms develop within 1 to 12 hours of exposure and include drooping of the eyelids, dry mouth, difficulty swallowing, difficulty talking, blurred vision, and double vision. The paralysis then moves downward from the face to the throat, chest, abdomen, and extremities. Ultimately, the muscles of respiration will be fully paralyzed and asphyxial death results.

Treatment consists of ventilatory assistance and the administration of an antitoxin. The antitoxin (trivalent botulinum antitoxin) should be administered as soon as possible once botulism is suspected. If treatment is not promptly administered, the paralysis will set in and may take several months for function to return. A vaccine is now available for many of the botulinum types.

Ricin

Ricin is a toxin derived from the processing of castor beans (*Ricinus communis*). It is easy to produce and stable. Ricin can be ingested, injected, or delivered as a toxic cloud (inhalation). Symptoms begin approximately 3 hours after inhaling ricin and include coughing, chest tightness, fever, dyspnea, nausea, and muscle aches. Symptoms following ingestion include nausea, vomiting, internal bleeding, liver failure, and, ultimately, multiple organ failure. If injected, ricin causes death of muscles and lymph nodes near the injection site. This can lead to organ failure and death.

No vaccine or antitoxin is available for ricin. Treatment is supportive. Fluid replacement is paramount. If ingested, lavage with activated charcoal may be beneficial.

Bacteria

Tularemia

Tularemia, also known as *rabbit fever* or *deer fly fever*, is caused by the bacteria *Francisella tularensis*. The bacteria are highly infective. In fact, a single bacterium has the potential to infect a human. It is contracted through inhalation and open wounds resulting in two forms: ulceroglandular tularemia and inhalational tularemia.

Ulceroglandular tularemia is usually contracted under natural conditions through inoculation by contact with the skin or mucous membranes of an infected animal or from the bites of infected deer flies, mosquitoes, and ticks. This results in the formation of an ulcer at the site of inoculation. Later, lymph nodes proximal to the ulcer become swollen and tender. The patient will usually develop fever and malaise.

Inhalational tularemia is characterized by the sudden onset of chills, fever, headache, muscle aches, fatigue, cough, and loss of body fluids. The incubation period is 1 to 21 days with 3 days being average. The illness can last up to 3 weeks. The mortality rate is approximately 30 percent.

A vaccine is available. Tularemia is treated with doxycycline, ciprofloxacin, gentamycin, or streptomycin.

Anthrax

Anthrax is caused by the bacterium *Bacillus anthracis.* Although rare in humans, this organism is often seen in veterinary practice. This bacterium produces specialized reproductive cells known as spores. Bacterial spores have thick walls and are able to withstand varying temperatures, humidity, and other unfavorable conditions. In fact, anthrax spores can survive in sunlight for several days and steam heat up to 318°F and can remain viable in soil or water for years. The anthrax bacteria (or its spores) can enter the body through inhalation, ingestion, or through breaks in the skin. The incubation period for anthrax is typically 1 to 6 days (although longer incubation periods have been documented). Anthrax cannot be spread person to person. A vaccine for anthrax is available

Anthrax can affect the skin, lungs, or gastrointestinal tract. When anthrax is limited to the skin, it is referred to as *cutaneous anthrax.* This form is usually contracted from tissues of infected animals (sheep, goats, cattle). Cutaneous anthrax can be treated with antibiotics including penicillin, doxycycline and ciprofloxacin (Cipro). Treatment usually last for at least 60 days because spores can take that long to germinate.

Inhalation anthrax, while more common in cattle, results from deposition of the bacterial spores in the lungs. This results in fever and fatigue (flu-like symptoms) within 1 to 7 days after exposure. This is often followed by a slight improvement. Then, there is an abrupt onset of respiratory distress (cough, dyspnea, tachycardia), shock and eventually death. The fatality rate for untreated inhalation anthrax is greater than 90 percent. Ciprofloxacin (Cipro) is the antibiotic of choice. It is given intravenously for 14 days and orally for at least 60 days. Persons possibly exposed to anthrax should be immediately started on antibiotic therapy and remain on it until tests have excluded or confirmed infection.

Intestinal anthrax has been reported and causes abdominal distress, vomiting, and, in some cases, bloody diarrhea. It takes a large spore load to cause intestinal anthrax, but the infection can lead to septicemia and death.

Plague

Plague, also referred to as the *black death,* killed millions of people in the pre-antibiotic area and still poses a threat as a WMD. Plague is cased by *Yersinia pestis* bacterium, which is not a spore former. The two types of plague infections are bubonic plague and pneumonic plague.

Bubonic plague is the most common and is transmitted from rodents to humans by the bite of an infected flea. The infection spreads through the lymphatic system, causing swollen lymph nodes in the groin (known as *buboes*). The infection can invade the bloodstream, causing septicemia.

Pneumonic plague can result from septicemia or inhalation of the organism. The bacteria spread rapidly in the lungs, causing a hemorrhagic pneumonia. This feature makes plague an attractive agent for biological warfare. Untreated pneumonic plague is usually fatal. The incubation period is 2 to 10 days. The patient with plague is highly infectious! The illness usually lasts 1 to 2 days. Symptoms include malaise, high fever, tender lymph nodes, skin lesions, chills, headaches, bloody sputum, pneumonia, circulatory failure, and death.

Persons exposed to plague should be treated with doxycycline or ciprofloxacin (Cipro). No vaccine is available. Pneumonic plague can be treated successfully if antibiotics are started within 24 hours of the onset of symptoms. Antibiotics used in pneumonic plague include streptomycin, doxycycline, chloramphenicol, and ciprofloxacin.

Brucellosis

Brucellosis, also known as *undulant fever*, is caused by bacteria in the *Brucella* species (*Brucella suis, Brucella melitensis, Brucella abortus*). The Brucella species is not a spore former. The infection is spread via inhalation. The incubation period is 5 to 21 days, but can occasionally take up to 2 months. Brucellosis tends to cause incapacitation rather than death in most cases. Initially the patient will develop flu-like symptoms (fever, chills, headache, loss of appetite, mental depression, extreme fatigue, aching joints, sweating, nausea, and vomiting). Brucellosis is treated with the antibiotics doxycycline and rifampin. Treatment is usually for a minimum of 6 weeks. The relapse rate is high.

Patients infected with smallpox, plague, and ebola are contagious. The key to exposure prevention is the use of appropriate PPE, which is used in EMS every day to control the spread of bloodborne pathogens.

Nuclear Agents

Nuclear agents are substances that emit ionizing radiation, which is harmful to all living creatures. These agents can be delivered though the use of nuclear weapons or through detonation of conventional weapons that disperse radioactive materials ("dirty" bombs). Exposure can occur in three ways. Persons can become contaminated, irradiated, or materials can be incorporated into the body. With contamination, radioactive materials get onto the body or clothing. Removal is accomplished through thorough decontamination and clothing removal. It is important to remember that exposure to radiation is reduced by (1) limiting the time of exposure, (2) increasing the distance from the source, and (3) shielding personnel from the source.

Irradiation

Nuclear radiation cannot be felt, seen, or otherwise detected by any of our senses. However, it damages the cells of the human body as it passes through them. Radiation passage changes the structure of molecules and essential elements of the cell. Damaged cells then go on to repair themselves, die, or to produce altered or damaged cells (cancer). As the intensity and duration of exposure increases, so do the degree and extent of cell damage and the risk to life.

Symptoms of radiation poisoning can vary, but include nausea, vomiting, severe burns, fatigue, and then death. Persons exposed to radiation should be decontaminated as soon as possible following accepted procedures. Patients with internal radiation exposure (ingestion or inhalation) are at increased risk for developing hypothyroidism or thyroid cancer. For persons with high levels of exposure, the early administration of stable potassium iodine (KI) will block thyroid uptake of radioiodine (90 percent blockage if KI is administered within 1 hour of exposure and 50 percent blockage if KI administered within 6 hours of exposure). KI administration should be continued for 1 to 2 weeks postexposure.

SUMMARY

EMTs and paramedics must be familiar with common WMDs. In dealing with a possible WMD attack, it is important to remain calm, put on personal protective equipment, and stay upwind and uphill until the scene has been deemed safe to approach. Always use the Incident Command System or Incident Management System as appropriate. When the agent is identified, apply treatment per local protocol. EMS personnel may be in particular demand when antidote administration is required. Therefore, EMS personnel must be familiar with the common WMD antidotes and treatments. Regardless, your personal safety and that of your crew should always be your first priority.

KEY WORDS

antidote. A remedy for counteracting a poison.

spore. An oval body, formed within certain species of bacteria. It is regarded as a resting phase during the life cycle of the cell and is extremely resistant to environmental factors.

vesicant. A blistering drug or agent.

GLOSSARY OF STREET DRUG NAMES

CENTRAL NERVOUS SYSTEM STIMULANTS[1]

A
Amp
Bam
Batu (methcathinone)
Beans (MDMA)
Benies
Bennie (Benzidrine)
Black and white
Black beauties
Black birds
Blue angels
Blue beauties
Bombido (injectable amphetamine)
Bombita (Spanish-speaking community)
Candy
Cartwheels
Cat (methcathinone)
Chalk
Chicken powder
Chocolate
Chris
Christine
Christmas eve

Christmas trees
Christy (smokable meth)
Coast to coast
Coke (cocaine)
Copilot
Crack (cocaine)
Crank
Crink
Cris
Crisscross
Crissroads
Croak (method and crack)
Crystal (methamphetamine)
Dexies
Disco pellets
Dominoes
Double cross
Eye openers
Fire (meth and crack)
Flake (cocaine)
Footballs
Glass
Go-fast
Gold dust (cocaine)
Granulated orange

Green and clears
Greenies
Hanyak
Head drugs
Hearts
Hiropon (smokable methamphetamine or methcathinone)
Ice
Inbetweens
Jam
Jelly baby
Jolly baby
Jugs
Kaksonjae
LA (long-acting amphetamines)
LA glass (smokable LA)
LA turnarounds
Leapers
Lid poppers
Lid proppers
Little bomb
Max (dissolved gamma hydroxy buterate mixed with amphetamine)

---

[1]A form of amphetamine unless otherwise stated.

Meth
Mexican crack
Minibennie
Nugget
Oranges
Peaches
Pep pills
Pink and green
Pinks
Quartz
Rippers

Rock (cocaine)
Rosa (Spanish-speaking community)
Roses
Shabu (methcathinone)
Snap
Snow (cocaine)
Speed
Speedball (heroin plus cocaine)
Toot
Truck drivers

Turnarounds
Uppers
Ups
Wake-ups
Whiffledust
Whites
X
XTC
Yellow jackets

PHENCYCLIDINE (PCP)

A Beam me up Scotty (PCP and crack)
Ace
Ad
Amoeba
Angel dust
Animal tranquilizer
Aurora
Black acid (PCP and LSD)
Bush
Bust bee
Cheap cocaine
Cosmos
Criptal
Devil's dust
Dipper
DOA
Domex (PCP and ecstasy)
Dummy mist

El Diablito (for combination of PCP, marijuana, cocaine, and heroin in Spanish-speaking community)
Frios (marijuana laced with PCP in Spanish-speaking community)
Goon
Green
Guerrilla
Hog
Jet
K
Kools (marijuana laced with PCP)
Lemon 714
Lovely
Magic dust
Mauve
Mist

Monkey tranquilizers
Mumm dust
Niebla (Spanish-speaking community)
Octane (PCP laced with gasoline)
Ozone
Peace pill
Purple
Rocket fuel
Shermans
Sherms
Special LA coke
Superacid
Supercoke
Supergrass
Superjoint
Trangs
Tranq[2]
Wack

HEROIN

Black tar
Brown
Chinese white
H
H and stuff

Horse
Junk
Mexican mud
Scat
Shit

Skag
Smack
Snow
Stuff
Tango and Cash

---

[2]Many drugs have the same name.

OTHER ANALGESICS

Black (opium)
Blue velvet (paregoric plus
    amphetamine)
Dollies (methadone)
M (morphine)

Microdots (morphine)
PG or PO (paregoric)
Pinks and grays
    (propoxyphene
    hydrochloride)

Poppy (opium)
Tar (opium)
Terp (terpin hydrate or cough
    syrup with codeine)

CENTRAL NERVOUS SYSTEM DEPRESSANTS[3]

Blue birds
Blue devil
Blue heaven
Blues
Bullets
Dolls
Double trouble
Downs
Goofballs

Green and whites
    (chlordiazepoxide)
Greenies
Ludes
Nembies
Peanuts
Peter (chloral hydrate)
Rainbows
Red Devils

Roaches (chlordiaepoxide)[2]
Seccy
Seggy
T-birds
Toolies
Tranqs[2]
Wallbangers
Yellow jackets
Yellows

HALLUCINOGENS

Acid (LSD)
Blue dots (LSD)
Cactus (mescaline)
Crystal[2]

Cube (LSD)
D (LSD)
Mesc (mescaline)
Mexico mushroom (psilocybin)

Owsleys (LSD)
Pearly gates (morning glory
    seeds)

CANNABINOLS

Acapulco gold
Bhang
Brick
Charas
Colombian
Gage
Ganja
Grass
Hash
Hay
Hemp

J
Jane
Jive
Joint
Key or Kee
Lid
Locoweed
Mary Jane
Mexican
MJ
Muggles

Pot
Reefer
Roach[2]
Rope
Sativa
Stick
Sweet Lucy
Tea
Texas tea
Weed
Yesca

---

[2]Many drugs have the same name.
[3]Moderate length of action, like secobarbital, unless otherwise noted.

SOLVENTS AND INHALANTS

Air blast
Ames
Amies
Aroma of men
Bang
Boopers
Bullet
Buzz bomb
Climax

Honey oil
Huff
Huffing
Jac aroma
Kicks
Laughing gas (nitrous oxide)
Locker room (isobutyl nitrate)
Medusa
Moon gas

Oz
Pearls (amyl nitrite)
Poppers (isobutyl or amyl nitrate)
Poppers (isobutyl or amyl nitrite)
Rush
Snappers
Sniffers
Whiteout

INHALANTS

Air blast
Ames
Amies
Amys
Aroma of men
Bang
Boppers
Bullet

Buzz bomb
Climax
Honey oil
Huff
Laughing gas (nitrous oxide)
Locker room (isobutyl nitrate)
Medusa
Moon gas

Oz
Pearls (amyl nitrite)
Poor man's pot
Poppers (isobutyl or amyl nitrate)
Whiteout

STREET DRUG LINGO

Abe's cape: $5 bill

Agonies: withdrawal symptoms

All star: user of many types of drugs

Amped out: fatigue after using methamphetamine

Baby habit: occasional user of drugs

Bad go: bad reaction to a drug

Bagging: using inhalants

Batt: hypodermic needle

Bedbugs: fellow addicts

Bender: drug party

Bone: $50 piece of crack

Boulder: $20 worth of crack

Cooker: one who manufactures methamphetamine

Deck: 1 to 15 g of heroin

Demo: sample size of crack

Deuce: $2 worth of drug

Eight ball: 1/8 ounce of any type of drug

Gluey: one who sniffs or inhales glue

Huffer: one who uses inhalants

Hype: an addict, most frequently refers to IV drug users

Lid: 1 ounce of marijuana

Meth head: regular meth user

Meth monster: one who gets a violent reaction to methamphetamine

Rolling: Getting high on Ecstasy

Snot: residue left after smoking amphetamines

Snotball: rubber cement rolled into balls and burned so the fumes can be inhaled

Speed freak: regular meth user

Spike: hypodermic needle

EMERGENCY INTRAVENOUS FLUIDS QUICK REFERENCE GUIDE

✳ Plasma Protein Fraction (Plasmanate)

Class	Protein colloid
Action	Plasma volume expander
Indication	Hypovolemic states (especially burn shock)
Contraindication	None when used in the management of life-threatening situations
Precautions	Hypertension
	Short shelf life
Side Effect	Edema
Dosage	Dosage should be titrated according to patient's hemodynamic response; follow accepted resuscitation formulas in the management of burn shock
	Adult: 250–500 mL (12.5–25 g protein) not to exceed 10 mL/min
Route	IV infusion
Pediatric Dosage	10–30 mL/kg at 5–10 mL/min

✳ Dextran

Class	Imitation protein (sugar) colloid
Action	Plasma volume expander
Indication	Hypovolemic shock
Contraindication	Patients with known hypersensitivity to the drug
	Patients receiving anticoagulants

Precautions	Severe anaphylactic reactions have been known to occur
	Monitor for circulatory overload
	Can impede accurate blood typing because dextran molecule coats the erythrocytes; draw tube of blood for blood typing before administering dextran
Side Effects	Nausea
	Vomiting
Dosage	Dosage should be titrated according to patient's hemodynamic response
	500 mL over 15–30 minutes
Route	IV infusion
Pediatric Dosage	Same as adult

✳ Hetastarch (Hespan)

Class	Artificial colloid
Action	Plasma volume expander
Indication	Hypovolemic states
Contraindication	Patients receiving anticoagulants
Precautions	Monitor for circulatory overload
	Large volumes of hetastarch may alter the coagulation mechanism
Side Effects	Nausea
	Vomiting
Dosage	Dosage should be titrated according to patient's hemodynamic response
	500–1000 mL, not to exceed 20 mL/kg/hr; total dose not to exceed 1500 mL in 24 hours
Route	IV infusion
Pediatric Dosage	Safety in children has not been established

✳ Polygeline (Haemaccel)

Class	Artificial colloid
Action	Plasma volume expander
Indication	Hypovolemic states
Contraindication	Patients with known hypersensitivity to the drug
Precautions	Allergic reactions (rare)
Side Effects	Urticaria, tachycardia, bradycardia, dyspnea
Dosage	Dosage should be titrated according to patient's hemodynamic response
Route	IV
Pediatric Dosage	Dosage should be titrated according to the patient's hemodynamic response

Lactated Ringer's Solution

Class	Isotonic crystalloid
Action	Approximates the electrolyte concentration of the blood
Indication	Hypovolemic shock
Contraindications	Congestive heart failure
	Renal failure
Precaution	Monitor for circulatory overload
Side Effects	Rare
Dosage	*Hypovolemic shock (systolic less than 90 mmHg):* Infuse "wide open" until a systolic of 100 mmHg is attained; once a systolic of 100 mmHg has been attained, infusion should be slowed to 100 mL/hr
	Other: As indicated by the patient's condition and situation being treated
Route	IV infusion
Pediatric Dosage	20 mL/kg repeated as required based on hemodynamic response

5 Percent Dextrose in Water (D_5W)

Class	Sugar solution
Action	Glucose nutrient solution
Indications	IV access for emergency drugs
	For dilution of concentrated drugs for IV infusion
Contraindication	Should not be used as a fluid replacement for hypovolemic states
Precautions	Monitor for circulatory overload
	Draw tube of blood before administering to diabetics
Side Effects	Rare
Dosage	Generally administered TKO
Route	IV infusion
Pediatric Dosage	Same as adult

10 Percent Dextrose in Water ($D_{10}W$)

Class	Hypertonic sugar solution
Action	Replaces blood glucose
Indications	Hypoglycemia
	Neonatal resuscitation
	Rarely used as an IV infusion; rather, as a bolus dose as needed

Contraindication	Should not be used as fluid replacement for hypovolemic states
Precautions	Monitor for circulatory overload
	Draw tube of blood before administering $D_{10}W$ to diabetics
Side Effects	Rare
Dosage	Dependent on patient's condition and condition being treated
Route	IV infusion
Pediatric Dosage	<3 months of age, 2–6 mL/kg IV/IO

✳ 0.9 Percent Sodium Chloride (Normal Saline)

Class	Isotonic electrolyte
Action	Fluid and sodium replacement
Indications	Heat-related problems (heat exhaustion and heat stroke)
	Freshwater drowning
	Hypovolemia
	Diabetic ketoacidosis
Contraindication	Congestive heart failure
Precaution	Electrolyte depletion (K^+, Mg^{2+}, Ca^{2+}, among others) can occur following administration of large amounts of normal saline
Side Effect	Thirst
Dosage	Dependent on patient's condition and situation being treated; in freshwater drowning and heat emergencies, the administration is usually rapid
Route	IV infusion
Pediatric Dosage	Dose is dependent on patient's size and condition

✳ 0.45 Percent Sodium Chloride (One-Half Normal Saline)

Class	Hypotonic electrolyte
Action	Slow rehydration
Indications	Patients with diminished renal or cardiovascular function for which rapid rehydration is not indicated
Contraindications	Cases in which rapid rehydration is indicated
Precaution	Electrolyte depletion can occur following administration of large amounts of one-half normal saline
Side Effects	Rare
Dosage	Dependent on patient's condition and situation being treated
Route	IV infusion
Pediatric Dosage	Dose is based on patient's size and condition

✳ 5 Percent Dextrose in 0.9 Percent Sodium Chloride (D₅NS)

Class	Hypertonic sugar and electrolyte solution
Action	Provides electrolyte and sugar replacement
Indications	Heat-related disorders
	Freshwater drowning
	Hypovolemia
	Peritonitis
Contraindications	Should not be administered to patients with impaired renal or cardiovascular function
Precaution	Draw tube of blood before administering to diabetics
Side Effects	Rare
Dosage	Dependent on patient's condition and situation being treated
Route	IV infusion
Pediatric Dosage	Dose is dependent on patient's size and condition

✳ 5 Percent Dextrose in 0.45 Percent Sodium Chloride (D₅1/2NS)

Class	Slightly hypertonic sugar and electrolyte solution
Action	Provides electrolyte and sugar replacement
Indications	Heat exhaustion
	Diabetic disorders
	For use as a TKO solution in patients with impaired renal or cardiovascular function
Contraindications	Situations in which rapid fluid replacement is indicated
Precaution	Draw tube of blood before administering to diabetics
Side Effects	Rare
Dosage	Dependent on patient's condition and situation being treated
Route	IV infusion
Pediatric Dosage	Dose is dependent on patient's size and condition

✳ 5 Percent Dextrose in Lactated Ringer's Solution (D₅LR)

Class	Hypertonic sugar and electrolyte solution
Action	Provides electrolyte and sugar replacement
Indications	Hypovolemic shock
	Hemorrhagic shock
	Certain cases of acidosis
Contraindications	Should not be administered to patients with decreased renal or cardiovascular function
Precautions	Monitor for signs of circulatory overload
	Draw tube of blood before administering to diabetics
Side Effects	Rare

Dosage	Dependent on patient's condition and situation be- ing treated
Route	IV infusion
Pediatric Dosage	Dose is dependent on patient's size and condition

✳ Pediatric Fluid Resuscitation

Bolus #1	20 mL normal saline or lactated Ringer's solution
Bolus #2	20 mL normal saline or lactated Ringer's solution
Bolus #3	10 mL/kg of colloid or blood

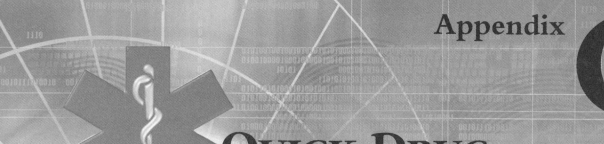

QUICK DRUG REFERENCE

INTRODUCTION

This appendix provides a quick reference to the most commonly used emergency medications. The dosages and indications have been taken from the most recent Advanced Cardiac Life Support (ACLS) standards of the American Heart Association. Drugs not covered in ACLS are taken from the American Medical Association's *Drug Evaluation*. It is important to remember that specific drugs, dosages, indications, and routes may vary by area. It is essential that paramedics be familiar with these variations and follow the guidelines established by the medical director of the system in which they work.

 Activated Charcoal

Class	Adsorbent
Action	Adsorbs toxins by chemical binding and prevents gastrointestinal adsorption
Indication	Poisoning following emesis or when emesis is contraindicated
Contraindications	None in severe poisoning
Precautions	Should only be administered following emesis in cases in which it is so indicated
	Use with caution in patients with altered mental status
	May absorb ipecac before emesis; if ipecac is administered, wait at least 10 minutes to administer activated charcoal
Side Effects	Nausea and vomiting
	Constipation
Dosage	1 g/kg (typically 50–75 g) mixed with a glass of water to form a slurry

Route	Oral
Pediatric Dosage	1 g/kg mixed with a glass of water to form a slurry

✳ Adenosine (Adenocard)

Class	Antidysrhythmic
Action	Slows atrioventricular conduction
Indication	Symptomatic PSVT
Contraindications	Second- or third-degree heart block
	Sick-sinus syndrome
	Known hypersensitivity to the drug
Precautions	Dysrhythmias, including blocks, are common at the time of cardioversion
	Use with caution in patients with asthma
Side Effects	Facial flushing
	Headache
	Shortness of breath
	Dizziness
	Nausea
Dosage	6 mg given as a rapid intravenous (IV) bolus over a 1- to 2-second period; if, after 1–2 minutes, cardioversion does not occur, administer a 12 mg dose over 1–2 seconds
Route	IV; should be administered directly into a vein or into the medication administration port closest to the patient and followed by flushing of the line with IV fluid
Pediatric Dosage	Safety in children has not been established

✳ Albuterol (Proventil)

Class	Sympathomimetic (β_2 selective)
Action	Bronchodilation
Indications	Asthma
	Reversible bronchospasm associated with chronic obstructive pulmonary disease
Contraindications	Known hypersensitivity to the drug
	Symptomatic tachycardia
Precautions	Blood pressure, pulse, and electrocardiogram (ECG) results should be monitored
	Use caution in patients with known heart disease
Side Effects	Palpitations
	Anxiety
	Headache
	Dizziness
	Sweating

Dosage	*Metered-dose inhaler:* One to two sprays (90 μg per spray)
	Small-volume nebulizer: 0.5 mL (2.5 mg) in 2.5 mL normal saline over 5–15 minutes
	Rotohaler: One 200 μg Rotocap should be placed in the inhaler and breathed by the patient
Route	Inhalation
Pediatric Dosage	0.15 mg/kg (0.03 mL/kg) in 2.5 mL normal saline by small-volume nebulizer

✳ Aminophylline

Class	Xanthine bronchodilator
Actions	Smooth muscle relaxant
	Causes bronchodilation
	Has mild diuretic properties
	Increases heart rate
Indications	Bronchial asthma
	Reversible bronchospasm associated with chronic bronchitis and emphysema
	Congestive heart failure
	Pulmonary edema
Contraindications	Patients with history of hypersensitivity to the drug
	Hypotension
	Patients with peptic ulcer disease
Precautions	Monitor for dysrhythmias
	Monitor blood pressure
	Do not administer to patients on chronic theophylline preparations until the theophylline blood level has been determined
Side Effects	Convulsions
	Tremor
	Anxiety
	Dizziness
	Vomiting
	Palpitations
	PVCs
	Tachycardia
Dosages	*Method 1:* 250–500 mg in 90 or 80 mL of D_5W infused over 20–30 minutes (approximately 5–10 mg/kg/hr)
	Method 2: 250–500 mg (5–7 mg/kg) in 20 mL of D_5W infused over 20–30 minutes
Route	Slow IV infusion
Pediatric Dosage	6 mg/kg loading dose to be infused over 20–30 minutes; maximum dose not to exceed 12 mg/kg over 24 hours

✳ Amiodarone HCL (Cordarone)

Class	Antidysrhythmic agent (group III)
Action	Prolongs action potential and refractory period
	Slows the sinus rate; increases PR and QT intervals
	Decreases peripheral vascular resistance
Indications	Life-threatening cardiac dysrhythmias such as ventricular tachycardia and ventricular fibrillation
Contraindications	Severe sinus node dysfunction
	Sinus bradycardia
	Second- and third-degree atrioventricular block
	Hemodynamically significant bradycardia
Precaution	Heart failure
Side Effects	Hypotension
	Nausea
	Anorexia
	Malaise, fatigue
	Tremors
	Pulmonary toxicity
	Ventricular ectopic beats
Dosage	*Adults:* Loading dose of 150 mg over 10 minutes (15 mg/min)
	Maintenance dose: 1 mg/min for 6 hours, then 0.5 mg/min until dysrhythmia is controlled or oral therapy begins
Route	IV, oral
Pediatric Dosage	5 mg/kg IV or IO; maximum dose: 15 mg/kg

✳ Amrinone (Inocor)

Class	Cardiac inotrope
Actions	Increases cardiac contractility
	Vasodilator
Indication	Short-term management of severe congestive heart failure
Contraindication	Patients with history of hypersensitivity to the drug
Precautions	May increase myocardial ischemia
	Blood pressure, pulse, and electrocardiogram (ECG) results should be constantly monitored
	Amrinone should only be diluted with normal saline or one-half normal saline; no dextrose solutions should be used
	Furosemide (Lasix) should not be administered into an IV line delivering amrinone
Side Effects	Reduction in platelets
	Nausea and vomiting
	Cardiac dysrhythmias

Dosage	0.75 mg/kg bolus given slowly over 2- to 5-minute interval followed by maintenance infusion of 2–15 mg/kg/min
Route	IV bolus and infusion as described earlier
Pediatric Dosage	Safety in children has not been established

✳ Amyl Nitrite

Class	Nitrate
Actions	Causes coronary vasodilation
	Removes cyanide ion via complex mechanism
Indication	Cyanide poisoning (bitter almond smell to breath)
Contraindications	None when used in the management of cyanide poisoning
Precaution	Has tendency for abuse
Side Effects	Headache
	Hypotension
	Reflex tachycardia
	Nausea
Dosage	Inhalant should be broken and inhaled; repeated as needed until patient is delivered to emergency department; effects diminish after 20 minutes
Route	Inhalation
Pediatric Dosage	Inhalant should be broken and inhaled; repeated until patient is delivered to emergency department

✳ Anistreplase (Eminase)

Class	Fibrinolytic
Action	Dissolves blood clots
Indication	Acute myocardial infarction
Contraindications	Persons with internal bleeding
	Suspected aortic dissection
	Traumatic cardiopulmonary resuscitation
	Severe persistent hypertension
	Recent head trauma or known intracranial tumor
	History of stroke in the past 6 months
	Pregnancy
Precautions	May be ineffective if administered within 12 months of prior streptokinase or anistreplase therapy
	Antidysrhythmic and resuscitative drugs should be available
Side Effects	Bleeding
	Allergic reactions
	Anaphylaxis
	Fever
	Nausea and vomiting

Dosage	30 units slow intravenously over 2–5 minutes
Route	IV (slow)
Pediatric Dosage	Not recommended

✳ Aspirin

Class	Platelet inhibitor and anti-inflammatory
Action	Inhibits platelet aggregation
Indications	New chest pain suggestive of acute myocardial infarction
	Signs and symptoms suggestive of recent stroke (cerebrovascular accident)
Contraindication	Patients with known hypersensitivity to the drug
Precautions	Gastrointestinal bleeding and upset stomach
Side Effects	Heartburn
	Nausea and vomiting
	Wheezing
Dosage	160 or 325 mg by mouth chewed
Route	Oral
Pediatric Dosage	Not recommended

✳ Atracurium (Tracrium)

Class	Nondepolarizing neuromuscular blocker
Action	Paralyzes skeletal muscles including respiratory muscles
Indication	To achieve paralysis for endotracheal intubation (rapid-sequence induction)
Contraindication	Patients with known hypersensitivity to the drug
Precautions	Should not be administered unless persons skilled in endotracheal intubation are present
	Endotracheal intubation equipment must be available
	Oxygen equipment and emergency resuscitative drugs must be available
	Paralysis occurs in 2 minutes and lasts 35–70 minutes
Side Effects	Prolonged paralysis
	Hypotension
	Bradycardia
Dosage	0.4–0.5 mg/kg IV
Route	IV
Pediatric Dosage	<2 years: 0.3–0.4 mg/kg; >2 years: 0.4–0.5 mg

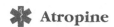 **Atropine**

Class	Parasympatholytic (anticholinergic)
Actions	Blocks acetylcholine receptors
	Increases heart rate
	Decreases gastrointestinal secretions
Indications	Hemodynamically significant bradycardia
	Hypotension secondary to bradycardia
	Asystole
	Organophosphate poisoning
Contraindication	None when used in emergency situations
Precautions	Dose of 0.04 mg/kg should not be exceeded except in cases of organophosphate poisonings
	Tachycardia
	Hypertension
Side Effects	Palpitations
	Tachycardia
	Headache
	Dizziness
	Anxiety
	Dry mouth
	Pupillary dilation
	Blurred vision
	Urinary retention (especially in older men)
Dosage	*Bradycardia:* 0.5 mg every 3–5 minutes to maximum of 0.04 mg/kg
	Asystole: 1 mg
	Organophosphate poisoning: 2–5 mg
Routes	Intravenous (IV)
	Endotracheal (endotracheal dose 2 to 2.5 times the IV dose)
Pediatric Dosage	*Bradycardia:* 0.02 mg/kg (minimum dose of 0.1 mg)
	Maximum single dose: child, 0.5 mg; adolescent, 1.0 mg
	Maximum total dose: child, 1.0 mg; adolescent, 2.0 mg

Bretylium Tosylate (Bretylol)

Class	Antidysrhythmic
Actions	Increases ventricular fibrillation threshold
	Blocks the release of norepinephrine from peripheral sympathetic nerves
Indications	Ventricular fibrillation refractory to lidocaine
	Ventricular tachycardia refractory to lidocaine
	PVCs refractory to first-line medications

Contraindications	None when used in the management of life-threatening dysrhythmias
Precautions	Postural hypotension occurs in approximately 50 percent of patients receiving bretylium
	Patient must be kept supine
	Dosage is decreased in patients being treated with catecholamine sympathomimetics
Side Effects	Hypotension
	Syncope
	Bradycardia
	Increased frequency of dysrhythmias
	Dizziness and vertigo
Dosage	5 mg/kg; may be repeated at dose of 10 mg/kg up to a total dose of 30 mg/kg
Route	Rapid intravenous (IV) bolus
Pediatric Dosage	5 mg/kg

✳ Bumetanide (Bumex)

Class	Potent diuretic
Actions	Inhibits reabsorption of sodium chloride
	Promotes prompt diuresis
	Slight vasodilation
Indications	Congestive heart failure
	Pulmonary edema
Contraindications	Dehydration
	Pregnancy
Precautions	Should be protected from light
	Dehydration
Side Effects	Few in emergency usage
Dosage	0.5–1.0 mg
Routes	IV, IM
Pediatric Dosage	Safety in children has not been established

✳ Butorphanol (Stadol)

Class	Synthetic analgesic
Actions	Central nervous system depressant
	Decreases sensitivity to pain
Indication	Moderate to severe pain
Contraindications	Patients with a history of hypersensitivity to the drug
	Head injury
	Use with caution in patients with impaired respiratory function
Precautions	Respiratory depression (naloxone should be available)
	Patients dependent on narcotics

Side Effects	Symptoms of withdrawal when administered to persons dependent on narcotics
	Nausea
	Altered levels of consciousness
Dosage	*Intravenous:* 1 mg
	Intramuscular: 2 mg
Routes	IV, IM
Pediatric Dosage	Rarely used

✳ Calcium Chloride

Class	Electrolyte
Action	Increases cardiac contractility
Indications	Acute hyperkalemia (elevated potassium level)
	Acute hypocalcemia (decreased calcium level)
	Calcium channel blocker (e.g., nifedipine, verapamil) overdose
	Abdominal muscle spasm associated with spider bite and Portuguese man-of-war stings
	Antidote for magnesium sulfate
Contraindication	Patients receiving digitalis
Precautions	IV line should be flushed between calcium chloride and sodium bicarbonate administration
	Extravasation may cause tissue necrosis
Side Effects	Dysrhythmias (bradycardia and asystole)
	Hypotension
Dosage	2–4 mg/kg of a 10 percent solution; may be repeated at 10-minute intervals
Route	IV
Pediatric Dosage	5–7 mg/kg of a 10 percent solution

✳ Chlorpromazine (Thorazine, Largactil)

Class	Major tranquilizer (Phenothiazine)
Actions	Blocks dopamine receptors in brain associated with mood and behavior
	Has antiemetic properties
Indications	Acute psychotic episodes
	Mild alcohol withdrawal
	Intractable hiccoughs
	Nausea and vomiting
Contraindications	Comatose states
	Presence of sedatives
	Presence of hallucinogens or phencyclidine-like compounds
Precautions	Orthostatic hypotension
	May cause extrapyramidal reactions (Parkinsonian), especially in children

Side Effects	Physical and mental impairment
	Drowsiness
Dosage	25–100 mg
Route	IM
Pediatric Dosage	0.5 mg/kg

✳ Dexamethasone (Decadron, Hexadrol)

Class	Steroid
Actions	Possibly decreases cerebral edema
	Anti-inflammatory
	Suppresses immune response (especially in allergic reactions)
Indications	Anaphylaxis (after epinephrine and diphenhydramine)
	Asthma
	Chronic obstructive pulmonary disease
Contraindications	None in the emergency setting
Precautions	Should be protected from heat
	Onset of action may be 2–6 hours and thus should not be considered to be of use in the critical first hour following an anaphylactic reaction
Side Effects	Gastrointestinal bleeding
	Prolonged wound healing
Dosage	4–24 mg
Routes	IV, IM
Pediatric Dosage	0.2–0.5 mg/kg

✳ Dextrose (50 Percent)

Class	Carbohydrate
Action	Elevates blood glucose level rapidly
Indication	Hypoglycemia
Contraindications	None in the emergency setting
Precaution	A blood sample should be drawn before administering 50 percent dextrose
Side Effect	Local venous irritation
Dosage	25 g (50 mL)
Route	IV
Pediatric Dosage	0.5 g/kg slow IV; should be diluted 1:1 with sterile water to form a 25 percent solution

✳ Diazepam (Valium)

Class	Tranquilizer (benzodiazepine)
Actions	Anticonvulsant
	Skeletal muscle relaxant
	Sedative

Indications	Major motor seizures
	Status epilepticus
	Premedication before cardioversion
	Skeletal muscle relaxant
	Acute anxiety states
Contraindication	Patients with a history of hypersensitivity to the drug
Precautions	Can cause local venous irritation
	Has short duration of effect
	Do not mix with other drugs because of possible precipitation problems
	Flumazenil (Romazicon) should be available
Side Effects	Drowsiness
	Hypotension
	Respiratory depression and apnea
Dosage	*Status epilepticus:* 5–10 mg intravenously (IV)
	Acute anxiety: 2–5 mg intramuscularly (IM) or IV
	Premedication before cardioversion: 5–15 mg IV
Routes	IV (care must be taken not to administer faster than 1 mL/min), IM, rectal
Pediatric Dosage	*Status epilepticus:* 0.1–0.2 mg/kg

✳ Digoxin (Lanoxin)

Class	Cardiac glycoside
Actions	Increases cardiac contractile force
	Increases cardiac output
	Reduces edema associated with congestive heart failure
	Slows atrioventricular conduction
Indications	Congestive heart failure
	Rapid atrial dysrhythmias, especially atrial flutter and atrial fibrillation
Contraindications	Any patient with signs or symptoms of digitalis toxicity
	Ventricular fibrillation
Precautions	Monitor for signs of digitalis toxicity
	Patients who have recently suffered a myocardial infarction have greater sensitivity to the effects of digitalis
	Calcium should not be administered to patients receiving digitalis
Side Effects	Nausea and vomiting
	Dysrhythmias
	Yellow vision
Dosage	0.25–0.50 mg
Route	IV
Pediatric Dosage	25–40 mg

✳ Diltiazem (Cardizem)

Class	Calcium channel blocker
Actions	Slows conduction through the atrioventricular mode
	Causes vasodilation
	Decreases rate of ventricular response
	Decreases myocardial oxygen demand
Indications	To control rapid ventricular rates associated with atrial fibrillation and flutter
	Angina pectoris
Contraindications	Hypotension
	Wide-complex tachycardia
	Conduction system disturbances
Precautions	Should not be used in patients receiving intravenous β-blockers
	Hypotension
	Must be kept refrigerated
Side Effects	Nausea and vomiting
	Hypotension
	Dizziness
Dosage	0.25 mg/kg bolus (typically 20 mg) IV over 2 minutes, followed by a maintenance infusion of 5–15 mg/hr
Routes	IV, IV drip
Pediatric Dosage	Rarely used

✳ Dimenhydrinate (Gravol, Dramamine)

Class	Antihistamine
Action	Antiemetic
Indications	Nausea and vomiting
	Motion sickness
	To potentiate the effects of analgesics
Contraindications	Comatose states
	Patients who have received a large amount of depressants (including alcohol)
Precautions	Use with caution in patients with seizure disorders
	Asthma
Side Effects	May impair mental and physical ability
	Drowsiness
Dosage	*Slow intravenous:* 12.5–25.0 mg
	Intramuscular or oral: 50–100 mg
Routes	IV, IM, oral
Pediatric Dosage	Pediatric data unavailable

✳ Diphenhydramine (Benadryl)

Class	Antihistamine
Actions	Blocks histamine receptors
	Has some sedative effects
Indications	Anaphylaxis
	Allergic reactions
	Dystonic reactions due to phenothiazines
Contraindications	Asthma
	Nursing mothers
Precautions	Hypotension
Side Effects	Sedation
	Dries bronchial secretions
	Blurred vision
	Headache
	Palpitations
Dosage	25–50 mg
Routes	Slow IV push, deep IM
Pediatric Dosage	2–5 mg/kg

✳ Dobutamine (Dobutrex)

Class	Sympathomimetic
Actions	Increases cardiac contractility
	Little chronotropic activity
Indication	Short-term management of congestive heart failure
Contraindication	Should only be used in patients with an adequate heart rate
Precautions	Ventricular irritability
	Use with caution following myocardial infarction
	Can be deactivated by alkaline solutions
Side Effects	Headache
	Hypertension
	Palpitations
Dosage	2.5–20 µg/kg/min
	Method: 250 mg should be placed in 500 mL of D_5W, which gives a concentration of 0.5 mg/mL
Route	IV drip
Pediatric Dosage	2–20 µg/kg/min

✳ Dopamine (Intropin)

Class	Sympathomimetic
Actions	Increases cardiac contractility
	Causes peripheral vasoconstriction

Indications	Hemodynamically significant hypotension (systolic blood pressure of 70–100 mmHg) not resulting from hypovolemia
	Cardiogenic shock
Contraindications	Hypovolemic shock in which complete fluid resuscitation has not occurred
	Pheochromocytoma
Precautions	Presence of severe tachydysrhythmias
	Presence of ventricular fibrillation
	Ventricular irritability
	Beneficial effects lost when dose exceeds 20 µg/kg/min
Side Effects	Ventricular tachydysrhythmias
	Hypertension
	Palpitations
Dosage	*Initial dose:* 2–5 µg/kg/min; increase as needed
	Method: 800 mg should be placed in 500 mL of D$_5$W, giving a concentration of 1600 mg/mL
Route	IV drip only
Pediatric Dosage	2–20 µg/kg/min

✳ Droperidol (Inapsine)

Class	Butyrophenone antipsychotic/antiemetic
Actions	Antagonizes the effects of drugs that act on the chemoreceptor trigger zone (CTZ)
	Reduces anxiety and produces sedation
Indication	Acute psychosis
	Nausea/vomiting
Contraindication	Patients with known hypersensitivity to the drug
Precautions	"Black box" warning regarding QT interval prolongation
	Use with caution in the elderly, debilitated, or poor-risk patients
	Monitor vital signs and ECG
Side Effects	Drowsiness
	EPS symptoms (dystonia)
	Dizziness
	Restlessness
	Hypotension
	Tachycardia
Dosage	2.5–10.0 mg IV
Route	IV
Pediatric Dosage	0.088–0.165 mg/kg IV (children >2 years)

✳ Edrophonium (Tensilon)

Class	Anticholinesterase
Actions	Inhibits action of enzyme cholinesterase, thus potentiating acetylcholine
	Increases parasympathetic tone
Indication	PSVT refractory to vagal maneuvers; considered a second-line agent to verapamil or adenosine
Contraindication	Patients with a history of hypersensitivity to the drug
Precautions	Respirations must be constantly monitored
	Bradycardia
	Hypotension
	Avoid exposure to dextrose solutions
Side Effects	Dizziness
	Syncope
Dosage	5 mg
Route	IV
Pediatric Dosage	0.1–0.2 mg/kg

✳ Enoxaparin (Lovenox)

Class	Anticoagulant (low molecular-weight heparin)
Action	Acts as effective anticoagulant
Indications	Unstable angina
	Non-Q-wave myocardial infarction
	Pulmonary embolism
	Deep venous thrombosis
Contraindication	Patients with a known hypersensitivity to the drug or heparin
Precaution	Do not use in patients with major bleeding or at increased risk of bleeding
Side Effects	Confusion
	Dizziness
	Edema
	Bleeding complications
Dosage	*Myocardial infarction/angina:* 1 mg/kg SC
	Pulmonary embolism: 0.5 mg/kg SC
Routes	SC, IV
Pediatric Dosage	1 mg/kg SC

✳ Epinephrine 1:1000

Class	Sympathomimetic
Action	Bronchodilation

Indications	Bronchial asthma
	Exacerbation of chronic obstructive pulmonary disease
	Allergic reactions
	Pediatric cardiac arrest (after initial epinephrine dosage)
Contraindications	Patients with underlying cardiovascular disease
	Hypertension
	Pregnancy
	Patients with tachydysrhythmias
Precautions	Should be protected from light
	Blood pressure, pulse, and electrocardiogram (ECG) results must be constantly monitored
Side Effects	Palpitations and tachycardia
	Anxiousness
	Headache
	Tremor
Dosage	0.3–0.5 mg
Route	Subcutaneous
Pediatric Dosage	0.01 mg/kg up to 0.3 mg

✳ Epinephrine 1:10 000

Class	Sympathomimetic
Actions	Increases heart rate and automaticity
	Increases cardiac contractile force
	Increases myocardial electrical activity
	Increases systemic vascular resistance
	Increases blood pressure
	Causes bronchodilation
Indications	Cardiac arrest
	Anaphylactic shock
	Severe reactive airway disease
Contraindications	Epinephrine 1:10 000 is for intravenous (IV) or endotracheal use; it should not be used in patients who do not require extensive resuscitative efforts
Precautions	Should be protected from light
	Can be deactivated by alkaline solutions
Side Effects	Palpitations
	Anxiety
	Tremulousness
	Nausea and vomiting
Dosage	*Cardiac arrest:* 0.5–1.0 mg repeated every 3–5 minutes; higher doses may be ordered by medical control
	Severe anaphylaxis: 0.3–0.5 mg (3–5 mL); occasionally an epinephrine drip is required

Routes	IV, IV drip, endotracheal (endotracheal dose 2 to 2.5 times IV dose)
Pediatric Dosage	0.01 mg/kg initially; with subsequent doses, epinephrine 1:1000 should be used at a dose of 0.1 mg/kg

✳ Esmolol (Brevibloc)

Class	Beta-blocker (β_1 selective)
Actions	Decreases heart rate
	Decreases atrioventricular conduction
Indication	Symptomatic supraventricular tachycardia (including atrial fibrillation and atrial flutter) as evidenced by chest pain, palpitations, or dizziness
Contraindications	Sinus bradycardia
	Heart block greater than first degree
	Cardiogenic shock
	Overt congestive heart failure
	Patients with bronchospastic disease (asthma)
Precautions	Hypotension is common and is usually dose related
	Patients with congestive heart failure may have worsening of their symptoms
	May worsen bronchospastic disease
Side Effects	Dizziness
	Diaphoresis
	Hypotension
	Nausea
Dosage	*Preparation:* Place two 2.5 g ampules in 500 mL of D_5W, yielding a concentration of 10 mg/mL
	Loading dose: 500 mg/kg/min for 1 minute, then reduce to maintenance dose
	Maintenance dose: 50 mg/kg/min; if ineffective after 4 minutes, repeat loading dose and increase maintenance dose to 100 mg/kg/min; may repeat as needed until a total maintenance dose of 200 mg/kg/min has been achieved
Route	IV infusion only
Pediatric Dosage	Safety in children has not been established

✳ Etomidate (Amidate)

Class	Sedative/hypnotic
Action	Creates an ultra-short-acting sedative/hypnotic effect
Indication	Induction agent for rapid-sequence induction
Contraindication	Known hypersensitivity to the drug
Precautions	Marked hypotension
	Severe asthma
	Severe cardiovascular disease

Side Effects	Myoclonic skeletal muscle movement
	Apnea
	Laryngospasm
Dosage	0.1–0.3 mg/kg IV over 15–30 seconds
Route	IV
Pediatric Dosage	>10 years: same as adult dose; <10 years: not indicated

✳ Fentanyl Citrate (Sublimaze)

Class	Narcotic
Actions	Central nervous system depressant
	Decreases sensitivity to pain
Indications	Severe pain
	Adjunct to rapid-sequence induction
	Adjunct to rapid-sequence sedation
	Maintenance of analgesia
Contraindications	Shock
	Severe hemorrhage
	Undiagnosed abdominal pain
	Patients with history of hypersensitivity to the drug
Precautions	Respiratory depression (naloxone should be available)
	Hypotension
	Nausea
Side Effects	Dizziness
	Altered level of consciousness
	Bradycardia
Dosage	25–100 µg
Route	IV
Pediatric Dosage	2–12 years: 1.7–3.3 µg/kg

✳ Flumazenil (Romazicon)

Class	Benzodiazepine antagonist
Action	Reverses the effects of benzodiazepines
Indication	To reverse central nervous system respiratory depression associated with benzodiazepines
Contraindications	Flumazenil should not be used as a diagnostic agent for benzodiazepine overdose in the same manner naloxone is used for narcotic overdose
	Known hypersensitivity to the drug
Precautions	Administer with caution to patients dependent on benzodiazepines because it may induce life-threatening benzodiazepine withdrawal
	Should not be used as part of a "coma cocktail"

Side Effects	Fatigue
	Headache
	Nervousness
	Dizziness
Dosage	0.2 mg IV over 30 seconds, repeated as needed to a maximum dose of 1.0 mg
Route	IV
Pediatric Dosage	Pediatric data unavailable

✳ Fosphenytoin (Cerebyx)

Class	Anticonvulsant
Actions	Converts to phenytoin
	Suppresses seizure activity
Indications	Major motor seizures
	Antidysrhythmic
Contraindication	Hypersensitivity to the drug or to the phenytoin (hydantoin) class of drugs
Precautions	Patients with impaired renal function
	Alcoholism
	Hypotension
	Heart block
Side Effects	Dizziness
	Somnolence
	Hypotension
	Heart block
Dosage	15–20 mg phenytoin equivalent/kg IV, IM
Route	IV, IM
Pediatric Dosage	15–20 mg phenytoin equivalent/kg IV/IM

✳ Furosemide (Lasix)

Class	Potent diuretic
Actions	Inhibits reabsorption of sodium chloride
	Promotes prompt diuresis
	Vasodilation
Indications	Congestive heart failure
	Pulmonary edema
Contraindications	Pregnancy
	Dehydration
Precautions	Should be protected from light
	Dehydration
Side Effects	Few in emergency usage
Dosage	40–80 mg
Route	IV
Pediatric Dosage	1 mg/kg

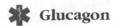 **Glucagon**

Class	Hormone (antihypoglycemic agent)
Actions	Causes breakdown of glycogen to glucose
	Inhibits glycogen synthesis
	Elevates blood glucose level
	Increases cardiac contractile force
	Increases heart rate
Indications	Hypoglycemia
	Beta-blocker overdose
Contraindication	Hypersensitivity to the drug
Precautions	Only effective if there are sufficient stores of glycogen within the liver
	Use with caution in patients with cardiovascular or renal disease
	Draw blood for glucose test before administration
Side Effects	Few in emergency situations
Dosage	*Intravenous:* 0.25–0.5 unit
	Intramuscular: 1.0 mg
Routes	IV, IM
Pediatric Dosage	0.03 mg/kg

Haloperidol (Haldol)

Class	Major tranquilizer (butyrophenone)
Actions	Blocks dopamine receptors in brain responsible for mood and behavior
	Has antiemetic properties
Indication	Acute psychotic episodes
Contraindications	Should not be administered in the presence of other sedatives
	Should not be used in the management of dysphoria caused by Talwin
Precaution	Orthostatic hypotension
Side Effects	Physical and mental impairment
	Parkinson-like reactions have been known to occur, especially in children
Dosage	2–5 mg
Route	IM
Pediatric Dosage	Rarely used

Heparin

Class	Anticoagulant
Action	Inhibits antithrombin III–thrombin complex

Indications	Unstable angina
	Non-Q-wave myocardial infarction
	Pulmonary embolism
	Deep venous thrombosis
Contraindication	Patient with known hypersensitivity to the drug or pork products
Precaution	Do not use in patients with major bleeding or thrombocytopenia
Side Effects	Confusion
	Dizziness
	Edema
	Bleeding complications
Dosage	5000 units IV followed by maintenance infusion
Routes	IV, SC
Pediatric Dosage	50 units/kg followed by maintenance infusion

✳ Hydralazine (Apresoline)

Class	Antihypertensive (potent vasodilator)
Actions	Relaxes vascular smooth muscle
	Decreases arterial pressure (diastolic greater than systolic)
	Increases cardiac output
Indications	Hypertensive emergency in which a prompt reduction in blood pressure is required
	Hypertension accompanying pregnancy
Contraindications	Patients with a known history of coronary artery disease
	Rheumatic heart disease involving the mitral valve
	History of hypersensitivity to the drug
Precautions	May induce angina
	May cause electrocardiogram (ECG) changes and cardiac ischemia
	Blood pressure, pulse rate, and ECG results should be constantly monitored
Side Effects	Headache
	Nausea
	Vomiting
	Tachycardia
	Palpitations
	Diarrhea
Dosage	20–40 mg given by slow IV bolus; may be repeated, if required
Route	IV
Pediatric Dosage	Safety in children has not been established

✳ Hydrocortisone (Solu-Cortef)

Class	Steroid
Actions	Anti-inflammatory
	Suppresses immune response (especially in allergic and anaphylactic reactions)
Indications	Severe anaphylaxis
	Asthma and chronic obstructive pulmonary disease
	Urticaria (hives)
Contraindications	None in the emergency setting
Precautions	Must be reconstituted and used promptly
	Onset of action may be 2–6 hours, and thus the drug should not be expected to be of use in the critical first hour following an acute anaphylactic reaction
Side Effects	Gastrointestinal bleeding
	Prolonged wound healing
	Suppression of natural steroids
Dosage	100–250 mg
Routes	IV, IM
Pediatric Dosage	30 mg/kg

✳ Hydroxyzine (Vistaril)

Class	Antihistamine
Actions	Antiemetic
	Antihistamine
	Antianxiety
	Potentiates analgesic effects of narcotics and related agents
Indications	To potentiate the effects of narcotics and synthetic narcotics
	Nausea and vomiting
	Anxiety reactions
Contraindication	Patients with a history of hypersensitivity to the drug
Precautions	Orthostatic hypotension
	Analgesic dosages should be reduced when used with hydroxyzine
	Urinary retention
Side Effect	Drowsiness
Dosage	50–100 mg
Route	Deep IM
Pediatric Dosage	1 mg/kg

✳ Insulin (Humilin, Novolin, Iletin)

Class	Hormone (hypoglycemic agent)
Actions	Causes uptake of glucose by the cells
	Decreases blood glucose level
	Promotes glucose storage
Indications	Elevated blood glucose
	Diabetic ketoacidosis
Contraindications	Avoid overcompensation of blood glucose level; if possible, administration should wait until the patient is in the emergency department
Precautions	Administration of excessive dose may induce hypoglycemia
	Glucose should be available
Side Effects	Few in emergency situations
Dosage	10–25 units regular insulin IV followed by an infusion at 0.1 units/kg/hr
Routes	IV, SQ
Pediatric Dosage	Dosage is based on blood glucose level

✳ Ipecac

Class	Emetic
Actions	Irritates the enteric tract
	Acts on vomiting center in the brain
Indication	Poisoning in conscious patient
Contraindications	Vomiting should not be induced in any patient with impaired consciousness
	Poisonings involving strong acids, bases, or petroleum distillates
	Antiemetic poisonings, especially of the phenothiazine type
Precautions	Monitor and ensure a patent airway
	The risk of aspiration is increased when using ipecac
Side Effects	Rare
Dosage	30 mL (1 oz) followed by 15 mL/kg of warm water
Route	Oral
Pediatric Dosage	*<1 year of age:* 10 mL
	1–12 years of age: 15 mL
	>12 years of age: 30 mL

✳ Ipratropium (Atrovent)

Class	Anticholinergic
Actions	Causes bronchodilation
	Dries respiratory tract secretions

Indications	Bronchial asthma
	Reversible bronchospasm associated with chronic bronchitis and emphysema
Contraindications	Should not be used in patients with history of hypersensitivity to the drug
	Should not be used as primary acute treatment of bronchospasm
Precaution	Monitor vital signs
Side Effects	Palpitations
	Dizziness
	Anxiety
	Headache
	Nervousness
Dosage	500 mcg placed in small-volume nebulizer (typically administered with a β-agonist)
Route	Inhaled
Pediatric Dosage	Safety in children has not been established

Isoetharine (Bronkosol)

Class	Sympathomimetic (β_2 selective)
Actions	Bronchodilation
	Increases heart rate
Indications	Asthma
	Reversible bronchospasm associated with chronic bronchitis and emphysema
Contraindication	Patients with history of hypersensitivity to the drug
Precautions	Blood pressure, pulse, and electrocardiogram (ECG) results must be constantly monitored
Side Effects	Palpitations
	Tachycardia
	Anxiety
	Tremors
	Headache
Dosage	*Hand nebulizer:* Four inhalations
	Small-volume nebulizer: 0.5 mL (1:3 with saline)
Route	Inhalation only
Pediatric Dosage	0.25–0.5 mL diluted with 4 mL normal saline

Isoproterenol (Isuprel)

Class	Sympathomimetic
Actions	Increases heart rate
	Increases cardiac contractile force
	Causes bronchodilation

Indications	Bradycardias refractory to atropine (when transcutaneous pacing is unavailable)
	Severe status asthmaticus
Contraindication	Should not be used to increase blood pressure in cardiogenic shock
Precautions	Can cause ventricular irritability
	Can be deactivated by alkaline solutions
	Should be used with caution for recent myocardial infarction
	External pacing, if available, should be used instead of isoproterenol
Side Effects	Tachydysrhythmias
	Tremors
	Palpitations
	Headache
Dosage	1 mg should be placed in 500 mL of D_5W and then slowly infused at 2–10 µg/min and titrated until the desired rate is obtained or until PVCs occur
Route	IV drip only
Pediatric Dosage	0.1 µg/kg/min

✳ Ketamine (Ketalar)

Class	Sedative/hypnotic and analgesic
Action	Causes dissociative state
Indication	Induction agent for rapid-sequence induction
Contraindications	Patients with hypersensitivity to the drug
	Significantly elevated blood pressure
Precautions	Hallucinations can occur with emergency, particularly on emergence
	Emergency airway and resuscitative equipment and drugs must be available
Side Effects	Hallucinations
	Increased skeletal muscle tone
Dosage	0.5–1.0 mg/kg IV
	2.0–4.0 mg/kg IM
Routes	IV, IM
Pediatric Dosage	0.5–0.3 mg/kg IV, IM

✳ Ketorolac (Toradol)

Class	Nonsteroidal anti-inflammatory agent
Actions	Anti-inflammatory
	Analgesic (peripherally acting)
Indication	Mild to moderate pain
Contraindications	Patients with a history of hypersensitivity to the drug
	Patients allergic to aspirin

Precautions	Gastrointestinal irritation or hemorrhage can occur
Side Effects	Edema
	Rash
	Heartburn
Dosage	*Intravenous:* 15–30 mg
	Intramuscular: 30–60 mg
Routes	IV, IM
Pediatric Dosage	Rarely used

✳ Labetalol (Trandate, Normodyne)

Class	Sympathetic blocker
Actions	Selectively blocks α_1-receptors and nonselectively blocks β-receptors
Indication	Hypertensive crisis
Contraindications	Bronchial asthma
	Congestive heart failure
	Heart block
	Bradycardia
	Cardiogenic shock
Precautions	Blood pressure, pulse, and electrocardiogram (ECG) results must be constantly monitored
	Atropine should be available
Side Effects	Bradycardia
	Heart block
	Congestive heart failure
	Bronchospasm
	Postural hypotension
Dosage	20 mg by slow IV infusion over 2 minutes; doses of 40 mg can be repeated in 10 minutes until desired supine blood pressure is obtained or until 300 mg of the drug has been given
	200 mg placed in 500 mL D_5W to deliver 2 mg/min
Route	IV infusion or slow IV bolus as described earlier
Pediatric Dosage	Safety in children has not been established

✳ Levalbuterol (Xopenex)

Class	Sympathetic agonist (β_2 selective)
Action	Bronchodilation
Indications	Asthma
	Reversible bronchospasm associated with chronic obstructive pulmonary disease
Contraindications	Known hypersensitivity to the drug
	Symptomatic tachycardia

Precaution	Blood pressure, pulse, and electrocardiogram (ECG) results should be monitored
Side Effects	Palpitations
	Anxiety
	Headache
	Dizziness
Dosage	0.63 mg in 3.0 mL normal saline every 6–8 hours
Route	Inhalation
Pediatric Dosage	0.31 mg in 3.0 mL normal saline 3 times a day

✳ Lidocaine (Xylocaine)

Class	Antidysrhythmic
Actions	Suppresses ventricular ectopic activity
	Increases ventricular fibrillation threshold
	Reduces velocity of electrical impulse through conductive system
Indications	Malignant PVCs
	Ventricular tachycardia
	Ventricular fibrillation
	Prophylaxis of dysrhythmias associated with fibrinolytic therapy
Contraindications	High-degree heart blocks
	PVCs in conjunction with bradycardia
Precautions	Dosage should not exceed 300 mg/hr
	Monitor for central nervous system toxicity
	Dosage should be reduced by 50 percent in patients older than 70 years of age or who have liver disease
	In cardiac arrest, use only bolus therapy
Side Effects	Anxiety
	Drowsiness
	Dizziness
	Confusion
	Nausea and vomiting
	Convulsions
	Widening of QRS complex
Dosage	*Bolus:* Initial bolus of 1.0–1.5 mg/kg; additional boluses of 0.5–0.75 mg/kg can be repeated at 3- to 5-minute intervals until the dysrhythmia has been suppressed or until 3.0 mg/kg of the drug has been administered; reduce dosage by 50 percent in patients older than 70 years of age
	Drip: After the dysrhythmia has been suppressed, a 2–4 mg/min infusion may be started to maintain adequate blood levels
Routes	IV bolus, IV infusion
Pediatric Dosage	1 mg/kg

✳ Lorazepam (Ativan)

Class	Tranquilizer (benzodiazepine)
Actions	Anticonvulsant
	Sedative
Indications	Major motor seizures
	Status epilepticus
	Premedication before cardioversion
	Acute anxiety states
Contraindication	Patients with a history of hypersensitivity to the drug
Precautions	Has short duration of effect
	Do not mix with other drugs because of possible precipitation problems
	Flumazenil (Romazicon) should be available
	Dilute with normal saline of D_5W prior to IV administration
Side Effects	Drowsiness
	Hypotension
	Respiratory depression and apnea
Dosage	0.5–2.0 mg IV; may be increased to 1.0–4.0 mg IV
Routes	IV, IM, rectal
Pediatric Dosage	0.05–0.10 mg/kg (maximum dose 4 mg)

✳ Magnesium Sulfate

Class	Anticonvulsant and antidysrhythmic
Actions	Central nervous system depressant
	Anticonvulsant
	Antidysrhythmic
Indications	*Obstetrical:* Eclampsia (toxemia of pregnancy)
	Cardiovascular: Severe refractory ventricular fibrillation or pulseless ventricular tachycardia, post–myocardial infarction as prophylaxis for dysrhythmias, and torsade de pointes (multiaxial ventricular tachycardia)
Contraindications	Shock
	Heart block
Precautions	Caution should be used in patients receiving digitalis
	Hypotension
	Calcium chloride should be readily available as an antidote if respiratory depression ensues
	Use with caution in patients with renal failure
Side Effects	Flushing
	Respiratory depression
	Drowsiness

Dosage	1–4 g
Routes	IV, IM
Pediatric Dosage	Not indicated

✳ Mannitol (Osmotrol)

Class	Osmotic diuretic
Actions	Decreases cellular edema
	Increases urinary output
Indications	Acute cerebral edema
	Blood transfusion reactions
Contraindications	Pulmonary edema
	Patients who are dehydrated
	Hypersensitivity to the drug
Precautions	Rapid administration can cause circulatory overload
	Crystallization of the drug can occur at lower temperatures
	An in-line filter should be used
Side Effects	Pulmonary congestion
	Sodium depletion
	Transient volume overload
Dosage	1.5–2.0 g/kg
Routes	IV slow bolus or infusion
Pediatric Dosage	0.25–0.5 g/kg IV over 60 minutes

✳ Meperidine (Demerol)

Class	Narcotic
Actions	Central nervous system depressant
	Decreases sensitivity to pain
Indication	Moderate to severe pain
Contraindications	Patients receiving monoamine oxidase inhibitors
	Undiagnosed abdominal pain
	Patients with history of hypersensitivity to the drug
Precautions	Respiratory depression (naloxone should be available)
	Hypotension
	Nausea
Side Effects	Dizziness
	Altered level of consciousness
Dosage	*Intravenous:* 25–50 mg
	Intramuscular: 50–100 mg
Routes	IV, IM
Pediatric Dosage	1 mg/kg

Metaproterenol (Alupent)

Class	Sympathomimetic (β_2 selective)
Actions	Bronchodilation
	Increases heart rate
Indications	Bronchial asthma
	Reversible bronchospasm associated with chronic bronchitis and emphysema
Contraindications	Patients with cardiac dysrhythmias or significant tachycardia
Precautions	Blood pressure, pulse, and electrocardiogram (ECG) results must be constantly monitored; occasional nausea and vomiting reported
Side Effects	Palpitations
	Anxiety
	Headache
	Nausea and vomiting
	Dizziness
	Tremor
Dosage	*Metered-dose inhaler:* Two to three inhalations; can be repeated in 3–4 hours if required
	Small-volume nebulizer: 0.2–0.3 mL diluted in 2–3 mL normal saline administered over 5–15 minutes
Route	Inhalation only
Pediatric Dosage	0.05–0.3 mL in 4 mL normal saline

Metaraminol (Aramine)

Class	Sympathomimetic (indirect acting)
Actions	Causes release of endogenous stores of norepinephrine
	Increases cardiac contractile force
	Increases cardiac rate
	Causes peripheral vasoconstriction
Indication	Hemodynamically significant hypotension not due to hypovolemia
Contraindication	Hypotensive states due to hypovolemia
Precautions	Constant monitoring of blood pressure is essential
	Not effective in catecholamine-depleted patients
Side Effects	Palpitations
	Tachycardia
	PVCs
	Hypertension
	Tremor
	Dizziness
Dosage	200 mg should be placed in 500 mL of D_5W; this gives a concentration of 0.4 mg/mL, which should

be slowly infused and titrated to blood pressure response

5–10 mg can be administered intramuscularly when an IV line cannot be placed

Routes	IV drip, IM
Pediatric Dosage	Safety in children has not been established

✳ Methylprednisone (Solu-Medrol)

Class	Steroid
Actions	Anti-inflammatory
	Suppresses immune response (especially in allergic reactions)
Indications	Severe anaphylaxis
	Asthma and chronic obstructive pulmonary disease
Contraindications	None in the emergency setting
Precautions	Must be reconstituted and used promptly
	Onset of action may be 2–6 hours, and thus the drug should not be expected to be of use in the critical first hour following an anaphylactic reaction
Side Effects	Gastrointestinal bleeding
	Prolonged wound healing
	Suppression of natural steroids
Dosage	*General usage:* 125–250 mg
Routes	IV, IM
Pediatric Dosage	30 mg/kg

✳ Metoclopramide (Reglan)

Class	Phenothiazine antiemetic
Actions	Antiemetic
	Reduces gastroesophageal reflux
Indications	Nausea and vomiting
	Gastroesophageal reflux
Contraindications	Gastrointestinal hemorrhage
	Bowel obstruction or perforation
	Patients with a history of hypersensitivity to the drug
Precaution	Extrapyramidal (dystonic) symptoms have been reported
Side Effects	May impair mental and physical ability
	Drowsiness
Dosage	*Intramuscular:* 10–20 mg
	Intravenous: 10 mg by slow IV push over 1–2 minutes
Routes	IV, IM
Pediatric Dosage	Rarely indicated

✳ Metoprolol (Lopressor)

Class	Sympathetic blocker (β_2 selective)
Action	Selectively blocks β_2-adrenergic receptors (cardioprotective)
Indication	Suspected or definite acute myocardial infarction in patients who are hemodynamically stable
Contraindications	Heart rate less than 45 beats per minute
	Systolic blood pressure <100 mmHg
	Heart block
	Shock
	History of asthma
Precautions	Blood pressure, pulse, and electrocardiogram (ECG) results must be constantly monitored
	Atropine and transcutaneous pacing should be available
Side Effects	Bradycardia
	Heart block
	Congestive heart failure
	Depression
	Bronchospasm
Dosage	Initial bolus of 5 mg slow IV injection
	May repeat 5 mg bolus in 5 minutes if vital signs are stable
	May repeat 5 mg bolus in 10 minutes if vital signs are stable
Route	Slow IV bolus
Pediatric Dosage	Safety in children has not been established

✳ Midazolam (Versed)

Class	Tranquilizer (benzodiazepine)
Actions	Hypnotic
	Sedative
Indications	Premedication before cardioversion
	Acute anxiety states
Contraindications	Patients with a history of hypersensitivity to the drug
	Narrow-angle glaucoma
	Shock
Precautions	Emergency resuscitative equipment must be available
	Flumazenil (Romazicon) should be available
	Dilute with normal saline of D_5W prior to intravenous administration
	Respiratory depression more common with midazolam than with other benzodiazepines

Side Effects	Drowsiness
	Hypotension
	Amnesia
	Respiratory depression and apnea
Dosage	1.0–2.5 mg administered IV
Routes	IV, oral, intranasal
Pediatric Dosage	0.03 mg/kg

✳ Morphine

Class	Narcotic
Actions	Central nervous system depressant
	Causes peripheral vasodilation
	Decreases sensitivity to pain
Indications	Severe pain
	Pulmonary edema
Contraindications	Head injury
	Volume depletion
	Undiagnosed abdominal pain
	History of hypersensitivity to the drug
Precautions	Respiratory depression (naloxone should be available)
	Hypotension
	Nausea
Side Effects	Dizziness
	Altered level of consciousness
Dosage	*Intravenous:* 2–5 mg followed by 2 mg every few minutes until the pain is relieved or until respiratory depression ensues
	Intramuscular: 5–15 mg based on patient's weight
Routes	IV, IM
Pediatric Dosage	0.1–0.2 mg/kg IV

✳ Nalbuphine (Nubain)

Class	Synthetic analgesic
Actions	Central nervous system depressant
	Decreases sensitivity to pain
Indication	Moderate to severe pain
Contraindication	Patients with a history of hypersensitivity to the drug
Precautions	Use with caution in patients with impaired respiratory function
	Respiratory depression (naloxone should be available)
	Patients dependent on narcotics may experience symptoms of withdrawal
	Nausea

Side Effects	Dizziness
	Altered mental status
Dosage	5–10 mg
Routes	IV, IM
Pediatric Dosage	Rarely used

✳ Naloxone (Narcan)

Class	Narcotic antagonist
Action	Reverses effects of narcotics
Indications	Narcotic overdoses including the following: morphine, Dilaudid, fentanyl, Demerol, paregoric, methadone, heroin, Percodan, and Tylox
	Synthetic analgesic overdoses including the following: Nubain, Stadol, Talwin, Darvon, and alcoholic coma
	To rule out narcotics in coma of unknown origin
Contraindication	Patients with a history of hypersensitivity to the drug
Precautions	May cause withdrawal effects in patients dependent on narcotics
	Short acting; should be augmented every 5 minutes
	Should never be used as part of a "coma cocktail"
Side Effects	Rare
Dosage	1–2 mg
Routes	IV, IM, endotracheal (endotracheal dose 2 to 2.5 times IV dose)
Pediatric Dosage	*<5 years old:* 0.1 mg/kg
	>5 years old: 2.0 mg

✳ Nesiritide (Natrecor)

Class	Natriuretic polypeptide
Actions	Vasodilation
	Sodium excretion
	Diuresis
Indication	Acutely decompensated congestive heart failure (CHF)
Contraindications	CHF secondary to valvular heart disease
	Patients with known hypersensitivity to the drug
Precautions	Use with caution in patients receiving ACE inhibitors
	Physiological monitors should be applied
Side Effects	Headaches
	Back pain
	Catheter/injection site pain
	Fever
	Leg cramps

Dosage	Initial bolus of 2.0 μg/kg over 60 seconds followed by continuous infusion of 0.01 μg/kg/min
Route	IV
Pediatric Dosage	Not indicated

✳ Nifedipine (Procardia)

Class	Calcium channel blocker
Actions	Relaxes smooth muscle, causing arteriolar vasodilation
	Decreases peripheral vascular resistance
Indications	Severe hypertension
	Angina pectoris
Contraindications	Known hypersensitivity to the drug
	Hypotension
Precautions	Blood pressure should be constantly monitored
	May worsen congestive heart failure
	Nifedipine should not be administered to patients receiving intravenous β-blockers
Side Effects	Dizziness
	Flushing
	Nausea
	Headache
	Weakness
Dosage	10 mg sublingually; puncture the capsule several times with a needle and place it under the patient's tongue and have him or her withdraw the liquid medication
Routes	Oral, sublingual
Pediatric Dosage	0.25–0.5 mg/kg

✳ Nitroglycerin (Nitrostat)

Class	Antianginal
Actions	Smooth muscle relaxant
	Reduces cardiac work
	Dilates coronary arteries
	Dilates systemic arteries
Indications	Angina pectoris
	Chest pain associated with myocardial infarction
Contraindications	Children younger than 12 years of age
	Hypotension
Precautions	Constantly monitor blood pressure
	Syncope
	Drug must be protected from light
	Expires quickly once bottle is opened

Side Effects	Headache
	Dizziness
	Hypotension
Dosage	One tablet repeated at 3- to 5-minute intervals up to three times
Route	Sublingual
Pediatric Dosage	Not indicated

✳ Nitroglycerin Paste (Nitro-Bid)

Class	Antianginal
Actions	Smooth muscle relaxant
	Decreases cardiac work
	Dilates coronary arteries
	Dilates systemic arteries
Indications	Angina pectoris
	Chest pain associated with myocardial infarction
Contraindications	Children younger than 12 years of age
	Hypotension
Precautions	Constantly monitor blood pressure
	Syncope
	Drug must be protected from light
	Expires quickly once bottle is opened
Side Effects	Dizziness
	Hypotension
Dosage	1/2 to 1 inch
Route	Topical
Pediatric Dosage	Not indicated

✳ Nitroglycerin Spray (Nitrolingual Spray)

Class	Antianginal
Actions	Smooth muscle relaxant
	Decreases cardiac work
	Dilates coronary arteries
	Dilates systemic arteries
Indications	Angina pectoris
	Chest pain associated with myocardial infarction
Contraindication	Hypotension
Precautions	Constantly monitor vital signs
	Syncope can occur
Side Effects	Dizziness
	Hypotension
	Headache

Dosage	One spray administered under the tongue; may be repeated in 3–5 minutes; no more than three sprays in 15-minute period; spray should not be inhaled
Route	Sprayed under tongue on mucous membrane
Pediatric Dosage	Not indicated

✳ Nitrous Oxide (Nitronox, Entonox)

Class	Gas
Action	Central nervous system depressant
Indications	Pain of musculoskeletal origin, particularly fractures
	Burns
	Suspected ischemic chest pain
	States of severe anxiety including hyperventilation
Contraindications	Patients who cannot comprehend verbal instructions
	Patients intoxicated with alcohol or drugs
	Head-injury patients who exhibit an altered mental status
	Chronic obstructive pulmonary disease; increased oxygen concentration may cause respiratory depression
	Thoracic injury suspicious of pneumothorax
	Abdominal pain and distension suggestive of bowel obstruction
Precautions	Use only in well-ventilated area
	Gas-scavenging system is recommended
	May not operate properly at low temperatures
Side Effects	Headache
	Dizziness
	Giddiness
	Nausea
	Vomiting
Dosage	Self-administered only using fixed 50 percent nitrous oxide and 50 percent oxygen blender
Route	Inhalation only
Pediatric Dosage	Self-administered only

✳ Norepinephrine (Levophed)

Class	Sympathomimetic
Action	Causes peripheral vasoconstriction
Indications	Hypotension (systolic blood pressure <70 mmHg refractory to other sympathomimetics)
	Neurogenic shock

Contraindication	Hypotensive states due to hypovolemia
Precautions	Can be deactivated by alkaline solutions
	Constant monitoring of blood pressure is essential
	Extravasation can cause tissue necrosis
Side Effects	Anxiety
	Palpitations
	Headache
	Hypertension
Dosage	0.5–30 µg/min
	Method: 8 mg should be placed in 500 mL of D_5W, giving a concentration of 16 µg/mL
Route	IV drip only
Pediatric Dosage	0.01–0.5 µg/kg/min (rarely used)

✳ Olanzapine (Zyprexia, Zyprexia Zydis)

Class	Atypical antipsychotic
Action	Sedative
	Antipsychotic
Indication	Acute psychosis
Contraindication	Patients with known hypersensitivity to the drug
Precaution	Patients with cardiovascular disease
Side Effects	Myalgias
	Somnolence
	Dizziness
	Postural hypotension
Dosage	5–15 mg PO
Route	PO (rapidly dissolving)
Pediatric Dosage	Not indicated

✳ Oxygen

Class	Gas
Action	Necessary for cellular metabolism
Indication	Hypoxia
Contraindications	None
Precautions	Use cautiously in patients with chronic obstructive pulmonary disease (COPD)
	Humidify when providing high-flow rates
Side Effect	Drying of mucous membranes
Dosage	*Cardiac arrest:* 100 percent
	Other critical patients: 100 percent
	COPD: 35 percent (increase as needed)
Route	Inhalation
Pediatric Dosage	24–100 percent as required

✳ Oxytocin (Pitocin)

Class	Hormone (oxytocic)
Actions	Causes uterine contraction
	Causes lactation
	Slows postpartum vaginal bleeding
Indication	Postpartum vaginal bleeding
Contraindications	Any condition other than postpartum bleeding
	Cesarean section
Precautions	Essential to ensure that the placenta has delivered and that there is not another fetus before administering oxytocin
	Overdosage can cause uterine rupture
	Hypertension
Side Effects	Anaphylaxis
	Cardiac dysrhythmias
Dosage	*Intravenous:* 10–20 units in 500 mL of D_5W administered according to uterine response
	Intramuscular: 3–10 units
Routes	IV drip, IM
Pediatric Dosage	Not indicated

✳ Pancuronium Bromide (Pavulon)

Class	Neuromuscular-blocking agent (nondepolarizing)
Actions	Skeletal muscle relaxant
	Paralyzes skeletal muscles including respiratory muscles
Indication	To achieve paralysis to facilitate endotracheal intubation
Contraindication	Patients with known hypersensitivity to the drug
Precautions	Should not be administered unless persons skilled in endotracheal intubation are present
	Endotracheal intubation equipment must be available
	Oxygen equipment and emergency resuscitative drugs must be available
	Paralysis occurs within 3–5 minutes and lasts for approximately 60 minutes
Side Effects	Prolonged paralysis
	Hypotension
	Bradycardia
Dosage	0.04–0.1 mg/kg; repeat doses of 0.01–0.02 mg/kg intravenously as required every 20–40 minutes
Route	IV
Pediatric Dosage	0.1 mg/kg

✳ Phenobarbitol (Luminal)

Class	Barbiturate
Actions	Suppresses spread of seizure activity through the motor cortex
	Central nervous system depressant
Indications	Major motor seizures
	Status epilepticus
	Acute anxiety states
Contraindication	History of hypersensitivity to the drug
Precautions	Respiratory depression
	Hypotension
	Can cause hyperactivity in children
	Extravasation may cause tissue necrosis
Side Effects	Drowsiness
	Children may become hyperactive
Dosage	100–250 mg
Routes	IV slowly, IM
Pediatric Dosage	10 mg/kg

✳ Phenytoin (Dilantin)

Class	Anticonvulsant and antidysrhythmic
Actions	Inhibits spread of seizure activity through motor cortex
	Antidysrhythmic
Indications	Major motor seizures
	Status epilepticus
	Dysrhythmias due to digitalis toxicity
Contraindications	Any dysrhythmia except those due to digitalis toxicity
	High-grade heart blocks
	Patients with history of hypersensitivity to the drug
Precautions	Should not be administered with glucose solutions
	Hypotension
	Electrocardiogram (ECG) monitoring during administration is essential
Side Effects	Local venous irritation
	Itching
	Central nervous system (CNS) depression
Dosage	*Status epilepticus:* 150–250 mg (10–15 mg/kg) not to exceed 50 mg/min
	Digitalis toxicity: 100 mg over 5 minutes until the dysrhythmia is suppressed or until a maximum dose of 1000 mg has been administered or symptoms of CNS depression occur
Route	IV (dilute with saline)
Pediatric Dosage	*Status epilepticus:* 8–10 mg/kg IV
	Digitalis toxicity: 3–5 mg/kg IV over 100 minutes

Physotigmine (Antilirium)

Class	Cholinesterase inhibitor
Actions	Inhibits cholinesterase
	Potentiates acetylcholine
Indications	Tricyclic antidepressant overdoses (Elavil, Tofranil, Triavil, Norpramin)
	Atropine (belladonna) overdoses
Contraindications	Asthma and chronic obstructive pulmonary disease
	Gangrene
	Diabetes
	Cardiovascular disease
Precautions	Monitor for bronchospasm and laryngospasm
	Seizures
Side Effects	Excessive salivation
	Bradycardia
	Emesis
Dosage	0.5–2.0 mg
Route	IV
Pediatric Dosage	0.5–1.0 mg over 5 minutes

Pralidoxime (2-Pam, Protopam)

Class	Cholinesterase reactivator
Actions	Reactivates cholinesterase in cases of organophosphate poisoning
	Deactivates certain organophosphates by direct chemical reaction
Indications	Severe organophosphate poisoning as characterized by muscle twitching, respiratory depression, and paralysis
Contraindications	Poisonings due to inorganic phosphates
	Poisonings other than organophosphates
Precautions	Always ensure safety and protection of rescue personnel
	Laryngospasm, tachycardia, and muscle rigidity have occurred following rapid administration
	Should only follow atropinization
Side Effects	Excitement
	Manic behavior
Dosage	1–2 g in 250–500 mL of normal saline infused over 30 minutes
Route	IV drip
Pediatric Dosage	20–40 mg/kg by the same method

✴ Procainamide (Pronestyl)

Class	Antidysrhythmic
Actions	Slows conduction through myocardium
	Elevates ventricular fibrillation threshold
	Suppresses ventricular ectopic activity
Indications	Persistent cardiac arrest due to ventricular fibrillation and refractory to lidocaine
	PVCs refractory to lidocaine
	Ventricular tachycardia refractory to lidocaine
Contraindications	High-degree heart blocks
	PVCs in conjunction with bradycardia
Precautions	Dosage should not exceed 17 mg/kg
	Monitor for central nervous system toxicity
Side Effects	Anxiety
	Nausea
	Convulsions
	Widening of QRS complex
Dosage	*Initial:* 20 mg/min until dysrhythmia is abolished, hypotension ensues, QRS complex is widened by 50 percent of original width, or total of 1.7 mg/kg has been given
	Maintenance: 1–4 mg/min
Routes	Slow IV bolus, IV drip
Pediatric Dosage	Rarely used

✴ Prochlorperazine (Compazine)

Class	Phenothiazine antiemetic
Action	Antiemetic
Indications	Nausea and vomiting
	Acute psychosis
Contraindications	Comatose states
	Patients who have received a large amount of depressants (including alcohol)
	Patients with a history of hypersensitivity to the drug
Precaution	Extrapyramidal (dystonic) symptoms have been reported
Side Effects	May impair mental and physical ability
	Drowsiness
Dosage	5–10 mg slow IV or IM
Routes	IV, IM
Pediatric Dosage	Not recommended

✳ Promethazine (Phenergan)

Class	Phenothiazine antihistamine (H_1 antagonist)
Actions	Mild anticholinergic activity
	Antiemetic
	Potentiates actions of analgesics
Indications	Nausea and vomiting
	Motion sickness
	To potentiate the effects of analgesics
	Sedation
Contraindications	Comatose states
	Patients who have received a large amount of depressants (including alcohol)
Precaution	Avoid accidental intraarterial injection
Side Effects	May impair mental and physical ability
	Drowsiness
Dosage	12.5–25.0 mg
Routes	IV, IM
Pediatric Dosage	0.5 mg/kg

✳ Propranolol (Inderal)

Class	Sympathetic blocker
Action	Nonselectively blocks β-adrenergic receptors
Indications	Ventricular tachydysrhythmias refractory to lidocaine and bretylium
	Recurrent ventricular fibrillation refractory to lidocaine and bretylium
	Tachydysrhythmias due to digitalis toxicity
Contraindications	Asthma and chronic obstructive pulmonary disease
	Patients dependent on sympathetic agonists
	Congestive heart failure
Precautions	Should not be given concurrently with verapamil
	Atropine and transcutaneous pacing should be readily available
Side Effects	Bradycardia
	Heart blocks
	Congestive heart failure
	Bronchospasm
Dosage	1–3 mg diluted in 10–30 mL of D_5W given slowly IV
Route	Slow IV bolus
Pediatric Dosage	0.01 mg/kg

✳ Racemic Epinephrine (MicroNEFRIN)

Class	Sympathomimetic
Actions	Bronchodilation
	Increases heart rate
	Increases cardiac contractile force
Indication	Croup (laryngotracheobronchitis)
Contraindications	Epiglottitis
	Hypersensitivity to the drug
Precautions	Vital signs should be constantly monitored
	Should be used only once in the prehospital setting
Side Effects	Palpitations
	Anxiety
	Headache
Dosage	0.25–0.75 mL of a 2.25 percent solution in 2.0 mL normal saline
Route	Inhalation only (small-volume nebulizer)
Pediatric Dosage	0.25–0.75 mL of a 2.25 percent solution in 2.0 mL normal saline

✳ Retaplase (Retavase)

Class	Fibrinolytic
Action	Increases plasmin by increasing the conversion of plasminogen
Indication	Acute myocardial infarction
Contraindications	Retaplase is absolutely contraindicated in the following cases:

1. Active internal bleeding
2. Suspected aortic dissection
3. Traumatic CPR (rib fractures, pneumothorax)
4. Severe, persistent hypertension
5. Recent head trauma or known intracranial tumor
6. History of stroke in the past 6 months
7. Pregnancy

It is relatively contraindicated in the following cases:

1. History of trauma or major surgery in the last 2 months
2. Initial blood pressure greater than 180 systolic or 110 diastolic that is controlled by medical treatment
3. Active peptic ulcer disease or blood in stool
4. History of stroke, tumor, brain surgery, or head injury
5. Known bleeding disorder of current use of warfarin (Coumadin)
6. Significant liver dysfunction or kidney failure

7. Known cancer of illness with possible thoracic, abdominal, or intracranial abnormalities

8. Prolonged CPR

Precautions	Emergency resuscitative drugs and equipment should be immediately available
	Antidysrhythmic medications should be readily available
Side Effects	Bleeding
	Allergic reactions
	Fever
	Nausea and vomiting
Dosage	10 units IV over 2 minutes. Repeat 10 units IV (over 2 minutes) in 30 minutes (20 units total)
Route	IV
Pediatric Dosage	Not indicated

✳ Rocuronium Bromide (Zemuron)

Class	Nondepolarizing neuromuscular blocker
Action	Prevents neuromuscular transmission by blocking the effect of acetylcholine
	Skeletal muscle paralysis
Indication	Induction of skeletal muscle paralysis
Contraindication	Hypersensitivity to the drug
Precautions	Underlying cardiovascular disease
	Dehydration or electrolyte abnormalities
Side Effect	Bronchospasm
Dosage	*Initial dose rapid-sequence induction:* 600 µg/kg
	Maintenance dose: 100–200 µg/kg continuous infusion
Route	IV, IV drip
Pediatric Dosage	*Initial dose:* 600 µg/kg
	Maintenance dose: 75–125 µg/kg continuous infusion

✳ Salbutamol (Ventolin)

Class	Sympathomimetic (β_2 selective)
Action	Bronchodilation
Indications	Asthma
	Reversible bronchospasm associated with chronic obstructive pulmonary disease
Contraindications	Known hypersensitivity to the drug
	Symptomatic tachycardia
Precautions	Blood pressure, pulse, and electrocardiogram (ECG) results should be monitored
	Use caution in patients with known heart disease

Side Effects	Palpitations
	Anxiety
	Headache
	Dizziness
	Sweating
Dosage	*Metered-dose inhaler:* One to two sprays (90 μg per spray)
	Small-volume nebulizer: 0.5 mL (2.5 mg) in 2.5 mL normal saline over 5–15 minutes
	Rotohaler: One 200 μg Rotocap should be placed in the inhaler and breathed by the patient
Route	Inhalation
Pediatric Dosage	0.15 mg/kg (0.03 mL/kg) in 2.5 mL normal saline by small-volume nebulizer

✺ Sodium Bicarbonate

Class	Alkalinizing agent
Actions	Combines with excessive acids to form a weak volatile acid
	Increases pH
Indications	Late in the management of cardiac arrest, if at all
	Tricyclic antidepressant overdose
	Severe acidosis refractory to hyperventilation
Contraindication	Alkalotic states
Precautions	Correct dosage is essential to avoid overcompensation of pH
	Can deactivate catecholamines
	Can precipitate with calcium
	Delivers large sodium load
Side Effect	Alkalosis
Dosage	1 mEq/kg initially followed by 0.5 mEq/kg every 10 minutes as indicated by blood gas studies
Route	IV
Pediatric Dosage	1 mEq/kg initially followed by 0.5 mEq/kg every 10 minutes

✺ Sodium Nitrite

Class	Nitrate/cyanide antidote
Action	Converts hemoglobin to methemoglobin for treatment of cyanide poisoning
Indication	Cyanide poisoning
Contraindication	Should not be administered to asymptomatic individuals
Precaution	Hypotension common with rapid IV administration
Side Effects	Exessive methemoglobinemia
	Hypotension

Dosage	300 mg IV; half-original dose repeated as needed (every 30 minutes) or if initial dose is ineffective
Route	IV
Pediatric Dosage	10 mg/kg IV; half-original dose repeated as needed (every 30 minutes) or if initial dose is ineffective

Sodium Nitroprusside (Nipride, Nitropress)

Class	Potent vasodilator
Actions	Peripheral arterial and venous vasodilator
	Decreases blood pressure
	Increases cardiac output in congestive heart failure
Indication	Hypertensive emergency
Contraindications	None when used in the management of life-threatening emergencies
Precautions	Bottle must be wrapped in foil to protect from light
	Should not be administered to children or pregnant women in the prehospital setting
	Reduce the dosage in elderly patients
	Blood pressure, pulse, and electrocardiogram (ECG) results must be diligently monitored
Side Effects	Nausea
	Retching
	Vomiting
	Palpitations
	Diaphoresis
	Tachycardia
	Dizziness
	Side effects often diminish as dosage is reduced
Dosage	0.5 mg/kg/min
Route	IV infusion only
Pediatric Dosage	Not indicated in prehospital setting

Sodium Thiosulfate

Class	Cyanide antidote
Action	Converts cyanide to thiocyanate where it can be eliminated by the body
Indication	Cyanide poisoning
Contraindication	None in the setting of cyanide poisoning
Precautions	None in the setting of cyanide poisoning
Side Effects	Nausea
	Vomiting
	Arthralgias
	Psychosis
Dosage	12.5 g IV; half-original dose repeated as needed
Route	IV
Pediatric Dosage	400 mg/kg IV; half-original dose repeated as needed

✳ Sotalol HCL (Betapace, Sotacor)

Class	Antidysrhythmic (group II) and β-adrenergic-blocking agent (nonselective)
Actions	Blocks stimulation of β_1 (myocardial) and β_2 (pulmonary, vascular, and uterine) adrenergic receptor sites
	Suppression of dysrhythmias
Indication	Management of life-threatening ventricular dysrhythmias
Contraindications	Uncompensated congestive heart failure
	Pulmonary edema
	Cardiogenic shock
	Bradycardia or heart block
Precautions	Renal impairment
	Hepatic impairment
Side Effects	Fatigue
	Weakness
	Anxiety
	Dizziness
	Drowsiness
	Insomnia
	Memory loss
	Mental depression
	Mental status changes
	Nervousness
	Nightmares
Dosage	80 mg twice daily; may be gradually increased to 160–320 mg/day in two to three divided doses up to 480–640 mg/day
Route	Oral
Pediatric Dosage	Not indicated

✳ Streptokinase (Strepase)

Class	Fibrinolytic
Action	Dissolves blood clots
Indication	Acute myocardial infarction
Contraindications	Persons with internal bleeding
	Suspected aortic dissection
	Traumatic cardiopulmonary resuscitation
	Severe persistent hypertension
	Recent head trauma or known intracranial tumor
	History of stroke in the past 6 months
	Pregnancy
Precautions	May be ineffective if administered within 12 months of prior streptokinase or anistreplase therapy
	Antidysrhythmic and resuscitative drugs should be available

Side Effects	Bleeding
	Allergic reactions
	Anaphylaxis
	Fever
	Nausea and vomiting
Dosage	1.5 million units over 1 hour
Route	IV drip
Pediatric Dosage	Not recommended

Succinylcholine (Anectine)

Class	Neuromuscular blocking agent (depolarizing)
Actions	Skeletal muscle relaxant
	Paralyzes skeletal muscles, including respiratory muscles
Indication	To achieve paralysis to facilitate endotracheal intubation
Contraindication	Patients with known hypersensitivity to the drug
Precautions	Should not be administered unless persons skilled in endotracheal intubation are present
	Endotracheal intubation equipment must be available
	Oxygen equipment and emergency resuscitative drugs must be available
	Paralysis occurs within 1 minute and lasts for approximately 8 minutes
Side Effects	Prolonged paralysis
	Hypotension
	Bradycardia
Dosage	1–1.5 mg/kg (40–100 mg in an adult)
Route	IV
Pediatric Dosage	1 mg/kg

Terbutaline (Brethine)

Class	Sympathomimetic
Actions	Bronchodilator
	Increases heart rate
Indications	Bronchial asthma
	Reversible bronchospasm associated with chronic obstructive pulmonary disease
	Preterm labor
Contraindication	Patients with known hypersensitivity to the drug
Precautions	Blood pressure, pulse, and electrocardiogram (ECG) results must be constantly monitored
Side Effects	Palpitations
	Tachycardia
	Premature ventricular contractions

Anxiety

Tremors

Headache

Dosage	*Metered-dose inhaler:* Two inhalations, 1 minute apart
	Subcutaneous injection: 0.25 mg; may be repeated in 15–30 minutes
Routes	Inhalation, Subcutaneous injection, IV drip (in preterm labor)
Pediatric Dosage	0.01 mg/kg subcutaneously

✳ Thiamine (Vitamin B₁)

Class	Vitamin
Action	Allows normal breakdown of glucose
Indications	Coma of unknown origin
	Alcoholism
	Delirium tremens
Contraindications	None in the emergency setting
Precautions	Rare anaphylactic reactions have been reported
	Should not be used as part of a "coma cocktail"
Side Effects	Rare, if any
Dosage	100 mg
Routes	IV, IM
Pediatric Dosage	Rarely indicated

✳ Tissue Plasminogen Activator (tPA, Activase)

Class	Fibrinolytic
Action	Dissolves blood clots
Indication	Acute myocardial infarction
Contraindications	Persons with internal bleeding
	Suspected aortic dissection
	Traumatic cardiopulmonary resuscitation
	Severe persistent hypertension
	Recent head trauma or known intracranial tumor
	History of stroke in the past 6 months
	Pregnancy
Precautions	Antidysrhythmic and resuscitative drugs should be available
Side Effects	Bleeding
	Allergic reactions
	Anaphylaxis
	Fever
	Nausea and vomiting
Dosage	*Front-loaded regimen:* 15 mg IV bolus over 1–2 minutes, followed by infusion of 50 mg over

the first hour and 35 mg over the second hour (total dose 100 mg)

Standard regimen: 10 mg IV bolus over 1–2 minutes, followed by 50 mg over the first hour, 20 mg over the second hour, and 20 mg over the third hour

Route	IV (slow) and IV infusion
Pediatric Dosage	Not recommended

✴ Trimethobenzamide (Tigan)

Class	Antiemetic
Action	Antiemetic with fewer sedative effects than other common antiemetic drugs
Indication	Nausea and vomiting
Contraindications	Children (injectable form only)
	Patients with a history of hypersensitivity to the drug
Precaution	Extrapyramidal (dystonic) symptoms have been reported
Side Effects	May impair mental and physical ability
	Drowsiness
Dosage	200 mg IM
Route	IM
Pediatric Dosage	Parenteral administration not recommended

✴ Vasopressin

Class	Hormone, vasconstrictor
Actions	Antidiuretic hormone
	Potent vasoconstrictor
Indication	Caridiac arrest
Contraindication	None when used in the emergency setting
Precautions	Few in emergency setting
Side Effects	Blanching of skin
	Hypertension
	Bradycardia
Dosage	40 units IV (single dose only)
Route	IV
Pediatric Dosage	Not indicated

✴ Vecuronium (Norcuron)

Class	Neuromuscular-blocking agent (nondepolarizing)
Action	Skeletal muscle relaxant
	Paralyzes skeletal muscles including respiratory muscles

Indication	To achieve paralysis to facilitate endotracheal intubation
Contraindication	Patients with known hypersensitivity to the drug
Precautions	Should not be administered unless persons skilled in endotracheal intubation are present
	Endotracheal intubation equipment must be available
	Oxygen equipment and emergency resuscitative drugs must be available
	Paralysis occurs within 1 minute and lasts for approximately 30 minutes
Side Effects	Prolonged paralysis
	Hypotension
	Bradycardia
Dosage	0.08–0.1 mg/kg
Route	IV
Pediatric Dosage	0.1 mg/kg

✳ Verapamil (Isoptin, Calan)

Class	Calcium channel blocker
Actions	Slows conduction through the atrioventricular node
	Inhibits reentry during paroxysmol supraventricular tachycardia (PSVT)
	Decreases rate of ventricular response
	Decreases myocardial oxygen demand
Indication	PSVT
Contraindications	Heart block
	Conduction system disturbances
Precautions	Should not be used in patients receiving intravenous β-blockers
	Hypotension
Side Effects	Nausea
	Vomiting
	Hypotension
	Dizziness
Dosage	2.5–5 mg; a repeat dose of 5–10 mg can be administered after 15–30 minutes if PSVT does not convert; maximum dose is 30 mg in 30 minutes
Route	Intravenous
Pediatric Dosage	*0–1 year:* 0.1–0.2 mg/kg (maximum of 2.0 mg) administered slowly
	1–15 years: 0.1–0.3 mg/kg (maximum of 5.0 mg) administered slowly

✳ Ziprasidone (Geodon)

Class	Atypical antipsychotic
Actions	Sedative
	Antipsychotic
Indication	Acute psychosis
Contraindications	Patients with known hypersensitivity to the drug
	Patients with prolonged QT syndrome
Precautions	History of seizures
	Stroke
	Alzheimer's disease
Side Effects	Myalgias
	Somnolence
	Dizziness
	Postural hypotension
Dosage	10–20 mg IM
Route	IM
Pediatric Dosage	Not indicated

ADULT ADVANCED CARDIAC LIFE SUPPORT ALGORITHMS

Bradycardia Algorithm

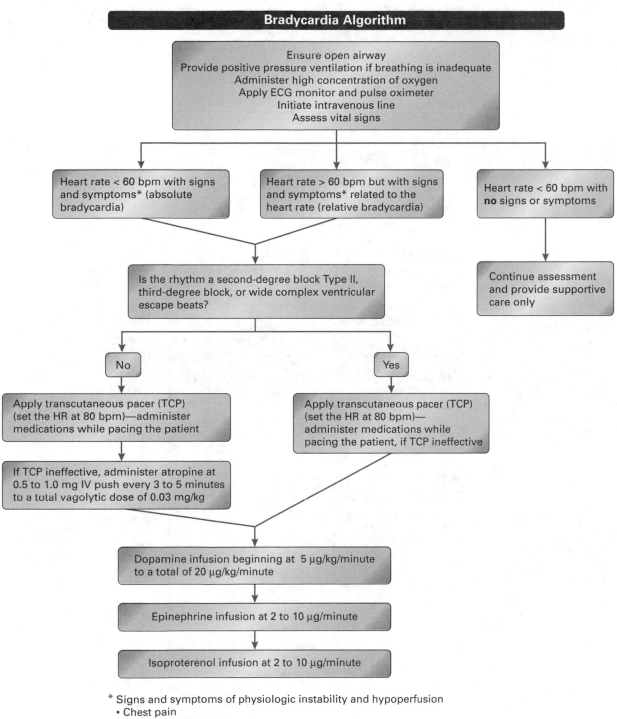

Ensure open airway
Provide positive pressure ventilation if breathing is inadequate
Administer high concentration of oxygen
Apply ECG monitor and pulse oximeter
Initiate intravenous line
Assess vital signs

Heart rate < 60 bpm with signs and symptoms* (absolute bradycardia)

Heart rate > 60 bpm but with signs and symptoms* related to the heart rate (relative bradycardia)

Heart rate < 60 bpm with no signs or symptoms

Continue assessment and provide supportive care only

Is the rhythm a second-degree block Type II, third-degree block, or wide complex ventricular escape beats?

No

Yes

Apply transcutaneous pacer (TCP) (set the HR at 80 bpm)—administer medications while pacing the patient

Apply transcutaneous pacer (TCP) (set the HR at 80 bpm)—administer medications while pacing the patient, if TCP ineffective

If TCP ineffective, administer atropine at 0.5 to 1.0 mg IV push every 3 to 5 minutes to a total vagolytic dose of 0.03 mg/kg

Dopamine infusion beginning at 5 µg/kg/minute to a total of 20 µg/kg/minute

Epinephrine infusion at 2 to 10 µg/minute

Isoproterenol infusion at 2 to 10 µg/minute

* Signs and symptoms of physiologic instability and hypoperfusion
- Chest pain
- Shortness of breath
- Decreased mental status
- Hypotension
- Evidence of poor perfusion and shock
- Weakness and fatigue
- Lightheadedness
- Syncope
- Diaphoresis
- Pulmonary congestion (crackles or rales)
- PVCs
- Acute myocardial infarction

Adult Advanced Cardiac Life Support Algorithms

Tachycardia Algorithm

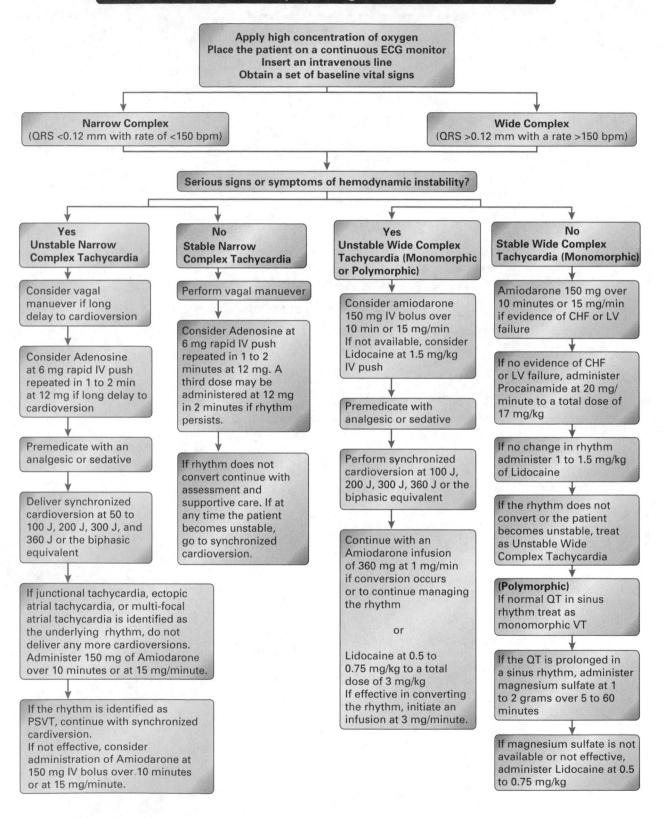

Apply high concentration of oxygen
Place the patient on a continuous ECG monitor
Insert an intravenous line
Obtain a set of baseline vital signs

Narrow Complex
(QRS <0.12 mm with rate of <150 bpm)

Wide Complex
(QRS >0.12 mm with a rate >150 bpm)

Serious signs or symptoms of hemodynamic instability?

Yes
Unstable Narrow Complex Tachycardia

Consider vagal manuever if long delay to cardioversion

Consider Adenosine at 6 mg rapid IV push repeated in 1 to 2 min at 12 mg if long delay to cardioversion

Premedicate with an analgesic or sedative

Deliver synchronized cardioversion at 50 to 100 J, 200 J, 300 J, and 360 J or the biphasic equivalent

If junctional tachycardia, ectopic atrial tachycardia, or multi-focal atrial tachycardia is identified as the underlying rhythm, do not deliver any more cardioversions. Administer 150 mg of Amiodarone over 10 minutes or at 15 mg/minute.

If the rhythm is identified as PSVT, continue with synchronized cardioversion.
If not effective, consider administration of Amiodarone at 150 mg IV bolus over 10 minutes or at 15 mg/minute.

No
Stable Narrow Complex Tachycardia

Perform vagal manuever

Consider Adenosine at 6 mg rapid IV push repeated in 1 to 2 minutes at 12 mg. A third dose may be administered at 12 mg in 2 minutes if rhythm persists.

If rhythm does not convert continue with assessment and supportive care. If at any time the patient becomes unstable, go to synchronized cardioversion.

Yes
Unstable Wide Complex Tachycardia (Monomorphic or Polymorphic)

Consider amiodarone 150 mg IV bolus over 10 min or 15 mg/min
If not available, consider Lidocaine at 1.5 mg/kg IV push

Premedicate with analgesic or sedative

Perform synchronized cardioversion at 100 J, 200 J, 300 J, 360 J or the biphasic equivalent

Continue with an Amiodarone infusion of 360 mg at 1 mg/min if conversion occurs or to continue managing the rhythm

or

Lidocaine at 0.5 to 0.75 mg/kg to a total dose of 3 mg/kg
If effective in converting the rhythm, initiate an infusion at 3 mg/minute.

No
Stable Wide Complex Tachycardia (Monomorphic)

Amiodarone 150 mg over 10 minutes or 15 mg/min if evidence of CHF or LV failure

If no evidence of CHF or LV failure, administer Procainamide at 20 mg/minute to a total dose of 17 mg/kg

If no change in rhythm administer 1 to 1.5 mg/kg of Lidocaine

If the rhythm does not convert or the patient becomes unstable, treat as Unstable Wide Complex Tachycardia

(Polymorphic)
If normal QT in sinus rhythm treat as monomorphic VT

If the QT is prolonged in a sinus rhythm, administer magnesium sulfate at 1 to 2 grams over 5 to 60 minutes

If magnesium sulfate is not available or not effective, administer Lidocaine at 0.5 to 0.75 mg/kg

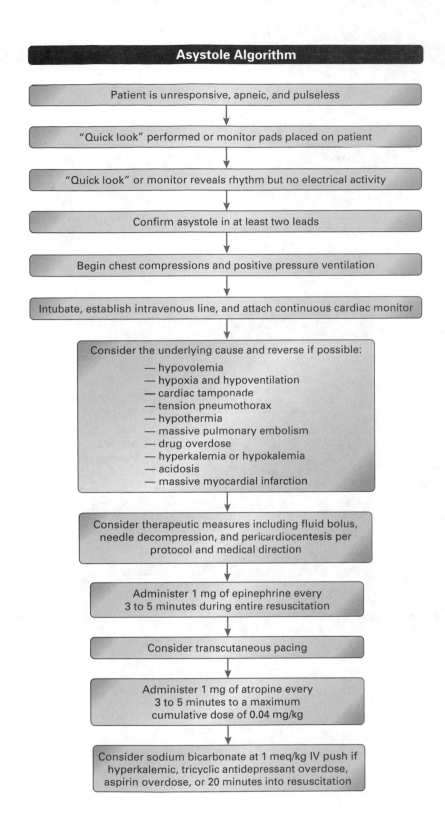

Asystole Algorithm

Patient is unresponsive, apneic, and pulseless

"Quick look" performed or monitor pads placed on patient

"Quick look" or monitor reveals rhythm but no electrical activity

Confirm asystole in at least two leads

Begin chest compressions and positive pressure ventilation

Intubate, establish intravenous line, and attach continuous cardiac monitor

Consider the underlying cause and reverse if possible:

— hypovolemia
— hypoxia and hypoventilation
— cardiac tamponade
— tension pneumothorax
— hypothermia
— massive pulmonary embolism
— drug overdose
— hyperkalemia or hypokalemia
— acidosis
— massive myocardial infarction

Consider therapeutic measures including fluid bolus, needle decompression, and pericardiocentesis per protocol and medical direction

Administer 1 mg of epinephrine every 3 to 5 minutes during entire resuscitation

Consider transcutaneous pacing

Administer 1 mg of atropine every 3 to 5 minutes to a maximum cumulative dose of 0.04 mg/kg

Consider sodium bicarbonate at 1 meq/kg IV push if hyperkalemic, tricyclic antidepressant overdose, aspirin overdose, or 20 minutes into resuscitation

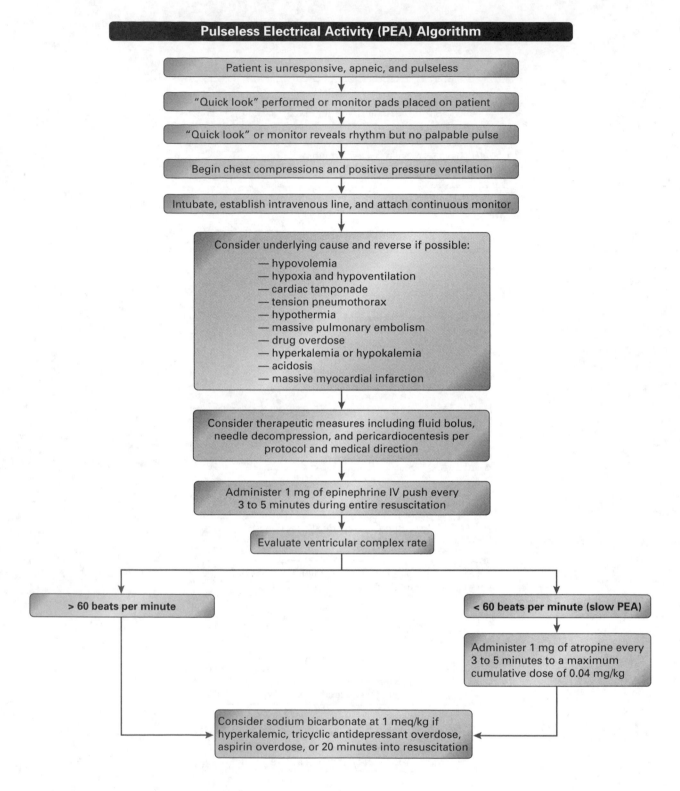

Pulseless Electrical Activity (PEA) Algorithm

Patient is unresponsive, apneic, and pulseless

"Quick look" performed or monitor pads placed on patient

"Quick look" or monitor reveals rhythm but no palpable pulse

Begin chest compressions and positive pressure ventilation

Intubate, establish intravenous line, and attach continuous monitor

Consider underlying cause and reverse if possible:

— hypovolemia
— hypoxia and hypoventilation
— cardiac tamponade
— tension pneumothorax
— hypothermia
— massive pulmonary embolism
— drug overdose
— hyperkalemia or hypokalemia
— acidosis
— massive myocardial infarction

Consider therapeutic measures including fluid bolus, needle decompression, and pericardiocentesis per protocol and medical direction

Administer 1 mg of epinephrine IV push every 3 to 5 minutes during entire resuscitation

Evaluate ventricular complex rate

> 60 beats per minute

< 60 beats per minute (slow PEA)

Administer 1 mg of atropine every 3 to 5 minutes to a maximum cumulative dose of 0.04 mg/kg

Consider sodium bicarbonate at 1 meq/kg if hyperkalemic, tricyclic antidepressant overdose, aspirin overdose, or 20 minutes into resuscitation

Synchronized Cardioversion Algorithm

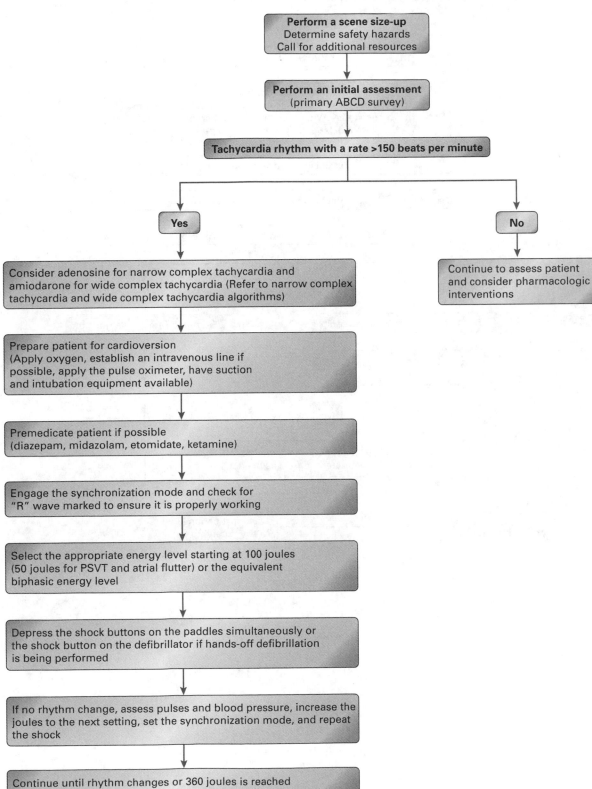

Perform a scene size-up
Determine safety hazards
Call for additional resources

Perform an initial assessment
(primary ABCD survey)

Tachycardia rhythm with a rate >150 beats per minute

Yes

No

Consider adenosine for narrow complex tachycardia and amiodarone for wide complex tachycardia (Refer to narrow complex tachycardia and wide complex tachycardia algorithms)

Continue to assess patient and consider pharmacologic interventions

Prepare patient for cardioversion
(Apply oxygen, establish an intravenous line if possible, apply the pulse oximeter, have suction and intubation equipment available)

Premedicate patient if possible
(diazepam, midazolam, etomidate, ketamine)

Engage the synchronization mode and check for "R" wave marked to ensure it is properly working

Select the appropriate energy level starting at 100 joules (50 joules for PSVT and atrial flutter) or the equivalent biphasic energy level

Depress the shock buttons on the paddles simultaneously or the shock button on the defibrillator if hands-off defibrillation is being performed

If no rhythm change, assess pulses and blood pressure, increase the joules to the next setting, set the synchronization mode, and repeat the shock

Continue until rhythm changes or 360 joules is reached

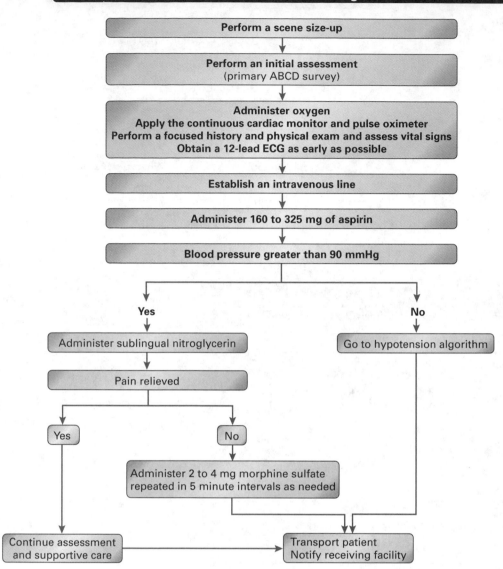

Acute Ischemic Chest Pain Algorithm

Perform a scene size-up

Perform an initial assessment
(primary ABCD survey)

Administer oxygen
Apply the continuous cardiac monitor and pulse oximeter
Perform a focused history and physical exam and assess vital signs
Obtain a 12-lead ECG as early as possible

Establish an intravenous line

Administer 160 to 325 mg of aspirin

Blood pressure greater than 90 mmHg

Yes → Administer sublingual nitroglycerin

No → Go to hypotension algorithm

Pain relieved

Yes → Continue assessment and supportive care

No → Administer 2 to 4 mg morphine sulfate repeated in 5 minute intervals as needed

Transport patient
Notify receiving facility

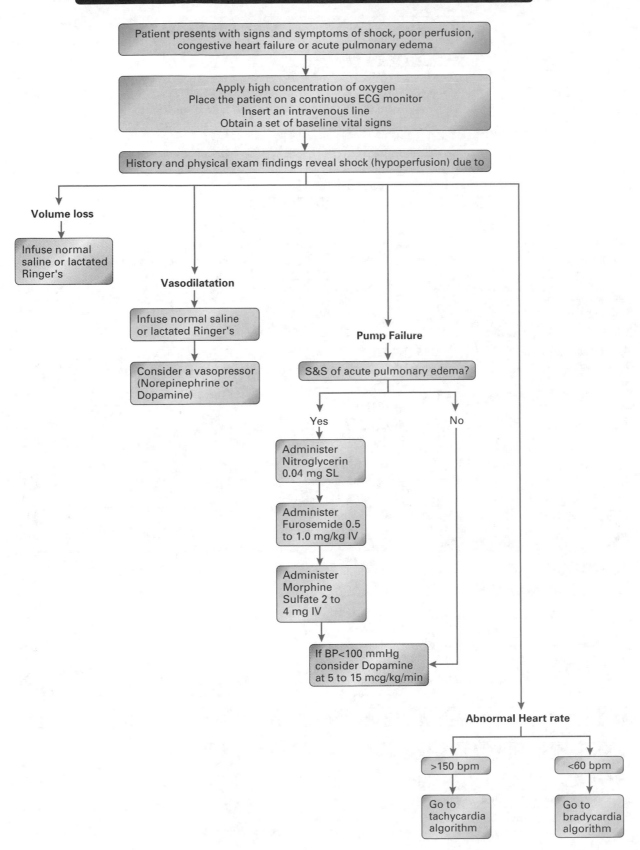

Shock/Hypotension/Acute Pulmonary Edema Algorithm

Patient presents with signs and symptoms of shock, poor perfusion, congestive heart failure or acute pulmonary edema

Apply high concentration of oxygen
Place the patient on a continuous ECG monitor
Insert an intravenous line
Obtain a set of baseline vital signs

History and physical exam findings reveal shock (hypoperfusion) due to

Volume loss

Infuse normal saline or lactated Ringer's

Vasodilatation

Infuse normal saline or lactated Ringer's

Consider a vasopressor (Norepinephrine or Dopamine)

Pump Failure

S&S of acute pulmonary edema?

Yes

No

Administer Nitroglycerin 0.04 mg SL

Administer Furosemide 0.5 to 1.0 mg/kg IV

Administer Morphine Sulfate 2 to 4 mg IV

If BP<100 mmHg consider Dopamine at 5 to 15 mcg/kg/min

Abnormal Heart rate

>150 bpm

<60 bpm

Go to tachycardia algorithm

Go to bradycardia algorithm

Adult Advanced Cardiac Life Support Algorithms

Ventricular Fibrillation/Pulseless Ventricular Tachycardia (VF/VT) Algorithm

Patient is unresponsive, apneic, and pulseless

↓

"Quick look" performed or monitor pads placed on patient

↓

"Quick look" or monitor reveals ventricular fibrillation or pulseless ventricular tachycardia

↓

Defibrillate at 200, 300, and 360 J or equivalent biphasic energy level

↓

Assess pulse and rhythm

Pulse absent ← → **Pulse present**

Pulse present
Assess breathing status
Assess rhythm
Treat patient according to post-resuscitation guidelines

Pulse absent

No change in rhythm

Change in rhythm
Go to appropriate algorithm or emergency cardiac care protocol (PEA or asystole)

No change in rhythm
Begin or resume chest compressions
Intubate patient
Establish intravenous line
Attach continuous monitor cables

↓

Administer
Epinephrine 1 mg IV push (repeat every 3 to 5 minutes for the entire resuscitation while patient is in cardiac arrest)
or
Vasopression 40 units IV push (administer only once followed by epinephrine in 10 to 20 minutes)

↓

Defibrillate
After 30 to 60 seconds at 360 J or biphasic equivalent after each drug bolus

→

Administer
*Amiodarone 300 mg IV push (repeat in 3 to 5 minutes at 150 mg IV push)

↓

Defibrillate
After 30 to 60 seconds at 360 J or biphasic equivalent after each drug bolus

↓

Administer
Lidocaine at 1.5 mg/kg IV push (repeat in 3 to 5 minutes at 1.5 mg/kg [1.0 to 1.5 mg/kg dose is acceptable with a repeat dose of 0.5 to 0.75 mg/kg]; total maximum cumulative dose is 3 mg/kg)

↓

Defibrillate
After 30 to 60 seconds at 360 J or biphasic equivalent after each drug bolus

↓

Consider administration of
- Procainamide at 50 mg/minute to a total dose of 17 mg/kg if VF/VT converts to another rhythm and then recurs
- Magnesium sulfate at 1 to 2 grams IV push if low magnesium levels are suspected (alcoholic, malnourished, hypomagnesemia) or torsades de pointes is rhythm
- Sodium bicarbonate 1 meq/kg IV push if hyperkalemia, tricyclic antidepressant overdose, aspirin overdose, or 20 minutes into the resuscitation attempt

↓

If at any time in algorithm rhythm changes, but patient remains pulseless and apneic, go to appropriate algorithm

↓

If at any time patient regains a pulse, assess breathing status, analyze the rhythm, continue with assessment, and administer an infusion of antidysrhythmic drug that was used just prior to the conversion as follows:
- Amiodarone: 360 mg IV infusion over 6 hours (1 mg/minute)
- Lidocaine: 1 to 4 mg/minute
- Procainamide: 1 to 4 mg/minute

*There is no evidence to suggest amiodarone has better discharge survival benefits in cardiac arrest over lidocaine; therefore, lidocaine can be used as a first-line antidysrhythmic drug prior to the administration of amiodarone.

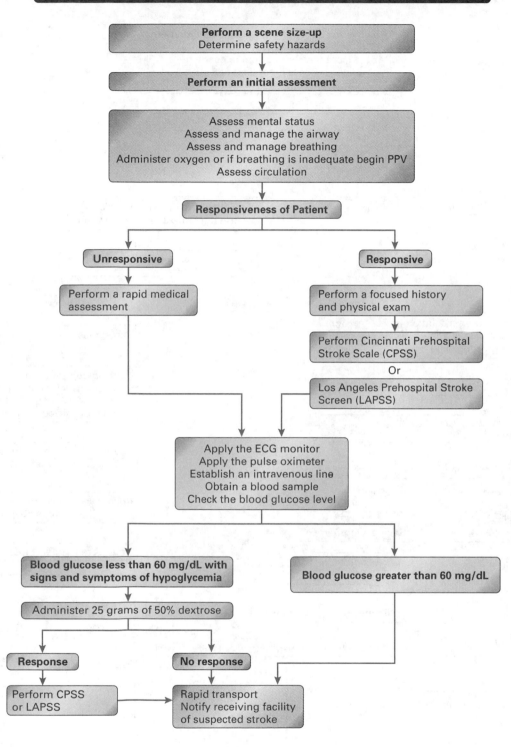

Suspected Stroke Algorithm

Perform a scene size-up
Determine safety hazards

Perform an initial assessment

Assess mental status
Assess and manage the airway
Assess and manage breathing
Administer oxygen or if breathing is inadequate begin PPV
Assess circulation

Responsiveness of Patient

Unresponsive

Perform a rapid medical assessment

Responsive

Perform a focused history and physical exam

Perform Cincinnati Prehospital Stroke Scale (CPSS)
Or
Los Angeles Prehospital Stroke Screen (LAPSS)

Apply the ECG monitor
Apply the pulse oximeter
Establish an intravenous line
Obtain a blood sample
Check the blood glucose level

Blood glucose less than 60 mg/dL with signs and symptoms of hypoglycemia

Administer 25 grams of 50% dextrose

Blood glucose greater than 60 mg/dL

Response

Perform CPSS or LAPSS

No response

Rapid transport
Notify receiving facility of suspected stroke

Hypothermia Algorithm

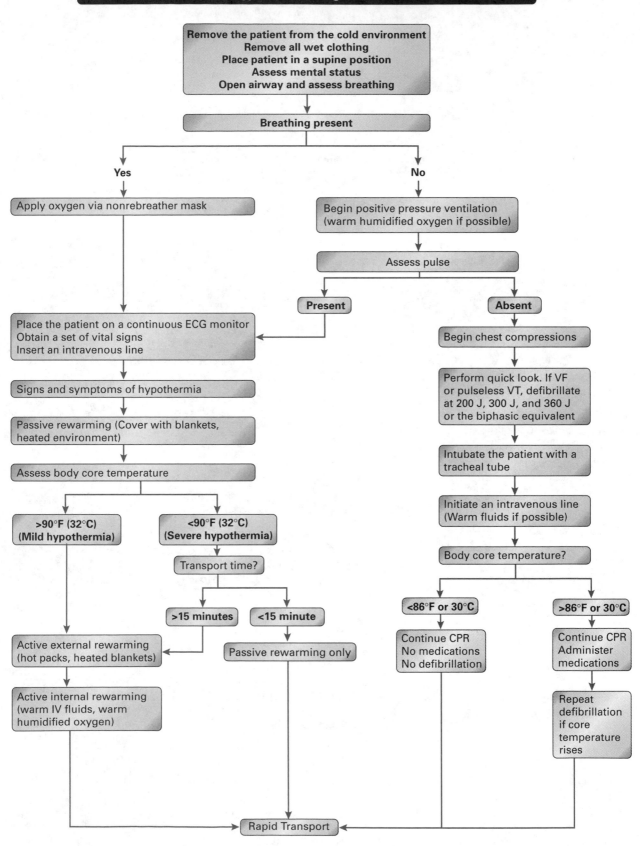

Remove the patient from the cold environment
Remove all wet clothing
Place patient in a supine position
Assess mental status
Open airway and assess breathing

↓

Breathing present

Yes → **No**

Yes: Apply oxygen via nonrebreather mask

No: Begin positive pressure ventilation (warm humidified oxygen if possible)

↓

Assess pulse

Present — **Absent**

Present → Place the patient on a continuous ECG monitor / Obtain a set of vital signs / Insert an intravenous line

↓

Signs and symptoms of hypothermia

↓

Passive rewarming (Cover with blankets, heated environment)

↓

Assess body core temperature

>90°F (32°C) (Mild hypothermia) — **<90°F (32°C) (Severe hypothermia)**

Severe: Transport time?

>15 minutes — **<15 minute**

>15 minutes: Active external rewarming (hot packs, heated blankets)

<15 minute: Passive rewarming only

Active external rewarming (hot packs, heated blankets) ↓ Active internal rewarming (warm IV fluids, warm humidified oxygen)

Absent: Begin chest compressions

↓

Perform quick look. If VF or pulseless VT, defibrillate at 200 J, 300 J, and 360 J or the biphasic equivalent

↓

Intubate the patient with a tracheal tube

↓

Initiate an intravenous line (Warm fluids if possible)

↓

Body core temperature?

<86°F or 30°C — **>86°F or 30°C**

<86°F or 30°C: Continue CPR / No medications / No defibrillation

>86°F or 30°C: Continue CPR / Administer medications

↓

Repeat defibrillation if core temperature rises

Rapid Transport

COMMON HOME PRESCRIPTION DRUG INFORMATION

The following information pertains to immediate prehospital emergencies. Some of these classifications cover a broad range of drugs. The information provided is very general and is intended only for use as a quick reference.

✳ Classification/Type

Type(s)	Therapeutic classification
Actions	The major mechanism or mechanisms of action and how the drug exerts its therapeutic effects
Indications	Condition or conditions for which the drugs are commonly prescribed
Adverse Effects	Any effect other than those that were therapeutically intended; usually undesirable, specific, and predictable; often a result of too much of the drug; may include any combination of those listed
Interactions	Presence of another drug or drugs may alter the effects of either drug or promote entirely different effects
How Supplied	Most common forms of the drug
Note	Miscellaneous relevant or nice-to-know information
Common Examples	A few examples (listed by trade name) of drugs in this class; when given, generic names are indicated by boldface type

✳ Antianginals

Type(s)	Nitrates and nitrites (primarily) (*see also* Beta-Blockers and Calcium Channel Blockers)

Actions	Nitrates and nitrites (coronary vasodilators)
	Vasodilation
	Decreases myocardial work and reduces MVO_2 by
	Reducing preload and afterload
	Improving coronary perfusion (including collateral)
	May relieve coronary vasospasm
Indications	Angina, acute myocardial infarction, congestive heart failure, and after myocardial infarction
	Coronary artery spasm and SVTs
	To increase exercise tolerance
Adverse Effects	*Cardiovascular system:* Hypotension, bradycardia, paradoxical angina, flushing, feeling of warmth, syncope, reflex tachycardia, palpitation, and possible reperfusion dysrhythmias (via relief of coronary vasospasm)
	Central nervous system: Transient or persistent headache, dizziness, weakness, and anxiety
	Other: N/V, may cause slight SL burning sensation
Interactions	Hypotensives, ETOH: May potentiate hypotension
How Supplied	Tablet, ointment or paste, aerosol, and transdermal patch
Note	These patients usually have coronary artery disease
	Tablets may lose potency within a few months
	Aerosols maintain potency for up to 3 years
	Tolerance and dependence may develop after prolonged use
	Paramedics should avoid (prolonged) contact with nitro paste (e.g., during chest compression) because it will be absorbed through their skin
	Canister should *not* be shaken; if it is, that dose is sprayed out and the next dose is administered to the patient

Common Examples		
	Cardilate	Nitrol
	Coronex	Nitrolingual spray
	Isordil	Nitrong
	Nitrobid	Nitrostablin
	Nitrogard	Nitrostat

✳ Anticoagulants

Type(s)	Warfarin or Coumadin derivatives
Actions	Decreases the ability of blood to clot:
	Prevents further extension of the clot
	Prolongs blood-clotting time
	May prevent clotting
Indications	Prophylaxis or treatment of blood clotting:
	Venous thrombosis, pulmonary embolism
	Adjunct in the treatment of coronary occlusion and transient ischemic accidents

	Home dialysis
	Recurrent problems with blood clots
	Treatment of embolization in A-fib
	Postfibrinolytic therapy
Adverse Effects	Hemorrhage (from any organ or tissue)
	Excessive bleeding from minor cuts, menstruation, or nosebleed
	Melena, petechiae
	N/V/D
Interactions	Salicylates, some antibiotics: May prolong clotting time and increase risk of hemorrhage
How Supplied	Tablet
Note	Also known as "blood thinners"
	Patients on home dialysis may take heparin intravenously
	Antiplatelet (e.g., aspirin Persantine) effects are similar to anticoagulant effects
Common Examples	Coumadin Minihep
	Hepalean Sintrom
	Heparin Warfilone

✳ ## Anticonvulsants

Type(s)	Benzodiazepines, barbiturates, hydantoins, and succinimides
Actions	Prevents and suppresses the spread of seizure activity in the motor cortex
	Elevates seizure threshold
	Skeletal muscle relaxation
Indications	Epilepsy
	Chronic seizures
	Generalized tonic-clonic seizures
	"Absence spells" seizures
	Simple partial, complex partial, or myoclonic seizures
Adverse Effects	*Cardiovascular system:* Hypotension and dysrhythmia
	Central nervous system: Respiratory depression, apnea, excessive central nervous system depression, ataxia, dizziness, drowsiness, fatigue, weakness, confusion, behavioral disturbances, sedation, coma, amnesia, irritability, nervousness, headache, tremor, and paradoxical seizure (from overdose)
	Other: N/V/D, anorexia, abdominal pain, indigestion, constipation, visual disturbances, and nystagmus
Interactions	Central nervous system depressants: Potentiate effects
How Supplied	Tablet, capsule, and syrup
Note	Many patients are on combination therapy

Common Examples	Celontin	Milontin
	Depakene	Mogadon
	Dilantin	Mysoline
	Epival	Rivotril
	Mebaral	Tegretol
	Mebroin	Zarontin
	Mesantoin	

✳ Antidepressants: Monoamine Oxidase Inhibitors

Type(s)	Monoamine oxidase inhibitors (psychotropics)
Actions	Affects mood and behavior:
	Blocks impulse transmission at the synapse
	Inhibits catecholamine breakdown
Indications	Moderate-severe depression (usually refractory to tricyclic antidepressants)
	Atypical depression and phobic disorders (drug of choice)
	Prevention of panic attacks
	Depressive disorders (atypical, neurotic, or reactive)
Adverse Effects	*Cardiovascular system:* Tachycardia, PVCs, VT, hypotension, and sweating
	Central nervous system: Respiratory depression, central nervous system depression, dizziness, headache, irritability, anxiety, paresthesia, tremor, seizure, coma, ataxia, fever, and insomnia
	Other: N/V, urine retention, constipation, stiff neck, and dry mouth
Interactions	Antihypertensives: May potentiate effects
	Sympathomimetics or tyramine-rich foods and drinks: May potentiate effects (may induce hypertensive crisis)
	Central nervous system depressants: May potentiate effects
How Supplied	Tablet
Note	Overdose effects may persist for days
Common Examples	Marplan Parnate
	Nardil

✳ Antidepressants: Tricyclic Antidepressants

Type(s)	Tricyclic antidepressants (psychotropics)
Actions	Mechanism of action is not exactly clear:
	Antidepressant effects
	Mild sedative effects
	Cholinergic blockade
	May inhibit catecholamine breakdown
	Peripheral α blockade

	Impairs cardiac depolarization and conduction (−) inotropy
Indications	Severe endogenous depression (drug of choice)
	Prevention of panic attacks
	Pain control (some benefit for patients with fibromyalgia)
Adverse Effects	*Cardiovascular system:* Orthostatic hypotension, bradycardia, (wide complex) tachycardia, dysrhythmia, PVCs, conduction defects (widened QRS complex, prolonged PR and QT intervals, ST and T wave abnormalities, and atrioventricular blocks) may precipitate congestive heart failure
	Central nervous system: Initially confusion, anxiety, sweating, ataxia, and vomiting are seen; may precipitate mania and psychosis. Later central nervous system depression, delirium, hallucinations, coma, muscle rigidity, seizure, respiratory depression, and apnea may be present
	Other: Anticholinergic effects (fever, hot flushed skin, dry mucous membranes, pupil dilation, urine retention) and anti-α effects (hypotension, sedation, cardiac depression)
Interactions	Sympathomimetics: May potentiate effects
	Central nervous system depressants: May potentiate effects
How Supplied	Tablet and capsule
Note	Ingestion of 1–2 g is potentially lethal and hard to treat
	Physostigmine (Antilirium), a cholinergic, may reverse some cholinergic symptoms
	Clinically related to phenothiazines
	Overdose effects may persist for days

Common Examples		
Adapin	Norpramin
Anafranil	Pamelor
Asendin	Pertofrane
Aventyl	Sinequan
Desyrel	Surmontil
Elavil	Tofranil
Etrafon	Triadapin
Limbitrol	Triptil
Ludiomil	Vivactil

 Antidiabetics: Insulins

Type(s)	Insulin (pancreatic hormone)
Actions	Facilitates glucose transmembrane transport and stimulates carbohydrate metabolism
	Facilitates glucose storage (as glycogen), primarily in the liver, muscle, and kidney

Insulin type	Time (hour)		
	Onset	Peak	Duration
Short acting			
Regular (Toronto)	0.5–1	2.5–5	5–8
Similente	1–1.5	5–10	12–16
Intermediate acting			
NPH	1.5–2	4–12	24–48
Lente	2–2.5	7–15	22–48
Long acting			
PZI	4–7	10–30	36+
Ultralente	4–7	8–30	28–36+

Indications	Diabetes that cannot be controlled by diet alone
	Diabetics who cannot produce or excrete adequate amounts of insulin: usually type I (insulin-dependent diabetes mellitus), or juvenile diabetics
	In place of oral hypoglycemic therapy in patients with complications
Adverse Effects	*Other:* Hypoglycemia, hypokalemia, and electrolyte depletion
Interactions	ETOH, β-blockers, monoamine oxidase inhibitors, anabolic steroids, salicylates: May potentiate hypoglycemic effects
	Corticosteroids, thiazides, catecholamines: May diminish hypoglycemic effects
How Supplied	Multidose vial and penfill (subcutaneous or intramuscular injection); some are combination products
Note	Epinephrine may reverse hypoglycemic effects
	May be on combination of different insulin preparations
	Extracted from beef or pork pancreas or produced from genetic engineering
	Insulin preparations differ primarily in onset, peak, and duration of action, which may vary slightly among manufacturers
	Insulin is a protein and is destroyed in the gastrointestinal tract. It must be given parenterally. The abdomen, thigh, and arm are common sites.
Common Examples	Humilin Novolin
	Iletin Velosulin

✳ Antidiabetics: Oral Hypoglycemics

Type(s)	Oral hypoglycemics (sulfonylureas)
Actions	Stimulates pancreatic beta cells to produce and secrete insulin
Indications	To control hyperglycemia in patients whose diabetes cannot be controlled by diet alone and when insulin therapy is inappropriate; usually type II (non-insulin-dependent diabetes mellitus or adult) diabetics

Adverse Effects	Severe and prolonged hypoglycemia (especially when accompanied by acute ETOH overdose); possible associated hypoglycemic seizure
Interactions	ETOH, anabolic steroids, monoamine oxidase inhibitors, oral anticoagulants, salicylates, sulfonamides, β-blockers: May potentiate hypoglycemic effects
	Corticosteroids, glucagon, thiazides, catecholamines: May diminish hypoglycemic effects
How Supplied	Tablet
Note	Provides an alternative to intravenous insulin
	Oral hypoglycemics differ primarily in onset, peak, and duration of action
	Hypoglycemia may persist despite intravenous dextrose or may recur (because oral hypoglycemics are longer lasting than dextrose)
Common Examples	Diabeta Euglucon
	Diabinese Mobenol
	Dimelor Orinase

Antidysrhythmics

Type(s)	Various (classes I–IV)
Actions	Various, depends on specific antidysrhythmic:
	(−) chronotropy
	(+) or (−) inotropy
	(−) dromotropy
	Depresses automaticity
	Reduces MVO_2
	Suppresses PVCs
	Suppresses reentry activity
	Vagolytic
	May elevate the threshold for VF
Indications	To maintain NSR (or a controlled or stable abnormal rhythm)
	To prevent chronic rhythm disturbances
Adverse Effects	*Cardiovascular system:* Dysrhythmia, conduction disturbances, hypotension, myocardial depression, may induce or exacerbate congestive heart failure or pulmonary edema, and may precipitate angina
	Central nervous system: Headache, central nervous system depression, altered level of consciousness
	Other: N/V
Interactions	Other antidysrhythmics: May potentiate or depress effects
How Supplied	Tablet and capsule
Note	Usually prescribed after some type of cardiac insult

Common Examples   Antidysrhythmics may be classified by their predominant electrophysiological effects (e.g., Vaughn-Williams-Singh Classification).

Class I	Class II	Class III
Biquin	*Primarily β-Blockers*	Bretylate
Dilantin	Betaloc	Bretylol
Mexitil	Biocadren	Cordarone (amiodarone)
Norpace	Corgard	
Procan	Inderal	
Pronestyl	Lopressor	
Prosedyl	Sotacor	
Quinate	Tenormin	
Quinidex	Visken	
Quinine		
Rhythmodan		
Tonocard		
Xylocaine		

Class IV

Calcium channel blockers
Adalat
Cardizem
Isoptin
Cardiac glycosides
Cedilanid
Crystodigin
Digitaline
Lanoxin
Norvasc
Novodigozin

✳ Antihypertensives

Type(s)	Various (vasodilators, sympatholytics, β-blockers, diuretics, and combination products)
Actions	Vasodilation (decreased blood pressure)
	ACE inhibitors (reduced vasoconstriction)
	Sympatholytics (reduced vessel tone)
	α-Blockade (reduced SVR)
	Diuresis (decreased volume)
Indications	Hypertension, congestive heart failure
	Sodium retention, edema, ascites
Adverse Effects	*Cardiovascular system:* Orthostatic to profound hypotension, syncope, flushing, rebound hypertension, reflex tachycardia, dysrhythmia, angina, and PVCs

Central nervous system: Drowsiness, dizziness, confusion, sedation, and headache

Other: Fluid and Na$^+$ retention, congestive heart failure, electrolyte imbalance, N/V/D, abdominal pain, and muscle cramps

Interactions	Monoamine oxidase inhibitors: May potentiate hypotensive effects
How Supplied	Tablet and capsule
Note	Some are combination products

Common Examples

Aldomet	Loniten
Capoten	Minipress
Catapres	Serparsil
Combipres	Viskazide

❋ Anxiolytics (Antianxiety)

Type(s)	Primarily benzodiazepines (minor tranquilizers) and carbamates
Actions	Central nervous system depressant, sedation Skeletal muscle relaxation

Indications	Excessive anxiety and tension (acute or chronic):
	   Stresses of everyday life
	   Emotional and physical disorders
	   Tension from insomnia
	Anticonvulsant
	Muscle spasms
	Adjunctive management of acute ETOH or opiate withdrawal

Adverse Effects	*Cardiovascular system:* Hypotension and tachycardia *Central nervous system:* Respiratory depression, apnea, excessive central nervous system depression or sedation, coma, drowsiness, dizziness, vertigo, confusion, ataxia, slurred speech, headache, amnesia, fatigue, weakness, occasional paradoxical irritability, excitability, aggression, hallucinations, and delirium *Other:* N/V, pupil dilation
Interactions	Central nervous system depressants, including ETOH: Potentiate effects
How Supplied	Tablet, capsule, and caplet
Note	This is probably the most widely prescribed class of drugs in the world There is potential for tolerance, abuse, and addiction A withdrawal syndrome may result from abrupt cessation after chronic use

Common Examples	Atarax	Multipax
	Ativan (lorazepam)	Serax
	Donnatal	Stelzine
	Lectopam	Tranxene
	Librium (chlordiazepoxide)	Valium (diazepam)
	Loftran	Vivol (diazepam)
	Mellaril	Xanax

✳ Antipsychotics

Type(s)	Primarily phenothiazines (major tranquilizers) (psychotropics)
Actions	Phenothiazines alter behavior in such a way as to enable the patient to cope with illness and function in daily activities without excessive sedation
	Some also have antiemetic or anticholinergic effects
Indications	Acute and chronic control of behavioral disorders resulting from mental illness:
	Schizophrenia, recurrent mania
	Psychotic disorders
	Anxiety disorders
	Prevention of N/V
Adverse Effects	*Cardiovascular system:* Hypotension, bradycardia, dysrhythmia, and atrioventricular blocks
	Central nervous system: Respiratory depression, central nervous system depression, sedation, drowsiness, confusion, dizziness, weakness, tremor, seizure, and coma
	Other: Extrapyramidal effects (primarily muscle spasms) and anticholinergic effects (dry mouth, nasal congestion, blurred vision, salivation)
Interactions	Opiates, barbiturates, ETOH, and other central nervous system depressants: May potentiate effects
	"Epi": May be ineffective in reversing hypotension (may in fact potentiate the hypotension)
How Supplied	Tablet, solution, suspension, syrup, and suppository
Note	Diphenhydramine (Benadryl) or benztropine (Cogentin) may counteract some
	Tranquilizers induce calmness and sedation without excessively depressing level of consciousness

Common Examples	Haldol	Peridol	Sparine
	Haloperidol	Permitil	Stelazine
	Mellaril	Quide	Trilafon
	Nozinan	Serentil	

Appendix E

✳ Beta-Blockers

Type(s)	Sympathetic blocker
Actions	Some selectively block β_1 (cardioselective) or β_2 (bronchoselective) receptors; some are nonselective
Indications	Mild to moderate hypertension
	Prevention of recurrent angina
	Prevention of recurring tachydysrhythmias
	Migraines
Adverse Effects	*Cardiovascular system:* May precipitate or aggravate chronic obstructive pulmonary disease, asthma, bronchospasm, increased airway resistance, hypotension, bradycardia, atrioventricular block, and congestive heart failure
	Central nervous system: Fatigue, headache, hallucinations, seizure, and coma
	Other: N/V, may induce hypoglycemia
Interactions	Sympathomimetics: Block β effects (patient may be unable to mount a tachycardic response to hypovolemia)
	Calcium blockers: Potentiate bradycardia and myocardial depression
	Cardiac glycosides: Potentiate bradycardia
	Epinephrine: Severe vasoconstriction
	Diuretics: May potentiate antihypertensive effects
How Supplied	Tablet
Note	Acute withdrawal may precipitate angina (due to increased sensitivity to catecholamines)
	Often used in combination therapy
	Selective β-blockers are usually dose dependent (tend to lose β selectivity in higher doses)
Common Examples	Betaloc Lopressor
	Blocardren Sotacor
	Corgard Tenormin
	Inderal Visken

✳ Bronchodilators: Sympathomimetics

Type(s)	Sympathomimetics
Actions	Most are β selective (some are not)
	Bronchodilation (via β_2 stimulation)
	Some β effects
	Little or no α stimulation
Indications	Prevention or treatment of bronchospasm caused by reversible obstructive airway disease (chronic obstructive pulmonary disease, asthma, bronchitis, and emphysema)

Adverse Effects	*Cardiovascular system:* Excessive cardiac stimulation, tachycardia, palpitation, and hypertension; may precipitate angina, acute myocardial infarction, PVCs, and dysrhythmia; possible hypotension, sweating
	Central nervous system: Excessive central nervous system stimulation (anxiety to seizure), headache, dizziness, drowsiness, weakness, fatigue, and paresthesia
	Other: N/V, heartburn, bad taste, muscle cramps, and dry nose and throat; may cause severe paradoxical bronchospasm from repeated excessive use
Interactions	β-blocker: May block effects
	Monoamine oxidase inhibitors, tricyclic antidepressants: May potentiate effects
How Supplied	Aerosol, tablet, suppository, and nebulizer solution
Note	Aerosolized drugs may not reach the smaller airways, especially in the presence of bronchospasm and thick mucous plugs (the nebulizer solution will be much more effective)
	Aerosol sympathomimetics have the potential for patient tolerance and abuse
	These patients may also be on steroids and antibiotics
	Some are combination products
	Overdose effects may be reversed by a β-blocker such as propranolol (Inderal)
	Some are catecholamines, and some are not; they differ primarily in their onset and duration
	There is also a long-acting salbutamol called Serevent; it is not to be used for the compromised patient due to its longer onset of action

Common Examples		
	Alupent	Bronkometer
	Berotec	Bronkosol
	Brethaire	Serevent
	Brethine	Vaponefrin
	Bricanyl	Ventolin
	Bronkaid	

✳ Bronchodilators: Theophyllines

Type(s)	Theophyllines
Actions	Bronchodilation and vasodilation
	Respiratory stimulation
	Diuresis
	(+) chronotropy, (+) inotropy
Indications	Prevention and treatment of bronchospasm caused by reversible obstructive airway disease (chronic

	obstructive pulmonary disease, asthma, bronchitis, emphysema) and related bronchospastic disorders
Adverse Effects	*Cardiovascular system:* Hypotension, angina, tachycardia, palpitation, dysrhythmia, PVCs, and flushing
	Central nervous system: Headache, nervousness, irritability, anxiety, excitement, dizziness, mild delirium, insomnia, fever, tremor, seizure, coma, and increased respiratory rate
	Other: N/V/D, anorexia, abdominal cramps, hematemesis, diuresis, dehydration, and visual or auditory disturbances
Interactions	β-blockers: May oppose effects
	Barbiturates, phenytoin: May decrease theophylline blood levels
How Supplied	Tablet, aerosol, elixir, syrup, and suppository
Note	Children are very sensitive: Toxic-to-therapeutic ratio is small
	Some are combination products
Common Examples	Choledyl Somophyllin
	Phyllocontin Tedral
	Quibron Theo-Dur

Calcium Channel Blockers

Type(s)	Antidysrhythmic, antihypertensive, and antianginal
Actions	Blocks entry of calcium into the cell (especially cardiac and vascular smooth muscle):
	(−) chronotropy
	(−) inotropy
	(−) dromotropy
	Vasodilation (including coronary)
	Bronchodilation
	Inhibits coronary artery spasm
Indications	Nifedipine, verapamil, and diltiazem: Angina from coronary artery spasm and chronic stable angina (effort associated)
	Verapamil: PSVT, A-fib, A-flutter
Adverse Effects	**Verapamil and Nifedipine:**
	Cardiovascular system: Conduction disturbances, dysrhythmia, hypotension, bradycardia, congestive heart failure, flushing, and peripheral edema
	Central nervous system: Headache, fatigue, drowsiness, dizziness, nervousness, central nervous system depression, confusion, and insomnia
	Other: N/V/D/ and rash
	Diltiazem

Interactions	Digoxin: May increase digoxin blood levels
	β-blockers: May potentiate some effects
How Supplied	Tablet and capsule (oral and sublingual)
Note	Often used in combination therapy
	Verapamil's most potent activity is electrophysiological, and nifedipine's most potent activity is hemodynamic; diltiazem acts like a less potent combination of the two
Common Examples	Adalat Isoptin
	Cardizem

✳ Cardiotonics: Cardiac Glycosides

Type(s)	Digitalis ("Dig") preparations
Actions	Promotes movement of calcium into the cell:
	(+) inotrope
	(−) chronotrope
	(−) dromotrope
	Improves atrial conduction
Indications	Congestive heart failure, after myocardial infarction
	A-fib, A-flutter
	SVTs
Adverse Effects	*Cardiovascular system:* May exacerbate congestive heart failure and almost any dysrhythmia or conduction defect (usually conduction disturbances, PACs, PVCs, SVTs); hypotension
	Central nervous system: Fatigue, weakness, agitation, hallucinations, behavioral changes, headache, dizziness, vertigo, confusion, anxiety, paresthesia, and insomnia
	Other: N/V/D/, anorexia, malaise, visual disturbances, and hypokalemia
Interactions	Diuretics, Ca^{2+}, quinidine, amiodarone, Ca^{2+} blockers, catecholamines: May precipitate digitalis toxicity
How Supplied	Tablet and capsule
Note	Toxicity is more frequent in patients with hypokalemia, hypocalcemia, or hypomagnesemia
	About 7 to 40 percent of patients on digitalis develop some symptoms of toxicity
	Digitalized patients may develop more serious and resistant dysrhythmias following cardioversion; use of very low energy levels and prophylactic lidocaine or phenytoin may prevent this
	Digitalis glycosides vary in potency, onset, and duration of action; they are generally long acting
Common Examples	Cedilanid Lanoxin
	Crystodigin Novodigoxin
	Digitaline

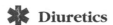 Diuretics

Type(s)	Various (primarily thiazides, loop, and combination products with antihypertensives, β-blockers, and aldosterone antagonists)
Actions	Diuresis
	Promotes sodium (Na^+) excretion
	Vasodilation
Indications	Hypertension
	Chronic fluid overload (congestive heart failure, pulmonary, peripheral edema)
	Liver cirrhosis with ascites and edema
	Decreased renal function (impairment)
	Edema (drug induced or from renal origin)
Adverse Effects	*Cardiovascular system:* Hypovolemia, hypotension, tachycardia, and dysrhythmia
	Central nervous system: Drowsiness, confusion, delirium, dizziness, weakness, seizure, and coma
	Other: Dehydration, electrolyte imbalance (most commonly K^+), hyperosmolality, dry mouth or thirst, cramps, N/V/D, and visual or auditory disturbances; may inhibit insulin release (hyperglycemia)
Interactions	Antihypertensives: Increased antihypertensive effects
How Supplied	Tablet, capsule, and suppository
Note	Also known as "water pills"
	These patients are often on potassium (K^+) supplements
	Electrocardiogram may show prominent P waves, diminished T waves, and presence of U waves
Common Examples	Aldactazide Dyazide
	Aldactone Lasix
	Duretic Moduret

✳ Narcotic: Analgesics

Type(s)	Narcotic (opiate) (natural, semisynthetic, synthetic)
Actions	Analgesia (increases pain threshold)
	Decreases anxiety, apprehension, fear
	Central nervous system depressant, sedation
	Cardiovascular (decreased anxiety reduces catecholamine release; vasodilation reduces preload)
Indications	Pain relief
	Cough suppression
	Sedation for anxiety, apprehension, and fear
	Antidiarrheal
Adverse Effects	*Cardiovascular system:* Hypotension, bradycardia, flushing, sweating, and pulmonary edema (noncardiogenic)

Central nervous system: Respiratory depression, apnea, central nervous system depression, euphoria, drowsiness, dizziness, weakness, excessive sedation, apathy, paradoxical central nervous system, stimulation, nervousness, anxiety, headache, seizure, coma, hallucinations, delusions, and mood change

Other: N/V, urine retention, may constrict or dilate pupils, and may suppress cough or corneal reflex

Interactions Central nervous system depressants, tricyclic antidepressants, and monoamine oxidase inhibitors: Potentiate effects

How Supplied Tablet, capsule, caplet, elixir, suppository, and intravenous

Note Narcotics have the potential for patient tolerance, abuse, and addiction

A withdrawal syndrome may result from abrupt cessation after chronic use

Common Examples

Ancasal	Morphine
Atasol	Numorphan
Codeine	Oxycocet
Darvon	Oxycodan
Demerol (meperidine)	Percocet
Dilaudid (hydromorphone)	Percodan
Empracet	Talwin
Exdol	Tylenol with codeine (Nos. 1, 2, 3, and 4)

✳ Sedatives and Hypnotics

Type(s) Primarily barbiturates, benzodiazepines; also piperidines, carbamates

Actions Sedatives induce central nervous system depression and sedation, and "calm the nerves"

Hypnotics induce and maintain sleep

Indications Some are for daytime use, some are for nighttime use

Anxiety, tension, stress, apprehension, irritability, excitement, and insomnia

Chronic behavioral disorders

Psychotherapy

Seizure disorders

Adverse Effects *Cardiovascular system:* Hypotension and pulmonary edema

Central nervous system: Central nervous system or respiratory depression, drowsiness, dizziness, weakness, confusion, delirium, headache, ataxia, slurred speech, hypnosis (paradoxical excitement in the elderly), possible paresthesia, seizure, coma, nightmares, and hangover

	Other: Extrapyramidal reactions, anticholinergic effects, Parkinson-like reactions (especially in children), N/V/D, rash, and withdrawal syndrome
Interactions	ETOH, other central nervous system depressants: Excessive central nervous system and respiratory depression
	Monoamine oxidase inhibitors: Inhibit barbiturate metabolism
How Supplied	Tablet, capsule, and suppository
Note	Some have potential for tolerance, abuse, and addiction from chronic use
	Some are combination products
	Duration of action varies with each drug; some may be extremely long acting

Common Examples

Amytal	Nembutal
Butisol	Nodular
Dalmane	Placidyl
Day-Barb	Plexonal
Doriden	Restoril
Halcion	Seconal
Mandrax	Tranxene
Mogadon	Tuinal

COMMON EXAMPLES OF HOME MEDICATIONS

Narcotic: Analgesics

Ancasal	Morphine
Atasol	Numorphan
Codeine	Oxycocet
Darvon	Oxycodan
Demerol	Percocet
Dilaudid	Percodan
Empracet	Talwin
Exdol	Tylenol with Codeine (Nos. 1, 2, 3, and 4)

Antianginals

Cardilate	Nitrol
Coronex	Nitrolingual Spray
Isordil	Nitrong
Nitrobid	Nitrostablin
Nitrogard	Nitrostat

Anxiolytics (Antianxiety)

Atarax

Ativan

Donnatal

Lectopam

Librium

Loftran

Mellaril

Multipax

Serax

Stelzine

Tranxene

Valium

Vivol

Xanax

Anticoagulants

Coumadin

Hepalean

Heparin

Minihep

Sintrom

Warfilone

Anticonvulsants

Celontin

Depakene

Dilantin

Epival

Mebaral

Mebroin

Mesantoin

Milontin

Mogadon

Mysoline

Rivotril

Tegretol

Zarontin

Antidepressants: Monamine Oxidase Inhibitors

Marplan

Nardil

Parnate

Antidepressants: Tricyclic Antidepressants

Adapin

Anafranil

Asendin

Aventyl

Desyrel

Elavil

Etrafon

Limbitrol

Ludiomil

Norpramin

Pamelor

Pertofrane

Sinequan

Surmontil

Tofranil

Triadapin

Triptil

Vivactil

Antidiabetics: Insulins

Humilin

Novolin

Iletin

Velosulin

Antidiabetics: Oral Hypoglycemics

Diabeta

Euglucon

Diabinese

Mobenol

Dimelor

Orinase

Antidysrhythmics

Antidysrhythmics may be classified by their predominant electrophysio-logical effects (e.g., Vaughn-Williams-Singh Classification).

Class I	Class II	Class III
Biquin	*Primarily β-blockers*	Bretylate
Dilantin	Betaloc	Bretylol
Mexitil	Biocadren	Cordarone
Norpace	Corgard	
Procan	Inderal	
Pronestyl	Lopressor	
Prosedyl	Sotacor	
Quinate	Tenormin	
Quinidex	Visken	
Quinine		
Rhythmodan		
Tonocard		
Xylocaine		

Class IV

Ca^{2+} *channel blockers*	*Cardiac glycoside*
Adalat	Cedilanid
Cardizem	Crystodigin
Isoptin	Digitaline
	Lanoxin
	Novodigozin

Antihypertensives

Aldomet

Loniten

Capoten

Minipress

Catapres

Serparsil

Combipres

Viskazide

Antipsychotics

Haldol	Peridol	Sparine
Haloperidol	Permitil	Stelazine
Mellaril	Quide	Trilafon
Nozinan	Serentil	

Beta-Blockers

Betaloc	Lopressor
Blocardren	Sotacor
Corgard	Tenormin
Inderal	Visken

Bronchodilators: Sympathomimetics

Alupent	Bronkaid
Berotec	Bronkometer
Brethaire	Bronkosol
Brethine	Vaponefrin
Bricanyl	Ventolin

Bronchodilators: Theophyllines

Choledyl	Somophyllin
Phyllocontin	Tedral
Quibron	Theo-Dur

Calcium Channel Blockers

Adalat	Isoptin
Cardizem	

Cardiotonics: Cardiac Glycosides

Cedilanid	Lanoxin
Crystodigin	Novodigoxin

Diuretics

Aldactazide	Dyazide
Aldactone	Lasix
Duretic	Moduret
Digitaline	

Sedatives and Hypnotics

Amytal

Butisol

Dalmane

Day-Barb

Doriden

Halcion

Mandrax

Mogadon

Nembutal

Nodular

Placidyl

Plexonal

Restoril

Seconal

Tranxene

Tuinal

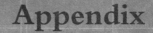 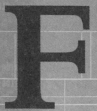

PEDIATRIC DRUG DOSAGES

PEDIATRIC EMERGENCY MEDICATION DOSAGES

✳ Activated Charcoal

Dose	1 g/kg
Maximum Dose	60 g No Max
Route	Oral, nasogastric
Remarks	If administered with ipecac, it will absorb the ipecac

✳ Adenosine

Dose	0.1 mg/kg first dose
	0.2 mg/kg second dose
Maximum Dose	12 mg
Route	Intravenous, intraosseous
Remarks	Rapid intravenous bolus

✳ Atropine

Dose	0.02 mg/kg
Route	Intravenous, intraosseous, endotracheal
Remarks	Minimum dose is 0.1 mg
	Maximum dose in child 0.5 mg; maximum total dose 1.0 mg
	Maximum dose in adolescent 1.0 mg; maximum total dose 2.0 mg

✳ Bretylium

Remarks   Not recommended for pediatric patients

✳ 10 Percent Calcium Chloride

Dose   20 mg/kg repeated once if necessary
Maximum Dose   500 mg No Max.
Route   Intravenous, intraosseous
Remarks   Give slowly (<100 mg/min)

✳ Dextrose

Dose   Neonates and infants up to 3 months old,
    $D_{10}W$ 2–6 mL/kg
    >3 months, $D_{25}W$ 2–4 mL/kg
Route   Intravenous, intraosseous
Remarks   If you do not have 25 percent, dilute $D_{50}W$ with sterile
    water 1:1.

✳ Diazepam

Dose   0.5 mg/kg rectal
    0.1–0.3 mg/kg intravenous, intraosseous
Route   Intravenous, intraosseous, rectal
Remarks   Maximum dose is 5 mg for children under the age of
    5 years and 10 mg for children over the age of 5 years

✳ Diphenhydramine (Benadryl)

Dose   1 mg/kg repeated once
Route   Intravenous, intraosseous, intramuscular
Remarks   Monitor blood pressure; maximum single dose is 50 mg

✳ Dobutamine

Dose   2–20 µg/kg/min
Route   Intravenous drip
Remarks   Titrate to desired effect

✳ Dopamine

Dose   2–20 µg/kg/min
Route   Intravenous drip
Remarks   Titrate to desired effect

❊ Epinephrine 1:1000 (Adrenalin)

Dose	0.01 mg/kg; 0.01 mL/kg
Route	Subcutaneous
Remarks	Do not exceed 0.5 mL

❊ Epinephrine 1:10 000

Dose	0.01 mg/kg (0.1 mL/kg) intravenous 0.1 mg endotracheal
Route	Intravenous, endotracheal, intraosseous
Remarks	Dose may be repeated at 5-minute intervals High dose: 0.1 mg/kg

❊ Fentanyl

Dose	1–3 µg/kg Repeat 0.5 µg/kg
Route	Intravenous, intraosseous
Remarks	Administer slow intravenous push

❊ Furosemide (Lasix)

Dose	1 mg/kg
Route	Intravenous, intraosseous
Remarks	Administer slow intravenous push over 5–10 minutes

❊ Glucagon

Dose	0.03 mg/kg
Route	Intravenous, intramuscular, subcutaneous
Remarks	Sufficient glycogen stores in liver are needed; increase in blood sugar maximum of 1 mg

❊ Lidocaine (Xylocaine)

Dose	1 mg/kg
Route	Intravenous, endotracheal, intraosseous
Remarks	Slow intravenous push; may be repeated at 8–10 minutes but total dose should not exceed 3 mg/kg

❊ Lorazepam (Ativan)

Dose	0.05 mg/kg
Route	Intravenous, intraosseous

Remarks   Administer slow intravenous push over 20–30 seconds
Maximum of 0.2 mg/kg
Dose may be repeated every 10–15 minutes.

✳ Midazolam (Versed)

Dose   0.07–0.3 mg/kg (usually 0.1 mg/kg)
Oral: 0.3–0.5 mg/kg
Intramuscular: 0.2 mg/kg
Rectal: 0.4–0.5 mg/kg
Route   Intravenous, intraosseous
Remarks   Administer slow intravenous push over 20–30 seconds

✳ Morphine

Dose   0.1 mg/kg
Route   Intravenous, endotracheal, intraosseous
Remarks   Monitor respirations and administer slow intravenous

✳ Naloxone (Narcan)

Dose   <5 years: 0.1 mg/kg
>5 years: 2.0 mg
Route   Intravenous, endotracheal, intraosseous, intramuscular
Remarks   Slow intravenous push; if desired response is not
achieved, subsequent dose of 0.1 mg/kg may be given

✳ Salbutamol (Ventolin)

Dose   <5 years: 1.25–2.5 mg
>5 years: 2.5–5.0 mg
Intravenous bolus 4 μg/kg over 2–5 minutes
Repeat once as needed
Infusion 0.2 μg/kg/min up to maximum 10 μg/kg/min
Route   Nebulizer mask
Remarks   Administer through a nebulizer mask using nonhu-
midified oxygen at approximately 8 L/min or until
mask starts to mist; administer drug with 2 mL of
normal saline if not premixed in nebules

✳ Sodium Bicarbonate

Dose   1 mEq/kg
Route   Intravenous
Remarks   Infuse slowly
Ensure adequate ventilations

PRECALCULATED PEDIATRIC DRUG DOSAGES

Drug Supplied and Dose		Atropine 0.1 mg/mL 0.02 mg/kg		Diazepam 5 mg/mL 0.2 mg/kg		Dextrose 25% or 50% 0.5 g/kg			Epinephrine 1:10 000 0.01 mg/kg	
Age	kg	mg	mL	mg	mL	g	%	mL	mg	mL
Birth	3	0.1	1.0	0.6	0.1	1.5	25	6	0.03	0.3
3 months	5	0.1	1.0	1.0	0.2	2.5	25	10	0.05	0.5
6 months	7	0.14	1.4	1.4	0.28	3.5	25	14	0.07	0.7
1 year	10	0.20	2.0	2.0	0.4	5	25	20	0.10	1.0
2 years	12	0.24	2.4	2.4	0.48	6	50	12	0.12	1.2
3 years	15	0.30	3.0	3.0	0.6	7.5	50	15	0.15	1.5
4 years	17	0.34	3.4	3.4	0.68	8.5	50	17	0.17	1.7
5 years	18	0.36	3.6	3.6	0.72	9	50	18	0.18	1.8
6 years	20	0.40	4.0	4.0	0.8	10	50	20	0.20	2.0
8 years	25	0.50	5.0	5.0	1.0	12.5	50	25	0.25	2.5
10 years	30	0.60	6.0	6.0	1.2	15	50	30	0.30	3.0
12 years	38	0.76	7.6	7.6	1.52	19	50	38	0.38	3.8
14 years	50	1.0	10.0	10	2	25	50	50	0.50	5.0

Drug Supplied Dose/kg		Lidocaine 20 mg/mL 1 mg/kg		Lorazepam 4 mg/mL 0.05 mg/kg		Naloxone 0.4 mg/mL 0.1 mg/kg		Bicarbonate 50 mEq/50 mL 1 mEq/kg	
Age	kg	mg	mL	mg	mL	g	mL	mEg	mL
Birth	3	3	0.15	0.15	0.038	0.3	0.3	3.0	3.0
3 months	5	5	0.25	0.25	0.06	0.5	0.5	5.0	5.0
6 months	7	7	0.35	0.35	0.088	0.7	0.7	7.0	7.0
1 year	10	10	0.5	0.5	0.125	1.0	1.0	10.0	10.0
2 years	12	12	0.6	0.6	0.15	1.2	1.2	12.0	12.0
3 years	15	15	0.75	0.75	0.188	1.5	1.5	15.0	15.0
4 years	17	17	0.85	0.85	0.21	1.7	1.7	17.0	17.0
5 years	18	18	0.9	0.9	0.225	1.8	1.8	18.0	18.0
6 years	20	20	1.0	1	0.25	2.0	2.0	20.0	20.0
8 years	25	25	1.25	1.25	0.313	2.0	2.0	25.0	25.0
10 years	30	30	1.50	1.5	0.375	2.0	2.0	30.0	30.0
12 years	38	38	1.9	1.9	0.475	2.0	2.0	38.0	38.0
14 years	50	50	2.5	2.5	0.625	2.0	2.0	50.0	50.0

PEDIATRIC MEDICATION INFUSIONS

An infusion pump is highly recommended.

✳ Aminophylline

How Supplied	Use 25 mg/mL solution
Dose	0.2 mL/kg in 100 D_5W, over 20–30 minutes
Maintenance	
Dose	0.5 mg/kg/hr
Remarks	To mix: Add 125 mg to 250 mL D_5W (or 50 mg in 100 mL D_5W)
Note	1 microdrop/kg/min of this solution = 0.5 mg/kg/hr

✳ Dobutamine

How Supplied	Use 25 mg/mL solution
Dose	2–12 μg/kg/min
Remarks	To mix: Add 30 mg to 250 mL D_5W
Note	1 microdrop/kg/min of this solution = 2 μg/kg/min

✳ Dopamine

How Supplied	Use 40 mg/mL solution
Dose	2–12 μg/kg/min
Remarks	To mix: Add 80 mg (2 mL) to 250 mL D_5W
Note	1 microdrop/kg/min of this solution = 5 μg/kg/hr

✳ Epinephrine

How Supplied	Use 1:1000 solution, 1 mg/mL
Dose	0.1–1.0 μg/kg/min
Remarks	To mix: Add 1.5 mg (1.5 mL) to 250 mL D_5W
Note	1 microdrop/kg/min of this solution = 0.1 μg/kg/hr

✳ Lidocaine

How Supplied	Use 2 percent solution, 20 mg/mL
Dose	20–50 μg/kg/min
Remarks	To mix: Add 300 mg (15 mL) to 250 mL D_5W
Note	1 microdrop/kg/min of this solution = 20 μg/kg/hr

Appendix G

Pediatric Advanced Cardiac Life Support Treatment Algorithm

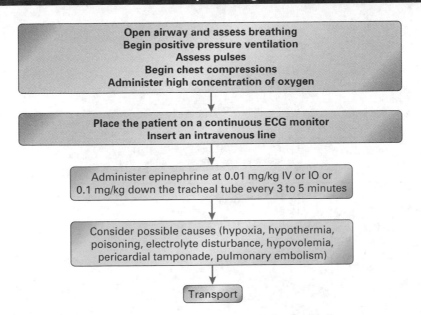

Pediatric Asystole Algorithm

Open airway and assess breathing
Begin positive pressure ventilation
Assess pulses
Begin chest compressions
Administer high concentration of oxygen

Place the patient on a continuous ECG monitor
Insert an intravenous line

Administer epinephrine at 0.01 mg/kg IV or IO or
0.1 mg/kg down the tracheal tube every 3 to 5 minutes

Consider possible causes (hypoxia, hypothermia,
poisoning, electrolyte disturbance, hypovolemia,
pericardial tamponade, pulmonary embolism)

Transport

FIGURE G–1 Pediatric asystole and pulseless arrest protocol.

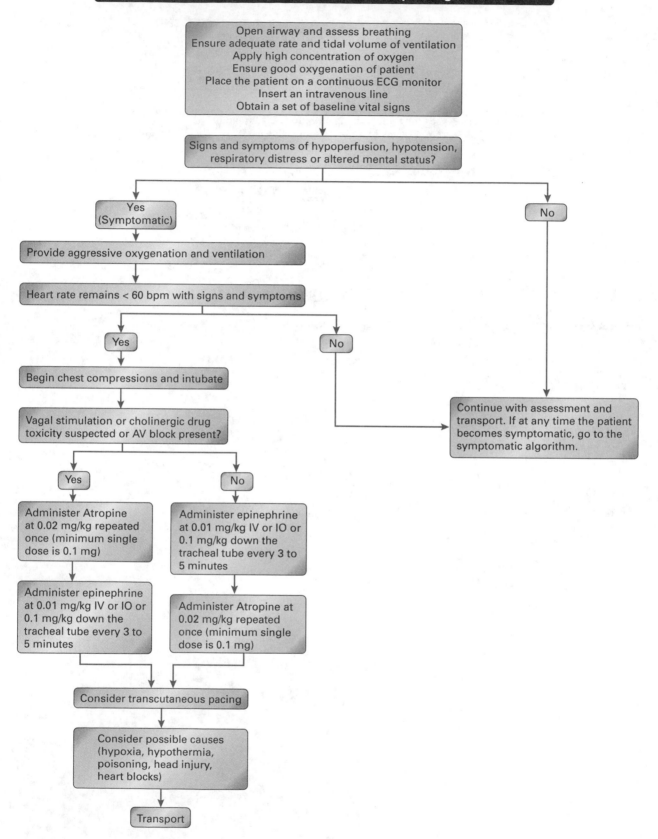

Pediatric Bradycardia (Heart rate < 60 bpm) Algorithm

Open airway and assess breathing
Ensure adequate rate and tidal volume of ventilation
Apply high concentration of oxygen
Ensure good oxygenation of patient
Place the patient on a continuous ECG monitor
Insert an intravenous line
Obtain a set of baseline vital signs

Signs and symptoms of hypoperfusion, hypotension, respiratory distress or altered mental status?

Yes (Symptomatic)

No

Provide aggressive oxygenation and ventilation

Heart rate remains < 60 bpm with signs and symptoms

Yes

No

Begin chest compressions and intubate

Continue with assessment and transport. If at any time the patient becomes symptomatic, go to the symptomatic algorithm.

Vagal stimulation or cholinergic drug toxicity suspected or AV block present?

Yes

No

Administer Atropine at 0.02 mg/kg repeated once (minimum single dose is 0.1 mg)

Administer epinephrine at 0.01 mg/kg IV or IO or 0.1 mg/kg down the tracheal tube every 3 to 5 minutes

Administer epinephrine at 0.01 mg/kg IV or IO or 0.1 mg/kg down the tracheal tube every 3 to 5 minutes

Administer Atropine at 0.02 mg/kg repeated once (minimum single dose is 0.1 mg)

Consider transcutaneous pacing

Consider possible causes (hypoxia, hypothermia, poisoning, head injury, heart blocks)

Transport

FIGURE G–2 Pediatric bradycardia protocol.

Appendix H

DRUG ADMINISTRATION SKILLS

SUBCUTANEOUS DRUG ADMINISTRATION

Subcutaneous injection is a method of administering drugs directly into subcutaneous or fatty tissue, where they are absorbed into the general circulation (see Procedure H–1). Medication injected subcutaneously is typically absorbed more slowly than through the intravenous routes but faster than through the oral route. The subcutaneous injection of epinephrine may be lifesaving in severe cases of asthma or allergic reactions. Glucagon can also be administered subcutaneously for the treatment of insulin shock. The medication must be administered into the subcutaneous tissue and not into the more superficial dermis or deeper muscle, connective tissue, or blood vessels.

Procedure H–1 Subcutaneous Administration

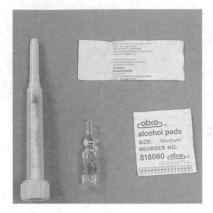

H–1a Prepare the equipment.

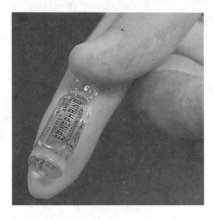

H–1b Check the medication.

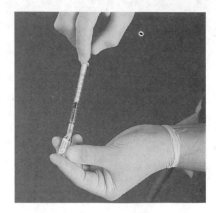

H–1c Draw up the medication.

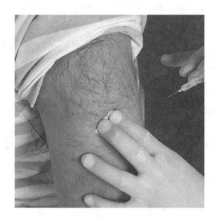

H–1d Prep the site.

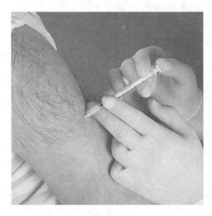

H–1e Insert the needle at a 45° angle.

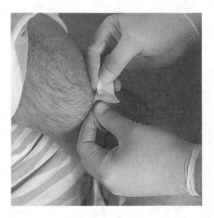

H–1f Remove the needle and cover the puncture site.

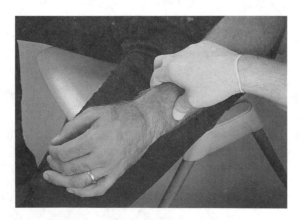

H–1g Monitor the patient.

Epinephrine 1:1000 is the emergency drug most frequently given subcutaneously. The procedure is as follows:

1. Receive order.
2. Confirm the drug order, amount to be given, and route and write the information down.
3. Prepare the necessary equipment and observe body substance isolation precautions (gloves):
   - 1-cc syringe
   - One needle (preferably 1 to $1\frac{1}{2}$ inches in length, 16 to 22 gauge) to withdraw medication
   - One needle (preferably $\frac{1}{2}$ to $\frac{5}{8}$ inch in length, 25 gauge) for drug administration
   - Alcohol or povidone-iodine preparation
   - 2 × 2 gauze pad
   - Medication
   - Sharps container
4. Explain to the patient what you are going to do and reconfirm that the patient is not allergic to the medication. Be sure to advise the patient of any complications that might result from the administration.
5. Examine the ampule of medication, including name and expiration date. Hold it up to the light and inspect for discoloration or particles in the solution. Do not administer if discolored or if particles are present.
6. "Shake down" the ampule. This will force the liquid to the lower portion of the ampule so that it can be broken without spillage of the drug.
7. Break the ampule using a 2 × 2 gauze pad to prevent injury.
8. Draw the medication into the syringe. Invert the syringe and expel any air present.
9. Choose a suitable site. The easiest and most accessible site is the subcutaneous tissue over the deltoid muscle in the arm.
10. Prepare the site by cleansing it with a povidone-iodine or alcohol preparation using a firm circular motion from the site outward.
11. Pinch up the skin and insert the needle into the tissue at a 45-degree angle.
12. Inject the medication into the subcutaneous tissue slowly.
13. Remove the syringe. Do not recap the needle.
14. Apply pressure to the site with sterile gauze pad.
15. Dispose of the syringe and medication container in appropriate sharps container.
16. Cover with an adhesive strip.
17. Confirm administration of the medication.
18. Closely monitor the patient for the desired therapeutic effect and possible side effects.
19. Document procedure and patient effects.

INTRAMUSCULAR INJECTION

Intramuscular (IM) injection is a method of administering drugs directly into muscle, where it is absorbed into the general circulation. Prehospital administration of IM drugs is relatively uncommon but is useful when other administration routes fail. Several prehospital drugs can be administered IM, the most common being diazepam, meperidine, morphine, and glucagon. Absorption by the IM route is slower than by the IV route; because it requires adequate perfusion, it may be ineffective in the hypotensive patient. IM injections may be contraindicated in patients with coagulopathies (a defect in the clotting mechanism of the body) or those who take anticoagulants.

Several sites are used for intramuscular injections (see Figure H–1).

The procedure for intramuscular medication administration is as follows (see Procedure H–2):

1. Receive order.

2. Confirm the drug order, amount to be given, and route and write the information down.

3. Prepare the necessary equipment and observe body substance isolation precautions (gloves):
   - Syringe of sufficient size to contain the medication
   - One needle (preferably 1 to 1½ inches in length, 16 to 22 gauge) to withdraw medication
   - One needle (preferably ¾ to 1 inch in length, 21 to 25 gauge) for drug administration
   - Alcohol or povidone-iodine preparation
   - 2 × 2 gauze pad
   - Medication
   - Sharps container

4. Explain to the patient what you are going to do and reconfirm that the patient is not allergic to the medication. Be sure to advise the patient of any complications that might result from the administration.

5. Examine the ampule of medication, including name and expiration date. Hold it up to the light and inspect for discoloration or particles in the solution. Do not administer if discolored or if particles are present.

6. "Shake down" the ampule. This will force the liquid to the lower portion of the ampule so that it can be broken without spillage of the drug.

7. Break the ampule using a 2 × 2 gauze pad to prevent injury.

8. Draw the medication into the syringe. Invert the syringe and expel any air present.

9. Choose a suitable site. The easiest and most accessible site is the deltoid muscle in the arm (see Figure H–1).

10. Prepare the site by cleansing it with a povidone-iodine or alcohol preparation using a firm circular motion from the site outward.

11. Insert the needle into the tissue at a 90-degree angle (see Figure H–2e).

12. Aspirate the syringe to ensure that you are not in a blood vessel. If you get any blood return, you should withdraw the needle and reattempt administration at another site.

13. Inject the medication slowly.

14. Remove the syringe. Do not recap the needle.

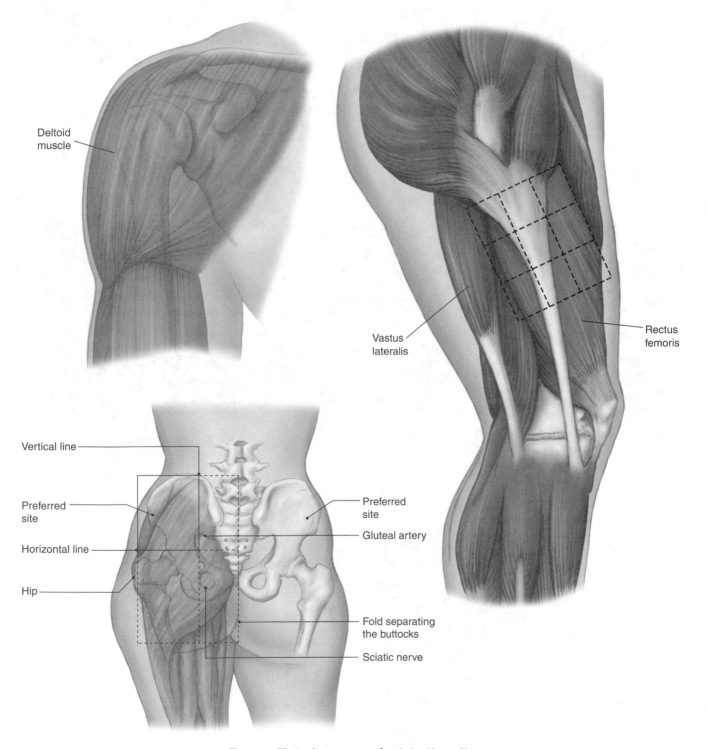

FIGURE H–1 Intramuscular injection sites.

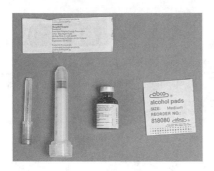

H–2a Prepare the equipment.

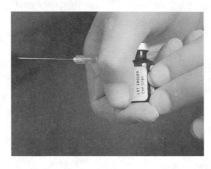

H–2b Check the medication.

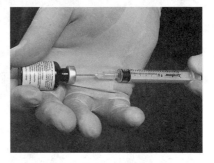

H–2c Draw up the medication.

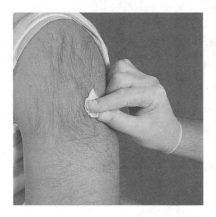

H–2d Prepare the site.

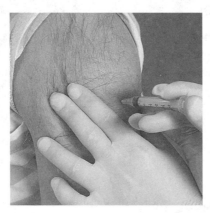

H–2e Insert the needle at a 90° angle.

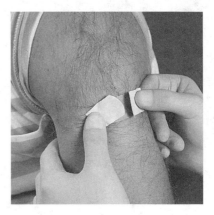

H–2f Remove the needle and cover the puncture site.

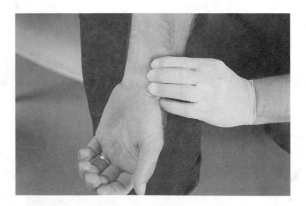

H–2g Monitor the patient.

15. Dispose of the syringe and medication container in appropriate sharps container.

16. Cover with an adhesive strip.

17. Confirm administration of the medication.

18. Closely monitor the patient for the desired therapeutic effect and possible undesired side effects.

19. Document procedure and patient effects.

INTRAVENOUS SETUP

1. Receive order.

2. Confirm the intravenous (IV) fluid, amount to be given, and route and write the information down.

3. Prepare the necessary equipment and observe body substance isolation precautions (gloves and goggles):
   - Appropriate IV fluid
   - Appropriate administration set

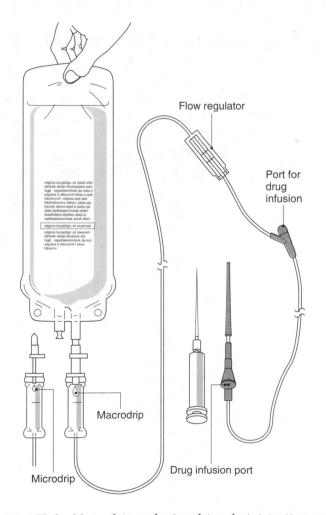

FIGURE H–2 Macrodrip and microdrip administration sets.

- Appropriate indwelling catheter
- Extension IV tubing if necessary

4. Remove the envelope from the IV fluid.

5. Inspect the fluid, making sure that it is not discolored and does not contain any particulate matter; check that it contains the correct amount of fluid. Do not administer if discolored, if particles are present, or if less than the indicated quantity of fluid is present.

6. Open and inspect the IV tubing.

7. Attach the extension tubing.

8. Close the clamp on the tubing.

9. Remove the sterile cover from the IV fluid and the administration set.

10. Insert the administration set into the IV fluid.

11. Squeeze the drip chamber to fill it with fluid.

12. Bleed all of the air out of the IV tubing.

13. Hang the bag on an IV pole (or have a bystander hold it) at the appropriate height.

PROCEDURE FOR INTRAVENOUS CANNULATION

The procedure is as follows (see Procedure H–3):

1. Receive order.

2. Confirm the drug order, amount to be given, and route and write the information down.

3. Prepare the necessary equipment and observe body substance isolation precautions (gloves and goggles):
   - Appropriate IV fluid and administration set (previously set up)
   - Appropriate indwelling catheter (18 gauge for lifelines and 12 to 16 gauge for fluid administration)
   - Tourniquet
   - Povidone-iodine or alcohol preparation
   - Antibiotic ointment
   - 2 × 2 gauze pad
   - 1-inch tape
   - Short arm board
   - Sharps container

4. Explain to the patient what you are going to do. Be sure to advise the patient of any complications that might result from the procedure.

5. Place the tourniquet (or inflate blood pressure cuff to 20 mmHg below systolic pressure) just above the elbow and place the arm in a dependent position.

6. Select a suitable vein and palpate it (see Chapter 5, Figures 5–6 and 5–7).

Procedure H–3   Peripheral Intravenous Access

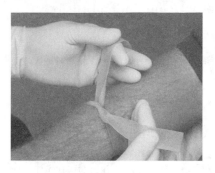

H–3a   Place the constricting band.

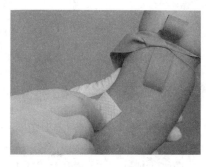

H–3b   Cleanse the venipuncture site.

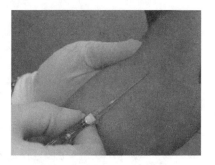

H–3c   Insert the intravenous cannula into the vein.

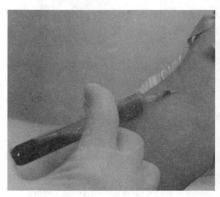

H–3d   Withdraw any blood samples needed.

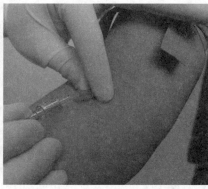

H–3e   Connect the IV tubing.

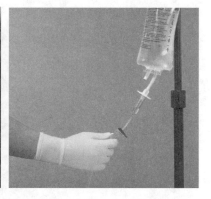

H–3f   Turn on the IV and check the flow.

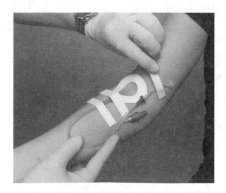

H–3g   Secure the site.

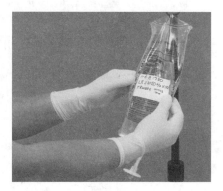

H–3h   Label the intravenous solution bag.

7. Select the most prominent vein on the hand, forearm, or antecubital space that is straight, on a flat surface, and not rolling. If possible, avoid veins over joints, using the antecubital veins as a last resort.

8. A vein may be distended for easier cannulation by gently tapping on it with the fingers.

9. Prepare the site by cleansing it with a povidone-iodine or alcohol preparation using a firm circular motion from the vein outward.

10. Apply traction on the skin below the venipuncture site and stabilize the vein.

11. Tell the patient there will be a quick, painful stick.

12. With the bevel of the needle upward, puncture the skin using a 30- to 45-degree angle. Enter the vein directly from above or from the side.

13. When the vein is entered, you should feel a "pop" and see flashback into the catheter (see Chapter 5, Figures 5–8 through 5–10).

14. Carefully lower the catheter and advance the needle and catheter approximately 2 mm to stabilize the needle in the vein.

15. Slide the catheter off the needle into the vein and then remove the needle. Dispose of the needle in a puncture-proof (sharps) container.

16. Remove the tourniquet.

17. Connect the IV tubing and slowly open the valve.

18. Confirm that the fluid is flowing freely without any evidence of infiltration.

19. Apply povidone-iodine ointment or an antibiotic ointment over the puncture and cover with a sterile 2 × 2 gauze pad or adhesive bandage.

20. Securely tape the IV catheter to the skin using any acceptable technique.

21. Make a loop with the infusion tubing and tape the loop to the arm.

22. Adjust the flow rate.

23. If the vein is over a joint, immobilize with a short arm board to prevent dislodgment of the catheter.

24. Document the successful completion of the IV.

25. Monitor the patient for the desired effects and any undesired ones as well.

EXTERNAL JUGULAR VEIN CANNULATION

Intravenous Access in the External Jugular Vein

The external jugular vein is a large peripheral vein in the neck, between the angle of the jaw and the middle third of the clavicle. It connects into the central circulation of the subclavian vein. Because it lies so close to the central circulation, cannulation here offers many of the same benefits afforded central venous access. Fluids and medications rapidly reach the core of the body from this site.

Consider the external jugular vein only after you have exhausted other means of peripheral access or when a patient requires immediate fluid administration. This is an extremely painful site to access, so you typically will reserve its use for patients with a decreased or total loss of consciousness.

1. Receive order.
2. Confirm the drug order, amount to be given, and route and write the information down.
3. Prepare the necessary equipment and observe body substance isolation precautions (gloves and goggles):
   - Appropriate intravenous (IV) fluid and administration set (previously set up)
   - Appropriate indwelling catheter (18 gauge for lifelines and 12 to 16 gauge for fluid administration)
   - Povidone-iodine or alcohol preparation
   - Antibiotic ointment
   - 2 × 2 gauze pad
   - 1-inch tape
   - Sharps container
4. Explain to the patient what you are going to do (if the patient is conscious). Be sure to advise the patient of any complications that might result from the procedure.
5. Position the patient supine with feet elevated (when possible).
6. Turn the head in the direction away from the side to be cannulated.
7. Select a suitable vein and palpate it.
8. Prepare the site by cleansing it with a povidone-iodine or alcohol preparation.
9. Apply traction on the vein just below the clavicle.
10. Attach a 10 mL syringe to an IV catheter. Align the catheter and point the tip of the catheter toward the feet.
11. Tell the patient there will be a quick, painful stick.
12. With the bevel of the needle upward, puncture the skin using a 30-degree angle. The needle tip should enter midway between the angle of the jaw and the clavicle and should be aimed toward the shoulder on the same side as the vein. Apply suction to the syringe. As the vein is entered, note a flashback of blood.
13. Carefully lower the catheter and advance the needle and catheter approximately 2 mm to stabilize the needle in the vein.
14. Slide the catheter off the needle into the vein and then remove the needle. Dispose of the needle into a puncture-proof (sharps) container.
15. Connect the IV tubing and slowly open the valve.
16. Confirm that the fluid is flowing freely without any evidence of infiltration.

17. Apply povidone-iodine ointment or an antibiotic ointment over the puncture and cover with a sterile 2 × 2 gauze pad or adhesive bandage.

18. Securely tape the IV catheter to the skin using any acceptable technique.

19. Make a loop with the infusion tubing and tape the loop to the neck.

20. Adjust the flow rate.

21. Document the successful completion of the IV.

22. Monitor the patient for the desired effects and any undesired ones as well.

INTRAVENOUS BOLUS

Intravenous bolus, or IV push, is a method of administering drugs directly into the bloodstream (see Procedure H–4). This method provides a rapid route for medications. Because this is a rapid method of drug administration, it is the most commonly used route for life-threatening emergencies. These emergencies include the following:

- Ventricular dysrhythmias
- Supraventricular tachycardia
- Symptomatic bradycardia
- Hypoglycemia
- Metabolic acidosis
- Seizures
- Acute pulmonary edema
- Cardiopulmonary arrest
- Narcotic overdose
- Pain control

1. Receive order.

2 Confirm the drug order, amount to be given, and route and write the information down.

3. Prepare the necessary equipment and observe body substance isolation precautions (gloves):
    - Syringe of sufficient size to contain the medication (or pre-filled syringe)
    - Needle (preferably 1 inch long, 18 gauge)
    - Alcohol or povidone-iodine preparation
    - 2 × 2 gauze pad
    - Medication
    - Sharps container

4. Explain to the patient what you are going to do and reconfirm that the patient is not allergic to the medication. Be sure to advise the patient of any complications that might result from the administration.

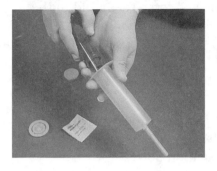

H–4a   Prepare the equipment.

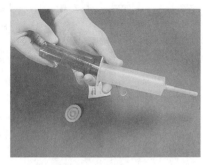

H–4b   Prepare the medication.

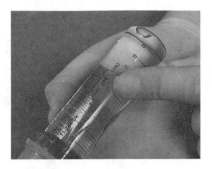

H–4c   Check the label.

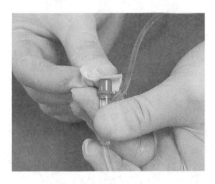

H–4d   Select and clean an administration port.

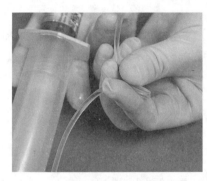

H–4e   Pinch the line.

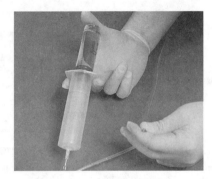

H–4f   Administer the medication.

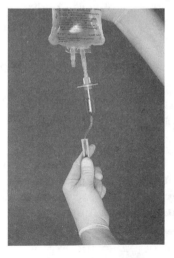

H–4g   Adjust the IV flow rate.

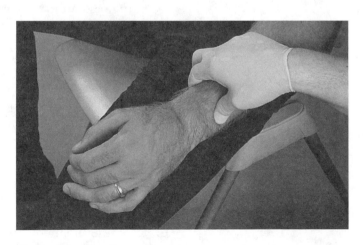

H–4h   Monitor the patient.

5. Examine the ampule of medication, including name and expiration date. Hold it up to the light and inspect for discoloration or particles in the solution. Do not administer if discolored or if particles are present.

6. "Shake down" the ampule. This will force the liquid to the lower portion of the ampule so that it can be broken without spillage of the drug.

7. Break the ampule using a 2×2 gauze pad to prevent injury.

8. Draw the medication into the syringe. Invert the syringe and expel any air.

9. Locate the medication port on the IV administration set and cleanse it with an alcohol swab.

10. Insert the needle into the medication port.

11. Pinch the IV line off above the medication port.

12. Administer the medication in a slow, deliberate fashion.

13. Remove the needle and wipe the medication port with an alcohol swab.

14. Release the pinched line.

15. Confirm administration of the medication.

16. Closely monitor the patient for the desired therapeutic effects as well as any undesired side effects.

INTRAVENOUS INFUSION ADMINISTRATION

Intravenous piggyback or IV drip infusion provides a route for continuous medication administration (see Procedure H–5). It offers the advantage of being easily titrated to increase or decrease the rate of flow or to discontinue the infusion based on the patient's response.

1. Receive order.

2. Confirm the drug order, amount to be given, and route and write the information down.

3. Prepare the necessary equipment and observe body substance isolation precautions (gloves):
   - Medication
   - Syringe to transfer the medication from the ampule to the diluent
   - Alcohol preparation or other antibacterial scrub
   - Two 18-gauge, 1-inch needles
   - Label for the bag
   - Sharps container

4. Explain to the patient what you are going to do and reconfirm that the patient is not allergic to the medication. Be sure to advise the patient of any complications that might result from the administration.

5. Examine the medication, including name and expiration date.

6. Assemble the equipment and attach the needle to the syringe if not preattached.

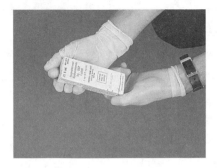

H-5a Select the drug.

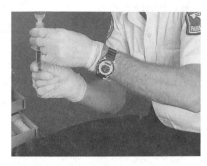

H-5b Draw up the drug.

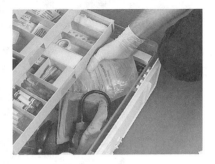

H-5c Select the IV fluid for dilution.

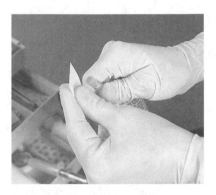

H-5d Clean the medication addition port.

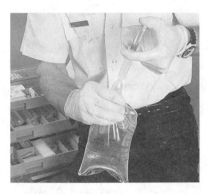

H-5e Inject the drug into the fluid.

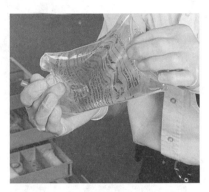

H-5f Mix the solution.

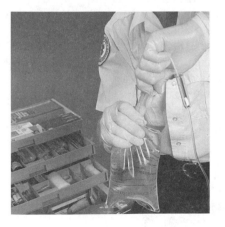

H-5g Insert an administration set and connect to main IV line with needle.

7. Calculate and draw up desired volume of drug into syringe.

8. Draw the medication into the syringe using aseptic technique. Invert and expel any air.

9. Cleanse the medication port on the IV bag into which the medication will be added.

10. Invert the bag and add the medication through the medication addition port.

11. Remove the needle and dispose of in sharps container and cleanse the medication addition port.

12. Invert the bag several times and place an administration set into it.

13. Bleed the air out of the administration set and attach a 1-inch, 18-gauge needle.

14. Cleanse the medication port on the administration set of the already established IV line and insert the needle.

15. Tape the needle securely.

16. Set the primary IV rate to TKO.

17. Adjust the flow rate of the piggyback infusion to the desired dose.

18. Label the bag.

19. Confirm establishment of the infusion.

20. Closely monitor the patient for the desired therapeutic effects as well as any undesired side effects.

ENDOTRACHEAL TUBE ADMINISTRATION

Endotracheal bolus is a procedure that allows the delivery of a medication directly to the tracheobronchial tree and lung tissue via an endotracheal tube. The number of drugs administered via an endotracheal tube (ETT) is limited, and it is generally used during cardiac arrest when intravenous access is not available. The three medications most commonly administered via an ETT are atropine, epinephrine, and lidocaine. Although Narcan can be given via the ETT, other routes are available and may be preferable. There is some debate as to the exact amount of drug to be administered. However, the dose of drug should be at least equal to the IV dose and should be delivered in a volume of 5 to 10 mL.

The procedure is as follows:

1. Receive order.

2. Confirm the order, amount to be given, and route and write the information down.

3. Prepare the necessary equipment and observe body substance isolation precautions (gloves):

   • Prefilled syringe and needle or 18- or 19-gauge needle with syringe

   • Sterile saline or water for dilution

   • Sharps container

4. Examine the ampule of medication, including name and expiration date. Hold it up to the light and inspect for discoloration or particles in the solution. Do not administer if discolored or if particles are present.

5. Hyperventilate the patient in anticipation of administration.

6. Remove the bag-valve-mask unit and inject the medication down the tube.

7. Replace the bag-valve-mask unit and resume ventilation.

8. Monitor the patient for the desired therapeutic effect and any possible undesired side effects.

9. Dispose of needle in sharps container.

INTRAOSSEOUS INFUSION

Intraosseous (IO) infusion is a puncture into the medullary cavity of a bone that provides the paramedic with a rapid access route for fluids and medications. Generally IO infusion is indicated for the pediatric patient up to 6 years of age. The IO site is for temporary use only. Once the child's condition has stabilized, another form of intravenous therapy should be initiated. Prolonged use of IO infusion has led to infection more often than traditional IV lines. IOs are indicated in the following cases:

- Cardiac arrest
- Multisystem trauma associated with shock and/or severe hypovolemia; severe dehydration associated with vascular collapse and/or loss of consciousness
- Any child who is unresponsive and in need of immediate drug or fluid resuscitation (burns, status asthmaticus, status epilepticus, and sepsis)

The procedure is as follows:

1. Receive order.

2. Confirm the order, amount to be given, and route and write the information down.

3. Prepare the necessary equipment and observe body substance isolation precautions (gloves):
   - Medication
   - Intravenous fluid and tubing
   - 10 mL syringe
   - Injectable saline
   - Intraosseous needle or 16- to 18-gauge spinal needle (see Figure H–3)
   - Povidone-iodine preparation
   - Antibiotic ointment
   - Several rolls of Kling

4. Examine the ampule of medication, including name and expiration date. Hold it up to the light and inspect for

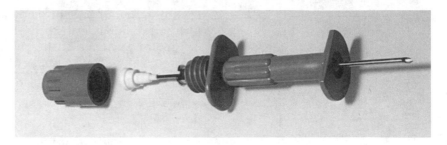

FIGURE H–3 Intraosseous needle or 16- to 18-gauge spinal needle.

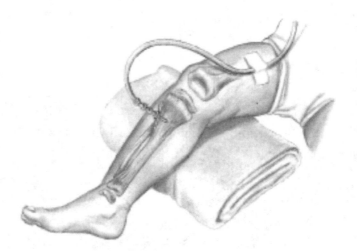

FIGURE H–4 Intraosseous infusion.

discoloration or particles in the solution. Do not administer if discolored or if particles are present.

5. Identify the landmark for insertion, preferably the anteromedial aspect of the proximal tibia, approximately 1 to 3 cm below the tibial tuberosity.

6. Prepare the area extensively with three povidone-iodine preparations in a circular fashion.

7. Replace your gloves with sterile gloves.

8. Take the sterile needle and insert it into the bone at a perpendicular angle or angled slightly inferior.

9. Using a twisting motion, introduce the needle using a 90-degree inferior puncture away from the joint and epiphyseal plate. There will be a decrease in resistance when the needle has been inserted. Stop insertion when a lack of resistance is felt (see Figures H–4 and H–5).

10. Remove the stylet, place a 10 mL syringe on the needle, and aspirate a small amount of marrow to verify the position of the needle.

11. Attach another 10 mL syringe filled with sterile saline. Inject 5 to 10 mL of saline to clear the lumen of the needle.

12. Attach the IV line and the desired fluid.

13. Place antibiotic ointment around the site and secure with tape.

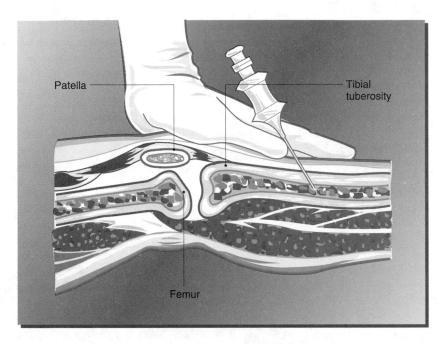

Patella

Tibial
tuberosity

Femur

FIGURE H–5 Intraosseous infusion.

14. Administer the medication.

15. Remove the syringe. Do not recap the needle. Dispose of the needle and syringe properly.

16. Following administration of a medication, 10 mL of saline should be administered to expedite absorption into the circulatory system.

17. Closely monitor the child for the desired effects as well as any side effects.

NEBULIZED INHALATION

Nebulized inhalation of drugs is a method of delivering medications via the tracheobronchial tree using a nebulizer. Nebulized inhalation mixes oxygen with a medication, which results in a vapor that the patient can inhale. Nebulized medication administration is used in the prehospital setting for asthma and chronic obstructive pulmonary disease (COPD). Commonly used medications include albuterol (Proventil), salbutamol (Ventolin), and metaproterenol (Alupent).

1. Receive order.

2. Confirm the order, amount to be given, and route and write the information down.

3. Prepare the necessary equipment and observe body substance isolation precautions (gloves, mask, and goggles):
   - Side-stream nebulizer
   - Oxygen tubing
   - Medication
   - Normal saline for dilution of the bronchodilator

4. Explain procedure to the patient.

5. Take the patient's vital signs and connect the patient to a cardiac monitor.

6. Assemble the nebulizer and place the bronchodilator and saline solution in the reservoir of the side-stream nebulizer.

7. Connect the device and administer oxygen at 6 to 12 lpm and start treatment.

8. Have the patient inhale normally through the mouthpiece or through the mask.

9. Have the patient take a deep breath every three to five inhalations.

10. Continue treatment until the solution is depleted.

11. Administer supplemental oxygen following treatment.

12. Reassess the patient's vital signs and monitor the electro-cardiogram results.

BAG-VALVE NEBULIZED MEDICATION ADMINISTRATION

Nebulized medication administration may be required in patients with serious airway compromise due to a severe asthma attack. In these situations, the intubated patient may receive nebulized ventolin via the bag-valve device. Commonly used medications include albuterol (Proventil), salbutamol (Ventolin), and metaproterenol (Alupent).

1. Receive order.

2. Confirm the order, amount to be given, and route and write the information down.

3. Prepare the necessary equipment and observe body substance isolation precautions (gloves, mask, and goggles):
   - Side-stream nebulizer
   - Oxygen tubing
   - Bag-valve-mask device
   - Intubation equipment
   - Medication
   - Normal saline for dilution of the bronchodilator

4. Take the patient's vital signs and connect the patient to a cardiac monitor and O_2 saturation monitor.

5. Assemble the nebulizer and place the bronchodilator and saline solution in the reservoir of the side-stream nebulizer.

6. Connect the nebulizer to the bag-valve device and administer oxygen at 6 to 12 lpm and start treatment.

7. Ventilate the patient 12 to 20 times per minute.

8. Continue treatment until the solution is depleted.

9. Continue to assist ventilations following treatment.

10. Reassess the patient's vital signs, and monitor the electro-cardiogram results.

11. Repeat treatment as necessary per protocol.

SELF-ADMINISTERED NITROUS OXIDE

A 50:50 nitrous and oxygen mixture allows the patient to regulate his or her pain control by self-administering the gas. This mixture has a rapid effect on the central nervous system and depresses cortical function with no direct effects on the respiratory system. It has an extremely short half-life. Nitrous oxide is indicated in the following situations:

- Musculoskeletal trauma
- Thermal burns
- Childbirth

Nitrous oxide is contraindicated in the following situations:

- Altered mental status
- Alcohol intoxication
- Head injury
- Abdominal or chest trauma
- Shock
- Pneumothorax
- Pulmonary disease (chronic obstructive pulmonary disease or asthma)
- Inability to comprehend or respond to verbal commands
- Inability to self-administer
- Abdominal distension suggestive of bowel obstruction

    1. Receive order.
    2. Confirm the drug order, amount to be given, and route and write the information down.
    3. Prepare the necessary equipment and observe body substance isolation precautions (gloves):
        - Medication tank(s)
        - Face mask
    4. Invert the nitrous tank several times to create vaporization and mix the gases.
    5. Open the pressure valves on the oxygen and nitrous tanks.
    6. Explain to the patient what you are going to do and reconfirm that the patient is not allergic to the medication. Be sure to advise the patient of any complications that might result from the administration.
    7. Instruct the patient on the use of the device.
    8. Place the patient in a sitting position (if possible) and instruct and assist the patient in creating a tight face mask seal.
    9. Coach the patient to inhale and exhale normally.

10. If the patient feels uncomfortable for any reason during the procedure, the patient should remove the mask and breathe normally.

11. No one should apply or hold the face mask to the patient except the patient.

12. Monitor the patient for changes in level of consciousness and other vital signs.

EPINEPHRINE AUTOINJECTORS (EPI-PEN)

Patients who experience severe allergic reactions now carry epinephrine in autoinjectors. These injectors deliver an intramuscular dose of 0.3 mg of epinephrine for adults or 0.15 mg for children. These injectors are indicated for severe allergic reactions due to insect stings or bites, foods, drugs, or other allergens.

1. Receive order.

2. Confirm the order, amount to be given, and route and write the information down.

3. Prepare the necessary equipment and observe body substance isolation precautions (gloves):
   - Epinephrine autoinjector
   - Personal protective equipment

4. Explain to the patient what you are going to do and reconfirm that the patient is not allergic to the medication. Be sure to advise the patient of any complications that might result from the administration.

5. Assess need for epinephrine administration.

6. Examine the autoinjector for name, dose, and expiration date.

7. Remove safety cap from autoinjector.

8. Place autoinjector on outer thigh.

9. Press hard until you hear the injector function.

10. Hold autoinjector in place for several seconds.

11. Gently massage the injection area for 10 to 15 seconds.

12. Take the patient's vital signs, connect the patient to a cardiac monitor, and watch for a change in the patient's condition.

UMBILICAL VEIN CATHETERIZATION

Umbilical vein catheterization (UVC) is a method of gaining access by placing a special catheter or tubing into the umbilical vein of the neonatal umbilicus. This procedure allows the paramedic to administer fluids or medications when percutaneous cannulation into a small vein is impossible. Indications include a neonatal patient, less than 1 week of age, in need of intravenous (IV) access but without accessible peripheral veins.

The procedure is as follows:

1. Receive order.

2. Confirm the drug order, amount to be given, and route and write the information down.

3. Prepare the necessary equipment and observe body substance isolation precautions (gloves and goggles):

   - Appropriate IV fluid and administration set (previously set up)
   - Appropriate indwelling catheter
   - Povidone-iodine or alcohol preparations
   - Antibiotic ointment
   - 2 × 2 gauze pad
   - 1-inch tape
   - Sharps container

4. Explain to the patient's parents what you are going to do. Be sure to advise the patient's parents of any complications that might result from the procedure.

5. Restrain the infant, if necessary.

6. Clean and drape the area. The umbilicus should be cleansed, using povidone-iodine solution.

7. Place a loose tie of umbilical tape around the base of the umbilicus.

8. Locate the two umbilical arteries and one umbilical vein. The vein has a thin wall and larger lumen compared with the thick walls and smaller lumen of the umbilical arteries. Trim the cord approximately 1 cm to provide a fresh opening.

9. Using a sterile hemostat, insert the tip of the hemostat into the lumen of the vein. Gently open the hemostat to dilate the vessel.

10. Introduce and advance a heparinized–saline flushed umbilical catheter approximately 2 to 4 inches. This will place the catheter into the inferior vena cava of the infant. You should note blood return after inserting the catheter. Do not force the catheter because severe hemorrhage or liver injury may occur.

11. Hook up the catheter to a three-way stopcock. Flush the catheter with 1 mL heparin solution.

12. Secure the catheter, using the piece of umbilical tape, by tying the tape around the umbilicus.

13. After securing the catheter, hook the IV tubing to the stopcock to allow for the administration of fluids and/or medications.

14. Monitor the umbilicus for bleeding. A dressing is usually not used in this situation, so that the umbilicus can be viewed.

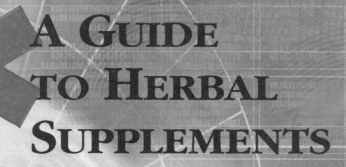
Herb	Source: medicinal ingredients	Classification	Suggested uses
Alfalfa (*Medicago sativa*)	**Leaves and flowers:** Vitamins, minerals, proteins, enzymes	Diuretic, tonic	Helpful in stomach ailments including aiding peptic ulcers; improves appetite; relieves urinary and bowel disorders; eliminates retained water
Aloe vera (*Aloe vera*)	**Leaves:** Polysaccharides, amino acids, vitamins, minerals, aloin	Emollient, purgative	Healing and soothing for the stomach; effective laxative; useful for bug bites, skin irritation, burns, minor cuts, and scratches; helps the body to eliminate waste material in adults with bronchial asthma
Bilberry (*Vaccinium myrtillus*)	**Fruit:** Anthocyanosides	Antiseptic, astringent	Improves nighttime vision, helps preserve eyesight, prevents eye damage, regulates bowel action, and stimulates appetite
Cascara sagrada (*Rhamnus purshiana*)	**Dried bark:** Hydroxianthracene derivative (HAD), free anthraquinone	Laxative, tonic	Acts on large intestine and stimulates peristalsis; useful in constipation, dyspepsia, and other digestive complaints; liver tonic *Caution: Contraindicated in lactating or pregnant women*

Herb	Source: medicinal ingredients	Classification	Suggested uses
Cat's claw (*Uncaria tomentosa*)	**Bark:** Proanthocyanidins, alkaloids, phytochemicals	Antiviral, antioxidant	Useful in stimulating the flow of gastric juices and pancreatic secretions; beneficial for irritable bowel syndrome and Crohn's disease; anti-inflammatory, immune system booster
Cayenne (*Capsicum frutescens*)	**Fruit:** Capsaicin, carotenoids, capsicidins heat value 40,000 scovill units per gram	Stimulant, digestive	Used to stimulate appetite and aid digestion; increases production of gastric juices and relieves gas and bowel pains or cramps; irritating to hemorrhoids *Caution: Do not use in gastrointestinal problems*
Chamomile (*Maticaria chamomilla*)	**Flower:** Volatile oil, bisabolols, flavonoids	Anti-inflammatory, antispasmodic, anti-infective, mild sedative, calmative	Calms the nerves and upset stomach; reduces anxiety, soothes ulcers, and reduces mucous membrane inflammations; good antibacterial action; rare cases of allergic reaction in those with severe hypersensitivity to ragweed pollen
Coltsfoot (*Tussilago farfara*)	**Leaves:** Flavonoids, mucilage, tannin	Expectorant, anticatarrhal, antispasmodic, demulcent	Pulmonary coughs and colds; used for asthma, bronchitis, and emphysema
Cranberry (*Vaccinium macrocrarpon*)	**Twig and fruit:** Anthocyanidins	Antioxidant, bacteriostatic effect	Cleanses and stops infections in the urinary tract
Damiana (*Turnera aphrodisiaca*)	**Leaves and flowers:** Volatile oil, flavonoids, hydroquinine, glycoside	Tonic, nervine, aphrodisiac, antidepressant	Recommended as a laxative and as a general tonic; helps relieve anxiety and may enhance sexual performance *Caution: Damiana interferes with iron absorption*
Dandelion (*Taraxacum officinale*)	**Leaves and Roots:** Sesquiterpenes, triterpenes, phenolic acids, carotenoids	Used in kidney and liver disorders; a natural diuretic and digestive aid; reduces blood pressure, may help prevent iron deficiency, anemia, chronic rheumatism, gout, and stiff joints	Used in kidney and liver disorders; a natural diuretic and digestive aid; reduces blood pressure and may help prevent iron deficiency, anemia, chronic rheumatism, gout, and stiff joints

Herb	Source: medicinal ingredients	Classification	Suggested uses
Devil's claw (*Harpagophytum procumbens*)	**Root:** Harpogoside, beta-sitosterol	Anti-inflammatory, antirheumatic, analgesic, sedative	For arthritis and rheumatism; helpful to reduce swelling, relieve pain, and improve mobility in the joints *Caution: Contraindicated during pregnancy*
Dong quai (*Angelica sinensis*)	**Root:** Volatile aromatic oil, polysaccharides	Tonic immuno-stimulant, antispasmodic	Used to treat all symptoms of menopause as an alternative to estrogen therapy; regulates the hormonal system; overall tonic for female reproductive system; reduces high blood pressure and premenstrual syndrome *Caution: Contraindicated in pregnancy*
Echinacea (*Echinacea angustifolia* and *E. purpurea*)	**Root:** Echinacosides, polysaccharides, phytosterols	Antibiotic, antifungal immunostimulant	Stimulates and boosts immune function; has cortisone-like activity that helps wound healing; fights bacterial and viral infections *Caution: Contraindicated in pregnancy*
Evening primrose (*Oenothera biennis*)	**Plant:** Gamma-linolenic acid (GLA), mixed tocopherols	Antispasmodic	Used in treatment of multiple sclerosis and premenstrual syndrome; helps prevent heart disease and stroke and maintains healthy skin *Caution: Excess consumption can result in oily skin*
Eyebright (*Euphrasia officinalis*)	**Herb:** Iridoid glycosides, tannins, phenolic acids, volatile oil	Astringent, tonic	Strengthens the eye and assists in aiding the body to dissolve cataracts, heal lesions, and heal conjunctivitis
Fenugreek (*Trigonella foenum-graecum*)	**Seeds:** Flavonoids, saponin, vitamins	Demulcent, expectorant	Helpful in stomach and intestinal problems; good expectorant for coughs and colds
Feverfew (*Tanacetum parthenium*)	**Leaves:** Sesquiterpene lactones (parthenolide)	Anti-inflammatory, emmenagogue	Helps prevent migraine headaches and also useful against swelling and arthritis; stimulates digestion and improves liver function *Caution: Contraindicated in lactating or pregnant women*

Herb	Source: medicinal ingredients	Classification	Suggested uses
Ginger (*Zingiber officinale*)	**Root:** Volatile oil, phenylalkylketones	Diaphoretic, cholagogue, carminative, stimulant	Relieves indigestion and abdominal cramping; benefit in relieving motion sickness, dizziness, nausea, and colds; ginger lowers blood clotting
Ginkgo biloba (*Ginkgo biloba*)	**Leaves:** Flavoglycosides (quercetin, proanthocyanidins); also contains terpenes	Antiasthmatic, bronchodilator, platelet activating factor (PAF) inhibitor	Increases blood flow to the brain; decreases memory loss, Alzheimer's disease, cerebral vascular insufficiency, and blood clotting; has the ability to neutralize free radicals and also beneficial for asthma, stress, vertigo, and tinnitus *Caution: Potential drug interaction with warfarin and aspirin; take with food*
Ginseng (*Panax schin-seng*)	**Root:** Ginsenosides (triterpene saponins), glycosides	Tonic, stimulant, demulcent, stomachache	Stimulates both physical and mental activity; antifatigue (insomnia, nervousness, poor appetite); enhances immune system, inhibits exhaustion of adrenal gland; antistress *Caution: If you are pregnant or if you have high blood pressure, consult with your physician or health practitioner before using*
Goldenseal (*Hydrastis canadensis*)	**Root:** Alkaloids (hydrastine), fatty acids, volatile oil	Anti-inflammatory, tonic, mild laxative	Strengthens the immune system to help cold and flu symptoms; acts as an anti-inflammatory; helpful in constipation and in stomach disorders such as indigestion *Caution: Contraindicated during pregnancy*
Guggulipids (*Commiphora mukul*)	**Stem:** Essential oil, guggulsterone, oleoresin	Anticholesterenic	Lowers blood cholesterol by 14 to 27 percent and can lower triglycerides by 22 to 23 percent; helps reduce atherosclerotic plaques; improves the heart metabolism and increases liver metabolism of low-density lipoprotein cholesterol *Caution: Contraindicated during pregnancy*

Herb	Source: medicinal ingredients	Classification	Suggested uses
Hawthorn (*Crategus oxyacantha*)	**Berries:** Flavonoids, glycosides, saponins, catechins, tannins, procyanidins	Cardiac tonic, hypotensive, antisclerotic	Alleviates hypertension and high blood pressure and reduces the severity of angina attacks; sedative and antispasmodic effects
Horsetail (*Equisetum arvense*)	**Herb:** Silicic acid, minerals, silica, flavoglucosides, saponins, alkaloids	Astringent, diuretic	Genitourinary complaints, mild diuretic, broken nails, hair loss, skin; stimulates an increase in white blood cells; used for arteriosclerosis and inflamed or enlarged prostate
Licorice (*Glycyrrhiza glabra*)	**Root:** Glycyrrhizin, flavonoids	Demulcent, diuretic, expectorant, laxative	Gastric ulcers, adrenal insufficiency, and hypoglycemia; good for coughs and other bronchial complaints *Caution: Contraindicated for those with high blood pressure or if pregnant*
Milk thistle (*Siybum marianum*)	**Seeds and Leaves:** Flavonoids (silymarin)	Hepatoprotective, cholagogue	Promotes flow of bile; tonic for spleen, stomach, kidney, and gallbladder; beneficial for liver disease (jaundice, hepatitis, and cirrhosis)
Oats (*Avena sativa*)	**Stems and seeds:** Proteins, c-glycosyl flavones, avenacosides	Antidepressant, cardiac tonic, nervine	Lessens debility, depression, stress, and menopause symptoms; good for skin disease; tonic for impotence
Parsley (*Petroselinum sativum*)	**Leaves and seeds:** Volatile oil, coumarins, flavonoids	Carminative, diuretic, expectorant, antispasmodic	Relieves gas and is a natural diuretic; good for coughs, asthma, and suppressed or difficult menstruation
Peppermint (*Mentha piperita*)	**Leaves:** Essential oil, flavonoids, carotenes	Diaphoretic, carminative, antispasmodic	Aids in digestion, flatulence, colds, influenza, and migraines
Pumpkin (*Cucurbita pepo*)	**Seeds:** Linoleic acid, cucurbitacins, zinc	Diuretic, demulcent, taeniacide, anthelmintic	Effective in reducing the size and symptoms of an enlarged prostate. Helps to expel tapeworms
Pygeum (*Pygeum africanum*)	**Bark:** Phytosterols (sitosterols), terpenoids, ferulic esters	Anti-inflammatory, diuretic, antiedema	Prostatitis, benign prostatic hypertrophy (BPH), incontinence, painful urination, dysuria, cancer of the prostate, and urinary tract disorders

Herb	Source: medicinal ingredients	Classification	Suggested uses
Rosehips (*Rosa species*)	**Fruit:** Bioflavonoids, vitamins (C, B-complex)	Astringent, diuretic, tonic	Excellent source of vitamin C for nervous and stressful situations; helps prevent infections; blood purifier
Saw palmetto (*Serenoa serrulata*)	**Berries:** Saponins, phytosterols, fatty acids, volatile oil	Tonic, diuretic, sedative, endocrine agent	Benign prostatic hypotrophy, antiallergic and anti-inflammatory; urinary tract disorders, impotence, and infertility in women
Slippery elm (*Ulmus fulva*)	**Inner bark:** Mucilage: galactose, galacturonic acid	Demulcent, emollient, astringent, mucilage	Gastric or duodenal ulcers; inflammation of stomach, colitis, coughs, sore throat, and soothes skin disorders
St. John's wort (*Hypericum perforatum*)	**Herb:** Essential oil, glycosides (hypericin), flavonoids	Sedative, anti-inflammatory, astringent	Antidepressant; stress and irritability; immune support, anti-inflammatory, antiviral, AIDS *Caution: Avoid excessive exposure to sunlight since hypericin may render the skin photosensitive; note: most resembles monoamine oxidase inhibitors*
Valerian (*Valeriana officinalis*)	**Root:** Valerinic acid, sequiterpenes, glycoside, essential oils	Sedative, hypnotic, nervine, hypotensive	Balancing agent for hyperexcitability and exhaustion; calms nervous disorders and acts as both sedative and tranquilizer; helps headaches, high blood pressure, and stomach and menstrual cramps *Caution: Contraindicated in pregnancy; high doses should be avoided over a long period of time*
White willow (*Salix alba*)	**Bark:** Salicin, tannins, flavonoid glycosides (quercetin)	Analgesic, anti-inflammatory, tonic	Soothes headaches and reduces fevers; helps stomach ailments and heartburn; mild analgesic for arthritic and rheumatic conditions
Wild yam (*Dioscorea villosa*)	**Root:** Diosgenins, saponins, glycosides	Anti-inflammatory, cholagogue, mild diaphoretic, spasmolytic	Menopause, menstrual cramps, ovarian pain; various types of rheumatism and intestinal colic

Herb	Source: medicinal ingredients	Classification	Suggested uses
Bee pollen	**Bee pollen:** Vitamins, minerals, enzymes, amino acids	Supplement	Provides energy and essential nutrients; helpful in stomach ailments, hormonal system, allergies, hay fever, and exhaustion and builds resistance to diseases *Caution: Some people may be allergic to bee pollen; try small amounts of doses daily*
Coenzyme Q10	**CO Q10 Ubiquinone:** Japanese source	Supplement	Vital role in energy production at the cellular level and recommended in the treatment of cardiovascular disease; revitalizes the immune system
Flaxseed	**Seed:** Alpha-linolenic acid (ALA), omega-3 series of essential fatty acids	Purgative, demulcent, emollient	Helps lower cholesterol and blood triglyceride levels and helps prevent clot formation; digestive and urinary disorders
Glucosamine sulfate	**Crab shell:** Glucose, amino and sulfate group, mucopolysaccharides, glycoproteins	Supplement	Stimulates the synthesis of cartilage in the joints; relief from pain and inflammation around joints associated with osteoarthritis
Pycnogenol	**Pine bark extract:** Proanthocyanidins, natural soluble organic acids, glucose, bioflavonoid	Antioxidant	Strengthens blood vessels and useful for allergies; anti-inflammatory and antiaging; neutralizes existing free radicals in the blood

COMMON USES OF HERBAL EXTRACTS

Note: The following information should not be used for the diagnosis, treatment, or prevention of disease in humans. The information contained herein is in no way intended to be a guide to medical practice or a recommendation that herbs be used for medicinal purposes. This information is presented here for its educational value and as information for medical personnel.

Condition	Common herbs
Allergy	Nettles, echinacea, goldenseal, bee pollen
Antibacterial	Echinacea, garlic, angelica, barberry
Anticatarrhal	Elder, goldenseal, sandalwood, hyssop
Antidepressant	Lavender, St. John's wort, oats, damiana, rosemary, schizandra
Antifungal	Garlic, propolis, cinnamon, black walnut
Anti-inflammatory	Oak bark, thyme, peppermint, propolis, sage
Antiseptic	Peppermint, thyme, propolis, sage, oak bark, black walnut
Antispasmodic	Valerian, passion flower, peppermint, red clover, catnip, rosemary, motherwort, thyme
Antiviral	St. John's wort, echinacea, garlic, astragalus
Aphrodisiac	Schizandra, ginseng, damiana
Arthritis or rheumatism	Devil's claw, alfalfa, wild yam, white willow, black cohosh, sarsaparilla, glucosamine
Asthma	Mullein, coltsfoot, goldenseal, ginkgo biloba, horehound, licorice, elecampane, blessed thistle, wild cherry, blue cohosh
Astringent	Nettles, plantain, red raspberry, oak bark, goldenseal, rhubarb, sage, true unicorn, yellow dock, wild cherry bark, wood betony
Blood purifiers	Red clover, blessed thistle, burdock, sarsaparilla
Bronchial support	Schizandra, mullein, coltsfoot, fenugreek, horehound, hyssop, licorice, elecampane, thyme, myrrh, goldenseal
Cardiovascular	Hawthorn, fo-ti, oats, reishi, motherwort
Cholesterol	Hawthorn, reishi, linden, guggulipids
Circulatory	Ginkgo biloba, garlic, ginger, gotu kola, capsicum, prickly ash, hawthorn, bioflavonoids
Colds or flu	Echinacea, catnip, peppermint, boneset, elder, zinc lozenge
Cough	Wild cherry bark, licorice (daytime usage), slippery elm, coltsfoot, horehound
Diarrhea (*also see* Astringent)	Oak bark, plantain, thyme, chamomile
Digestive aids	Barberry, true unicorn, yellow dock, wild cherry bark, wood betony
Diuretics	Parsley, corn silk, couch grass, dandelion (also natural potassium source), buchu, uva ursi, rosehips, sandalwood
Earache	Mullein oil, garlic, sage (to swab in and around ear)
Eczema	Nettles, chickweed, goldenseal, red clover, burdock
Expectorant	Elecampane, fenugreek, plantain, thyme, horehound, hyssop, licorice, sage, mullein, garlic
Eyes	Eyebright, chamomile (eyewash)
Fever	Sage, thyme, echinacea, white willow, nettles, wild indigo, yarrow
Flatulence	Fennel, peppermint, ginger, sage
Hay fever	Nettles, echinacea (*see* Allergy)
Headache	White willow, peppermint, lavender, passion, flower, wood betony, linden, ginger, rosemary, valerian
High blood pressure	Garlic, hawthorne, yarrow
Immune support	Astragalus, reishi, nettles, shiitake, schizandra, echinacea, propolis, garlic, Pau D'Arco, cat's claw
Impotency	Oats, ginseng, damiana, sarsaparilla
Kidney or bladder	Couch grass, meadowsweet, uva ursi, cranberry
Laxative	Cascara sagrada, rhubarb
Liver	Yellow dock, milk thistle, boneset, fo-ti, blessed thistle, barberry, lipoic acid
Lymphatics	Echinacea, red clover
Male hormonals	Sarsaparilla, ginseng, damiana, oats
Menopause or premenstrual syndrome	Dong quai, evening primrose, licorice, black cohosh
Mental alertness	Ginkgo biloba, rosemary, gotu kola, periwinkle (helpful with senility)

Migraine headaches	Feverfew
Nausea	Peppermint, gingerroot, red raspberry
Nervine	Oats, passion flower, hops, chamomile, valerian, linden, reishi, rosemary, skullcap
Oral (mouthwash or antiseptics)	Myrrh gum, oak bark, goldenseal, chlorophyll
Pain (reduction)	Hops, white willow, valerian (also add immune herbal)
Prostate	Saw palmetto, pygeum, pumpkin seed
Psoriasis	Burdock, red clover, echinacea, chickweed, yellow dock, sarsaparilla
Respiratory	Horehound, mullein, myrrh, astragalus, goldenseal, elecampane
Shingles	Passion flower, echinacea, oats (proper nutritional and stress support)
Sore throat	Sage, slippery elm, wild indigo, red raspberry, echinacea
Stomachache	Fennel, ginger, peppermint, chamomile
Thyroid	Bladderwrack
Tonic	Ginseng, reishi, schizandra, gotu kola, fo-ti, nettles, oat
Ulcers	Marshmallow, licorice, slippery elm (gastric peptic), meadowsweet, red clover

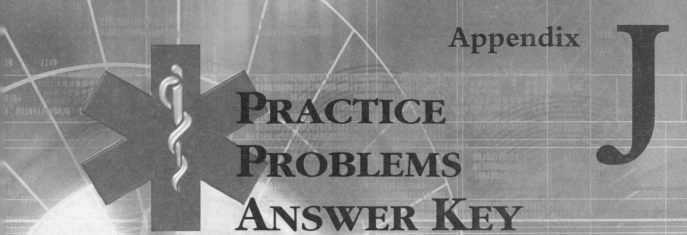

PRACTICE
PROBLEMS
ANSWER KEY

SECTION 1

1.	1 g	=	1000 mg
2.	1 mg	=	1000 μg
3.	1 mg	=	0.001 g
4.	0.8 mg	=	800 μg
5.	1.5 L	=	1500 mL
6.	400 000 mg	=	400 g
7.	800 mg	=	0.8 g
8.	500 mL	=	0.5 L
9.	37°C	=	98.6°F
10.	104°F	=	40°C
11.	1/4 gr	=	16.25 mg
12.	2 Tbsp	=	30 mL
13.	180 lb	=	82 kg
14.	7 lb	=	3.2 kg
15.	25 kg	=	55 lb

SECTION 2

1. 10 mL
2. 4 mL
3. 5 mL
4. 100 mL
5. 2 mL

6. 0.33 mL
7. 1.5 mL
8. 2 mL
9. 8 mL
10. 50 mL

SECTION 3

1. 3.4 mL *This could be approximated to 3.5 mL. Check with your medical control.*
2. 6.8 mL
3. 0.59 mL *This could be approximated to 0.6 mL. Check with your medical control.*
4. 72 mL or 73 mL
5. 0.2 mL

SECTION 4

1. 800 mg/mL
2. 9 g
3. 5 mg/mL
4. 50 mg
5. 100 mg
6. 4 mg/mL
7. 1600 mg/mL
8. 3 mL
9. 4 μg/mL
10. 2 mg/mL

SECTION 5

1. 30 gtt/min
2. 60 gtt/min
3. 30 gtt/min
4. 30 gtt/min
5. 30 gtt/min
6. 5 gtt/min

7. 15 gtt/min
8. 23 gtt/min
9. 6 gtt/min
10. 60 gtt/min

SECTION 6

1. 30 gtt/min
2. 15 gtt/min
3. 30 gtt/min
4. 45 gtt/min
5. 45 gtt/min
6. 90 gtt/min
7. 15 gtt/min
8. 51–52 gtt/min
9. 10 mg/kg/min
10. 4 mg/kg/min

SECTION 7

1. 100 gtt/min
2. 50 gtt/min
3. 15 gtt/min
4. 100 gtt/min (first hour)
   25 gtt/min (over 8 hours)
5. 38 gtt/min

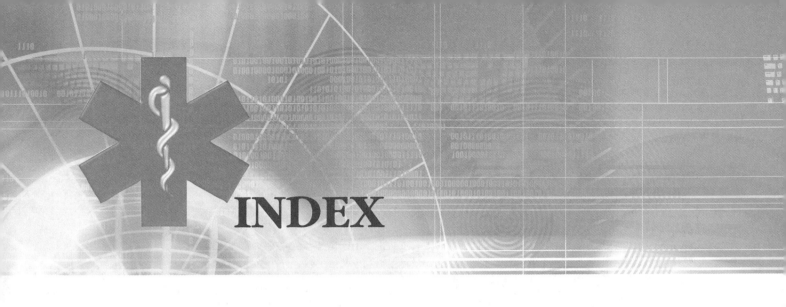

INDEX

Inocor, 148–149, 416–417
Inotrope, 128, 218
Insertion of indwelling IV catheter, 111–115
Insulin, 3, 270–274, 435, 481–482, 495
Insulin shock, 269–270
Internal environment, 87
International controls, 13
International System of Units (SI), 65
Interstitial fluid, 87
Intestinal anthrax, 400
Intracardiac, 63
Intracellular, 117
Intracellular fluid (ICF), 87
Intradermal, 63
Intramuscular (IM) injection, 57–58, 61, 510–513
Intraosseous (IO) infusion, 58–59, 523–525
Intravascular fluid, 87
Intravenous bolus administration, 518–520
Intravenous cannulation, 112–115
Intravenous fluids. *See* Fluids, electrolytes and IV
   therapy
Intravenous (IV) injection, 58, 513–522
   external jugular vein cannulation, 516–518
   IV bolus, 518–520
   IV piggyback, 520–522
   macrodrip/microdrip, 513
   pediatric patients, 62
   peripheral IV access, 514–516
   setup, 513–514
Intravascular, 117
Intropin, 143–145, 425–426
Investigational new drug (IND), 6
IO infusion, 58–59, 523–525
Ipratropium, 239–240, 435–436
Iron, 333–334
Irreversible antagonism, 35
Irritant gases, 394–395
Ischemic chest pain algorithm, 472
Islets of Langerhans, 266
Isoetharine, 234–235, 436
Isopropyl alcohol, 335
Isoproterenol, 141–143, 436–437
Isoptin, 170–171, 464
Isotonic solutions, 95
Isuprel, 141–143, 436–437
IV bolus administration, 518–520
IV cannulation, 112–115
IV injection. *See* Intravenous (IV) injection
IV piggyback, 520–522
IV push, 518–520
IV therapy, 94–115. *See also* Fluids, electrolytes
   and IV therapy

Jenner, Edward, 2

Ketalar, 256–257, 437
Ketamine, 256–257, 437
Ketoacidosis, 267, 268–269
Ketones, 268
Ketorolac, 387–388, 437–438

KI, 401
Korsakoff's psychosis, 279
Kussmaul respirations, 266, 269

L, 66
Labeling, 11
Labetalol, 155–156, 438
Laboratory-produced drug sources, 4–5
Lactated Ringer's solution, 103–104, 409
Lactic acid, 133
Lanoxin, 181–182, 423
Largactil, 357–358, 421–422
Lasix, 201–202, 431, 500
Leukocytes, 92
Levalbuterol, 230–231, 438–439
Levophed, 140–141, 449–450
Lewisite, 394
Licorice, 534
Lidocaine, 160–163, 439, 500, 502, 503
Lilly Cyanide Antidote Kit, 324
Lipid-soluble drugs, 30
Liquid drugs, 18–20
Listings. *See* Quick reference
Liter (L), 66
Lithium, 335–336
Loading dose, 33
Local, 63
Lopressor, 153–154, 444
Lorazepam. *See* Ativan (lorazepam)
Lovenox, 184–185, 427
Luminal, 296, 298, 452

m³, 66
Magnesium, 89
Magnesium sulfate
   cardiovascular system, 176–177
   obstetrical/gynecological emergencies,
      304–305
   quick reference, 440–441
   respiratory system, 240–241
Maintenance dose, 33
Mannitol, 36, 285–286, 441
Marburg virus, 398
Margin of safety, 44
Mark I kit, 395, 396
Mechanism of action, 34–36
Medical asepsis, 54–55
Medical control, 12–13
Medical control protocols and guidelines, 12–13
Medical director, 11–12
Medical oversight, 11–17
   controlled drugs, 14, 15
   drug names, 16–17
   drug standards, 16
   international controls, 13
   medical control, 12–13
   medical director, 11–12
   narcotics, 14
   U.S. controls, 13–14
Medically clean techniques, 54

Xeriscape™ Gardening

X·E·R·I·S·C·A·P·E™
G·A·R·D·E·N·I·N·G

Water Conservation for the American Landscape

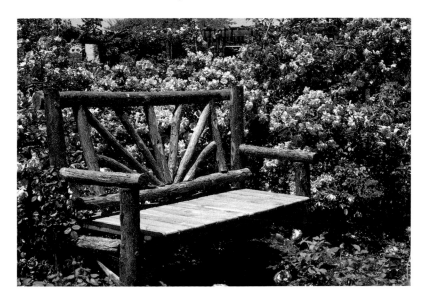

Principal Photography by Connie Lockhart Ellefson

Connie Lockhart Ellefson,
Thomas L. Stephens,
and Doug Welsh, Ph.D.

MACMILLAN PUBLISHING COMPANY
NEW YORK

MAXWELL MACMILLAN CANADA
TORONTO

MAXWELL MACMILLAN INTERNATIONAL
NEW YORK OXFORD SINGAPORE SYDNEY

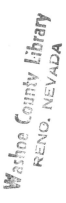

In selecting plants look for time-tested favorites. Old-fashioned or antique roses have a place in any Xeriscape landscape because of their inherent durability and drought tolerance.
(PHOTO: DOUG WELSH)

Macmillan Publishing Company   Maxwell Macmillan Canada, Inc.
866 Third Avenue   1200 Eglinton Avenue East, Suite 200
New York, NY 10022   Don Mills, Ontario M3C 3N1

Macmillan Publishing Company is part of the Maxwell Communcation Group of Companies.

Library of Congress Cataloging-in-Publication Data

Ellefson, Connie Lockhart, 1954–
    Xeriscape gardening: water conservation for the American
landscape / Connie Ellefson, Tom Stephens, and Doug Welsh.
        p.   cm.
    Includes index.
    ISBN 0-02-614125-6
    1. Xeriscaping—United States.   2. Drought-tolerant plants—United
States.   I. Stephens Thomas (Thomas L.)   II. Welsh, Douglas F.
III. Title.
SB475.83.E45   1992
635.9′5—dc20   91-32779   CIP

Macmillan books are available at special discounts for bulk purchases for sales promotions, premiums, fund-raising, or educational use. For details, contact:
Special Sales Director
Macmillan Publishing Company
866 Third Avenue
New York, NY 10022

10 9 8 7 6 5 4 3 2 1

Printed in the United States of America

To my grandfathers, Bruce Hixson and
Cecil Lockhart, who gave me my green thumb.
—Connie Lockhart Ellefson

This book is gratefully dedicated to the memory of my parents, Clyde and
Dorothy Stephens, and my grandparents, Ralph and Laura Nolin, who
taught me the significance of plants and the environment in which we
live, the value of hard work and persistence, and the importance of serving
God through serving others with my life.
—Thomas L. Stephens

To my wife, Julie, for her encouragement and support.
—Doug Welsh, Ph.D.

Contents

Acknowledgments

I would like to thank all of the terrific people who cheerfully shared their ideas and gardens with me. Getting acquainted and working with you was the best part of this project.

Northeast: Bonnie Lee Appleton, Elizabeth Brabec, Ruth Dyckman, Jeff Featherstone, Al Frank, Robert Griffith, Bruce Hamilton, Jeff Licht, Bruce and Cindy McGranahan, Don Rakow, Justin Schwartz, Jan Shaw, Manny Shemin, Richard Weir.

Southeast: Bruce Adams, Diane Culver, Pat Dailey, Steve and Yvonne Havas, Andy Hull, Gary Knox, Preston Lewis, Fox McCarthy, Brian Smith, Todd Tibbitts, Gary Wade.

Central: Bonnie Arnold, Lucia Athens, Bill Ball, Ken Ball, James Beard, Fawn Bell, Don Buma, Elizabeth Burst, Betty and Frank Cordiner, Wilbur Davis, David Draper, Gary Finstad, Dale Greenwood, Bonnie Harper-Lore, May and Randolph Harris, Diane Henderson et al., Gary Hightshoe, Dick Hildreth, Greg Hurst, Panayoti Kelaidis, Jim Knopf, Martha Latta, Terry Lewis, Dick and Rollande Lockhart, Alvis McFarland, Robert McNeil, Mike Miller, Sandy Snyder, Anna Thurston, Bob Vilotti, Sally Wasowski, Carl Whitcomb, Mark Widrlechner, Mary Witt, Ben Wofford, Dan and Amber Wofford, Suzanne Wuerthele.

Southwest: Cathy Conner, Ali Davidson, Steven Davis, Lynn Ellen Doxon, Pete Ellefson, Polly Fukuhara, Bob Haggard, David Harbison, Ken Harrison, Jean Heflin, Gerry Kiff, John Olaf Nelson, Kent Newland, Judith Phillips, Jane Ploeser, Kay Stewart, Tom Stille, Lariene Treat, Jan Tubiolo, John White.

Northwest: Dan Borroff, Nota Lucas, Gil Schieber, Cathy Wright.

Hawaii: Denise DeCosta, Chester Lao, Paul Weissich.

Special thanks to those master long-sufferers, Jerry, Ben, and Ian Ellefson, and to my editor, Pam Hoenig.

CONNIE LOCKHART ELLEFSON

I would like to thank
— My teachers, from elementary through graduate school—particularly Mrs. Bernice Wright and Miss Goldie Jenkins of Mt. Pleasant School—who believed in me and taught me to read, design, and think for myself;
— My many students, clients, and employees through the years—especially Byron Pursiful and Kim Folks—who have challenged me to get the best from them and from myself, whether teaching, writing, designing, or constructing a landscape project;
— My wonderful wife, Sandy, and our super children, Scott, Jason, and Edie Jane, who have continually encouraged and supported me throughout my professional and teaching careers, but especially during the develoment of this book.

And special thank yous to Connie Ellefson, my coauthor, and Pam Hoenig, our editor, for their hard work in completing this book and for their efforts at keeping me on track, which was often a mighty challenge.

THOMAS L. STEPHENS

The Xeriscape landscape movement has brought together two dynamic groups of people: the gardeners (amateur and professional) and the water providers (utilites, authorities, and agencies). These groups, referred to as the "green" and "blue" industries, have the common goal of preserving our water resources and enhancing landscape beauty within our concrete cities. Through their combined efforts, these groups have made, and continue to make, a difference. As a horticultural educator and past president of the National Xeriscape Council, Inc., I have been privileged to circulate among Xeriscape enthusiasts across the nation. Some of my most cherished relationships have resulted from my professional activities in Xeriscape landscaping.

This book represents the collective efforts of more than just the three authors. However, without the efforts of Connie Lockhart Ellefson this book would not have been completed. I would like to acknowledge the sacrifice, dedication, and expertise that Connie brought to the book.

I would also like to acknowledge my valued colleagues in the Extension Service at Texas A&M University. Their shared knowledge is overwhelming and a resource that I draw upon often.

And, finally, I wish to recognize my children, Katherine and John, for they are my selfish reason for working to preserve water resources and protect the environment for the future.

DOUG WELSH, PH.D.

Preface

This book is dedicated to the home landscaper who wishes to improve the environment, extend the relaxing influence of the natural beauty of the region, and/or simply save money and time while enjoying the landscape.

It was conceived out of my own frustration at having no idea what to do next after being inspired by Xeriscape lectures by the Denver Water Department. This book is intended to be an informative manual that will make it abundantly clear what your next step should be, no matter the degree to which you want to reduce your landscape watering.

A Note About Xeriscape™ Gardening

The drought of 1977 across California, the Great Plains, and the Rocky Mountains left little doubt that we must seriously rethink our assumptions about endless supplies of fresh water for landscapes. The word "Xeriscape" was created in 1981 by a task force consisting of members of the Denver Water Department, Colorado State University, and the Associated Landscape Contractors of Colorado to focus on a new way to look at landscaping: water conservation through creative landscaping.

The concept of Xeriscape landscaping was an attempt to begin the process of change in landscaping which would lessen the effects of water shortages experienced in future droughts. Its purpose was to focus attention on the amount of water used in landscaping and to publicize ways it could be reduced without sacrificing quality of surroundings.

The task force felt so strongly that the word "Xeriscape" should always be associated with their carefully developed "Seven Principles of Xeriscape Landscaping" that the Denver Water Department trademarked the word to remind people that the two go hand in hand.

In 1986 the trademark was given to the National Xeriscape Council, Inc. (NXCI), a nonprofit organization founded to promote and ensure the integrity of Xeriscape landscaping. It serves as a clearinghouse for information about Xeriscape landscaping and supports the development of Xeriscape demonstration gardens all over the United States.

NXCI has reviewed this book for adherence to the Xeriscape principles, found it acceptable, and has, thus, licensed the book.

We gratefully acknowledge NXCI for providing hundreds of pages of information and sources of information in the preparation of this book, and for reviewing the manuscript.

The term Xeriscape and the Xeriscape logo are trademarks of the National Xeriscape Council, Inc., P.O. Box 767936, Roswell, GA 30076.

P·A·R·T O·N·E

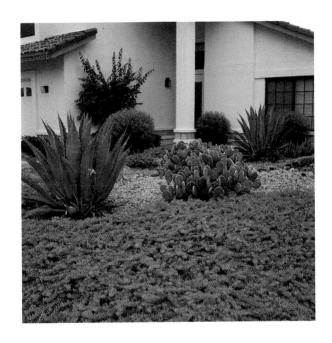

The Xeriscape
Principles

Xeriscape Landscaping:

*Quality Landscaping That Conserves
Water and Protects the Environment*

XERISCAPE LANDSCAPING... What it is not:
- Vast seas of gravel and concrete
- A few forlorn cacti surrounded by gravel
- More brown than green
- All dry and dusty
- "Zero-scape"

What it is: A charming, disarming, compelling, and often lush solution to an age-old problem that has become an urgent one as we move into the twenty-first century: how to create a beautiful, restful outdoor environment without pouring thousands of gallons of expensively purified water down the drain in the process.

"Xeriscape™" is a sleek new word that represents a sensible old idea: Let the outdoor environment you create around your home echo the natural world of your region, and you'll reap countless rewards, including simplifying your life and adding restful beauty. This approach has come into its own in recent years with the wide welcome given to such ideas as low-maintenance landscaping, natural landscaping, and the like.

With Xeriscape landscaping, however, there is a new and compelling twist—the designing or redesigning of a landscape to eliminate some of the estimated fifty percent of domestic or residential water usage that goes into maintaining landscapes in the United States. That is, nearly half of the water employed for domestic use ends up on your lawn or garden. And approximately half of *that* amount is considered to be applied unnecessarily or wasted.

Coined from the Greek word *xeros*, meaning "dry," and *landscape*, Xeriscape landscaping has come to mean "quality, water-efficient landscaping." The creation of a Xeriscape landscape involves a series of specific and interconnected steps, from planning to maintenance, which can result in an estimated twenty to eighty percent savings in landscape water usage.

Xeriscape landscaping does *not* mean, as one might suspect, prickly visions of cactus and yucca, nor does it mean expanses of bone-dry gravel and plastic. Instead, picture a landscape that requires little, if any, additional water save for what falls from the sky as rain or snow or mist—the desert Southwest in spring or the open grasslands of the Great Plains in summer, for example. Every region has its own lushness when left to its own devices, and this is our model for Xeriscape landscapes.

In Xeriscape landscaping we take our cue from the natural world by emphasizing the use of plants for our landscapes which require only the amount of rainfall we have available in our specific region. In Colorado this is an average of fourteen inches per year; in California, eight to eighty inches, depending on the part of the state you're in; in Texas, sixteen to sixty inches; in Florida, fifty-five; and so forth. It often means the use of native plants, or plants adapted to the area's level of natural rainfall.

It may take up to three years to wean a new or changed landscape to a minimum of applied water, but with careful planning, in most parts of the country it's quite possible to reduce or completely eliminate the need for added water above natural precipitation.

Xeriscape landscaping can mean anything from simply paying closer attention to an existing plantscape's site-specific water needs to designing a whole new landscape based on Xeriscape guidelines. It can be as simple as replacing a steeply sloped turf area with lavender or low-growing junipers, or as intricate as renovating an entire existing landscape.

From the beginning, Xeriscape landscaping was meant to show that we can effect dramatic decreases in landscape water usage with no sacrifice in beauty. An important point to understand is that Xeriscape landscaping is adaptable to virtually any style of landscaping, from the most rustic wildflower meadow or rock garden to the most formal groomed lawn with accent plants. There are different degrees of Xeriscape landscaping, too, in that some may require irrigation, but significant water savings are still possible if the water is applied efficiently.

A well-executed Xeriscape landscape may appear indistinguishable from other landscapes on the block. They are often far more beautiful, with sunny displays of sturdy, uncommon flowers and intriguing collections of shrubs and trees—a far cry from the forlorn moonscapes passed off as "low-water, low-maintenance." In fact, in our opinion, if it isn't beautiful, then it isn't a Xeriscape landscape.

Nationwide we pump out an average of 82 billion gallons of water each day from groundwater, and

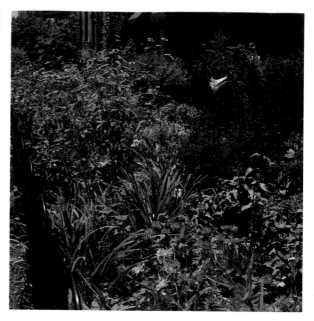

A historic building in Washington, D.C., renovated into office space, provides a home for this courtyard "cottage garden," featuring (clockwise from front) Stokes' aster (Stokesia laevis), orange daylilies (Hemerocallis spp.), black-eyed Susans (Rudbeckia hirta), white garden lily (Lilium spp.), and Japanese barberry (Berberis thunbergii var. atropurpurea).

Sweet-smelling lavender (Lavandula spp.) makes a beautiful addition to any Xeriscape garden, serving as a perennial flower, a low-growing hedge, or a richly textured ground cover.

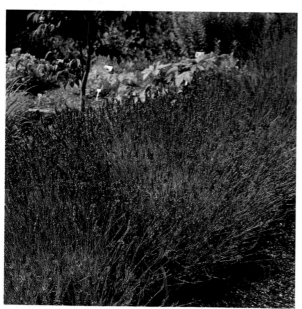

only 61 billion gallons are replaced each day through rainfall and runoff. When we hear of Kentucky bluegrass, which requires thirty-five to forty inches of water (including natural precipitation) each year, blanketing cities that receive fourteen inches of rainfall per year, we know there must be a better way. Large estates in southern Florida, an area that struggles to fill its freshwater needs, may use 600 or more gallons of water per capita (person) per day (gpcd), compared to the national average of 100 to 150 gpcd. Much of that 600 gpcd may be wasted, the victim of poor irrigation.

Even on the modest scale of a residential landscape, the numbers can be an eye-opener. In the Denver area a summertime rise in the monthly water bill of $20 represents about 25,000 gallons that are going to the landscape. Envision a typical 1,800-square-foot house with water nearly two feet deep in it and you have about the amount being poured onto the landscape each summer month in addition to any rainfall.

In nearly every region of the country there is a need for Xeriscape landscaping. The map of drought potential that appears below shows that most of the country may be subject to at least occasional drought, lasting from one to several growing seasons. This contradicts a common misconception about Xeriscape landscaping—that it is necessary only in the arid West, where rainfall is almost invariably less than that required for traditional landscape plants.

In fact, even in parts of the country where rainfall is what we in the West would consider utterly lavish (thirty to forty-five inches per year compared to our eight to fourteen), people still water their yards, not only through the occasional dry spell, but year-round. In those areas, as in any area of the country, proper irrigation management as well as better choices of plants and lawn grasses could eliminate much of that extraneous watering while still maintaining a lush, appealing landscape.

It's jokingly said that a drought in Georgia is when it doesn't rain for three days. In areas of the country such as Georgia or western Washington around Seattle, where the climate is more consistent, with less extremes of temperature and rainfall, it's hard to feel the urgency for Xeriscape landscaping.

Still, there is a two-month rainless period during the summer in Atlanta when water demand shoots up as people water to keep alive landscape plants that can't survive the dry season on their own. In many cases the increased watering is due more to people's strange, innate desire to water in hot weather than the plants' needs for it. The "people pressure" of the rapidly expanding Atlanta area creates peak water demands that local water authorities are sometimes hard-pressed to meet; as a result, Xeriscape landscaping is being actively promoted as "drought insurance." Plants adapted to Atlanta's seasonal variation in precipitation will survive the dry spell without being watered.

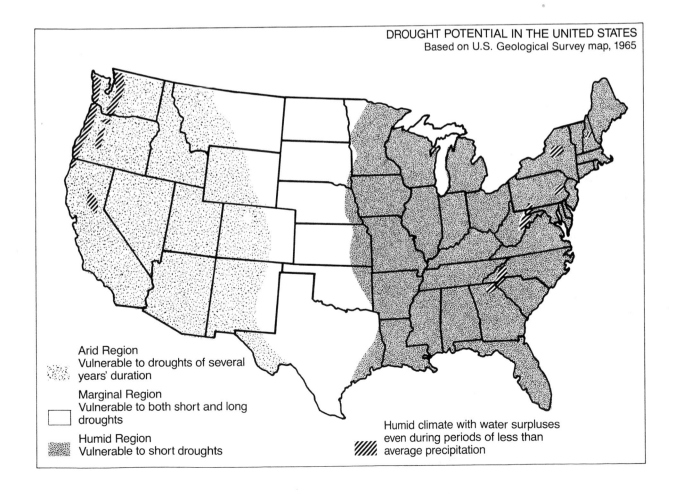

DROUGHT POTENTIAL IN THE UNITED STATES
Based on U.S. Geological Survey map, 1965

Arid Region
Vulnerable to droughts of several years' duration

Marginal Region
Vulnerable to both short and long droughts

Humid Region
Vulnerable to short droughts

Humid climate with water surpluses even during periods of less than average precipitation

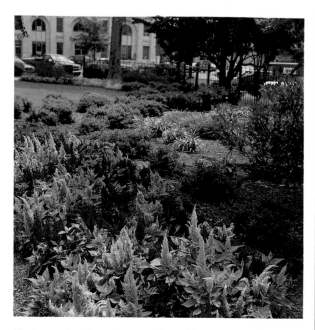

Xeriscape landscaping is adaptable to any style of landscaping, everything from formal to casual. This city center park in Marietta, Georgia, features drought-tolerant celosia (Celosia spp.) *and yaupon holly* (Ilex vomitoria) *laid out in precise beds. (Design: Post Landscape)*

In many areas of Texas alarming decreases in groundwater levels have led to a renewed emphasis on water conservation. In El Paso, where underground wells are virtually the city's only source of water supply, levels have lowered so much that the water has become increasingly brackish, or salty. The Edwards Aquifer underground supply underlying five counties in central Texas (which includes San Antonio) has drawn down so much that even with the exceptionally high 1990 rainfall, the water levels remain at least twenty to thirty-five feet below normal.

In Florida greater demands for water from an increasing population have created problems not only with seawater infiltration of freshwater supplies, but also with drastic alterations to the ecology of the Everglades. Pond levels are sometimes lowered so much that many species of plants and animals are left high and dry, unable to survive.

In 1991, California experienced its fiercest drought in recent history. In some instances farmers as well as residents faced being cut back to as little as one-quarter of their normal water supply. A spate of heavy spring rains brought some relief, but it was noted that six weeks of such rains would be needed to restore normal moisture levels. San Diego entered its fifth consecutive year of drought.

What all this means for the average American are higher water prices, for the resources to improve existing systems or to *motivate* conservation. Water costs rose as much as thirty-seven percent in two years in the late 1980s in some cities and are expected to continue to rise. Even with increases such as this, water is still relatively cheap for Americans. This may change in the near future.

Xeriscape landscaping was a concept born of desperation. It initially conjured up visions of sternly set limitations, but over the years it has proved to be not a severely limiting framework for design, but a very liberating one, freeing us from the shackles of a water-thirsty landscape—the endless hours of watering, mowing, trimming, edging, clipping, and weeding we've come to expect in landscaping.

Granted, it will take work and thought to develop the true Xeriscape landscape, a landscape that never needs watering. But it will all be worthwhile even if, for no other reason, we'll be assured of never having to worry about watering restrictions such as those shown on the next page, endured by residents of Nassau County (Long Island), New York, in 1990 and beyond.

Xeriscape Plants

In this book the term "Xeriscape plant" doesn't refer to the intrinsic differences between a desert plant and a bog plant. It refers to the appropriate plant choices and design that make them Xeriscape plants *in your region and within the specific microclimates of your site.*

With some very adaptable exceptions, the drought-tolerant plant palette for Maryland will not be the same as for Colorado. Here is where the regional nature of Xeriscape landscaping is evident. The rainfall distribution in one section of the country may be quite different from that of another section receiving the same amount of total annual

**NASSAU COUNTY WATER REGULATIONS
LAWN SPRINKLING**

1. All water sprinkling for lawns and shrubbery is prohibited between the hours of 10 am and 4 pm.

2. Houses with even-numbered street addresses may sprinkle on even-numbered calendar days. Houses with odd-numbered street addresses may sprinkle on odd-numbered calendar days. Houses with no street numbers may sprinkle on even-numbered calendar days. The hours for sprinkling are from midnight to 10 am and 4 pm to midnight.

THE COUNTY ORDINANCE APPLIES IN ALL CASES, BUT MANY WATER DISTRICTS HAVE REGULATIONS *IN ADDITION TO* THE COUNTY ORDINANCE.

Village of Bayville—No sprinkling Sat or when raining.

Village of East Williston—Sprinkling 6 pm–9 pm ONLY. No car washing.

Village of Farmingdale—East of Main Street, Sun & Thurs ONLY, West of Main Street, Sat and Wed ONLY.

Garden City Park Water District—No sprinkling 9 am–6 pm.

Manhasset/Lakeview Water District—Automatic sprinklers 3 am–5 pm. MUST HAVE RAIN SENSORS. Manual sprinklers, any two hours between 6 pm and 9 pm.

Old Westbury Water District—North of LIE [Long Island Expressway] mornings Sun, Tues & Thurs.

precipitation. A plant that can thrive on twenty inches of annual rainfall in Texas may not survive in another twenty-inch region where a large portion of the precipitation occurs as snowfall.

This distinction is more subtle than the better-known cautions about cold hardiness; it invites us to be even more aware of the nuances of our climate and to admire the tenacity of certain plant groups that can grow and produce seed even in a year when not a drop of rain falls after spring. Wild grasses are best adapted to withstand a summer-long drought, but many perennial flowers, shrubs, and trees are equally resilient. Some western trees can endure droughts of up to five years before they are taxed beyond their resources. Obviously, we won't purposely subject our trees to such a test, but it's easy to underestimate how truly tough they are.

Drought Tolerance Versus Drought Avoidance

Several terms are mistakenly used interchangeably when talking about water-conserving plants. "Drought tolerance" actually means the ability of a plant to withstand drought without dying. It makes no inference as to the plant's appearance when water-stressed. Another term, "drought avoidance," refers to a plant's ability to withstand drought without showing signs of stress.

Thus, much maligned in Colorado, Kentucky bluegrass has low drought avoidance—that is, it

Scarlet bugler penstemon (Penstemon barbatus) *and mixed prairie grasses make a luxuriant and natural hillside meadow.*

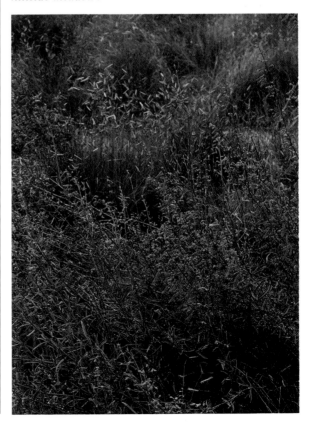

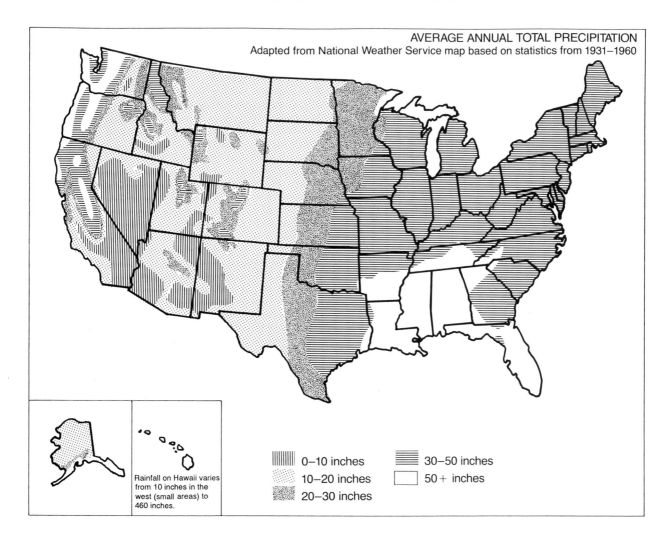

AVERAGE ANNUAL TOTAL PRECIPITATION
Adapted from National Weather Service map based on statistics from 1931–1960

Rainfall on Hawaii varies from 10 inches in the west (small areas) to 460 inches.

0–10 inches
10–20 inches
20–30 inches
30–50 inches
50+ inches

begins to look brown and pathetic shortly after being stressed, but it takes a very long time to die. (In fact, it will often go dormant until moisture conditions improve long before it succumbs.) Therefore, it has good drought tolerance, despite its bad reputation.

By contrast, in Colorado, tall fescue has high drought avoidance (stays green long into drought), but low drought tolerance (dies quickly after showing signs of water stress).

To put it another way, plants either tolerate or avoid drought. They may avoid drought by restricting water loss through their stomata (leaf openings); by rolling, folding, or shedding their leaves during drought spells (drought deciduous, common in native plants of the Southwest); or by several more intricate adaptations such as absorbing and storing

carbon dioxide at night for use in photosynthesis during the day. Some plants have thicker, leathery or finely divided leaves, or are covered with masses of tiny hairs that retain moisture and reflect light and heat. These plants are called water savers.

Other plants are water spenders. They avoid drought by increasing their uptake of water during drought to keep a high leaf-water content. This is done at the expense of soil moisture. If a plant can't avoid drought by maintaining a high leaf-water content, then it must be able to survive the dehydrating effects of drought. Dormancy is a primary means of tolerating drought.

Other plants are water efficient, which refers to plant growth per unit of water. Prairie grasses are more water efficient than desert plants because they grow a lot on a certain amount of water, whereas

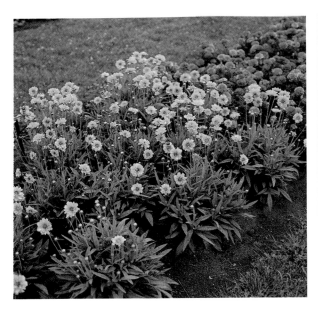

Dependable perennial Coreopsis lanceolata *flowers profusely even in its first season, and is extremely drought tolerant.*

desert plants continue to grow relatively slowly even when "ample" (for them) water is available. However, prairie grasses require about three times as much water as cacti do to remain healthy.

Recognizing these distinctions, I searched for definitive research detailing exactly which category each plant fits into, and found that there really isn't that much information available yet. That is, there is information about the moisture needs of a few species, but not of the hundreds of plants listed in this book. I have often had to fall back on the oversimplified term "drought tolerant," which throughout this book will mean "survives drought after establishment and still looks reasonably attractive."

How to Xeriscape Landscape

This book is divided into two major sections: the first addresses the fundamental principles involved in developing a Xeriscape landscape; and the second provides information, plant lists, and success stories/advice from home Xeriscape gardeners in different parts of the country (see Part Two: The Plants).

You may be starting from scratch, creating a new Xeriscape design, or you may have an existing water-thirsty landscape and want to effect a partial or complete renovation.

If you're not ready to make any changes in your existing plantscape, you can still begin the Xeriscape process by becoming a little more knowledgeable about the local climate and the small piece of the earth entrusted to your care. This involves gathering a little data (see the planning and design chapter) and making a few changes in your routine (see the irrigation and maintenance chapters).

Seven Xeriscape Landscaping Principles

The cornerstone of Xeriscape landscaping is the seven basic principles essential to a good Xeriscape design. Note that successful landscaping for water conservation incorporates all of these steps; changing turf areas without changing watering routines is hardly useful, as is planting lower-water-demanding plants without understanding how they need to be maintained in order to become established and thrive.

1. Planning and design
2. Soil analysis and improvements
3. Practical turf areas
4. Appropriate plant selection
5. Efficient irrigation
6. Mulching
7. Appropriate maintenance

Each of these steps will be covered in detail in the chapters that follow. Because of his background as a landscape architect, Tom Stephens wrote the chapters on planning, design, and maintenance; Doug Welsh, Ph.D., an expert in landscape water management, wrote extensively in the irrigation chapter, and provided technical assistance and editing throughout the book. Connie Ellefson wrote the remaining chapters.

Planning and Design

IN THIS chapter the complete planning and design process for a Xeriscape project is laid out in an easy-to-follow checklist fashion. Putting everything on paper in a systematic way (which seems to be the part that intimidates many of us) serves as a long-range guide to total site or individual project development. It also simplifies the calculations of quantities and costs of plant materials, and helps you to determine the water costs and savings gained by Xeriscape landscaping. The key point to remember is that planning and design can help you achieve a more environmentally sound and water-efficient landscape.

There are three good methods to complete a creative Xeriscape design.

The read and research do-it-yourselfer. First, for the self-motivated do-it-yourselfer, there are several good books (in addition to this one) and magazines on the market and at local libraries that can help you accumulate ideas and information on landscape and Xeriscape design, construction, and maintenance techniques. Xeriscape demonstration gardens in most regions of the country show how the basic fundamentals can be applied in a wide variety of situations.

Do-it-yourselfer courses. The second method is to attend a do-it-yourself home landscaping or Xeriscape course, workshop, or seminar taught by knowledgeable local landscape professionals at one of the universities or community colleges in your area, the local botanic garden or arboretum, adult education or vocational programs in your community, or landscape nurseries, garden centers, or building supply businesses. In some communities these seminars are sponsored by water utilities de-

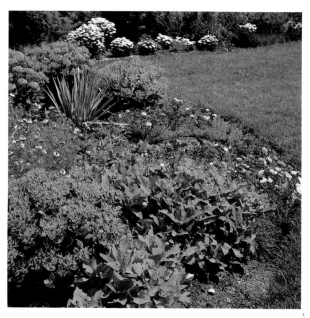

A curving flower bed makes a bright counterpoint to the turf-type tall fescue lawn at the Cornell Cooperative Extension Xeriscape Water-Conservation Garden (Long Island, New York). Clockwise from the right are portulaca (Portulaca grandiflora), *Melampodium 'Medallion', Sedum 'Indian Chief', variegated yucca* (Yucca filamentosa), *and spent tulip foliage* (Tulipa spp.). *Shasta daisies* (Chrysanthemum maximum) *are in the distance. (Design: Krall/Rakow/Weir)*

partments, and you might receive flyers announcing them in the mail with your water bill. These courses may range in length from a three- to four-hour seminar that covers only the basics without much detail, to a full ten- to twelve-week intensive course that covers the various facets of landscape design, construction, and maintenance. I've taught over 150 such courses to more than 1,500 students in the past twenty years and have seen many very successful results from such "coached" do-it-yourself projects.

Using a design professional. The third method, for the busy homeowner or the less creatively inclined, is to contact one or more of the many professionals in the landscape industry, such as landscape architects, landscape designers, landscape contractors, nursery growers, gardeners, and lawn maintenance contractors, for help in completing an effective Xeriscape project with the most economical expenditure of time and money.

The landscape architect or landscape designer is generally the lead design professional with four to seven years of college-level education and training in an accredited design program who provides a design service for a fee.

Quite often the landscape architect/designer can assist you in the master planning, detailed construction drawings, specification writing, bidding and negotiating, contract preparation and administration, project layout and staking, inspection of materials and methods, and supervision and coordination of the total project. An experienced landscape architect or designer will help you develop a realistic budget, establish priorities and phasing, and get you the most from your investment.

Many landscape architects are members of the national professional organization, the American Society of Landscape Architects (ASLA). To determine a landscape architect's affiliation and specialty, you can contact the local or regional chapter or the national organization, or check the Yellow Pages listing under landscape architects. Many states have licensing laws that are intended for the protection of the public. Selecting a licensed landscape architect can provide a level of assurance as to his or her competence and experience.

Before you select any landscape professional, you should investigate two or more firms or individuals, looking at their qualifications, references, and experience with projects similar in nature to what you have in mind.

The fees for landscape architectural and design services are usually based on one of the following four methods: an hourly rate (usually ranging from $35 to $100 per hour, sometimes not to exceed a given ceiling amount); a lump sum fixed fee per project or phase of a project; a fixed percentage of the budget or the total landscape project construction, planting, and irrigation costs; or a retainer basis for a specified period of time.

These fees should be discussed and agreed to in a contract form or letter of proposal by all parties before the design process begins. Any outside work by other professionals, such as a topographic site survey or a soils analysis and report, should be determined and specified as to who is responsible for their costs.

PLANNING AND DESIGN

Planning and design are actually two ends of a continuum, with planning being general and design, specific. Planning is the long-range look at your site or project, with the land regarded as a resource to be considered in relationship to your needs, wants, and desires. In Xeriscape landscaping, one of the primary overarching goals is to reduce the amount of water applied to the landscape, so looking at the project over several years and seasons makes good sense. Planning and thinking ahead will minimize the discouragement that can occur when the homeowner sees an increase in water usage during the first year (because newly installed plants need additional water to become established). It may take two to three years to achieve the goal of eliminating or markedly reducing the water applied to your landscape through good planning.

Design is the arrangement and definition of areas of your property and the elements in your landscape that have been set aside in the planning process. It is concerned with the selection of elements in the landscape, the specifying of materials (both hardscape and plantscape), and their arrangement in the landscape in a way that solves the problems and meets the challenges of your needs and budget range and of the site.

In site planning, the first step in the planning process, we define use areas in the landscape. Site planning is concerned with the location of physical objects and activities and structures. Practical use of turf areas (the third Xeriscape principle) is determined, and plans are made for the remaining areas.

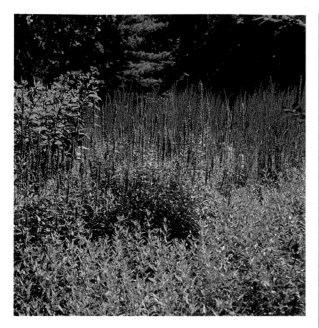

Featherreed grass (Calamagrostis acutiflora) *provides a background and color contrast for spike gayfeather* (Liatris spicata) *while echoing its form.*

An important part of site planning is circulation or traffic pattern planning, in which you create a workable system for the movement of vehicles and pedestrians, and determine how utilities fit into the system—on, below, and above the ground. This includes parking areas, driveways, walks, landings, paths, patios, and underground and overhead utility lines and equipment, and how these elements cross and connect with each other and tie into the property. It typically deals with the "hardscape" elements of landscaping, most of which do not need water and usually do best without excessive water. Concrete paving surfaces, for instance, will crack and flake when water is applied to them or finds its way beneath them, causing heaving during rapid freezing and thawing cycles in colder climates.

Beginning the Planning and Design Process

For a beautiful yet functional landscape project that minimizes water use, become familiar with all of the planning and design considerations presented in this chapter. Regardless of whether you work it

all out on paper or in your head, you will end up with a far better and more complete design. You may even find that you want to commit more of your planning to paper, perhaps by starting with the worksheets and diagrams that follow.

I can vouch for the importance of doing at least a minimum of planning and design on paper. I have been called into many projects as a professional designer by students and clients who have not engaged in some basic planning and design. As a result they have wasted valuable time and large sums of money on mistakes that are often hard to

*This dramatic Xeriscape landscape in California highlights several Xeriscape principles, such as good design, appropriate plant selection, and practical turf areas. Rather than covering this steep hillside with barely usable turf, the designers used junipers (*Juniperus spp.*) and heavenly bamboo (*Nandina domestica*) to draw people down to the deck area. (Design: Creative Landscape Consultants, Santa Clara, California. Photo: Saxon Holt)*

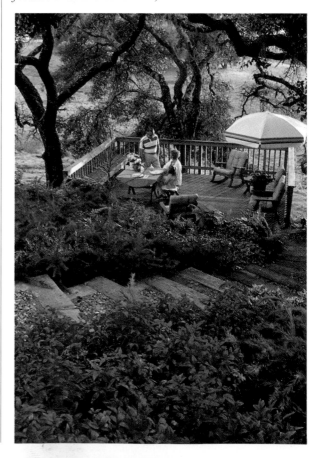

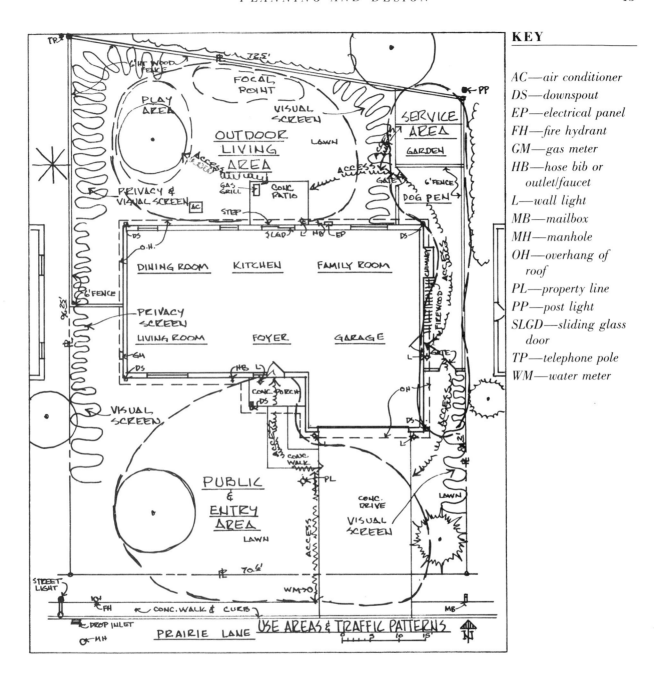

AC—air conditioner
DS—downspout
EP—electrical panel
FH—fire hydrant
GM—gas meter
*HB—hose bib or
    outlet/faucet*
L—wall light
MB—mailbox
MH—manhole
*OH—overhang of
    roof*
PL—property line
PP—post light
*SLGD—sliding glass
    door*
TP—telephone pole
WM—water meter

correct satisfactorily or economically. I strongly recommend, at the very minimum, that you use either a spiral or ring-bound notebook or sketchbook with sections set aside for designs, favorite plants, and hardscape materials to be considered, or a pocket folder to carry loose sketches in one side and brochures or lists of plants and hardscape materials in the other.

The thought of surveying your own property, determining your water pressure, and outlining a budget and phasing plan may instantly send you into the fetal position. Wandering dreamily through the botanic gardens or arboretum, staring at the trees in the nearest park or open space, or paging idly through a picture book or catalog on wildflowers may be as organized as you get.

If this is more your style, please take heart. The observation and study side of planning and design is just as important as the measuring and calculating. Chances are you love the plant selection side of landscaping. You know which plants you want to have in your landscape, you've noticed which ones grow readily in the wild near your home, and you've been absorbing the artistic elements of design without consciously realizing it.

In addition, your mind is probably processing planning information all the time. For instance, you are doing "traffic pattern" planning when you notice what a hassle it is to have all the garden tools stored in the garage, and the only way to get them to the garden is to haul them three-quarters of the way around the house. This may lead to a modification of your utility area design and circulation plan.

If you feel more comfortable laying out your design in your yard with garden hoses and wooden stakes, if you prefer to keep rough designs, budgets, and schedules in your head, if you'd rather make one well-thought-out change at a time, or if you can't bring yourself to draw more than a simple sketch of what you'd like your landscape to ultimately look like, that's fine! You can still have a beautiful Xeriscape garden. It may take longer, and possibly cost more in time and money, but it's better to go at your own pace than to forgo the Xeriscape process altogether.

The planning and design process I have used professionally and taught for several years consists of four basic steps. They are the program of needs and budget range, the site survey and inventory, the project analysis, and the design or synthesis.

STEP #1: THE PROGRAM OF NEEDS AND BUDGET RANGE

The first step is to determine the *program* or scope of your project, your objectives or goals. With my clients and students I use a form I have developed called Program of Needs and Budget Range, which enables a designer, client, or student to check off those items or elements to be incorporated into the design project. Going through this checklist will help you determine what you really want included in your Xeriscape project, how much effort and change you want to make, and your approximate budget and phasing plan.

First, you should answer the following questions:
• What are the ages, sexes, primary activities, and hobbies of the members of your family who will be using your outdoor spaces?
  • How important are each of the following to you?
—gardening
—maintenance of the landscape
—the quality of your surroundings
—outdoor entertaining (would you prefer a formal or informal atmosphere, and how many people do you usually entertain at once?)
  • What are some of your general outdoor needs?
—How much off-street parking is required?
—What types of walks, landings, and steps are required, and made of what "hardscape" materials?
—Is there a need for active game and play areas and structures?
—Do you need areas for quiet relaxation?
—What sports and games do you and your family play?
—Are there hobbies that must be accommodated in the landscape?
—Is privacy important and where is it most needed?
  • What is the goal for your Xeriscape landscape?
—A total elimination of watering or simply an improvement in overall water use?
  • Will your Xeriscape project require minimal changes or major renovations to achieve the goal?

This simple, yet striking ornamental grass, Miscanthus sinensis *'Gracillimus', provides nearly hedgelike privacy for the park bench in this Washington, D.C., public garden. (Design: Oehme, van Sweden & Associates)*

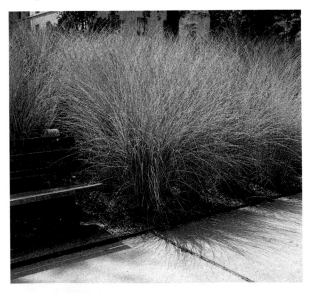

Budgeting
. . . .

One of the most critical and often most difficult decisions you must make when considering Xeriscape landscaping is the amount of the family budget that will be allocated to the project, both in the immediate future for a one-time project and over several years for a multiphased project. Whether you are planning a new Xeriscape landscape to go in all at one time or are renovating an older established landscape in bits and pieces, it is important to define the budget you are willing to commit to the project. Two general rules of thumb have been used for many years for developing budgets for a landscape project.

The first method is to allow ten to fifteen percent of the *value* (not cost) of your house and property for the general landscaping needs of a project. Included in such a project would be the soil preparation, sodding or seeding of the lawn areas, the planting of shade and ornamental trees, the basic foundation and other shrub and flower plantings, mulches for the planting beds, a basic irrigation

If a swimming pool is desired, balance its high water use with no-water hardscape and drought-tolerant plants. Crape myrtle (Lagerstroemia indica) *and ornamental grasses* (Miscanthus sinensia 'Gracillimus') *are good Xeriscape choices for the Southwest. (Design: Post Landscape)*

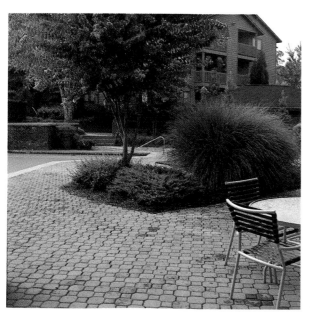

system, and a small entrance walk and patio (approximately 400 square feet each). Not included are such hardscape elements as fencing, decks, spas, pools, play structures, major retaining or screen walls, and other amenities that are like the extras on a new car—nice to have, but not necessary to minimum outdoor living.

The second method is not as precise or reliable and often is not as easy to determine. You must estimate the approximate area of the total site that will be landscaped, and figure $2 per square foot for a minimal project, scaling upwards to $5 or more per square foot for an elaborate hardscape and plantscape project. The wide variation depends on the size of the total area, including the footprint, or outline and area, of the house, the quality of the surroundings you prefer, and the various elements you have specified in your program of needs and budget range.

Usually I recommend that you use both methods to check one against the other to be sure you have considered everything and have a firm idea of the approximate dollars in the budget for the total Xeriscape project and for its various phases.

These two budgeting methods will give you an approximate idea of the cost of having a contractor do all or a major part of the total project. You can figure that by doing much of the labor yourself and by smart and timely buying of materials, you can save forty to fifty percent of the cost of the project. I have had numerous do-it-yourselfers as clients and as students, and many of their projects are as good or better than a professional landscape contractor or nursery grower could have done.

The size of the budget does not dictate the quality of the Xeriscape project. Some of the smallest and least expensive projects I have completed for my clients and my students have done are some of the best in quality, and have included in them all of the seven basic Xeriscape principles.

The Value of Landscaping and Xeriscape Landscaping

Some of the most frequent questions from clients and students are whether Xeriscape landscaping is a good investment, if there is any return on the investment, how long it takes to appreciate any return on the investment, and if it will help them

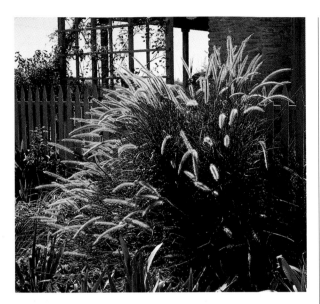

Many ornamental grasses, such as this purple fountain grass (Pennisetum setaceum), *offer both drought tolerance and aesthetic richness by adding texture to the landscape design. (Photo: Doug Welsh)*

sell their home. Most of us who use the Xeriscape principles are most interested in saving water and other natural resources, but it is also reassuring to know that a well-designed Xeriscape project can help us sell our homes if and when it is necessary.

These are all valid questions and have been addressed in the results of the Gallup Landscaping Survey, a national survey conducted in 1986 for Trendnomics and the National Gardening Association:

• Overall, new home buyers and buyers of previously owned homes estimate that landscaping, on the average, adds *14.87* percent to the value or selling price of their home.

• Prospective home buyers are interested in more than just the home itself. They are looking for a total living package and that includes landscape features. Trees and shrubs that reduce living costs by reducing energy (and water) costs are taken into account. The attractiveness of the landscaping can be a deciding factor between two similar properties. Landscaping and Xeriscape landscaping contribute to the overall salability of a house.

In the report *The Value of Landscaping*, put out by the Weyerhauser Company in 1986, real estate appraisers were asked to prioritize the factors they consider in appraising the value landscaping adds to real estate. It's significant to note that landscaping to conserve energy and landscaping to conserve water were numbers four and five on that list.

The fact that water conservation was included at all in the list of priorities is heartening, considering how recently it has gotten national attention. This information indicates that landscaping the home is indeed a good investment; however, it presents a real challenge to those of us in the green industry to educate the public and the real estate appraisal industry about the value of Xeriscape landscaping.

From my own experience I have found that Xeriscape landscaping is slightly more costly initially than the average landscape project, primarily because of the additional costs of proper soil preparation (which in many parts of the country is essential to any type of landscaping), and the scarcity of good-quality and larger sizes of Xeriscape and native plants in the nurseries. The availability factor is slowly being overcome by farsighted nursery growers who see the potential for providing quality products to a fast-growing segment of the market. The value of Xeriscape landscaping is only just beginning to be understood by the public and the green industry.

Phasing a Project

Once the overall budget is determined, you should decide if the project is to be phased in over an extended period of time and approximately how many dollars are to be available for each phase and when that phase will take place. At this point the budgeting and phasing is often akin to gazing into a crystal ball and is usually not very reliable, but can be used as a guideline in the development of a design and the completion of the project in a timely and cost-effective way.

You should also determine how much of the project is to be done by contractors and craftspeople and how much you will try to do yourself. I have seen many projects start out to be do-it-yourself types and end up either completed or redone by a contractor. It is very easy to be too ambitious as a do-it-yourselfer. It is best to start with small projects that you feel comfortable doing, then build up to

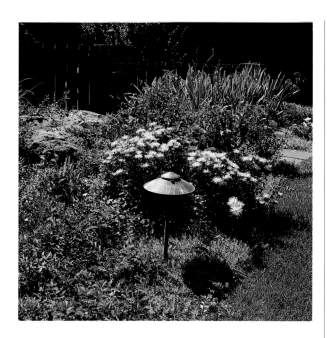

Careful planning allows you to add elegant touches such as garden lighting easily. Garden chrysanthemums (Chrysanthemum × morifolium) star in this late summer vignette, and spent iris foliage adds interest to the background. (Design: Thomas L. Stephens)

more technically difficult projects as your confidence and abilities grow and develop.

I recommend that you not attempt any project, no matter the size, without carefully thinking through each step of the construction or planting process. Planning ahead with an installation can save time, money, materials, plants, backaches, and tempers.

In addition to how much they can expect as a return on their investment, many clients and students want to know how soon they can recoup their investment. Unlike hardscape items, plants appreciate with new growth and therefore will become more valuable as time passes and they begin to mature. After five years you can expect five to ten percent appreciation, and after ten years, as much as ten to twenty percent.

If return on investment in less than five years is your primary goal, I recommend that you not budget or spend over the ten percent range and often much less. I sometimes recommend that unless you plan to live in a home for more than two to three years you not landscape at all.

Plants and Hardscape Elements in the Xeriscape Landscape

At the Program of Needs phase you should consider the general types of plants you want to use—whether shade, ornamental, or evergreen trees; evergreen, broadleaf evergreen, flowering and deciduous shrubs; ground covers; vines; flowers, either annual or perennial, wildflowers, spring or summer bulbs, or roses; and grasses, both turf-type and ornamental.

In addition to being as specific as possible about the plants you want to use, it is a good idea to attempt to focus on some of the hardscape materials to be used for driveways, walks, and paths; retaining and screen walls; fences and gates; and decks and patios. When selecting hardscape materials, decide whether the construction will be a do-it-yourself project or one done by skilled craftspeople or contractors. Knowing this helps to determine the degree of difficulty that can be designed into the project.

STEP #2: SITE SURVEY AND INVENTORY

Much as a doctor would run a series of tests to determine the exact condition of a patient, so also must you survey and inventory your existing site conditions to know exactly what you have to work with. The complexity of your Xeriscape project will dictate the extent of your site survey and inventory. If you plan a partial or total renovation of an existing high-water-consuming landscape or if you want to Xeriscape landscape a new home, I recommend a thorough survey of existing conditions on your site. This survey is used to develop a "base plan" on which you do the rest of your planning and design work. If you're modifying an existing landscape, but not extensively, you can skip this section altogether.

A survey can begin from scratch with only a simple freehand sketch of a site, a plot plan that may have been done by a land surveyor during the building permit stage, or a complete topographic survey by a professional land surveyor, a professional designer, or you.

A plot plan may have been a part of the mortgage closing papers you received when you purchased the house or property. It is a small drawing, usually eight-and-a-half by eleven or fourteen inches, that shows the property lines of the lot (sometimes with dimensions and bearings); any easements for utilities or accesses; the footprint, or outline, of the house, frequently with major dimensions; and sometimes the location of the driveways, patios, and walks. Occasionally spot elevations indicating the relative differences in height from a given fixed point are shown. The scale and north arrow direction are also usually shown and are important to record on a base plan.

A topographic survey by a professional land surveyor should indicate all of the pertinent existing site information necessary for designing the Xeriscape project. If your property is anything other than rectangular or square in shape, or has unusual features such as large changes in elevation or numerous trees of various sizes, it might be advisable to hire a professional land surveyor to do your survey.

If you are doing the survey and inventory as the beginning of a do-it-yourself project, securely tape your sketch of the house and site or the plot plan to a rather stiff board, such as illustration board, smooth-surfaced plywood, or particle board, so you can take it to the site and make measurements and record dimensions and notes as you go.

Begin with a team of at least two people, since it's much easier to survey with two than to try to hold or maneuver both ends of a measuring tape by yourself. For convenience use at least one hundred-foot measuring tape and one or two shorter carpenter's tapes of ten to twenty-five feet in length.

In measuring the house itself, it is important to measure the overall dimensions of the walls to arrive at the general shape of the building; then measure all windows, doors, and other openings and appurtenances (such as electric and gas meters, downspouts, and hose bibs), starting from one corner and moving around the house. Always add up all of these smaller dimensions to be sure they total the overall dimension of the walls.

If you have a wedge-shaped or oddly shaped (other than rectangular) lot, it is easier to begin with measurements of the house and then measure from known corners, windows, or other openings to property lines, easements, utilities, streets, trees and shrubs, etc.

If you are doing your own topographic survey, you will need either an engineer's level or, for less technical (but more time-consuming) yet adequate information, a string level and a long string, or a carpenter's level and a long two-by-four or two-by-six on edge and a yardstick or tape measure.

Using one of the level methods, measure vertical changes of elevation or height from a known point, such as the finished floor on the main level of the house. Be sure to measure and record all major changes in elevation; all ditches and swales; high and low points; and all locations of trees and shrubs, patios, walks, and drives. It is important to know this topographic information to be able to accurately design and provide for the drainage of water on the site. These horizontal and vertical measurements should all be recorded on the base plan.

Be as accurate as you can with your measurements and in recording them for future use in drawing the base plan, planning and designing the project, calculating areas and quantities, and designing the irrigation system.

A Checklist of Survey and Inventory Information

You should accurately measure and record the following items:

Man-made Elements

1. Legal and physical boundaries and utility and access easements. If you don't know where your easements are, you may have received a plot or survey plan at the closing of your mortgage, or you can call your local utility or planning department and ask them to look up your location in their recorded plats. They may be able to tell you the location of any easements on your property and rules about crossing them.

2. Buildings—their locations on the site and their lengths, widths, and heights, including doors, windows, rooflines, and roof overhangs, and groundlines; and other physical structures, such as fences,

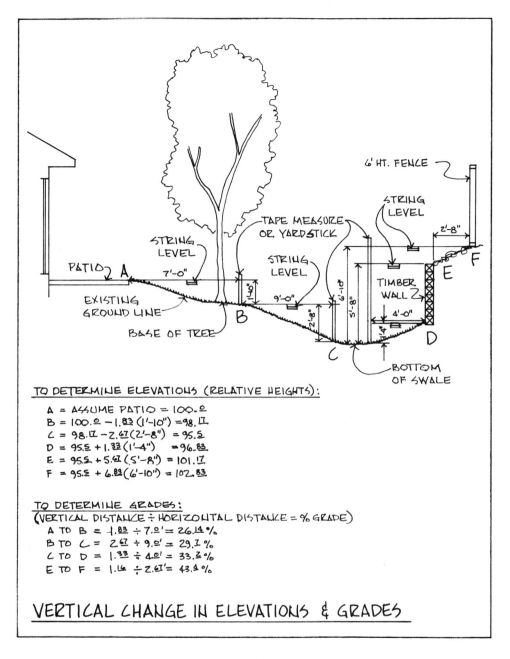

TO DETERMINE ELEVATIONS (RELATIVE HEIGHTS):

A = ASSUME PATIO = 100.0
B = 100.0 − 1.83 (1'-10") = 98.17
C = 98.17 − 2.67 (2'-8") = 95.5
D = 95.5 + 1.33 (1'-4") = 96.83
E = 95.5 + 5.67 (5'-8") = 101.17
F = 95.5 + 6.83 (6'-10") = 102.83

TO DETERMINE GRADES:
(VERTICAL DISTANCE ÷ HORIZONTAL DISTANCE = % GRADE)
A TO B = 1.83 ÷ 7.0' = 26.14 %
B TO C = 2.67 ÷ 9.0' = 29.7 %
C TO D = 1.33 ÷ 4.0' = 33.2 %
E TO F = 1.16 ÷ 2.67' = 43.4 %

VERTICAL CHANGE IN ELEVATIONS & GRADES

gates, and walls. Note the general room arrangement within the house. You may want to "extend" these areas into the outdoors with your design.

3. Circulation systems and traffic patterns such as roads, driveways, parking areas, walks, landings, paths, steps, and ramps, and the surfacing and paving materials. It is important to know the location on the ground as well as the changes in elevation and slope of the paved surfaces.

4. Utilities. It is vitally important to determine and record as accurately as you can the location of all utilities as early in the design process as possible to avoid potential conflicts with elements you have included in your plans. You could have a problem, for instance, if you designed a major structure such as a swimming pool, spa, gazebo, or patio over a utility line or easement. It could potentially be destroyed should the utility company need to excavate large areas to repair a broken water, sewer, or other major utility line.

In many communities firms subsidized by utility companies provide utility-locating services to home-

DETERMINING WATER PRESSURE AND FLOW RATES AT YOUR HOME

Pinpointing the exact static water pressure at your house can have a significant effect on planning a Xeriscape project. Many sprinkler components are designed to work best at 30 to 50 pounds per square inch (psi). Most drip irrigation components are designed to operate at very low pressures and flow rates (gpm or gph). Knowing the water pressure and flow rate will be important when you or your professional irrigation designer or installer is designing and laying out the irrigation system.

In some new subdivisions the water pressure may be as high as 90 psi. This causes the too-familiar "misting" of sprinkler heads, which leads to massive water loss through wind dispersal and evaporation. In this case a pressure-reducing valve (PRV) may be a necessary part of the sprinkler system. The high pressure may be lessened as the area is built up in the future, but if additional development is unlikely within one or two years, installing a PRV may be worthwhile and cost-effective in water savings.

If you are not on public water service but have a well, you may be faced with a problem of low water pressure. If so, you may have to install a pressure tank along with your pump system which will increase the pressure at the point of delivery to adequately operate the sprinkler system.

You can usually find out the water pressure in your area by contacting the water department. They usually have maps of the town showing mainline water pressures, and they can help you calculate the water pressure at your service line. However, since this isn't always the same as what's actually coming out of your faucet or hose bib, you may need to buy or borrow from a friend or a plumber a water pressure gauge. Attach the gauge to an outdoor faucet or hose bib, then turn on full force the outside faucet the gauge is attached to, and at least one other faucet either inside or outside the house (since we often use the water elsewhere while the sprinklers are on). The pressure gauge will tell you the working water pressure available for landscaping and irrigation.

Directly related to water pressure is the flow in gallons per minute (gpm) of water delivered to your house. In older parts of a town mineral deposits in galvanized service lines (the water lines running from the main water pipe in the street or utility easement to the house) may have reduced the carrying capacity to as little as twenty-five percent of what it was meant to carry. In a typical subdivision, delivery rates will be 15 to 30 gpm, whereas in a very old area it might be only 5 to 6 gpm. This means that, whereas in a newer area you might be able to run four sprinklers at once, in an older part of town you may be able to run only one. This may require the installation of a complicated system of valves in the sprinkler system or the replacement of the service line to the house, an expensive procedure in most areas.

Another way of estimating the water delivery rate is to look at the size of the lines coming into and out of the water meter (usually located in the yard of an older house and in the basement or utility crawl space in a newer house). A ¾-inch-diameter meter supply line delivers roughly 30 gpm and a ⅝-inch line, 20 gpm.

You can also take a five-gallon bucket and a stopwatch, place the bucket under the faucet, turn it on full force, and time how long it takes to fill the bucket. By simple math you can calculate the gallons per minute.

An alternative to all this is to plan a true Xeriscape landscape that needs so little additional watering that it can be taken care of with an occasional hand-held hose or portable sprinkler, or with the simpler drip-type irrigation system. If you are considering forgoing an automatic sprinkler system, please read the chapter about efficient irrigation beginning on page 103 before you continue your planning and design. It lists the pros and cons on the subject.

owners and contractors before they begin digging or excavating on a project. Sometimes the utililty companies provide such services directly. Check your local phone directory for the phone number of the locator service or utility company in your area. The following are the important utilities to accurately locate and record (including location and vertical depth):

• Natural gas mains and meters, or LP (liquid petroleum gas) tanks and feeder lines.
• Electrical
  —Both overhead and underground lines, meters, transformers, and breaker or fuse panels.
  —Lights, both line (110) voltage and low (12) voltage fixtures, transformers, and cable.
• Water mains, laterals, meters, hose connections (hose bibs), fire hydrants, and wells.
• Telephone lines, overhead and belowground, and any pedestals and connection boxes in the yard or attached to the house.
• Cable television lines and pedestals. (With these last two utilities, the lines are usually very shallow and are the most likely to be cut during construction, planting, and irrigation installation.)
• Downspouts and gutter outlets from roof drains.
• Sewers, both storm and sanitary, or septic tank and tile fields. These are important, even though they are usually several feet deep, as the potential need for major repairs could damage your landscape structures and plantings.
• Irrigation and sprinkler systems, main lines, taps, valves, controllers, moisture sensors, lateral lines and spray heads, driplines and emitters, drains, and blowouts.

5. Miscellaneous elements such as air conditioners, gas grills, firewood storage, flagpoles, and mailboxes.

6. Existing uses of the property or site.
• Recreational
• Circulation, hard or soft surface.
• Open space, fields, meadows, wood lots, or forests.
• Vegetable garden, pasture, garden, berry patch, or orchard.

Natural Resources

1. Topography, or the lay of the land: the high and low points, the ditches and swales for drainage, the slopes and grades and the degree of steepness of both, whether steep, moderate, or flat, and the drainage patterns and sources of drainage that cross or originate on the site. Often topography is indicated by contour lines or spot elevations at specific points, giving the relative height above or below a certain point called a benchmark, such as the fin-

ished floor elevation of the main or ground level of the house.

2. Soil types:
• the physical structure of the soil—is it clay, silt, or sand?
• the relative acidity and alkalinity, or pH.
• the major nutrient levels for nitrogen, phosphorus, and potassium.

3. Water bodies such as streams, ponds, lakes, or potentially dangerous dry gulches that might become a problem during flash flooding.

4. Subsurface materials, underlying layers of hardpan clay, sand and gravel, or bedrock. This information is available as part of the soils survey done by the Soils Conservation Service or from the U.S. Geological Survey maps of your area. These reports and maps can be found in most large libraries or ordered from government publications offices.

5. Vegetation:
• Location—accurately measure and record the location of all plants to within six inches.
• Diameter of trunk or stem—for large existing trees over twelve inches in diameter, measure at about forty-eight to fifty-four inches above the ground, or the diameter at breast height (dbh); for trees less than twelve inches, measure at six to twelve inches above the ground surface.
• Height of all plants—either measured or estimated.
• Spread of all plants—measure or estimate the diameter of the area covered by the branches, or dripline, and record the approximate circumference or coverage of the dripline or spread of the branches.
• Elevation or relative height of plants above the finished floor elevation of the house or a benchmark.
• Condition of the plants—whether to save, remove, or transplant to a new location or for future replanting in its same location after grading and hardscape construction are completed.
• Ecology—the surrounding environment and plant associations, whether natural or manmade.

6. Wildlife and pets—wild or domestic animals and birds that might have an effect on the survival of newly planted plants and lawns.

This information is some of the most vital if your goal is the absolute minimum of landscape watering. With it you can design your plant groupings to take full advantage of surface water flow (drainage) patterns. You'll put the higher-water-requiring plants in hollows or low spots, downstream of irrigated turf, or in lightly shaded areas that are protected from heat and wind. You'll locate the drier-adapted plants in sunny, open areas, on slopes, and next to hot pavement.

This planning and planting design process, coupled with the water-harvesting techniques discussed in the irrigation chapter, leads to one of the key Xeriscape concepts: *zoning*. Zoning refers to the grouping of plants so that their water needs are as nearly identical as possible. Whatever other stylistic or planning decisions you make, it is important to keep zoning in mind. You won't mix roses with cacti, moisture-loving perennials with rock garden flowers, or willows with sagebrush, for the simple reason that the water that must be lavished on the one will be wasted on, or may even kill or seriously injure, the other.

With the concept of zoning, it's possible to include a few high-moisture-loving plants in your landscape and still have a water-efficient design. You just group them together so you can water them together. In Xeriscape demonstration gardens this is often called the oasis zone, the moderate water zone, or the "needs regular watering" zone. For maximum impact and ease of watering, this zone is often placed near the house or main entry, but other locations may be just as suitable.

You may also have a low-water or a no-water zone farther out from your house. If possible, use no more than two or three different zones in your design, because each zone will have a different set of suitable plants and water requirements, and you don't want to create a hodgepodge design.

Soil Analysis. For Xeriscape landscaping, as well as more conventional landscaping, knowing your soil is extremely important because it will directly affect your plant selection during the planting design process (see soil improvements chapter for more detail). A soil analysis kit can usually be obtained from a County Cooperative Extension Office or a nursery or garden center. These tests are

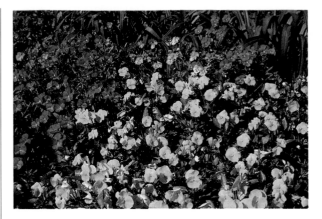

*Annual flowers such as these pansies (*Viola *spp.) can be incorporated into most Xeriscape landscapes. Simply group those plants that require regular watering in the same area of the garden. (Photo: Doug Welsh)*

relatively fast, inexpensive, and reliable, and can give you specific information on nutrient deficiencies and pH level you might need to correct in your yard.

You can also test the soil texture by squeezing a handful of moist soil in the palm of your hand. If the soil retains the squeezed shape completely, it is a heavily clay soil. If it slumps slightly, it is a loamy silt soil, and if it flattens out considerably, it is a sandy soil. You may wish to take samples from several areas of your site or yard if a favored plant or plant association you wish to use requires a soil texture different from the dominant soil type.

Natural Forces

We must be concerned with both the macro- and microclimatic conditions of a site:

1. Temperature—record normal ranges and extremes that will influence the survivability of plants. Note areas such as walls, fences, or plants that might alter the microclimatic conditions by reflection of sunlight or heat or might provide shade for plants, plant beds, or hard surfaces.

2. Precipitation:
•Averages and extremes of rainfall and snowfall.
•Rainfall and snowfall patterns for your area.

In planning a Xeriscape landscape it is good to know not only the annual precipitation of the area, but also the pattern of precipitation. In Colorado, for instance, the average annual precipitation is twelve to fourteen inches, but because of the presence of the Rocky Mountains, the pattern of precipitation varies considerably over the state. Western Pacific air masses are warmer and drier when they come over the mountains because they tend to drop their moisture along the Western Slope.

As a result, the Western Slope has a more even (and frequently higher) precipitation pattern through the spring and summer than the Eastern Slope, or the Front Range, which has a sharp peak of precipitation in May and much less the rest of the year. Thus plants that are adapted to the drier climate of the Front Range must also be able to get the moisture they need in May, not being able to count on receiving much more rainfall later in the year. Western Slope plants can rely on a more even supply. This is why it is helpful to study plants that grow wild very near where you live, rather than those that thrive several hundred miles away.

3. Wind direction and intensities—prevailing and seasonal changes that influence the moisture availability and wind protection required.

4. Sun angles:

• Horizontal sweep of the sun across the site in relationship to the north orientation (north arrow), the structures and areas on it, and the angle it makes in relationship to the horizontal surface of the earth.

• Daily and seasonal changes and variations.

5. Sun and frost pockets—hot and cold spots that might affect the survival of plants or make a space more or less usable. To determine these areas you will have to visit the site at different times of the day and night and during different seasons or rely on information from your neighbors or local weather station operator. Generally speaking, low areas will be cooler and high areas warmer, especially those with southern or southwestern exposures.

Perceptual Characteristics

1. Views, both into and out of a site. Locate both the desirable and undesirable views so you can decide how to frame the desirable views and screen the undesirable ones.

2. Smells and sounds, on and off the site. Locate sources and intensities of both so you can attempt to mitigate the effect they have on your project.

3. Dominant features, mountain views, ocean front views, sculptural features, unusual or specimen plants, or special hardscape elements.

4. General impressions of the site as to its potential and shortcomings, and of the elements on or off the site.

Drawing the Base Plan to Scale

The final procedure in the site survey and inventory step is to draw up a base plan indicating all of the data at a scale that you can use in the design studio or den, or on the dining room table. Plot plans and improvement surveys are usually at a plan scale of 1 inch = 20 feet, which is too small to work with for a Xeriscape design. This base plan is used for several different purposes in the design and implementation procedures, so pick a method and scale that will give you flexibility. Here are two possible methods:

1. Buy a large piece (twenty-four by thirty-six inches minimum) or a roll (twenty-four inches minimum width) of vellum or transparent tracing paper with a blue nonreproducible grid of eight by eight small squares per inch, and tape it down to a table or drawing board. It is best to use a large scale such as ⅛ inch = 1 foot (1 small square = 1 foot) or ¼ inch = 1 foot (two small squares = 1 foot). A one-hundred- by sixty-foot lot would take up twelve and a half by seven and a half inches at ⅛-inch scale and twenty-five by fifteen inches at ¼-inch scale. With ⅛- and ¼-inch scales, you can use a regular foot ruler, which is usually marked off in ¹⁄₁₆-inch increments, or use an architect's scale. Also buy several sheets or a twenty-yard roll of inexpensive transparent sketching paper to use for site analysis overlays and preliminary conceptual sketches and plans.

2. You can also buy grid vellum or tracing paper in ten by ten small squares per inch that can be used at a scale of 1 inch = 10 feet (an engineer's scale). It might be easier to translate an engineer's or surveyor's topographic survey drawing (usually drawn at 1 inch = 20 feet or less) using this scale. The engineer's scale is very easy to work with once you become used to it. A hundred- by sixty-foot lot

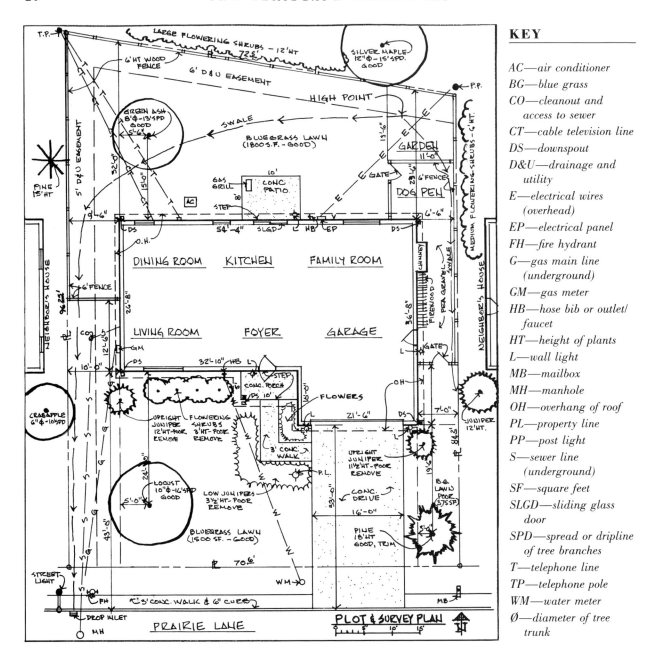

KEY

AC—*air conditioner*
BG—*blue grass*
CO—*cleanout and access to sewer*
CT—*cable television line*
DS—*downspout*
D&U—*drainage and utility*
E—*electrical wires (overhead)*
EP—*electrical panel*
FH—*fire hydrant*
G—*gas main line (underground)*
GM—*gas meter*
HB—*hose bib or outlet/ faucet*
HT—*height of plants*
L—*wall light*
MB—*mailbox*
MH—*manhole*
OH—*overhang of roof*
PL—*property line*
PP—*post light*
S—*sewer line (underground)*
SF—*square feet*
SLGD—*sliding glass door*
SPD—*spread or dripline of tree branches*
T—*telephone line*
TP—*telephone pole*
WM—*water meter*
Ø—*diameter of tree trunk*

will fit on a standard eight-and-a-half by eleven-inch piece of paper.

I find it best to use the ⅛- or ¼-inch scales for base and design plans because most carpenter's tape measures and carpenter's squares in the United States are in increments of ¹⁄₁₆ inch; therefore it is easier for you or your contractors to interpret a drawing at either of these scales. However, in a country that uses the metric system, you would be advised to use a metric scale and vellum in metric scale squares.

Whichever scale you choose, begin to graphically translate the field survey and analysis data onto a base plan. Be as accurate as possible in making this drawing since it will be the basis of your entire design process. Inaccurate base plans can cause troublesome and expensive problems in the design and implementation steps. Use a red pen or Hi-

Liter pen to mark off the information from your field notes as you transfer it onto the base plan. Be systematic in this process to avoid errors and oversights.

Once the base plan is drawn to scale, it is advisable to make at least one photocopy or print for use in the next two steps, the analysis and synthesis.

Photo and Video Surveys

Another important way to record the existing site conditions is with panoramic still photos or slides or with videotape. For many years we have used still on-site sketches and panoramic photo mosaics in the landscape architecture profession, but with the advent of small video cameras and camcorders, it is easier to videotape a site and replay it during the conceptual and final design process.

I first saw this video survey method used by one of my students in an adult education home landscaping course. For the past few years we have become more and more dependent on the videotaping of the existing site conditions and use it almost exclusively.

Not all of the items listed in the survey and inventory checklists here are important to every landscape project; however, you should at least be aware of the many influences that come to bear on a specific site and project. I recommend that new or inexperienced designers at least use the preceding information as a checklist to ensure that nothing important has been overlooked.

STEP #3: PROJECT ANALYSIS

Again, as with a doctor, once the patient's vital signs have been checked and the lab workups are in hand, an analysis of the data is performed and a diagnosis of the patient's health is made. The third step in the design process, then, is the detailed analysis of the two previous steps, the Program of Needs and Budget Range and the Site Survey and Inventory.

The first step in the program analysis is to prioritize the needs, wants, and desires of your family and to determine if these fit into your budget range and phasing plan. If you are remodeling an existing landscape, you may wish to make your highest priority the modification of the area that uses the most water. If designing a new Xeriscape landscape, you may want to give top priority to practical goals, such as creating shade to aid in energy conservation, reducing wind with a screen planting, or increasing privacy with lattices or vines on a trellis.

At this point it becomes a real challenge to try to zero in on the situation, and to clarify and set realistic priorities for those items on the program, but it *must be done*! If attention is not given to being as specific as possible at this stage, the project will never be as successful as it could be.

The next step is site analysis, and it is done in two distinctly different procedures—the aimless search and the systematic testing. They can be done in any order, but I usually recommend the aimless search first. In this step you are trying to determine the essential character of the site, the visual qualities and liabilities of the site, and any clues to possible uses of areas and existing elements of the site that might be helpful in developing your design.

This aimless search should be done with a notepad or sketch pad, a hand-held audio tape recorder and a still camera, or a video camera. It is best to walk around the site at several different times of the day and night and during the various seasons of the year, if possible, to be able to experience and accurately record the influences that time and weather have on the site and on you, the ultimate user.

The photo or video survey should be analyzed at this time and can be helpful in recording the data from the aimless search. Become familiar with the elements, objects, and areas of the site by reviewing the panoramic photos or the videotape over and over again. All too often I find my students omitting the aimless search on their projects because they think they can remember these conditions and factors without the extra effort of physically walking and experiencing the site. This is a good way to "miss the forest for the trees." You are most likely to overlook an important factor that can make a major influence on the design and the final outcome of the project.

The second procedure of site analysis is a sys-

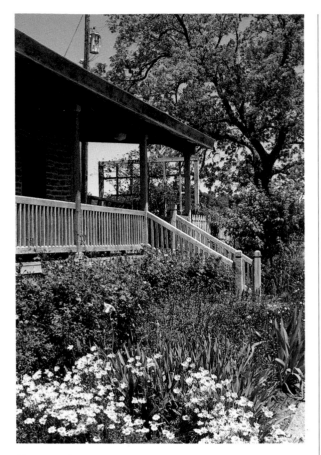

The revival of the "cottage garden" reminds us that the principles behind Xeriscape landscaping have been around for a long time. This garden in Independence, Texas, features Shasta daisies (Chrysanthemum maximum), bearded iris (Iris spp.), mealycups (Salvia farinacea), and roses (Rosa spp.). The old-fashioned flowers are an ideal complement to the rustic cottage. (Photo: Doug Welsh)

Some of the systematic site analysis considerations are:

• How many square feet or acres are included in the total site, and how much of that is covered already by the house, driveways, walks, patios, etc., leaving how much area for additional landscaping?

• What is the condition of the house, the siding, the trim, the windows and doors, shutters, etc.? This information is important so that if major repairs and maintenance are necessary, you can do this before introducing any plants that might get damaged in the maintenance process.

• What is the condition of the existing circulation or traffic paving elements, such as the driveways, walks, and patios? Does the existing paved surface drainage work or are there wet areas and puddles that could cause slick spots during rainy or winter conditions?

• What are specific areas suited for in the way of plants—that is, dry-soil or adapted plants or higher-water-demand plants?

• If there is an existing irrigation or sprinkler system, does it meet the needs of the existing landscape, and will it accommodate or easily be modified for the new Xeriscape design?

• Is the ground surface relatively flat, rolling hills, steep, rock outcroppings, etc.? Does the existing drainage meet the minimum of ¼ inch per foot (two

A large site could support the inclusion of an area of tallgrass prairie species such as side oats grama (Bouteloua curtipendula) *and prairie sand reed (Calamofilua longifolia) with an inviting pathway.*

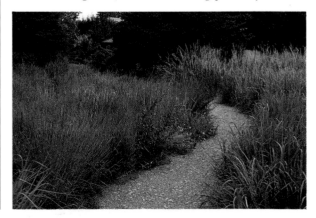

tematic testing of the site conditions. By determining and calculating square footages of areas, percentages and ratios of slopes, ditches and drainage areas, high and low points, heights of structures, plants, and elements, and establishing the distances across the site from one property line to another and from the house to either property line or easement, to the street, or to the neighbor's house, you will become familiar with the physical conditions and statistics of your property. By knowing this data, you can determine whether your program requirements will fit the physical character of the site.

percent) away from the house and other structures and paved surfaces? I will explain grading and drainage design later in this chapter.

Analyzing the various tests is another step in the systematic procedure. Soil tests will tell you whether the existing soil will support the proposed plants or if it is necessary to do extensive soil conditioning and improvement to ensure proper plant growth.

Water quality, pressure, and flow tests need to be analyzed to determine what, if anything, can be done to provide adequate water for the proposed plantings. At this time you might determine if an irrigation system is essential and if the water quality, pressure, and flow are adequate to provide an efficient irrigation system. For further information on irrigation design, refer to the chapter on efficient irrigation.

A thorough and comprehensive analysis of your program, budget, and site may be the most critical step in this design process. Hard testing and decision making are what the analysis step is all about. At this stage you are questioning the feasibility of your project. Identification and understanding of possible problems, concerns, and challenges are the first steps in the design process.

STEP #4: THE DESIGN OR SYNTHESIS

The final step of the design process is the synthesis or combination of all the data accumulated in the previous steps. A Xeriscape design should be organized for a pleasant environment, provide easy accessibility to and from the interior and exterior of the home, be dynamic and ever-changing throughout the seasons and the years, be simple and easily understood, be as economical as possible in both the initial installation and the continuing maintenance, be appropriate for the neighborhood, your budget, and your lifestyle, and be durable and long-lasting.

At this point in the planning and design process, you must keep in mind the other six principles of Xeriscape landscaping: soil improvements, practical use of turf areas, appropriate plant selection,

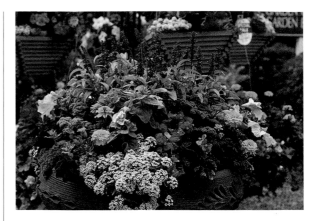

An easy and water-efficient way to add color to any Xeriscape garden is to use containers of annual flowers. This container filled with alyssum (Lobularia maritima), salvia (Salvia spp.), wax begonias (Begonia semperflorens), marigolds (Tagetes spp.), and petunias (Petunia spp.) is arranged in the typical English garden style. (Photo: Doug Welsh)

efficient irrigation, use of mulches, and appropriate maintenance. Becoming familiar with them now will help guide you toward a more complete Xeriscape plan and design. Separate chapters will deal with these topics in greater detail.

Where to Start?

The preliminary design begins with site planning, which includes the defining of use areas; understanding of the three-dimensional planes (the ground, walls, and ceiling planes); circulation or traffic pattern planning (the connecting links and surfaces between and through the use areas); and in a Xeriscape project, the definition of water-use zones, through to the detail design of all elements and areas of the site. You will be considering the problems, concerns, and challenges of the program, the budget range, the site survey and inventory, and the project analysis steps to put all of the pieces of the puzzle together to form a functional and beautiful Xeriscape project.

I recommend that you do two or more alternative preliminary solutions (on inexpensive transparent tracing paper) in the preliminary stage with different approaches to solving these problems, concerns,

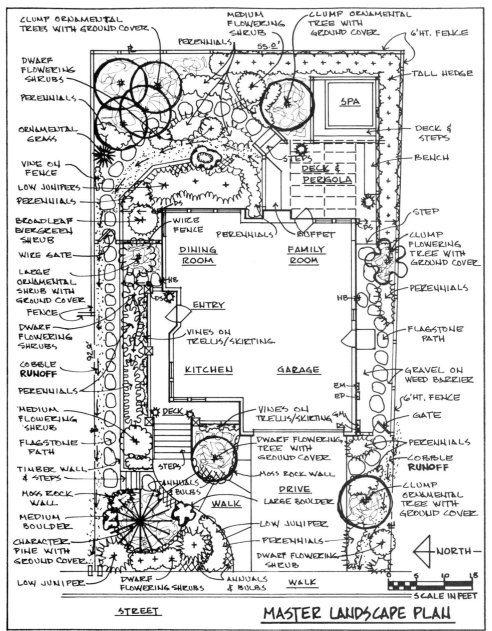

KEY

DS—downspout
EM—electrical meter
EP—electrical panel
GM—gas meter
HB—hose bib or
      outlet/faucet

and challenges. The more alternatives you explore for solutions to your specific program of needs, budget range, and site problems, the better able you will be to make an intelligent decision as to the best and most cost-efficient solution for the final design.

In a residential landscape there are three main areas to be considered individually and collectively along with the connections (circulation) among them. They are the public or entrance area, the service or utility area which includes storage structures, and the private or outdoor living area which includes spaces for play and relaxation.

Site planning is a three-dimensional process in which you consider the horizontal, ground, or *floor* plane; the vertical or *wall* plane; the overhead or *ceiling* plane; with strong consideration given to the fourth dimension of *time*. For a Xeriscape project, the floor plane is the most important, but you should be aware of and carefully consider the impact of the other two planes and how they influence the use of the site.

Horizontal, ground, or floor plane. is the first dimension to be considered, and quite often the one that is most costly in the overall landscape, and can benefit the most from the use of Xeriscape fundamentals. The landscape elements to be considered are:

•grading and drainage, with the necessary retaining walls, steps, ramps, and drainage structures, such as drop inlets, catch basins, culverts, and headwalls.

• soil conditioning—this important operation will be discussed in considerable depth in the chapter on soil improvements.

•paving surfaces for circulation, parking, sports, and play.

•plant surfaces and beds, such as grasses, whether turf or ornamental; ground covers other than grasses; and flowers such as perennials, annuals, and bulbs. Once we have defined these high-use and often high-visibility areas of grass, we can then define the other planting-bed-related ground plane surfaces.

•mulches, whether organic (bark) or inorganic (gravel).

•subsurface and surface irrigation, whether drip-type, porous pipe, or pop-up spray-type.

Vertical or wall plane. The enclosure elements of the landscape are important parts of this dimension. With these elements you can define spaces, create privacy and a feeling of being safe and cozy, and control access into and/or out of a space. Included are:

•fences and gates for definition of space and control of access.

•screens and screen walls for visual and climate control.

•plants for visual effect or climate control screens as with hedges and windbreaks.

Overhead or ceiling plane. The open sky is the ultimate ceiling, but often you must consider the inclusion of such elements as:

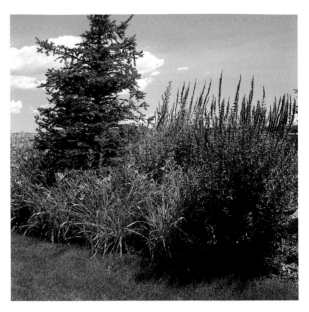

Late summer growth of purple loosestrife (Lythrum salicaria) *and daylilies* (Hemerocallis spp.) *completely screens a transformer. (Note: Do not plant purple loosestrife in the East; it's very invasive of wetlands—okay in semiarid climates.)*

•solid roofs for protection from the extremes of the weather.

•pergolas or trellises for shade and a feeling of enclosure overhead.

•tree limbs and branches, leaf canopies, and vines on trellises for a natural, as opposed to man-made ceiling.

Beginning the Site Planning Process

The first step in site planning, then, would be to define the general use of subareas and spaces of the project, keeping the Xeriscape principles in mind. A rough bubble diagram of the three main areas and the various subareas should be done on tracing paper. At this point the exact size and shape of the areas are not important, but the general size and shape are.

Other alternative uses for typical turf areas are:

•enlarged parking and driveway areas

•functional and more accessible walks and landings

• generous patios, decks, and gazebos for entertaining and relaxation

• hard surface play, sport, and game areas

• larger vegetable and flower gardens, berry patches, and fruit orchards

• shrub beds and flower beds for perennials, annuals, and ground covers

• areas for native grasses and wildflowers

• areas covered with organic (bark) or inorganic (gravel) mulches

• swimming and ornamental pools, waterfalls and streams, hot tubs and spas, or fountains and sculpture.

Circulation and Traffic Pattern Planning

After providing for the general shapes and locations of the alternative-use areas, you must develop the circulation and traffic patterns that link the use areas together and to the main areas of the project. Hard-surface paving materials used for this purpose do not normally require heavy use of water except for an occasional hosing down for cleaning.

When designing circulation and traffic patterns, you should always provide for the optimum and functional use of the walks, landings, driveways, and parking facilities. Front entrance walks should be of sufficient width for two adults to walk side by side comfortably, preferably four to five feet. On the other hand, a garden walk or a walk to a pet pen or barn can be a minimum of three feet wide.

Main driveways should be a minimum of ten feet wide to accommodate the vehicle, and allow for getting in and out of it without walking in the grass or plant or flower beds. A parking space for a single car should be a minimum of nine by eighteen feet, and preferably ten by twenty feet.

The minimum inside turning radius for a driveway should be fifteen to seventeen feet and the outside edge of pavement or curb radius, thirty to thirty-two feet. A dropoff area on a circular drive should be a minimum of twenty-one feet wide to allow one car to be parked dropping off passengers on the right while allowing enough room for another car to pass by on the left side.

All hard-surface elements should have a minimum cross grade of ¼ inch per foot for adequate drainage and to minimize standing water on the surface, which is both a safety hazard and a cause of long-term damage to the surface from infiltration into the surface material and freezing and thawing in cold climate areas. In addition, the drainage of water from hard-surface paving areas can contribute considerable amounts of water for planting beds adjacent to the surfaces and to the harvesting of water for future use. We will elaborate on water harvesting in the irrigation chapter.

The maximum grade for walks or ramps in areas of heavy snow and ice is eight-and-one-third percent (one foot rise vertically for twelve feet run horizontally). Steeper than this will become a safety hazard and dangerous to pedestrians. This grade is also recommended as maximum for handicapped walks and ramps.

When selecting hard-surface materials and elements, it is best if you try to avoid a glaring, cold, and commercial appearance. Use subdued colors and pleasant and safe textures (not slick and smooth), and provide a good scale (make the space comfortable to walk through or to be in for any length of time). The cost of hard-surface elements may account for better than fifty percent of the total cost of the project, so keep it simple and economical, yet bear in mind the long-term durability and ease of maintenance of the surface.

Development of Grading and Drainage Patterns

Once the major use areas, traffic patterns, and circulation surfaces have been determined, it is important to develop the drainage patterns and the necessary grading plan to achieve a satisfactory flow of water on the site.

Grading is any change in the existing slope or ground surface by mechanical means, no matter how slight. The three major purposes of grading are to shape the ground so water will flow (drainage), to fit elements into the site, such as decks and patios, and to create pleasing aesthetic appearances and effects, such as berms and terraces.

Drainage is the movement of water over the surface, below surface, and between the particles of earth. It is always necessary and is most often overlooked by developers, realtors, and home buyers.

Surface drainage is most important in a Xeriscape project. The speed of water movement on the surface depends on the steepness of the slope and the

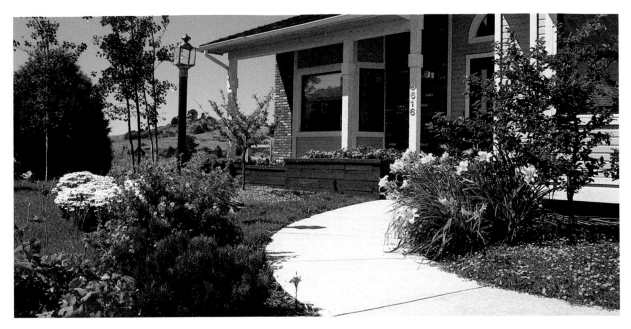

Perennials in this Colorado Xeriscape landscape provide year-round interest. In midsummer yellow predominates, with daylilies (Hemerocallis spp.) *and creeping potentilla* (Potentilla crantzii) *accenting the Sargent crab apple* (Malus sargentii) *on the right and* Potentilla fruticosa 'Setter's Gold' *next to dwarf mugo pine* (Pinus mugo) *on the left. Selecting plants with the right scale, and not crowding them in the landscape, is important in avoiding an overgrown look in a few years. (Design: Thomas L. Stephens. Photo: Scott Stephens)*

smoothness of the surface. The recommended minimum slope for hard surfaces, grass, and mulch areas is two percent. This is the same as the ¼ inch per foot mentioned in the section on circulation planning.

Water will create ponds or bogs if not moved or if moved too slowly. It will make gullies and create erosion if moved too fast. It is best not to use hard-surface ditches for drainage; it is better to allow the water to soak into the soil to provide for enhanced growth of plants and grasses.

Rather than use mechanical means of subsurface drainage, such as solid pipes and hard-surface ditches that carry the water off the site, I recommend that you "harvest" the water that Mother Nature provides you free of charge by rainfall and snowfall, and use it in your Xeriscape garden. It is wise conservation to collect and retain as much of this free water as you can, especially since water prices continue to rise and the availability becomes scarce, no matter the price. In Xeriscape projects, sometimes this free water is all that is needed to sustain low-water-demand plants. Water harvesting is explained in detail in the irrigation chapter.

Location and Selection of Plant Types

Now that the drainage patterns and grading plan are designed, it is time to consider the location of plant types. In the preliminary design step, I recommend that you not be too specific about the exact genus and species of plants, but that you concentrate on:

• what you want the plant to do—that is, shade, flower, cover the ground, produce edible fruit, etc.

• the form of plant you have in mind—that is, spreading, weeping, columnar, etc.

• the space available for the particular plant type—that is, open lawn, border planting, narrow side yard, etc.

• the life support conditions—that is, sun, soil, and moisture—that are available on the site.

You should consider these factors and select two or more plants that will fill the bill in the preliminary design stage. Then during the final design you can make the final selection, depending on the exact qualifications of a particular plant species. Become as familiar with your selections as you can before including them in your planting plan or buying and

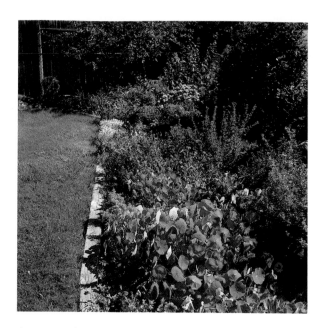

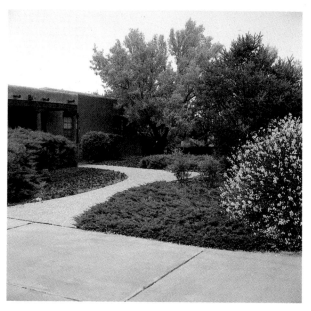

A strong edge gives this flower garden almost a planter box importance as well as ensuring that the grass won't creep into the flowers. Annual nasturtiums (Tropaeolum majus) *are prominent here, and garden chrysanthemums* (Chrysanthemum × morifolium) *light up the corner. (Design: Thomas L. Stephens/Joan Hartman)*

A simple design is often the most pleasing, as evidenced by this mature Albuquerque landscape. The trees and shrubs, including Russian olive (Elaeagnus angustifolia), *Spanish broom* (Spartium junceum), *and junipers* (Juniperus spp.), *are watered once a week for twenty minutes with a bubbler system. Only the petunias* (Petunia spp.) *receive more frequent hand-watering, as needed.*

planting them in your Xeriscape landscape, so you can be more positive of the ultimate results you will achieve.

Avoid selecting or buying a plant just because it is in flower at the time you see it in the nursery or because it is on sale or inexpensive at the time. You always get what you pay for, and sometimes that does not necessarily mean quality. Remember that a plant will become an important part of your project, and that it will change significantly over the seasons and over the years. You should be aware of these changes and how they will effect the ultimate results when you finalize your design.

I have attempted to outline the many important factors and considerations involved in the planning and design of a Xeriscape project. The process is complex and should not be considered otherwise. To be able to create a good design, you do not need every one of these items, but you should at least be aware of them and how they might affect your project.

There are numerous good books and courses on the subject of planning and design that can be more specific than I have been. If you are interested in learning more about these important principles of Xeriscape landscaping, pursue your interest by learning more about them through books, seminars, classes, and personal involvement in the process.

Any good teacher will tell you that the best way to learn and retain the most information about any subject is to immediately use the information in a real-life situation or to teach someone else about what you have just learned. I recommend, then, that you start your own Xeriscape planning and design project as soon as possible, and share your newfound excitement and information with a friend or neighbor, thereby helping yourself and your neighbor, and improving the environment around you.

Soil Analysis and Improvement

I RECENTLY picked up the book *The Dry Garden* (London: J. M. Dent & Sons, Ltd., 1983) by English author Beth Chatto. Though it's well known and popular in Xeriscape circles, I had never looked at it before, because I couldn't imagine what I could learn on the subject from someone who lives in a country that drips constantly (or so I thought). I was delighted to find that she lives in an area that receives an annual rainfall of about twenty inches, not much higher than the fourteen or so inches a year I work with in Colorado. Furthermore, she says she often gardens through a summer-long drought and on such poor soil that "even the native weeds sometimes curl up and die."

I was much struck by the simplicity of her statement, "I really don't hold with watering." A typical American, if more water-conservation-conscious than average, I realized such a straightforward position on how to structure landscape watering had never occurred to me.

Although Chatto, of course, waters in new plants to get rid of air pockets and to help them get established, even the severe drought experienced in Britain in 1976 failed to weaken her resolve not to water. Some of the newer plants died, but many looked remarkably good, she said.

Her secret is soil improvement. Every one of the hundreds of plants she has installed in her country gardens gets an ample measure of moisture-retentive organic material mixed into the planting hole. Organic material eventually breaks down, and in a more recent book, *Green Tapestry* (New York: Simon & Schuster, 1989), she explains that after six or seven years she sometimes rejuvenates a perennial bed that's looking a little tired, actually digging up the plants, mixing in organic matter again, and dividing and replanting the plants.

Plant choice figures in, too. Chatto notes that early in her gardening career she was occasionally given bog-loving plants, which she attempted to raise. But no matter how much organic material she mixed into their planting holes, they would die, and rather than change her determination not to keep watering, she evolved a plant palette more adaptable to the climate and soil.

Soil analysis and improvement is the second principle of Xeriscape landscaping. It's futile to say any one principle is more important than the others, but if there's one as nearly essential as planning and design, it's soil improvement. An appropriately improved soil will go further than anything else in helping the plant use all the moisture available to it, promoting the plant's vigor and water-use efficiency.

SOIL

A plant's growth is governed by what's called in agriculture the "principle of limiting factors"—that is, it's limited by the least available among six external factors: light, mechanical support (for the plant to be rooted in), heat, air, water, and nutrients. Soil supplies either completely or in part all but light.

A good soil is one that supports healthy plant life and also conserves moisture. Soil improvements take two forms: those designed to improve its physical structure and those designed to change its chemistry.

Physical changes include loosening tightly compacted soil, creating structure in structureless soil, and eliminating the drainage problems associated with a thin soil layer over a hardpan. These changes allow nutrients, water, and air to be better distributed through the soil and more available for the plant's use.

Chemical changes that may be needed include the addition of nutrients and minerals, alteration of pH (the acidity or alkalinity of the soil), or reduction of salinity (the concentration of soluble salts, especially sodium). These changes are usually made in order to favor the growth or survival of desired landscape plants. Giving the plants the nutrients and pH they need will help them to thrive and compete with weeds.

Xeriscape landscaping, even more than other types of landscaping, demands an intimate knowledge of the kind of soil you have to work with. (When water conservation is an objective, "chemical support" used to promote plant growth, weed exclusion, etc., is undesirable.) The type of soil you have will factor into your thinking as you consider what plants you want to grow. In addition to getting your soil analyzed or doing some homemade tests (which are less accurate), it's helpful to think about how certain soils develop.

We all know, for instance, that the soil affects which plants grow in an area, but what is less obvious is that plant cover affects soil. Trees shed an annual layer of leaf mulch and have a deep or (in most cases) shallow but not especially fibrous root system. Thus, the soil under heavily forested areas has rich organic soil just below the surface, but perhaps poor soil farther down. This is why when rain forests are cleared for crops, the farming is not always successful—the rich soil layer may be very thin.

Prairie grasses in the Midwest have amazingly fibrous root systems that may reach down six feet or even more for some short grasses. (Note: Lawn grasses have shallow roots primarily because we mow the tops of the grass short.) As the years pass the roots die and are replaced, leaving a legacy of humus, which makes prairie soil some of the richest in the world. As you move farthur west into semiarid and arid environments, vegetative cover gets progressively thinner, and the soil gets correspondingly poorer.

Conscientious garden primers always talk about "ideal soil." It has, they point out, a balance of solids (clay, sand, and silt) and pore spaces. It has as much as fifty percent by volume of pore space consisting of roughly half water and half air (after drainage), forty-five percent minerals (clay, silt, and sand particles), and five percent organic matter.

Furthermore, we learn the "ideal" mixture of soil mineral solids is roughly equal parts of clay, silt, and sand. This is called "loam" and is a soil classification in itself. It balances the disadvantages of the more extreme soils, draining well, but not drying out too fast, holding plenty of plant-available water, and having enough airspace for healthy plant growth.

Lastly, we learn that, unfortunately, ideal soil is very rare. Gardeners have to contend much more often with soil not only damaged by grading (which compacts soil and changes drainage patterns) and the stripping of nutritive topsoil, but also poor to begin with, containing too much clay or sand.

My question is, is this supposed to be news? I think all this talk about "ideal soil" is a little trifling and oversimplified because it assumes we all want to grow the same thing. The great news is that there's no such thing as "ideal soil," because it all depends on what you want to grow. If you want to grow jewel-

All yarrows are drought tolerant when established, and easy to grow. Fern-leaf yarrow (Achillea filipendulina) is the tallest yarrow, reaching three to five feet. Most species survive in poor soil.

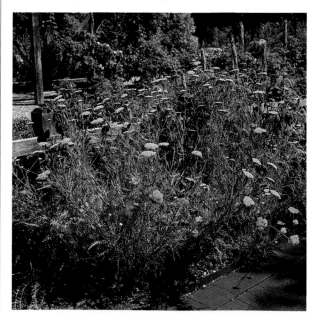

like alpine flowers, the "ideal" soil is gravelly and low in nutrients (poor). If you want to grow back-east perennials, then you need well-drained, humus-rich soil. If you want a cactus garden, your plants will blossom in dry, alkaline soil.

The point I try to make more than once in the following discussion about soils is that it's much easier to grow something appropriate to the soil you already have than to try to *significantly* change the soil. I've gone into extra detail on some of the topics, trying to explain the whys behind much of the standard brief information given about soils. If it's more information than you want or can bear about the subject right now, please at least "get" that one idea: that it's a real trial to alter the texture, pH, structure, salinity, etc., of the soil in a big way. So if it can fit into your concept of what you want your Xeriscape landscape to be, select plants that will thrive in your existing soil.

PHYSICAL STRUCTURE

In well-structured topsoil, individual soil particles tend to group together into granules or crumbs called aggregates. This is the soil's structure, and it's this structure that allows water and air to penetrate to the roots. Roots of plants grow through the spaces between the granules or crumbs, not through the soil itself, and the better the soil is structured the faster and deeper roots can grow in it. Therefore, turfgrasses will have a deeper root system in a loam than a clay. Sand, because of the large size of its particles, has little cohesion (the particles don't cling together) and cannot maintain a structure. Clay when wet and compacted is also structureless (we are advised not to work in clay soil when it's very wet to avoid compacting it further).

The mineral solids of unimproved soil govern the "behavior" of the soil, and the percentage of clay influences the properties of the soil far more than sand and silt. Clay consists of minute platelike particles that arrange themselves in a series as shown below. The plates are covered with negatively charged ions that attract and hold water (this is why certain clay soils are expansive) as well as positively charged ions such as calcium, potassium, and ammonium. It's the clay in soil that serves as a

reservoir for nutrients, holding them for the plant's use.

Clay soil has very tiny pores, and because of high surface tension between the water and the thin plates, as well as the small pore size, it's hard for air and water to move through the soil. As a result, plant roots may be denied moisture, suffer oxygen starvation, or even drown. Clay soil may hold up to four inches of water in the top foot, but only two inches may be available to the plants because the water is held more tightly in the soil than the plant can withdraw it.

This sketch shows how water applied over a square yard area moves through clay soil:

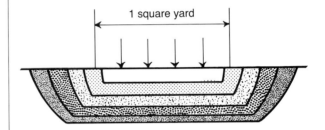

By contrast, sandy soil has lots of airspace. Because it has large particles, there is little surface area to hold the water, and because they're rounded, there isn't the adhesion between particle and water that there is with clay. A sandy soil tends to lose water rapidly, along with nutrients that are leached out below the root zone. Water applied to the same square yard would tend to move through the soil in this way, very quickly, too quickly for plant roots to make good use of it:

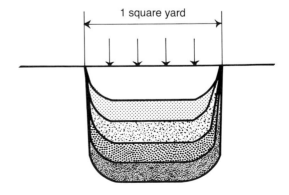

Silt is an intermediate particle size. It may be formed from the breakdown of sand particles, or may come from the same parent material as clay, eventually becoming clay after continued chemical and physical weathering. Silt, however, is more like sand in how it behaves in the soil, consisting of round particles, but much smaller than those of sand. Silt is not a very satisfactory soil material unless it's balanced by adequate sand, clay, and organic matter.

With either extremely sandy or extremely clayey soil, improvement can be made by adding soil amendments, either organic or inorganic. Traditional advice has held that the addition of organic amendments was the best and nearly universal answer to the problem of how to improve these types of soils.

In clay soils bits of decomposed organic matter (humus) provide a base for soil particles to gather onto, forming aggregates and adding structure to the soil. They also serve as wedges to open up pores. In sandy soil, humus acts as tiny reservoirs for holding water and dissolved nutrients, so the soil stays moist longer. In any soil the breakdown of the organic matter is accomplished by microorganisms that produce, in the process, humic acid. This chemical is believed to help bind particles of soil together, further enhancing the structure-building process of the soil.

In most instances the amending of soil with organic matter will prove beneficial, helping the plants in the predicted ways, but recent research and experiences with Xeriscape plantings have brought up some interesting exceptions:

•Where a plant naturally thrives in an area of poor soil, the addition of nutrients may cause it to "grow itself to death"—that is, it may experience such accelerated growth because of the extra nutrients provided by the organic matter that it becomes "leggy," and may die prematurely from being "spent." Certain flowers such as gaillardias will produce more blooms in poor soil or during drought because their flowering is a way to carry on the species in the face of impending death (by starvation or dehydration).

•In parts of the country where heat and humidity are high, such as in the extreme Southeast, microbial action in the soil uses up soil amendments so quickly that they're of little long-term value to the

plant. Organic amendments are recommended only for plants where the soil will be reworked regularly, such as in gardens and annual flower beds.

One of the drawbacks of organic materials is that they break down sooner or later, sometimes within a few months. Especially in sandy soils, as the microbial action breaks down the organic matter it eventually becomes small enough to be washed away and must be renewed periodically.

•Several universities around the country conducted long-term studies on the impact of adding organic soil amendments to the planting holes of trees and shrubs. It was found at each site that trees and shrubs planted without organic amendments developed more extensive root systems and stronger topgrowth than those planted with amendments. Apparently the struggle the "unamended" trees had to go through to become established led to their increased vigor later on.

A more recent study by Dr. Carl Whitcomb of Oklahoma State University confirmed this finding. Side-by-side comparisons showed a substantial increase in the size of trees grown without organic soil amendments compared to those grown with amendments. Looking at the seedlings grown with amendments alone you wouldn't see that they had been hindered, because they appeared healthy and well shaped. But compared to the test group, they were about half the size after a few years.

Organic amendments can cause other problems in the planting holes of large plants. These amendments may hold too much moisture, which most roots don't tolerate. When the roots begin to grow into the soggy amended soil, they suffocate. Conversely, when the amendments dry out they can be difficult to rewet, so even though the soil outside the planting hole may be moist, within the hole it may become too dry. If the quality of soil in the planting hole is enriched too much compared to the surrounding soil, or if the artificial medium container-grown plants are raised in is very different from the soil they're planted in, a barrier is created; roots then have difficulty moving out into the poorer soil, and there is reduced soil volume available for absorbing water and nutrients.

The problem, Dr. Whitcomb explains, comes when we amend *only* the planting hole for a tree or

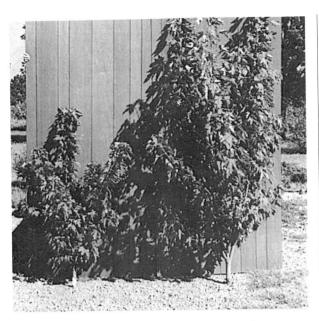

These two silver maples (Acer saccharinum) *were part of a test to determine the usefulness of adding organic soil amendments to the planting holes of new trees. After two years the tree* without *the soil amendments was nearly twice as large. The key is to incorporate soil amendments over a fairly large area, rather than just into the planting hole. If this isn't possible, it's better to eliminate soil amendments.*

shrub. The plant roots tend to remain in the hole, thus limiting the size of the plant. If you have the opportunity to amend the *entire planting bed* for a group of trees or shrubs, then the plants *can* benefit from the organic amendments.

There is some debate about the quantities of organic soil amendments needed when they *are* used, such as in shrub and flower beds, gardens, or new turf. Some experts recommend that no more than three cubic yards of material be added per 1,000 square feet per year, especially if manure is used (this corresponds to a 1¼- to 1½-inch layer). In clay soil too much introduced organic matter may create a salt problem. If possible, plan to amend poor soil every year and build up its quality gradually.

However, with turf, building up the soil slowly isn't very practical, so it's best to do a thorough job of improving the soil structure initially, since you have only one chance. Tom Stephens has been using a three-way mix consisting of three yards of manure, three yards of peat moss (or completed compost), and three yards of topsoil per 1,000 square feet as

soil improvement for nine years in the projects he's worked on in Colorado's alkaline clay soils. Though nine yards per 1,000 square feet is much higher than the usual recommended rate, he hasn't had any problems as a result of it. He includes this on all plantings, including turf, flower beds, ground covers, prairie gardens, and as a general improvement of the planting areas around trees and shrubs.

For many turf lawns in Georgia, Florida, and other places where the climate allows very large lawns to be installed without excessive water use, this extensive type of soil improvement is not economically feasible. In that case it's best to choose species that can tolerate native soils.

When incorporating organic amendments, always try to spread about one-third of the amendment over the soil, till that in to a depth of four to six inches, then spread the remainder of the amendment and till it in. This way a sharp line of unmixed layers won't form between the existing and improved soil; there will be a more gradual transition.

Inorganic amendments can also be used to improve the structure of clay or sandy soil. In the past, sand was sometimes recommended as a way to loosen tight clay soil. However, experience has shown this to be futile because you have to add *tremendous* quantities of sand in order to counter the effect of the clay and get anything but adobe. It's better to select another soil amendment to lighten clay soil, overexcavate (remove soil from a planting hole substantially larger than the root ball and replace with another soil blend that better suits the plant), or use plants that do well in clay soil.

Other inorganic amendments used to open up clay soil include perlite (heat-treated limestone), vermiculite (heat-treated mica), and cross-linked polyacrylamide. All of these, except cross-linked polyacrylamide, are relatively expensive and therefore impractical for amending more than small areas or using in potting soil.

Cross-linked polyacrylamide, also called water-absorbing polymer, hydro-gel, soil polymer, and soil enhancer, is an inert rock-salt–sized granule when dry that swells to a ¼- to ½-inch-wide gel particle, soaking up and storing as much as four hundred times its weight in pure water (rainwater and snowmelt). It stores two to three hundred times its weight in irrigation water because salts present in the water temporarily limit the absorption until the salts are flushed out by rainwater. Root hairs grow right into the gel particles and draw out water as needed.

The polymer helps loosen clay soil because it is always making minute expansions and contractions as it absorbs water and the plant roots draw it out. This provides aeration and improved drainage. It also improves the water-holding capacity of sandy soils by reducing evaporation from the soil and by providing "storage space" that doesn't dry out quickly.

I've been working with cross-linked polyacrylamide for nearly three years, primarily researching what it can be used for, after hearing about it at a Xeriscape conference in Denver. (The Colorado State Forest Service had already been using it for three years for their seedling tree program, finding they were able to increase the seedling survival rate substantially, at a cost of just a few cents a tree.)

The polymer's main value was originally thought to be savings in watering since it stores water in

soil for weeks and sometimes months, but I've come to think its ability to loosen clay soil and to store nutrients may become just as important. In a two-year study at Kansas State University, turf expert Dr. Jeff Nus found a definite relationship between the polymer's presence and the looseness of the soil. The study was made to determine if it might be possible to create a "softer" athletic field in order to reduce injuries.

Other inorganic soil amendments can achieve some but not all of these results, and cross-linked polyacrylamide's long life (an application may last ten years or longer), low cost, and safety (rated nonhazardous by the Occupational Safety and Health Administration) may make it a very useful soil amendment for Xeriscape landscaping. (Make sure the product you're using is labeled "94% cross-linked polyacrylamide." Many companies have produced inferior-quality polymers and are passing them off as the same product.)

Hardpan

Sometimes topsoil may have a tough, compacted soil layer a few inches down that is very difficult for plant roots to penetrate and that can cause extremely poor drainage. It may be a natural formation, or it may have been caused by heavy equipment compacting the subsoil during construction or even by foot traffic on moist clay soil. If a subsoil is clayey and gets wet while exposed, it can dry to a rocklike hardness. If the hardpan layer is not too thick, you may be able to break it up by having your soil plowed to a depth of eighteen inches or more. (If a Rototiller bounces off the existing soil, you know you have a hardpan and may want to call in professional help. The landscape contractor may scarify the surface first with the ripper teeth of a front-end loader, then do the plowing or tilling.)

If the layer is thicker, you may be able to improve the situation by installing a system of drain tiles. It may be necessary to have the entire planting area excavated with heavy equipment to a depth of about twenty-four inches, then have organic matter thoroughly mixed in.

If correcting the problem is more difficult or

Globe amaranth (Gomphrena globosa) *is a very colorful and drought-tolerant annual. Connie Ellefson's plants grew about fifteen inches tall in Colorado with virtually no watering (they were treated with water-absorbing polymers). The plants in this Atlanta photo, where rainfall is much higher, grew about two feet tall.*

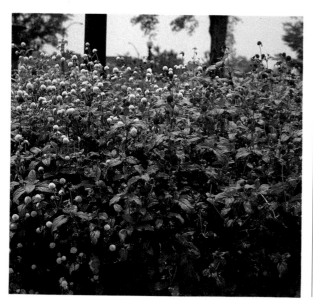

costly than it's worth, you may want to use raised beds for your plantings, filling the beds with good-quality soil and making sure they are deep enough for plant growth. This is often done in the Southwest where some soils are almost impossible to work with because of structural and chemical problems as described in the next section.

CHEMISTRY

A Del Rio, Texas, woman had to have a garden full of azaleas such as those she had loved in her youth back east. The soil of the area she has to work with has a pH of approximately 9.0, compared to azaleas' preference for slightly acid soil (5.5 to 6.5). Her landscape contractor had to replace all the soil in planting holes several feet deep and wide with peat moss. The azaleas are lovely, but they regularly die off after a few years and must be replaced when they start to outgrow their planting holes.

In Xeriscape landscaping, as in any other low-maintenance gardening, it's far better to select plants that can grow in the range of your soil's existing pH than to try to alter it substantially.

The soil's pH (its alkalinity or acidity) is one of the chemical variables in soil that home landscapers need to be concerned with, because it dictates to some extent whether you will or will not be able to grow certain plants. Fortunately, many plants are tolerant of a wide range of pH, as shown on the list, but there are limits, and although it's relatively simple to add sufficient amounts of humus to improve the soil as needed, you're fighting an uphill battle in trying to permanently and significantly alter the pH of the soil. You can't control the factors that made the soil the way it is, such as the underlying material, the amount of rainfall, and the chemical reading of your rainfall or irrigation water.

The pH of the soil affects plant growth because it influences the availability of essential nutrients. When the soil pH is between 6.0 and 7.5, nutrients such as phosphorus, calcium, potassium, and magnesium are most available to plants. As the pH drops below that range into an acidic condition, they become insoluble and less available for uptake by the plant, while iron, trace minerals, and some toxic elements such as aluminum become more available. Phosphorus, iron, and many trace minerals become insoluble and unavailable when the soil alkalinity rises above pH 8.0.

Soil pH also affects the availability of nitrogen because the nitrogen is actually bound up in organic matter and must be converted by several species of soil bacteria into forms usable by the plants. When the pH is too high or too low this bacterial activity decreases dramatically and little nitrogen is made available to the plants.

Remember that pH, like decibels, is a logarithmic scale, so a soil with a pH of 5.0 is ten times more acidic than one with a pH of 6.0. Turfgrasses prefer neutral soil (6.5 to 7.5) whereas many wildflowers and pines prefer a slightly acid soil (except in the West). If you live in an area with acid soil, you will very likely be amending the soil where you will be installing turfgrass to make it more neutral. Particularly in this situation it's better to separate turf from other planting areas because changing the pH to give one type of plant the best conditions may cause the other to perform poorly or even die, no matter how much care you lavish on it. This chart shows the quantities of chemical soil amendment needed to raise or lower pH to the neutral level. Again, it's better to select a turfgrass adaptable to the existing pH because even your irrigation water may be acid or alkaline and may hasten the soil's return to its original pH.

To lower pH to 6.5 (pounds sulfur or ammonium sulfate per 1,000 square feet by soil type)

Soil pH	Sand	Clay
7.0	10	20
7.5	30	45
8.5	45	70

To raise pH to 6.5 (pounds limestone per 1,000 square feet by soil type)

Soil pH	Sand	Loam	Clay
6.0	15	40	55
5.5	30	80	110
5.0	40	105	155
4.5	50	135	195

To lower the pH for individual plants or planting areas one-half to one point, say from 7.5 to 7.0 or

6.5, add ½ pound of ground sulfur or three pounds of iron sulfate per hundred square feet. To raise the pH by one point, use five pounds of ground limestone per hundred square feet. If done at planting time, the powder can be spaded into the soil and the water will carry it down to treat the lower soil. You can also spread the powder on the ground and water it in. It's helpful to leave the fallen needles from acid-loving conifers on the ground rather than clean them up because the acid in the needles leaches into the soil and helps maintain pH. Take soil pH readings every few years, especially if the plants begin to develop pale green leaves with dark veins, and add soil amendment as needed.

If you've had your soil tested by a cooperative extension service or other soil lab, the result will give you the pH reading of the sample as well as the levels of many common nutrients, and may give recommendations as to how to correct nutrient deficiencies. It's best to follow this local advice. For example, in some parts of the country, gypsum (calcium sulfate) added to an acidic pH clay soil helps aggregate the soil because of the chemical reaction between the calcium and the soil. But in arid environments the clay soil is often high in calcium already, so the resulting reaction produces a calcium salt and a marked decline in the soil.

Salinity

In arid parts of the West soils may have high concentrations of salts. They develop from the weathering of the minerals that are naturally found in the soils, but their levels may be compounded by the use of well water or softened water for irrigation, inorganic fertilizers, chemical amendments, and manures high in salt. Poor drainage is another culprit, either within the soil itself or on the surface.

Plant symptoms of high-salt soils include poor germination and growth, scorched and yellow leaves or browned and withered leaf margins (salt burn), and sometimes a dark, bluish green color. The presence of salt in the soil results in water moving out of the roots and creating water deficiency in the plants.

Strategies to combat this condition include improving internal drainage in the soil by adding or-

ganic amendments, making surface drainage better with drain tile systems, and avoiding the use of high-salt amendments.

In terms of real numbers, the high end of low-salt concentrations in soil is listed at roughly 2.0 milimhos (the unit for measuring soil salinity) per centimeter. Above this level, sensitive plants such as roses, most maples, pines, most viburnums, and other plants show symptoms of salt burn. Bluegrass grows poorly at 4.0 mmho/cm or above, and most landscape plants will show injury when the reading is between 4.0 and 8.0.

You can also choose plants tolerant of high-salt soils or, in extreme caes, do all plantings on berms of low-salt soil brought into your site. These raised beds are underlaid with a gravel and/or fabric barrier to prevent capillary action from drawing the salt up into the new soil.

The lists that follow are of some particularly salt-tolerant plants.

Trees with Moderate Salt Tolerance
(4–6 mmho/cm)

Acer negundo	Box elder
Betula populifolia	Gray birch
Celtis occidentalis	Hackberry
Fraxinus excelsior	European ash
F. quadrangulata	Blue ash
Juniperus scopulorum	Juniper
J. virginiana	Eastern red cedar
Koelreuteria paniculata	Goldenrain tree
Maclura pomifera	Osage orange
Robinia pseudoacacia	Black locust
Sophora japonica	Japanese pagoda tree, Chinese scholar tree
Ulmus pumila	Siberian elm

Trees with High-Salt Tolerance
(6–8 mmho/cm)

Ailanthus altissima	Tree-of-heaven
Amelanchier canadensis	Shadblow serviceberry
Crataegus crus-galli	Cockspur hawthorn
Elaeagnus angustifolia	Russian olive
Pinus thunbergii	Japanese black pine
Ptelea trifoliata	Water ash
Thuja occidentalis	American arborvitae

Shrubs with Moderate- to High-Salt Tolerance
(4–8 mmho/cm)

Caragana arborescens	Siberian pea shrub
Elaeagnus commutata	Silverberry
E. multiflora	Cherry elaeagnus
Juniperus chinensis	
'Pfitzerana'	
J. conferta	Japanese shore juniper
Lonicera tatarica	Tatarian honeysuckle
Rhamnus frangula	Glossy buckthorn
Spiraea vanhouttei	Vanhoutte spirea

Shrubs with Very High–Salt Tolerance
(above 8 mmho/cm)

Atriplex canescens	Four-wing saltbush
Baccharis halimifolia	Groundsel
Cytisus scoparius	Scotch broom
Halimodendron	Salt tree
halodendron	
Hippophae rhamnoides	Sea buckthorn
Myrica pensylvanica	Bayberry
Rhamnus cathartica	Common buckthorn
Rosa rugosa	Rugosa rose
Shepherdia canadensis	Buffaloberry
Tamarix gallica	Tamarisk
T. parviflora	

Grasses
(ranked from lowest to highest, 8–18 mmho/cm)

Agrostis palustris	Creeping bentgrass
Agropyron Smithii	Western wheatgrass
A. elongatum	Tall wheatgrass
Elymus canadensis	Canada wildrye
Cynodon dactylon	Bermudagrass
Puccinellia airoides	Alkaligrass
Distichlis stricta	Saltgrass
Sporobolus airoides	Alkali sacaton

Source: Dr. James Feucht and Jack Butler, *Landscape Management* (New York: Van Nostrand Reinhold Company, 1988)

These plants are common to temperate climates. Coastal areas also experience salt problems in soil because of saltwater intrusion into the groundwater. A list of salt-tolerant trees and shrubs for seashore plantings appears in the Appendix on pages 305–306.

Nutrients

People need vitamins, amino acids, and minerals to grow, and plants need chemical elements. At least fifteen elements (new research indicates the total may be sixteen to eighteen) are essential for plant growth:

• Carbon, oxygen, and hydrogen make up about ninety to ninety-five percent of the dry weight of the plant and are obtained from the carbon dioxide of the air and the water of the soil. They make up the plant structure.

• Nitrogen, phosphorus, and potassium, which are obtained from the soil, are used in the metabolism of plant structure, especially in forming proteins and chlorophyll. This is why nitrogen availability affects the greenness of plants.

• Calcium and magnesium are usually deficient in acid soils. They increase root hair growth and aid in photosynthesis.

• Sulfur is obtained from soil, especially organic matter, irrigation water, and gypsum. It heightens green color in grass, improves cold tolerance, and helps in metabolism.

• Iron, zinc, manganese, copper, boron, and molybdenum are micronutrients. Usually none are needed on acid soil, though iron may be needed on alkaline soils. The function of these elements is not completely understood, but they are thought to be part of enzymes that regulate plant metabolism. Deficiencies usually cause slow growth, but, except for iron, deficiencies in the soil are uncommon.

The soil test results from a lab should note any deficiencies that need correcting and recommend solutions.

Several inorganic amendments have been discussed here for improving soil chemistry. In most instances they are simply mixed into the planting hole or bed, or spread over the top of the soil and watered in. Cross-linked polyacrylamide may again prove useful, especially in sandy soils, because of its ability to hold in suspension whatever dissolved nutrients or chemicals are in solution. It may be possible to substantially reduce the application rates of those chemicals because they are stored in the polymer, not leached beyond the plant's reach. The National Fertilizer and Environmental Research Center (under the Tennessee Valley Authority) is researching this possibility.

ORGANIC AND INORGANIC SOIL AMENDMENTS

The following is a partial list of soil amendments that may prove useful for Xeriscape landscaping. They fall into two categories—organic and inorganic. Each has its uses in improving soils of various types.

Organic Soil Amendments

Formerly touted as being the cure-all for any type of poor soil, organic soil amendments have been found to be only a partial answer—that is, they work for some types of plantings (vegetable and flower gardens, shrub beds), but may be detrimental in others (native plants, trees and shrubs planted in individual planting holes). The important thing to remember about them is that they are a temporary measure. The nutrients and bulk available in them will eventually be broken down by the organisms that digest them. In dry climates this will happen more slowly than in hot, humid climates because the soil organisms are sparser and/or suppressed by the chemistry of the soil. They will get lawns off to a good start, but can't be relied on indefinitely. However, they are invaluable in the right setting to provide nutrients and improve soil structure.

Organic amendments (in general)

Advantages: Change chemistry of soil. Change physical structure. Add nutrients. Hold water. Are fairly inexpensive.

Disadvantages: Microbial action breaks substances down over time. Plant eventually uses nutrients.

Compost

Compost is the most cost-effective soil amendment because you simply recycle organic matter from your own landscape, thereby keeping the nutrients on-site instead of hauling them away. It's also avail-

able nationwide. Composting allows microbes to break down plant trimmings sufficiently so that the nutrients in them are released for the use of living plants. It basically speeds up what nature does already with all dead organic material.

The idea is to layer (or mix, for faster results according to latest research from *Organic Gardening*) various types of organic materials that will break down fairly easily (within two to six months) in a heap or bin of some type up to three to four feet tall, keep the pile suitably moist but not too soggy, and turn the material every other week with a pitchfork or spading fork to aerate, which keeps the pile "working" aerobically instead of anaerobically (much less smelly).

Manure

Barnyard manure has long been a favorite soil amendment. The type of manure is not important, though poultry manure will be much higher in nitrogen, but it should have been aged for at least a year. Fresh manure is too high in ammonia, so it should be avoided or allowed to lie fallow in the soil for several months before using or you run the risk of burning the plant roots. Heat-treating kills weed seeds that may be in manure. (Heat-treated, dried manure is available in bags for home garden use.)

Dairy barnyard manure may be available free from a commercial stable but may be moderately salty; it should be composted thoroughly before use. Steer manure is often very salty.

Leaf Mold

Leaf mold is especially useful for woodland wildflower gardens since it helps build soil similar in structure to the plant's native environment. Leaves may take up to two years to decompose into soft, spongy leaf mold suitable for amending the soil. A quick way to create leaf mold is to chop the leaves up by running over them with a lawn mower that has a bag attatchment to catch the small pieces. Create a bin by driving four five-foot grooved metal posts one foot into the ground in the shape of a square and surrounding the posts with four-foot-wide, one-inch-square chicken wire. Layer chopped-up leaves with acid soil, if available, hollowing out the top each time to hold water.

This method makes turning the leaf mold easier and can be used for regular compost piles, too. You simply lift the wire cage off and set it to one side, fork the material to aerate it, and return it to the cage.

Sawdust and Other Wood Products

Clay soils are helped by the addition of sawdust or bark chips, which open the soil without holding water. Nitrogen must be added when raw wood products are used because they use up a lot of nitrogen in their decomposition. If you're using raw wood products, add two to three pounds of high-nitrogen fertilizer to each one-inch layer spread over one hundred square feet *or* add ½ pound of actual nitrogen per ten cubic feet of wood product. Most commercial sources of wood products for soil amendment have been fortified with nitrogen to prevent this problem. Bark products have less of a nitrogen-robbing effect on the soil, and therefore are recommended highly.

If not chopped small enough, wood chunks will take a long time to decompose, which may suit your needs.

Shredded Newspapers

These break down fairly quickly to provide nutrients in a compost pile when mixed with manure, but will take longer when mixed in regular soil. Birdcage linings may have the proper mix of "materials." Avoid using shredded newspapers in food gardens because the ink may be taken up by the roots of the plants.

Peat Moss

The nutrient value of peat moss is very low; it's used primarily as a water-holding and soil-loosening agent. Sphagnum, not mountain meadow, peat is recommended because mountain peat moss decomposes too rapidly and may be more than fifty percent mineral solids, not just peat, and mountain meadows, sometimes thousands of years old, are destroyed to mine it.

Peat moss comes dry in bundles and should be thoroughly wetted before being incorporated into the soil.

Pure Humic Acid

Pure humic acid (leonhardite) is a byproduct found in the soil layer overlaying coal deposits that are stripped from coal mining areas. The material decomposes in sunlight to produce humic acid, which is taken into the soil by precipitation. It helps soil structure and soil chemistry, being the material produced by bacteria in the breakdown of organic matter. This is the chemical that is said to bind soil particles together, forming aggregates.

Surfactants

Also called wetting agents (or soaps), these additives break down the surface tension of water to help it move easily into the soil. They are either sprayed on as a liquid or spread on top of existing soil as a granule.

Ben Wofford's Worm Bed

Apparently worm beds are common in many parts of the country, but when Ben Wofford told me how he conquered red clay Oklahoma soil with a worm bed, it was the first I had heard of it. He set off an area in his backyard about eight feet by ten feet, digging in lime to neutralize the mild acidity to worms' favorite pH of 6.8 to 7.2 and gypsum to loosen the clay to a depth of ten to twelve inches. He added all the coffee grounds that accumulated at his office plus some spoiled bulk cornmeal supplied by a friend. To this he introduced a canful of fishing worms dug from his parents' farm in the Ozarks. He kept the bed covered with leaves and branches for about six months. The worm bed remained in place and after five years the worms had apparently spread to every corner of his average-sized suburban lawn, aerating and improving the soil to the point where Wofford rarely had to water his lawn, even when his neighbors were watering every other day. He had the greenest, healthiest lawn on the block.

Worms are especially popular in Seattle, too, where worm bins are promoted as part of Seattle's massive recycling effort. One bin holds thousands of manure worms that can easily digest the average eight pounds or so a week of kitchen scraps generated by two adults. The compost they produce is very rich and black.

Inorganic Soil Amendments

It's a rare soil that cannot use some improvement in physical structure. Colorado soils, with their high clay content, are generally regarded as very poor soil that should be amended organically at every opportunity. Yet Dr. James Feucht, professor of landscape plants at Colorado State University, reports that most of the soil samples sent to his department for testing contain adequate nutrition; it's their structure that gives a poor showing. Inorganic soil amendments are used to open up heavy soils and increase their water-holding capacity.

Inorganic amendments (in general)

Advantages: Improve soil structure without adding nutrients where not wanted. Are long-lasting: are not broken down by microbial action.

Disadvantages: Don't add nutrients. Expensive compared to organic amendments.

Vermiculite and Perlite

Vermiculite and perlite are inert, very lightweight, hollow particles used to increase aeration in soil. Their cost is such that they're only practical for use in potting soil for seedlings.

Sand

Sand is not really a practical soil amendment because it would only be used to lighten up heavy soils (high in clay), but should *not* be used in clay soil, as previously discussed (see page 37). Some companies have had success with builder's sand which is very coarse and doesn't turn clay to adobe.

Cross-Linked Polyacrylamide

Cross-linked polyacrylamide has been used successfully for several years to help establish stands of grass and reduce the transplant shock of trees and shrubs by providing them with a ready source of water. It appears to increase yields of certain crops such as tomatoes and other garden produce.

So far it seems to be most helpful during periods of drought or in dry parts of the country, where Xeriscape landscaping has a much lower margin for error. It may make less difference when and where plenty of water is available.

It is applied either dry or wet (hydrated) at the general rate of two pounds per cubic yard of soil. In flower and vegetable gardens this translates to about four pounds per hundred square feet when tilled six inches deep. In lawns the recommended rate is fifteen to thirty pounds per 1,000 square feet. For trees and shrubs the polymer may be incorporated at low rates for survival (a half to one teaspoon dry volume/one to two cups wet) for a small seedling, or at higher rates for added water storage and faster growth. One dry ounce stores roughly one to three gallons of water. Never put more than one dry ounce per half cubic foot of backfill volume when transplanting, because the swelling of the crystals may push the plant back out of the hole. Like fertilizer, cross-linked polyacrylamide is a material where more is definitely not better!

For small quantities, especially when transplanting seedlings or bedding out a few flowers, it's advisable to soak the polymer in water first (one pound will generally soak up the water needed to fill a typical thirty-three-gallon garbage pail, or one cup dry polymer—five ounces—per five-gallon bucket of water). Let the solution soak for at least one to one and a half hours.

The polymer can be used to help native grasses get started in large areas. If it's drilled in with the seed and watered in afterward (or rained on), rates as low as fifteen to forty pounds per acre may be used.

Topsoil

In the arid and semiarid West commercial topsoil may be said to be "nice work if you can get it." Given the extreme thinness of topsoil in general, it's hard to imagine that companies are able to locate sources of tons of real topsoil per year. The only time true surplus topsoil might be made available is when an area is being excavated for paving over, or for a building. Some companies may produce a reasonable facsimile out of soil and composted manure mixed together, but in the West, anyway, be a little skeptical about claims of "true topsoil." Inquire particularly where it came from. If the excavated area was formerly farmland or industrial area, it may have some unwanted chemical residues or weed seed.

Practical Turf Areas

As LAWNLIKE turf is generally the highest user of applied water in the landscape, in Xeriscape landscaping we try to plan the amount of turf so that the investment in water will be repaid in use and beauty. In many instances grass *is* the best choice. For play areas, playing fields, and areas for small pets, grass is often the only ground cover that will stand up to the wear. Turf also provides unity and simplicity when used as a design component.

Well-established turf reduces noise, air, and water pollution and is an excellent form of erosion control. It is second only to virgin forest in its ability to harvest water and recharge groundwater resources. Green lawn grass provides an oasis on a summer day, cooling the home and soothing the hot, tired soul in a time-tested fashion. If one is predisposed to roll around in a lush green lawn from time to time, no other ground cover will do.

Early in the history of Xeriscape landscaping this step was listed as "limited turf area." The thought was that since lawn grass is the highest and usually most visible user of applied water, it would behoove us to wipe out as much of it from our landscapes as possible. This made sense in the arid West where Xeriscape landscapes were born, because the discrepancy between the water needs of the most popular lawn grass (Kentucky bluegrass at thirty-five to forty inches per year) and the local rainfall amounts (eight to twenty inches per year) was so excessive.

But the Xeriscape concept has spread across the country, and the amount of water needed to maintain turf varies widely from region to region. Reducing the amount of turf in an area that receives fifty or more inches of rainfall each year won't lower water requirements as much as it does in the West. For this reason it is impractical to make a blanket recommendation about the reduction of turf area.

When deciding how much area you want in turf, consider the type of maintenance you're willing to do. You may prefer picking a few weeds from shrub and flower beds (though this can be more in the neighborhood of hundreds of weeds if you don't mulch and/or maintain adequately to shut them out) over the alternative of mowing and watering grass. Or you might prefer to run the mower around occasionally and be done with it (a thick stand of turf resists weed invasion), yet still hate the watering.

In Xeriscape landscaping you can have your grass and enjoy it, too. Much can be done by observing the other principles of Xeriscape landscaping to reduce necessary lawn watering.

PLANNING

When planning your lawn, realize that the shape of it affects water use. The narrow areas between houses are rarely large enough to be used for recreation, and they are difficult to water efficiently. John Olaf Nelson of the North Marin Water District (California) made a study of the water requirements of areas based on shape. He found that areas with the same square footage need increasingly more water as the perimeter increases. For instance, a ten- by fifty-foot area (the typical area between houses) contains five hundred square feet and has a perimeter of 120 feet. A twenty-three- by twenty-three-foot square area has a little over five hundred square feet and a perimeter of ninety-two feet. Nelson found that more irrigation water was applied to the rectangular area than the square area to keep it green. This is because traditional irrigation system components—sprinklers—are engineered to work best in an overlapping layout, for complete coverage. Trying to fit such a system into a narrow area leads to overwatering.

For Xeriscape landscaping try to plan turf areas large enough to be functional but with the smallest possible perimeter.

Other peripheral areas that could be replaced with very low-water-requiring designs include narrow planting strips between the driveway and property line, between the sidewalk and street, and behind fences adjacent to sidewalks. If it's still necessary to use turf in these narrow strips, try to use a lower-water-requiring grass, install efficient underground drip irrigation, and/or grade them with a slight depression. Don't berm them up because most of the water will run off and be wasted. (Unless it will pose a safety hazard, depressing all turf areas slightly next to walks helps conserve water that would otherwise run off over the pavement.)

Sloping areas are hard to water. If possible, turf areas should be on level ground. On slopes either replace turf with an alternative ground covering or with a low-water grass.

Remember that grass and other plant ground covers absorb water and return it to the atmosphere, while *porous* hardscape covers allow water to be absorbed into the ground and kept there. This makes more water available for nearby tree and

An example of an "impractical turf area." Avoid using long, narrow areas of turf because they are nearly impossible to irrigate without wasting water. (Photo: Doug Welsh)

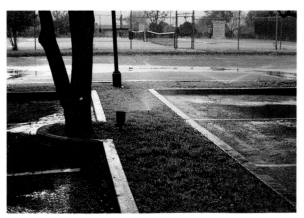

shrub roots. (Early unsuccessful water-conserving landscapes zeroed in too much on this idea, thus giving birth to not only the "acres of gravel" misconception about Xeriscape landscaping, but the descriptive term "zero-scape" as well. Fortunately, economics get in the way of most of us making the same mistake, because a gravel layer thick enough to exclude weeds is very expensive.)

The chapter on appropriate plant selection has information on alternative plant coverings (also dubbed "softscape"). Information on using "hardscape" features such as decks, walkways, and brick, stone, and concrete patios is included in the planning and design chapter.

In Xeriscape landscaping your goal should be to give as much thought to the amount of turf you really need in your landscape as you do to the hardscape. Realize that the low up-front cost of grass masks many years of ongoing maintenance costs, not only in terms of water, but also mowing time, fertilizer, and gas for mowers. Rather than blanketing your lot with turf because you can't think of anything else to cover it with, try to have a specific purpose you can state to yourself for each section of turfgrass in your design.

EFFICIENT IRRIGATION

Decisions you make about irrigation of turf are at the bottom line of Xeriscape landscaping. How you decide to handle the question of irrigation determines whether your water savings will be substantial or insignificant. Irrigation is covered in greater detail in chapter 6, but an overview as it relates to turf is given here. Basically, you have four options:

1. Eliminate turf completely and replace it with alternative ground coverings. Whether you opt for this depends on personal choice and what you want from the landscape. It has the potential to save the most water over traditional "lawnscapes" (unless you have already adopted water-conserving irrigation practices) and may be a very viable option for a small yard.

2. Install turf but don't irrigate it. Select a turfgrass whose water needs best match the natural

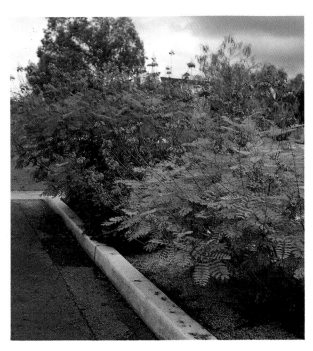

Red bird-of-paradise (Caesalpinia pulcherrima) *brightens up this commercial median strip, providing visual screening and high interest, and avoiding the pitfalls of a tiny, difficult-to-water turf area.*

rainfall amount and accept the fact that although it may turn brown (which means it's gone dormant) under drought conditions, it will green up again when rainfall occurs. Many species are drought tolerant and will live through extreme drought.

3. Install turf with an automatic sprinkler system. For large turf areas this is the most efficient method in terms of saving time, but it also gives the biggest opportunity for abusive use of irrigation water. The most wasteful practice is setting the timer to run the sprinklers at regular intervals throughout the growing season, regardless of the weather. The setting is usually calibrated to ensure the grass stays green during the driest, hottest spell, thus leading not only to a tremendous amount of overwatering, but conditioning the grass to depend on frequent watering. It's best to use the manual setting of a sprinkler system, taking time to learn how the soil in your yard correlates to watering frequency and just how much drought your lawn can take before being overstressed. Use the automatic timer only when you will be away from your yard for an extended period.

In his excellent book *Chemical-Free Lawn* (Emmaus, Pa.: Rodale Press, 1989), Warren Schultz recommends waiting as long as possible in the spring before you begin regular irrigation of your grass. He says you should even go so far as to dig up a shovelful of sod down to a depth of about nine inches, and not begin watering until the soil is dry to that depth. This forces the roots to reach down in their search for water, which in turn helps tide them over later in the summer when drought conditions are more severe. He also advises thoroughly wetting the soil to that depth and then not watering again until it reaches dryness there. This not only saves water but also discourages warm-season weeds that just *love* light and frequent irrigation (as well as frequent fertilization). The only caution about using this method is that heavy clay soil holds water in tension, and even though the soil may be moist, the grass roots may not be able to use all of it.

With automatic sprinklers take care to plan the system so that turf zones are separate from zones that water tree and shrub areas. Try to create separate zones for sloping areas so they may be given additional water as needed during drought without having to water areas not under stress. You may even want to zone shaded areas separately, because they are likely to need considerably less watering than sunny areas.

4. Use manual hose-end sprinklers rather than automatic systems. If your turf area is not too large, you may be able to water efficiently without a sprinkler system. Make sure you invest in sufficient hoses, quick-couple devices to make hooking up hoses a breeze, and shutoff timers to attach to the spigot and prevent accidentally leaving the sprinkler on for hours. Using this inexpensive option you are likely to be very conservative with watering, since the effort involved will make you think twice before dragging out hoses and setting them up, as opposed to simply pushing a button to start automatic sprinklers. Furthermore, manual sprinklers deliver water much more slowly, so if you have high water pressure in your area you won't be losing as much water to evaporation through misting.

SOIL IMPROVEMENT

Although efforts are being made to develop strains of turfgrass with deeper root systems to help them better withstand drought, lawn grass tends to remain relatively shallow-rooted because of poor soil, poor watering practices, and/or the fact that mowing grass short promotes shallow roots. Improving the soil is well worth the effort because it helps the grass fully utilize the water that reaches it, both in the form of precipitation and irrigation water.

General guidelines for improving soil under turfgrass are given in the previous chapter.

APPROPRIATE GRASS SELECTION

Select a lower-water-requiring turfgrass for your region or a drought-resistant cultivar. This is simpler than it sounds because the number of different grasses used for lawns in the United States is remarkably limited. In general the most common grasses in the northern and central areas of the United States are Kentucky bluegrass, fescues, bentgrasses, and ryegrasses, which are all cool-season grasses (meaning their best growth occurs during the cooler seasons of spring and fall). In southern states Bermudagrasses and zoysiagrasses are most common, with St. Augustinegrass, Bahiagrass, centipedegrass, and carpetgrass being grown in certain areas. These are warm-season grasses, which have their best growth during the summer.

If you want a grass with the closest appearance to traditional turfgrasses but with a lower water requirement, you will generally use turf-type tall fescues in place of Kentucky bluegrass and improved Bermudagrasses or zoysiagrasses in warmer regions. In the Gulf states and Hawaii, where rainfall is high and the growing season is nearly year-round, Bahiagrasses as well as Bermudagrasses and zoysiagrasses resist drought best. The next few years should see the development of much-improved cultivars of many of these species because breeding new strains of grass for drought tolerance is one of the highest priorities and a subject of intense research, not only at seed companies, but also at several universities.

Dr. James Beard, who researches and writes about turfgrass at Texas A&M University, notes that the drought-tolerance range among cultivars of one type of grass may be wider than the difference between species. For instance, in one test at College Station, Texas, several cultivars were left unirrigated for five months during which only three inches of rainfall fell. The cultivars 'NuMex Sahara' (Bermudagrass), 'Floratam' and 'Floralawn' (St. Augustinegrass), and 'Adalayd' (seashore paspalum) remained green the whole time. He emphasizes the importance of paying attention to cultivar as well as species when selecting a grass.

In addition, the climate of a region can affect the drought tolerance of turfgrass species. For example, in the hot, humid environment of central Georgia, tall fescues have shown much higher drought tolerance compared to when they're grown in more arid, high light intensity climates (*i.e.*, Phoenix, San Antonio). The level of drought tolerance of any given turfgrass material may rely heavily on the local environment.

The result of all the turfgrass research is that literally hundreds of strains of grass are released each year. (Often many other characteristics are being selected for—everything from height and width of blades to resistance to specific diseases and insects). Don't panic, though, because it isn't necessary to go crazy trying to evaluate them all yourself. In many instances the biggest improvement is between the original, or "common," strain and many of the cultivars. (The exception to this is Kentucky bluegrass, which in the past has not usually been improved for drought tolerance, though this is changing. The common strain is usually more tolerant of drought, but is also more susceptible to lawn diseases and insect pests such as sod webworms.)

The best strategy is to contact your county extension agent, whose job it is to keep up on just this type of research, and request the names of two or three strains of different grasses for your area that are highly rated with respect to drought tolerance. This way you'll have a couple of options when trying to obtain seed from a dealer, in case one strain isn't available.

Dr. Roch Gaussoin, turfgrass researcher at the University of Nebraska, favors the use of grass mixtures primarily of cool-season grasses. One of the major advantages of using mixtures for any turfgrass installation is that the planting is no longer a monoculture, so if a disease hits one strain it may not affect the other one(s) and will have greater difficulty spreading. Another benefit is that the shortcomings of one type of grass may be balanced by the strengths of another. For instance, fescue is a bunch-forming grass with higher wear tolerance and a lower water requirement than Kentucky bluegrass. However, it doesn't form a tightly knit sod unless it is sown very thickly. It might be mixed with a grass with a sod-forming habit of growth to create a better turf.

Appearance of Grasses

In traveling around the country to gather material for this book I made an astonishing discovery. In Kentucky bluegrass–mad Colorado the *only* way a Xeriscape advocate can make any headway with a Xeriscape skeptic is to show that it *is* still possible to have a bluegrasslike lawn. Efforts to promote the more water-thrifty grasses like fescue and blue grama grass were met with the perennial wail, "But it doesn't look like *real* grass!"

Imagine my surprise, then, in visiting south Texas and Florida to see people actually living with and seeing no shame in lawns of St. Augustinegrass and Bahiagrass which have blades up to 1/4 inch thick! My feeling is if these people can bravely hold their heads up and not think anything amiss with a nonbluegrass look, perhaps we, in other parts of the country, might be able to rethink our prejudices in this respect.

One of the most exciting things about Xeriscape landscaping is that many of the native American grasses are being scrutinized for adaptation to turfgrass (most of the traditional turfgrasses are imports). Names such as blue grama grass, beachgrass, alkaligrass, and especially buffalograss may be added to the palette of turfgrasses in the nineties. These and many other wild grasses, including species introduced from Eastern Europe and Russia, have been used for years in lowmaintenance areas such as roadside parks and highway rights-of-way. They have been long valued for their extreme drought tolerance and ability to survive untended.

The drawbacks in terms of landscape use have been that some of the grasses are coarse, have low wear tolerance, and are more of a gray-green than deep green color. With increasing interest in prairie restoration and native grasses, these species are beginning to be appreciated in their own right despite, or perhaps because of, their different appearances, and are showing up in urban landscapes. One way to use them in large yards is to raise two separate lawn areas, one a more traditional turf area close to the house or in the front yard, used intensely for recreation or decoration, and a section farther out or in the backyard given over to the lower-maintenance grasses, for a more natural look.

Part of the varying appearance of native grasses stems from the fact that they are often warm-season grasses—that is, they are green only during the growing season when temperatures rise above freezing. The rest of the year they are a warm, tan color, very beautiful in the right setting, but rather startling to eyes accustomed in northern climates to seeing cool-season turfgrasses greenest in spring and fall. So to switch, for instance, from bluegrass

Color differences in cool- and warm-season grasses are seen in this early October photo in Colorado. Warm-season buffalograss has already started changing from summer green to its dormant tan color; cool-season bluegrass may turn brownish in the summer if water is scarce, but greens up with fall rains.

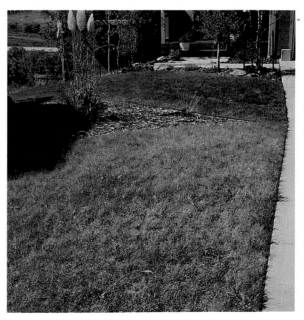

to buffalograss requires some adjustments in what we consider acceptable in grass. Buffalograss may turn brown in midsummer; it's possible to keep it green during that time, but it requires extra watering.

It's also possible to overseed a warm-season grass with a cool-season grass, but this increases water use, not only to help the seeds sprout, but also to maintain the grass. Sandy Snyder of Littleton, Colorado, found a perfect solution for her warm/cool-season dilemma by planting hundreds of spring-flowering bulbs in her warm-season buffalograss lawn. Her experience is described on page 55.

If you're interested in being more adventurous in your choice of lawn grasses, the sections that follow give more information about the ranges and uses of several alternative, as well as traditional, grasses.

Lawn Grasses for Xeriscape Landscaping

The following maps illustrate the grasses most often used for lawns in various areas of the United States, as well as alternative lawn grasses for Xeriscape landscapes.

As mentioned earlier, grasses are either warm or cool season, depending on the type of weather they grow best in. Warm-season grasses are adapted, not surprisingly, to southern climates because they come out of dormancy only when the temperature is above 50 degrees Fahrenheit, and grow vigorously when the temperature is between 80 and 95 degrees, withstanding even temperatures above 100 degrees. When the temperature drops below 50 most warm-season grasses start to turn tan; when it drops below freezing, they turn brown (signifying they are now in cold dormancy).

Cool-season grasses grow best in northern climates in the spring and fall when daytime temperatures range from 60 to 75 degrees. They may turn brown in the heat of summer, but they stay green through much colder temperatures in the winter because they don't lose chlorophyll when the temperature dips below 50 degrees the way warm-season grasses do.

A transition zone exists at the dividing line between where cool- and warm-season grasses are best adapted. In the transition zone neither type of grass is at its best because the winters may get too cold for warm-season grasses, and the summers too hot for the cool-season grasses. Overseeding a cool-season grass on top of a warm-season grass is sometimes done to give winter color to the lawn, but this takes extra water, so for Xeriscape landscaping it's best to pick a season that you can bear to see brownish lawn and go with the best locally adapted warm- or cool-season grass as needed.

Bunchgrasses grow as individual plants that spread over time. They may fill in the grass area if the seed is sown thickly enough. By contrast, sod-forming grasses send out runners aboveground (stolons) or belowground (rhizomes) that colonize, forming new plants at nodes along their length, and knit the grass tightly together.

To help you find a grass that might survive on your natural rainfall, I have indicated approximate rainfall ranges for each of the various grasses, including (where known) the optimum range. The optimum range is generally best for establishing a lawn. The grasses may survive on less water; they just won't be your "velvet greensward" (for sure). If you choose a grass that requires more rainfall than your area receives, you'll have to water it. Even if you pick an appropriate grass, you'll still have to water it to get it established, and also water if you live where ninety percent of the precipitation occurs as snowfall, and ninety percent of the heat comes in the summer, or any of the other conditions that factor in when you take a plant out of its native range. Some of the native grasses have a maximum optimum rainfall because when they receive too much moisture they start to get "leggy" and the turf becomes weedy.

Please keep in mind that the suggested water requirement is based on the best available information. Although there is a lot of research on turfgrass tolerance to drought (much more so than for trees and shrubs), the limits for each species and cultivar haven't yet been defined. There will probably always be surprises in that respect because it won't be possible to pin down how every grass adapts to every set of conditions.

One example is centipedegrass. A thick-bladed warm-season grass adapted only to the Gulf coastal plain in the United States, it needs regular watering. For that reason you might say no to this grass for

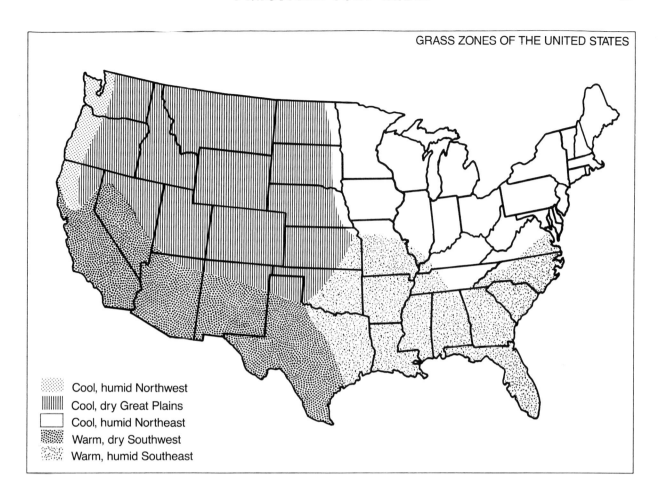

GRASS ZONES OF THE UNITED STATES

Cool, humid Northwest
Cool, dry Great Plains
Cool, humid Northeast
Warm, dry Southwest
Warm, humid Southeast

Xeriscape landscaping at first glance. But, because of its low cold tolerance, this grass will not grow out of its adapted range, which is an area that receives regular high amounts of rainfall. And, within its range, it *does* have a high degree of drought tolerance because it recovers quickly from drought stress. Given that it needs little mowing and fertilization, and is very wear tolerant, centipedegrass might make a good grass for Xeriscape landscaping after all, in the right situation.

The grasses are arranged in order of roughly lowest to highest water use. The advantages and disadvantages of each in general, and with respect to Xeriscape landscaping, are given along with propagation and mowing information. The term "PLS" (Pure Live Seed) crops up in the seeding rates for a few of the grasses. The reason for this designation is explained on pages 70–71 in the next section. For now just realize that it has to do most often with native grass seed that doesn't always have one

hundred percent germination and purity. The PLS quantity will give you the right amount of seed needed to establish a good stand of grass.

To choose a grass you need to look at what you want from your lawn, whether it be a traditional turf or an "all native" look. Reading through these descriptions may broaden your thoughts on that, leading you to consider trying some of the native grasses that you hadn't heard of. I wondered recently what would happen if I just let part of my bluegrass yard grow without mowing it, if it would die out after setting seed. I asked Bob Vilotti, grass expert at Denver's Arkansas Valley Seed Company, and he said, "Your grass would grow about a foot tall and just maintain itself. Bluegrass, when not mowed, is actually fairly drought tolerant."

This could be a simple way to get the prairie garden effect without too much effort. Just mow the grass with a curving edge for lawn area and let the rest go. Obviously this will be more effective if your weed population in the grass isn't too high (mowing once in the fall will help with this, says Vilotti). In addition, if you want the grass to stay green all summer, you may still have to irrigate it to a limited extent, though not as much as if it were maintained as a turf.

The grasses for which this idea would work best are buffalograss, blue grama grass, crested wheatgrass, bluegrass, and fine fescues. The introduced (not native) warm-season grasses such as Bermudagrass, St. Augustinegrass, and Bahiagrass will not produce the same "grasslands" effect. Bermudagrass, as well as cool-season bentgrasses, are too invasive. Cool-season grasses such as tall fescue, bromegrass, and perennial ryegrass will tend to develop too much leaf area and not enough of the attractive seed heads. Their growth is more "rank" (weedy-looking) than ornamental. Grass allowed to go to seed should be thought of as ornamental grass. It can withstand some traffic, but not continual wear, such as when a large dog is kept in the area.

For suitable grasses I have included the mature height if left unmowed. Each entry has a map of its native or adapted range, depending on the available information. The adapted range of the native grasses is not yet known, but given the toughness of most grasses, the limits could probably be extended considerably. As always, the microclimate for the plant is the key.

Dr. James Beard ranks turfgrasses as follows with respect to drought tolerance (again, this is a general guideline—as noted earlier, improvements in specific cultivars may rearrange this ranking).

Cool Season		Warm Season
Excellent	None	Blue grama grass
		Buffalograss
		Bermudagrass
		Zoysiagrass
		Bahiagrass
Good	Crested wheatgrass	None
	Hard fescue	
	Chewings fescue	
	Sheep fescue	
	Tall fescue	
	Red Fescue	

Cool Season		Warm Season
Medium	Kentucky bluegrass	None
	Canada bluegrass	
Fair	Perennial ryegrass	St. Augustinegrass
	Meadow fescue	
	Colonial bentgrass	
Poor	Rough bluegrass	Centipedegrass
	Creeping bentgrass	Carpetgrass
	Velvet bentgrass	

In general, the deeper a grass's roots, the more drought tolerant it will be. Because of poor irrigation and mowing practices, most lawn grasses never reach their potential root depth, but it's interesting to see the correlation between drought tolerance and the root depths that can theoretically be reached by the different grasses, as indicated by this table.

GRASS	ROOT DEPTH
Bentgrasses	1–8 inches
Kentucky bluegrass	8–18 inches
Red fescue	"
Ryegrasses	"
St. Augustinegrass	"
Zoysiagrass	to 5 feet
Bermudagrass*	"
Tall fescue	"
Blue grama grass	5–7 feet
Buffalograss	5–7 feet

*Note: Bermudagrass roots are typically only six inches deep in clay soil. Its drought tolerance comes from numerous rhizomes (underground stems), which are able to seek out soil moisture.

Researchers have evaluated mowing heights for years with regard to turf density, appearance, and pest resistance; the traditional lists of mowing heights have reflected these findings. The mowing heights listed in this book (usually slightly higher) provide the optimum mowing height balancing both appearance and water-efficiency considerations. Basically, you should mow your lawn, whatever the species, at the highest height possible that will still give you a nice-looking lawn.

Lowest- to Highest-Water-Use Grasses Used for Lawns

··

Warm-Season Grasses

Blue grama grass *(Bouteloua gracilis)*
Bunchgrass, South/Sod-forming, North

RAINFALL RANGE: 12 to 24 inches optimum, 8 to 50 inches possible

SOIL: Sandy to clayey optimum, sand to clay possible

pH: Neutral to alkaline soils, tolerates saline soils

PROPAGATION: Seed at 1 to 1½ pounds Pure Live Seed (PLS) per 1,000 square feet

GERMINATION TIME: 15 to 30 days

Sod occasionally available

MOWING HEIGHT: May be left unmowed (12 to 18 inches maximum height) or mowed at 3 inches periodically after sod is well established to encourage a dense cover. For a more meadowlike look, suggested mowing height is 5 inches

ADAPTED RANGE:

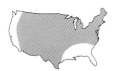

Blue grama is a native American grass, often seen in native stands with buffalograss. It has a bluish purple cast and is very drought tolerant, with an exceptional ability to go dormant during drought, then recover when more moisture is available. It is a bunch-forming grass in the South and a sod former in the North, at higher elevations, or when mowed (or grazed) regularly. Although it isn't shade tolerant, its roots can grow five to seven feet deep, and it's often used for erosion control.

Blue grama grass is well adapted to the windy, arid areas of the Great Plains, tolerates wide temperature and soil variations, from sandy to clayey, and does well in alkaline soil, though it rarely grows wild on even weakly acid soil. It is best used for lawns in cool, dry areas and can be left unmowed, since its seed heads are ornamental (resembling downward-curving combs about an inch long) and weediness is not a problem. Mature height is twelve

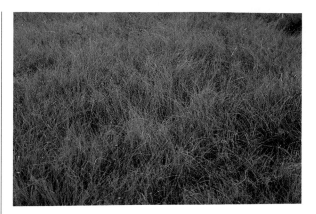

Blue grama grass makes a feathery-appearing lawn when left unmowed. It is very wear and drought tolerant, and has interesting seed heads resembling short curved combs in late summer.

to eighteen inches, but it may remain as low as six to eight inches if water is scarce.

The best way to establish a lawn of blue grama grass is to seed when night temperatures drop to 60 degrees Fahrenheit, but the soil is still warm (between 60 and 90 degrees). It can be started with plugs, but coverage is faster and more uniform with seeds. Keep soil moist until germination is mostly complete, then allow it to dry out between deep waterings to encourage deep rooting. Blue grama grass is drought tolerant, but will turn brown (go dormant) during prolonged droughts.

Dr. Robin Cuany is attempting to propagate improved strains of blue grama grass at Colorado State University, selecting for improved appearance while maintaining the grass's drought tolerance.

Buffalograss *(Buchloe dactyloides)*
Sod-forming

RAINFALL RANGE: 12 to 24 inches optimum, 10 to 35 inches possible

SOIL: Silty to clayey optimum, fairly sandy to clay possible

pH: 6.0 to 7.5 ('Prairie' cultivar: 4.7 to 8.0)

PROPAGATION: Seed at 1½ to 3 pounds PLS (burs) per 1,000 square feet

GERMINATION TIME: 7 to 10 days for treated seed; up to 3 years for untreated

Sod and plugs occasionally available

MOWING HEIGHT: May be left unmowed (6 to 8

inches maximum height) or mowed at 3 to 5 inches monthly or less frequently

ADAPTED RANGE:

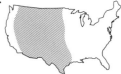

Buffalograss is one of the outstanding native and Xeriscape grasses, and it could become a major player in the turf field by the mid-1990s. Able to survive on as little as ten to twelve inches of rainfall per year, it adapts to sites receiving thirty inches or more per year. It is well adapted to heavy clay, alkaline soil; in fact, it grows in a wide range of soil conditions, though it doesn't thrive in sandy soil or shade. It can be mowed two or three times a summer, or left unmowed for a prairie look.

Buffalograss has soft, light green foliage and interesting seed heads. About half the plants are female and produce seed burs near the ground. The other half are male plants that produce comblike seed heads held above the plants. These are so pretty that some people grow buffalograss just for that effect.

Buffalograss is native to much of the upland Great Plains, and is the most northerly surviving of warm-season grasses, growing as far north as Montana. The first turf-type buffalograss was released through Texas A&M in 1989. Called 'Prairie', it is vegetatively propagated, meaning no seeds are available, and it must be produced from existing sod through sprigs or plugs.

Other types of buffalograss may be seeded or sodded, though sod is sometimes hard to locate and expensive because it must be cut fairly thick. Whereas bluegrass sod is cut ¾ inch thick, buffalograss sod is cut 1½ inches thick to include more of its root system. It can't be rolled, so it must be cut into squares. This extra weight adds to the transportation costs.

Denver gardeners Suzanne and Bill purchased and installed buffalograss sod in early June. Suzanne first used a spade to cut a rounded edge around their roughly square lawn, then Bill thoroughly rototilled the existing bluegrass lawn (the rounded edge helped keep the tiller from going into the adjacent flower bed). Suzanne systematically screened the top layer of soil from the whole yard over a wheelbarrow, composting the grass leaves and roots and returning the soil to the yard. This way the organic matter in the soil was retained.

On her 1,200-square-foot area Suzanne spread six bales of peat moss and twenty wheelbarrow loads of compost from the stockpile she had been working on for several years. She raked it smooth and firmed it by walking on it in a circular pattern. She didn't use fertilizer because it can kill new grass if applied incorrectly, and she didn't want to risk it.

Because the sod came in eighteen-inch squares, Suzanne cut a piece of plywood slightly larger than that to carry the sod. (She deems this the most backbreaking work she has ever done.) To avoid making permanent footprint depressions in the lawn, Suzanne put down boards as paths to move around on and fill cracks between the pieces with dirt and peat moss.

She drenched the lawn with water when all this was completed, then soaked it five days after that, then one week later, then two weeks later. After that she watered the lawn every one to two weeks. The grass grew very well and so did weeds, wildflowers, and other grasses. She realizes there may have been seeds in the existing soil and in the compost, but speculates there were probably some in the sod, too. Suzanne spent the summer picking out these intruders, gathering several bushelsful, but says there were none left by the end of the summer.

The grass wasn't cut till the end of the summer, then was cut as tall as possible. The male seed heads appeared in mid to late July. Suzanne says at least fifty people walking by her corner lot stopped to comment on how much they enjoyed seeing her beautiful, unusual lawn. The grass gradually started going dormant in September, with some green, some tan color. By first frost it was all tan.

Sandy Snyder, gardening consultant in Littleton, Colorado, has put in buffalograss in no less than three different ways. In 1984, wanting to replace a 2,000-square-foot vegetable garden with a low-maintenance, low-water grass, she and her husband decided to seed buffalograss. They used two and a half pounds of "Sharps New Improved" seed per 1,000 square feet, keeping the seedbed moist till the grass sprouted about two weeks later. They didn't use any soil amendments because the ground had already been improved during its "agricultural" phase when it was a garden, and she reasoned that the grass was adapted to heavy clay soil anyway.

Sandy spent so many hours hand-weeding that summer that if she had it to do again she would let the ground lie fallow for a year, killing weed seeds with a pre-emergent herbicide and killing sprouts with a contact herbicide. She would also sow the seeds at twice the rate to give them a better chance against the weeds.

The following spring Sandy discovered the difference between warm- and cool-season grasses in Denver. Her lawn was still brown two months after the neighbors' yards had greened up. Her friend Panayoti Kelaidis of the Denver Botanic Garden suggested she plant spring-flowering bulbs in the lawn to add spring color and greenery. (The flowers and leaves die down before the grass starts growing in early summer, so the spent bulb foliage can be mowed without harming the plants.) That fall she and her family planted 2,000 crocus, iris, tulip, and other bulbs. The result the next spring was so spectacular that Sandy has turned another area of her yard over to buffalograss specifically to provide more room for bulbs. The bulbs have multiplied

fortyfold over the years, giving a better show each year. (Note: It's important to use species, rather than hybrid, bulbs for this technique. The foliage of the hybrid bulbs remains green and tall too far into the summer, while the species bulb foliage dies down in a timely fashion with no sacrifice in the beauty of the blooms.)

Sandy feels that if a person wants to leave the grass unmowed and has the time to keep up with the weeding, it would be possible to do such "naturalizing" with bulbs flowering all summer, perhaps on a smaller area.

Even though weeds continue to be a problem, Sandy says she still spends far less time maintaining her lawn than any of her neighbors. Although buffalograss is said to be the most wear tolerant of the native grasses, and certainly the most compaction tolerant (remember how all those buffaloes tromped

These lovely Iris reticulata *bulbs brighten up Sandy Snyder's buffalograss lawn during spring months, when the grass is still dormant (tan). Later the flowers and foliage die back discreetly before it's time to mow the lawn in June. (Design and photo: Sandy Snyder)*

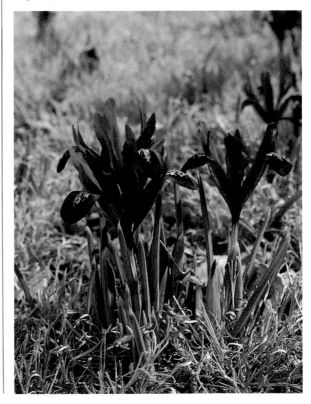

Summer shot of buffalograss maintained as a regular lawn.

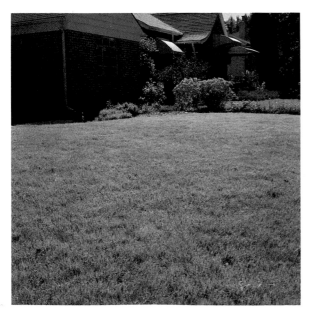

through the prairies), Sandy found that it doesn't take wear well when dormant because it is brittle then. She fertilizes just once a year during midsummer at one-quarter the rate recommended for bluegrass. She waters only during very hot or dry spells and just enough to keep the grass its normal light green color, not enough to encourage the weeds. She especially tries to avoid watering during spring and fall to discourage the cool-season weeds.

In late spring of 1990, Sandy converted another area to buffalograss by installing two-inch plugs of grass eight inches apart in all directions. One section had bare ground to start with, and the other was prepared with the very novel approach of killing the existing sod with glysophate (Roundup®), waiting a decent interval, and simply planting the plugs in the dead sod. She says both methods gave a complete coverage by July 1, but she had far less trouble with weeds in the grass planted in the dead sod.

Bermudagrass   (*Cynodon dactylon*)
Sod-forming

RAINFALL RANGE: 16+ inches optimum, 14 inches minimum
SOIL: Somewhat sandy to silty optimum; very sandy and clayey possible
pH: 5.5 to 7.5
PROPAGATION: COMMON BERMUDAGRASS: Seed at 2 to 3 pounds per 1,000 square feet
GERMINATION TIME: 7 to 14 days
IMPROVED BERMUDAGRASS: Sprigs
MOWING HEIGHT: 1 to 1½ inches
ADAPTED RANGE:

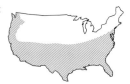

Bermudagrass is a warm-season sod-forming grass introduced from Africa in 1751 or earlier. Best adapted to fertile soils in the humid South, it is used in the Southwest as well on moist sites or irrigated land.

Bermudagrass is very drought and heat tolerant, disease resistant, and has outstanding wearability. In the South common Bermudagrass is seen in home lawns as often as Kentucky bluegrass is seen in the North. It has medium to fine texture, depending on the strain. It can be started from seed, with the seedbed kept moist until germination takes place. Although drought tolerant, it needs added water during dry spells to be kept green. For Xeriscape gardening, be prepared to tolerate some temporary browning during drought.

Bermudagrass (including improved strains) needs regular fertilization (one pound actual nitrogen per 1,000 square feet biannually, up to twice as much for hybrid Bermudagrasses) and regular mowing to maintain an attractive turf.

Andy Hull of Post Landscape, designers and builders of showcase commercial Xeriscape landscapes in Atlanta, says his firm uses Bermudagrass for any unirrigated site as well as for some irrigated ones, and they use it in full sun and partial shade settings.

Bermudagrass, being a warm-season grass, turns an off color during cool weather and brown after frost. It is more susceptible to disease when dormant. It can also be very invasive and difficult to eradicate where not wanted.

Zoysiagrass   (*Zoysia* spp.)   Sod-forming

RAINFALL RANGE: Approximately 30+ inches
SOIL: Well-drained, fine-textured (clayey)
pH: 5.0 to 7.0
PROPAGATION: Sprigs every 2 inches in rows 6 inches apart
Plugs at 6 inches apart
MOWING HEIGHT: 2 inches or left unmowed
ADAPTED RANGE:

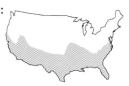

Three species of zoysiagrass are used for lawns in southern regions of the United States, varying in their texture and cold hardiness. All three are warm-season grasses. Sometimes zoysiagrasses rather than cool-season grasses are planted in the transition zone (where neither warm- nor cool-season grasses have ideal climatic conditions) since the zoysias are better able to muscle out crabgrass and other warm-season weeds. However, the zoysias turn brown because of cool temperatures through fall, winter, and spring, so the appearance is not much improved.

Zoysiagrasses are very wear tolerant. They form a dense sod that chokes out weeds, but they establish very slowly from sprigging (sod is still too expensive), and may take two to three years to fill in. They are drought and heat tolerant, though they must be irrigated in dry areas because of their shallow root systems. Because they are slower-growing than Bermudagrasses, they don't need mowing as often. Zoysiagrasses are resistant to most pests except billbugs.

Zoysia japonica (Japanese or Korean lawn grass) is the coarsest, most vigorous, and most winter hardy of the zoysias. It's the only zoysiagrass that can be established from seed (one to two pounds hulled seed per 1,000 square feet—germination time ten to fourteen days). It does well in heavy soils and requires fertilization for good growth and color. Post Landscape in Atlantic uses 'Meyer' zoysia, a variety of *Z. japonica*, on their irrigated areas. Andy Hull reports that it produces a lush turf and withstands some shade, but prefers full sun.

Zoysia matrella (Manila grass) is a medium-textured and medium-hardy species. It is very resistant to wear, weeds, and insect and disease damage, and is shade tolerant, but requires more fertilizer to stay dark green. Hardy only in Zones 9 to 11, *Z. tenuifolia* (mascarene grass) is sometimes listed as a ground cover, implying that it will accept a little but not very much foot traffic. Adapted to very few areas in the United States, it has nevertheless been hybridized with *Z. japonica* to produce a fine-textured, dark green, dense-growing grass called 'Emerald', which has proved superior to 'Meyer' in the southern United States.

Bahiagrass *(Paspalum notatum)* Bunchgrass

RAINFALL RANGE: Approximately 35+ inches
SOIL: Sandy to clayey
pH: 6.5 to 7.5
PROPAGATION: Seed at 2 to 3 pounds per 1,000 square feet; for quick cover, use up to 10 pounds per 1,000 square feet

GERMINATION TIME: 21 to 28 days
MOWING HEIGHT: 3 inches
ADAPTED RANGE:

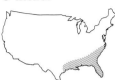

Introduced from Brazil in 1913, Bahiagrass is a coarse-textured, slow-growing grass that spreads slowly but is aggressive and forms a thick, thatch-resistant turf. It makes a dense, rather uneven turf, whose tough blades require a sharp mower to cut. Frequent mowing is required to remove seed heads.

Bahiagrass has some drought tolerance, but grows best with abundant water. It recovers well from drought. It is the most shade tolerant of the warm-season grasses. It may be planted in the spring or fall, and is sometimes mixed with fine fescue in the fall for quick cover.

Bahiagrass grows best on the southern coastal plain, adapting well to sandy or infertile soils. It has an extensive, deep root system, and is sometimes used for erosion control. Bahiagrass stays green longer in winter than other warm-season grasses. It is often used on low-maintenance, low-use areas where quality of turf is less important.

Seashore paspalum (*Paspalum vaginatum*) is a fine-textured Bahiagrass, tolerant of both salt and drought. Vegetatively propagated, it was introduced from Australia as an alternative to Bermudagrass in dry coastal areas. It is more drought tolerant than Bahiagrass, but needs more water than Bermudagrass.

St. Augustinegrass *(Stenotaphrum secundatum)*
Sod-forming

RAINFALL RANGE: 30 to 35+ inches
SOIL: Optimum: Well-drained, fertile, sandy loam
pH: 6.0 to 7.5
PROPAGATION: Sprigs at 12 inches apart
MOWING HEIGHT: 3 inches
ADAPTED RANGE:

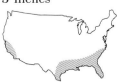

St. Augustinegrass is a coarse-textured, sod-forming, shade-tolerant grass grown in the mid South (coastal areas, Gulf states, Florida) and southern California. It needs fertile, well-drained soil rich in organic matter. A rather high-maintenance grass, it produces thick turf that crowds out weeds and other grasses when given the right conditions. It's also tolerant of salt spray and steady traffic.

St. Augustinegrass needs lots of moisture and fertilizer unless it's in the shade, where it's more drought tolerant. It is damaged by leaf spot, brown patch, and chinch bugs.

Centipedegrass   *(Eremochloa ophiuroides)*
Sod-forming

RAINFALL RANGE: 40+ inches
SOIL: Wide range. Optimum: Moderately acid soils of fine texture and low fertility. Doesn't do well in coarse-textured sands.
pH: 4.5 to 5.5
PROPAGATION: 30 ounces to 1 pound per 1,000 square feet
GERMINATION TIME: 14 to 20 days
Sprigs, plugs, sod
MOWING HEIGHT: Needs little mowing, as mature height is 3 to 4 inches
ADAPTED RANGE:

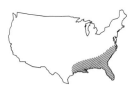

Centipedegrass was introduced from China in 1916. It is a medium-coarse (similar to St. Augustinegrass, but finer textured), sod-forming grass, considered one of the best low-maintenance grasses in the Deep South. It can be grown as far north as North Carolina and northern Alabama. In the upper South it can survive, but will be discolored by frost. It has low wear tolerance, though it recovers well from drought stress.

Centipedegrass resists weed invasion because of the thickness of the turf. It tolerates shade better than Bermudagrass and is disease resistant. It can take poor soils, though it may turn chlorotic if the soil is too alkaline.

Centipedegrass establishes slowly from seed. The first year the lawn may appear to be all crabgrass, but in the second the grass gradually takes over.

Carpetgrass   *(Axonopus affinis)*   Sod-forming

RAINFALL RANGE: 35 to 40+ inches
SOIL: Wet, acidic, sandy loam of low fertility optimum
pH: 4.5 to 5.5
PROPAGATION: Seed at 3 to 4 pounds per 1,000 square feet
GERMINATION TIME: 21 days
Sprigs, sod
MOWING HEIGHT: 1 inch
ADAPTED RANGE:

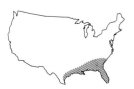

Carpetgrass is a poor choice for Xeriscape landscaping because it has little or no drought tolerance. It grows well in sandy soils, but not where the weather is dry during part of the growing season. It's best adapted to the lower coastal plain of the United States, though it won't tolerate salt spray and is very cold sensitive (it's not hardy north of Augusta, Georgia). It turns brown in winter even farther south. Carpetgrass is a coarse, rapidly spreading sod former that produces a dense, compact turf under low mowing. In fact, it must be kept low to prevent the formation of ugly seed heads.

Carpetgrass establishes quickly, but needs a slightly acidic soil in order to get enough iron.

Northern Grasses—Cool Season

'Fairway' crested wheatgrass   *(Agropyron cristatum* 'Fairway')   Bunchgrass

RAINFALL RANGE: 10 to 16.5 inches optimum, 8 to 19 inches possible
SOIL: Somewhat sandy to somewhat clayey; tolerates saline soil
pH: Adapted to weakly acid soil
PROPAGATION: Seed at 5 pounds PLS per 1,000 square feet

GERMINATION TIME: 21 days
MOWING HEIGHT: 3 + inches
If left unmowed, height is 12 to 18 inches
ADAPTED RANGE:

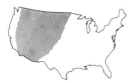

'Fairway' crested wheatgrass is a low-maintenance grass sometimes used as a Kentucky bluegrass look-alike, though it makes a better meadow grass. It is easily established from seed, but it requires the same care as any other lawn grass to get going. 'Fairway' crested wheatgrass won't germinate if the ground is dry, so it's best to start it in the spring when the weather is cooler and it's easier to keep up with the watering. After it germinates, taper off the watering as quickly as possible without killing the sprouts, in order to discourage weed growth.

'Fairway' crested wheatgrass is very drought tolerant, though it may go dormant during hot dry summer weather, and it tolerates cold well (it's native to Siberia), so it's well adapted to the mountainous regions of the West and the Great Plains. Although its roots may go as deep as two to three feet, it also has a dense root system close to the surface that enables it to compete easily with weeds.

This is one grass that thins out if watered too much because, as a bunchgrass, it's less able to withstand the invasion of water-loving, sod-forming grasses. Keep irrigation to a minimum and don't plant it in regions that get more than about twenty inches of precipitation annually.

'Ephraim' crested wheatgrass (Agropyron cristatum 'Ephraim') Bunchgrass

RAINFALL RANGE: 10 to 14 inches optimum, 8 to 25 inches possible
SOIL: Somewhat sandy to somewhat clayey; tolerates saline soil
PH: Wide range, moderately high alkaline tolerance
PROPAGATION: Seed at 5 pounds PLS per 1,000 square feet
GERMINATION TIME: 21 days

MOWING HEIGHT: 3 + inches
If left unmowed, height is 6 to 16 inches (6 inches if water is very scarce)
ADAPTED RANGE:

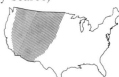

'Ephraim' crested wheatgrass was originally a native of the dry gravelly, clay soil in Ankara, Turkey. It was tested and developed near Ephraim, Utah, specifically because of its sod-forming characteristics. Many crested wheatgrasses are bunchgrasses, so they lack the erosion prevention capability of a sod-forming grass. 'Ephraim' has been tried as a lawn "substitute grass," but because it is very slow to fill in (rhizomes take a year to develop), it may still be better suited for low-maintenance, little-used grass areas. "It might spread faster if maintained as a traditional lawn grass," notes Bob Vilotti, "but then it takes as much water as fescue. 'Ephraim' is better for nonirrigated areas because it comes back readily from drought."

Says Boulder, Colorado, landscape architect Jim Knopf, "If what you want is a bluegrass look-alike, you might as well use turf-type tall fescue. Because of the way it grows, 'Ephraim' will never be as thick a turf when it's mowed."

Ephraim crested wheatgrass (Agropyron cristatum 'Ephraim') is a very drought-tolerant grass which can be maintained as a somewhat coarse lawn (though this takes more watering), or left unmowed and unirrigated. It will survive on as little as eight inches of rainfall per year, though it may turn brown in midsummer heat without supplemental irrigation.

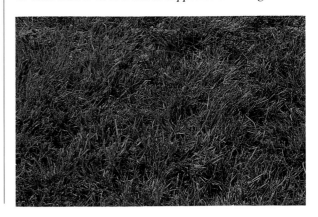

Smooth bromegrass *(Bromus inermis)*
Sod-forming

RAINFALL RANGE: 17 inches minimum for survival of pasture grass (the natural look); 25+ inches for lawns

SOIL: Silty to clayey; tolerates salt fairly well; not very vigorous on sandy or dense clay soils

pH: Neutral to slightly alkaline

PROPAGATION: Seed at 6 to 7 pounds PLS per 1,000 square feet

GERMINATION TIME: 10 to 14 days

MOWING HEIGHT: 4 inches

ADAPTED RANGE:

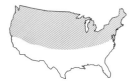

Native to Siberia, Europe, and China, smooth brome is a coarse-textured grass, often used for erosion control on highway rights-of-way. It has fairly good drought resistance, and can withstand heat and cold well, though its tolerance to wear is low. It goes dormant in drought and renews growth with the presence of moisture.

In order to stay green, smooth brome needs some irrigation in areas that receive less than about seventeen inches of rainfall per year. In seed mixtures with crested wheatgrasses it often dominates the low-lying areas that get more moisture, while the wheatgrasses congregate at the tops of slopes or other dry areas. Bromegrass has naturalized in Missouri where the rainfall rate ranges from thirty to forty-eight inches. Since it makes a very dense turf it can be hard to get rid of once it is started with too much irrigation or in higher rainfall areas.

Smooth bromegrass is best raised on deep, fertile prairie soils, but will grow on coarse-textured sands if fertilized.

Fine fescues Bunchgrasses
Hard fescue *(Festuca ovina* var. *duriuscula)*

RAINFALL: 13 inches minimum for survival of pasture grass, 25 to 30+ inches for lawns

UNMOWED HEIGHT: 8 to 16 inches

ADAPTED RANGE:

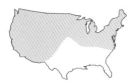

Sheep fescue *(F. ovina)*

RAINFALL: 9 inches minimum for pasture, 20 to 30 inches for lawns

UNMOWED HEIGHT: 8 to 16 inches

ADAPTED RANGE:

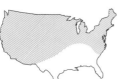

Chewings fescue *(F. rubra* var. *commutata)*

RAINFALL: Approximately 20+ inches for survival, 30 inches for lawns

UNMOWED HEIGHT: 16 to 40 inches

ADAPTED RANGE:

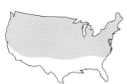

Red fescue *(F. rubra)* Sod-forming

RAINFALL: Same as chewings fescue

UNMOWED HEIGHT: 16 to 40 inches

ADAPTED RANGE:

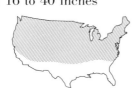

SOIL: Silty to clay optimum; will tolerate sandy to heavy clay

pH: 5.5 to 6.5

PROPAGATION: Seed at 3 to 5 pounds per 1,000 square feet

GERMINATION TIME: 10 to 21 days

MOWING HEIGHT: 2½ inches

Fine fescues are fine-textured grasses that cover much the same range, and respond to the same regimen of maintenance, as Kentucky bluegrass. They are better adapted than bluegrass to shade, poor soil, and dry locations, but are less wear tolerant. Often used in mixtures with bluegrass, they tend to be more aggressive when these harsher conditions are present, and are dominated by bluegrass when the soil is more fertile and conditions are more favorable.

Fine fescues are often planted for bank stabilization and, when left unmowed, have a delicate, windblown appearance. The chewings type is the best-looking for lawns, though the average person would have a hard time telling them apart. Red fescue is the most shade tolerant of the good "lawn" grasses, but is more susceptible to disease when overwatered. It makes a thick ground cover in naturalized areas. Hard fescue is favored for its deep green color, and hard fescue and sheep fescue are often found in wildflower mixes because they make good, resilient meadow grasses.

All fine fescues do less well in hot, humid weather than bluegrass, so their range doesn't extend quite as far south. They also resent too much fertilization; if overfertilized, they are more prone to disease (same with high humidity). The rate of fertilization should be about half that of Kentucky bluegrass.

Tall fescue *(Festuca arundinacea)*
Bunchgrass

RAINFALL RANGE: 18 inches minimum for survival, 21 to 25+ inches for lawn grass

SOIL: Silty to clay optimum, sandy to heavy clay possible

pH: 4.7 to 8.5

PROPAGATION: Seed at 10 to 12 pounds per 1,000 square feet

GERMINATION TIME: 7 to 12 days

Sod

MOWING HEIGHT: 3 inches

ADAPTED RANGE:

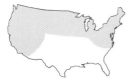

Tall fescue is a cool-season bunchgrass from Europe. It is easily established and grows well in irrigated soils or in areas receiving average annual precipitation of about eighteen inches or more. It performs best on clayey and clay soils and tolerates salt. Turf-type fall fescues gave the best performance and bluegrasslike appearance at the Denver Water Department's Xeriscape Demonstration Garden over the first five years of their test of five different turfgrasses (including mixtures).

Many of the newest strains of fescue have been developed specifically for wearability. For best turf appearance fescue should be seeded generously to fill in because it is a bunch-type grass. Where it gets thin, it tends to become thick-bladed and to have bare spaces between the "bunches" where weeds easily gain a foothold. Try to avoid mowing at less than the recommended height because this, too, can encourage bunchiness.

Fescue is more tolerant of shade than either bluegrass or buffalograss. It is used in the East for mined-land reclamation, in part because of its wide range of pH tolerance (in fact, it has naturalized and about taken over some areas), but in arid and semiarid regions it requires moist or irrigated sites. Occasionally smooth bromegrass (which is sod-forming) will be mixed with fescue to create a more tightly knit turf.

Tall fescue has a dense root system concentrated in the top twelve inches of soil, but if irrigation is

This turf-type tall fescue was seeded in April 1989 (photographed in August 1990) as part of a water-absorbing polymer test. A very high rate of polymer (forty-five pounds per thousand square feet) was incorporated into the soil before seeding. The backyard was equally lush with thirty pounds of polymer per thousand square feet. The owner estimated he saved about $190 in watering costs the first year over similarly sized and maintained yards. The only place where the grass became thin and bunchy (a problem with bunchgrasses) was next to the driveway where people get in and out of cars. This could be easily overcome by widening the driveway three to four feet with a gravel, wood chip mulch, or brick landing area.

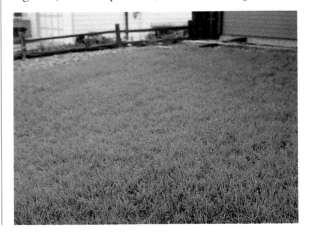

deep and infrequent it may send roots down as far as four feet, which helps it to survive drought. Fescue is interesting because it actually has a higher evapotranspiration rate (the rate at which it removes moisture from the soil through evaporation and transpiration) than Kentucky bluegrass, yet it is often touted as the answer to bluegrass for water-thrifty lawns. Because of its deeper root system, tall fescue may use substantially less applied water; it's better able to "mine" deeply for the water it needs.

Bob Vilotti raised a tall fescue lawn from seed in his backyard. He finds that it holds its deep green color much better than the bluegrass in his front yard. As of the end of June in its third growing season, the fescue still hadn't been fertilized, and had been watered only once (the bluegrass needed fertilizer twice and had been watered several times). He finds it a very fast-growing grass and says, "If you wait too long between mowing, you might as well get out there with a scythe." Overall, Vilotti has found that "as long as you get it mowed once a week, tall fescue makes an attractive turfgrass."

Kentucky bluegrass   *(Poa pratensis)*
Sod-forming

RAINFALL RANGE: 35 to 56 inches optimum, 20 inches minimum (enough for survival only)

SOIL: Moist, well drained, fertile, medium-textured

pH: 6.0 to 7.0

PROPAGATION: Seed at 1½ pounds per 1,000 square feet

Sod

GERMINATION TIME: 6 to 30 days

MOWING HEIGHT: 2½ to 3 inches, unmowed height 12 to 36 inches

ADAPTED RANGE:

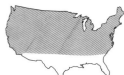

Kentucky bluegrass is the fine-bladed cool-season favorite of the northern United States and Canada. It is also grown in cool, humid areas along the West Coast, and in the mountainous and cool-weather areas of the South and Southwest. Most varieties of Kentucky bluegrass available today orig-

inated in the cool, humid regions of the world. Bluegrass is popular not only because of its texture, color, and excellent wearability, but also because of its ease of handling for sod growers. The sod can be rolled up easily, and new grass will grow from the exposed roots after the top sod layer is cut. Kentucky bluegrass seed is usually sold as mixtures of two or more varieties; mixtures that include other types of turf, such as bentgrass and rough-stalk bluegrass, often produce a turf that lacks uniformity.

If the intended grass area will be used for children's play or athletic activities, it may be worth the investment in water to maintain it in bluegrass. Otherwise, for areas that receive less than thirty inches of rainfall per year, or not much rainfall in the summer, there are probably better choices for a Xeriscape yard than Kentucky bluegrass.

Much of the landscape water use and abuse in semiarid climates comes from trying to keep Kentucky bluegrass green through the summer. Because it's a cool-season grass with low drought *avoidance* (turns brown quickly when drought occurs), the natural tendency for Kentucky bluegrass is to turn brown in summer's heat. We lose our faith in its ability to revive when cool weather/more precipitation comes along, and it's hard, hard, hard to resist the temptation to give it lots of water when it starts going dormant. And the fact is that Kentucky bluegrass does need at least eighteen to twenty inches of water per year to survive, so if you live in an area that gets less than that you'll have to water some. If you keep it mowed (which most of us will be doing, of course), it will need more watering to keep it thick and resistant to weed invasion. Just try to keep the waterings deep and infrequent, and try not to panic if it gets a little brown in between.

Perennial ryegrass is often mixed with bluegrass to improve the drought avoidance of the lawn (meaning its ability to stay green during drought). This also improves disease resistance because grass is not a "one-crop field." If disease invades, it will be more isolated.

These cultivars of Kentucky bluegrass are said to be low-water-using, though they may or may not be drought tolerant: 'Adelphi', 'Aron', 'A-20', 'Banff', 'Cheri', 'Cougar', 'Glade', 'Enoble' (low-water-using), 'Entopper', 'Galaxy' (low-water-using), 'Newport', 'Plush', 'S-21', 'Touchdown'.

Annual bluegrass *(Poa annua)* Bunchgrass

Not recommended for lawns because its low-growing tufted habit makes it unattractive.

Annual ryegrass *(Lolium multiflorum)*
Bunchgrass

RAINFALL RANGE: 18 inches and up
SOIL: Tolerates a wide range
pH: 6.0 to 7.0
PROPAGATION: Seed at 9 pounds per 1,000 square feet
GERMINATION TIME: 3 to 7 days
MOWING HEIGHT: 1 inch
ADAPTED RANGE:

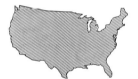

Annual ryegrass has little going for it in Xeriscape landscaping, needing frequent watering and having poor drought tolerance. Although it has some usefulness as a fast-germinating cover crop that can provide protection for slower-to-start perennial grass seed when planted together, it's not generally recommended for home lawns. Annual ryegrass is just that, an annual, which will die out over the winter in the North and succumb to summer heat in the South. If it constitutes more than twenty percent of a grass seed mixture, bare spots will result when the grass dies. It is sometimes overseeded in the South on top of warm-season grasses to maintain a green grass through the winter. This requires additional water, however, to start and maintain the grass.

The clever Xeriscape gardener might use annual ryegrass the way the pros (reclamation experts) do, as a temporary cover crop to prevent erosion in anticipation of a permanent seeding the following growing season, or as a "green manure" crop to be turned under and allowed to lie fallow for several weeks to add nitrogen to the soil before a permanent ground cover is planted.

Perennial ryegrass *(Lolium perenne)*
Bunchgrass

RAINFALL RANGE: Approximately 15+ inches
SOIL: Wide range, best on neutral to slightly acidic, fertile
pH: 6.0 to 7.0 (the cultivar 'Norlea' performs well up to pH 8.5)
PROPAGATION: Seed at 9 pounds per 1,000 square feet
GERMINATION TIME: 3 to 7 days
MOWING HEIGHT: 2½ to 3 inches
ADAPTED RANGE:

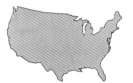

Perennial ryegrass is a rapid-developing grass. It has a finer texture than annual ryegrass and is also often used to overseed warm-season grasses. It has excellent wearability and tolerates some shade, but requires frequent watering and has only fair drought resistance.

Perennial ryegrass is interesting in that, in the 1980s, it was discovered that certain fungi called endophytes, which the grass hosted without harm to itself, actually repelled some grass-infecting insects such as weevils, bluegrass billbugs, and sod webworms. These endophytes are contained within the cells of the grass and are passed to the new generation of grass through the seeds. Some perennial ryegrasses have multiple disease resistance.

Because of their poor drought tolerance, they are not highly recommended for Xeriscape landscaping, but work well in the cool-climate areas of the West and Midwest, and northeastern coastal areas. Perhaps their most useful contribution is their endophytes, which are now being bred into strains of the more drought-tolerant tall fescues.

Colonial bentgrass *(Agrosti tenuis)*
Bunchgrass
Creeping bentgrass *(A. palustris)*
Sod-forming

RAINFALL RANGE: 35 inches and up
SOIL: Moist, fertile
pH: 4.5 to 6.7

PROPAGATION: Seed at ½ to 1 pound per 1,000 square feet

GERMINATION TIME: 4 to 12 days

MOWING HEIGHT: ¼ to 1 inch

ADAPTED RANGE:

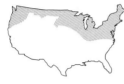

Colonial bentgrass

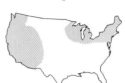

Creeping bentgrass

Warren Schultz says bentgrasses don't belong in home lawns. Beloved for putting greens, they not only tolerate short mowing heights, they require it, or a thick layer of thatch builds up. To keep them looking good, they need frequent watering as well, and all bentgrasses are susceptible to several diseases. Colonial bentgrass is more drought tolerant than creeping bentgrass, but still it thrives without constant care only in the coastal areas of the Northeast, the Pacific Northwest, and other northern areas where moist soils are prevalent.

Bentgrasses do best in full sun but will tolerate some shade. They are so aggressive that they can't be mixed with lower-maintenance grasses because they'll crowd them out. Colonial bentgrass does have the advantages of being able to survive in soils too acid for Kentucky bluegrass (as low as 4.5 to 5.0) and of being tolerant of fine-textured, poorly drained soils. It is often used in bank stabilization for grassy waterways, ditchbanks, and flood channels in the Pacific Northwest because of its ability to withstand prolonged winter flooding. Creeping bentgrass is able to thrive in poor, wet soils where nothing else might survive. Aside from these special uses, bentgrasses don't belong in a Xeriscape landscape, either.

Rough bluegrass *(Poa trivialis)* Sod-forming

RAINFALL RANGE: 25 to 30 inches and up

SOIL: Wet, clayey, poorly drained

pH: 6.0 to 7.0

PROPAGATION: Seed at 1 to 1½ pounds per 1,000 square feet

GERMINATION TIME: 21 days

MOWING HEIGHT: 1 to 2 inches

ADAPTED RANGE:

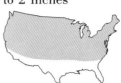

Also called rough-stalk bluegrass, this bluegrass is noted primarily for its shade tolerance. It has the bright green color and fine texture of Kentucky bluegrass, but requires frequent watering and is not drought tolerant. It also has poor wearability and can become weedy. It's probably not a good choice for Xeriscape landscaping unless you have a shady area that naturally receives a lot of water.

Shade Tolerance

In the past home landscapers were advised to pick among fine fescues, St. Augustinegrasses, zoysiagrasses, and bentgrasses if they had excessive shade in their yards. However, a four-year study at Rutgers University showed that some improved cultivars of Kentucky bluegrass (notably 'A-34', 'Nugget', 'Park', and 'Glade'), tall fescue ('Rebel' and 'Kentucky 31'), and perennial ryegrass ('Pennfine' and 'Linn') performed in heavy shade as well as, or better than, some of the more shade-tolerant species. With shade tolerance, as with drought tolerance, it's best to consult with a county extension agent or other local expert as to the best varieties for your area.

This list shows some generally recommended species for shade tolerance for different parts of the country:

Northern—cool climate:	Red and chewings fescue
Northern—warm climate:	Zoysiagrass
Humid Pacific Northwest:	Colonial bentgrass
Transition zone:	Tall fescue
Southern—warm climate:	Bahiagrass and St. Augustinegrass

INSTALLING NEW XERISCAPE LAWNS

You've *thoughtfully* decided on the size, shape, location, and type of grass you're going to use in the lawn areas in your Xeriscape landscape, and now must decide how to grow them. Seeding and sodding are most common, with plugging and sprigging being used less often. Depending on your choice of grass, you may not need to make a decision; some grasses are available only as seed or sod, etc. But some of the most popular grasses for Xeriscape landscaping, such as fescue and buffalograss, can be propagated in two or more ways.

There are pros and cons for choosing either to sod or to seed. For the adventurous Xeriscape gardener, seeding adds dozens of grass varieties and strains to choose from, allowing you to tailor the lawn not only to your own taste, but also to varying conditions on the site. Grasses available for sod are sharply limited. Seeding is *usually* less expensive initially than sod, and, with the right equipment, it can spread quickly over a large area.

However, there is one key point to remember for Xeriscape landscaping: *If* what you want is lawn-grass growth that will cover the ground in a reasonably short amount of time, say within a few weeks, seeding, in general, takes more water. It takes water not only to keep the ground constantly moist until germination (it may need sprinkling one to four times a day for two to three weeks), but also to keep the tender sprouts from drying out (more watering for another week or two). Then it must be watered for several more weeks till it is fully established. A sod lawn, by contrast, may need only two or three weeks of twice to thrice weekly watering to become established. (Sometimes the cost of the seed added to the cost of the water and the time to water equals or exceeds the initial cost of sod.)

Sod has additional advantages in that it can be installed on slopes without washing away, it provides instant cover, it can be installed almost any time during the growing season, and it smothers weeds near the surface.

Weeds are almost always a discouraging, though not unnatural presence in the seeded lawn. They are not only the "plants with the greater will to live," they are actually part of an orderly plant succession in the establishment of a mature grassland. If left to itself, an area of bare ground will be thick with annual weeds the first year or two, followed by perennial weeds that crowd out the annuals, and finally perennial grasses that eventually eliminate the perennial weeds. By establishing and maintaining

a lawn, we are actually keeping the ground in a suspended and somewhat "immature" state, reducing the perennial grasses' dominance, so those childish annual weeds just keep on appearing.

New lawn seedings will often contain annual weeds, including weedy grasses that sprout not only from the ground but also from weed seeds contained in the grass seed. After the turf becomes established and is mowed several times, most of these will usually disappear. However, perennial grass weeds should be removed before the grass is seeded (if you're trying to establish a new buffalograss lawn, for instance, Kentucky bluegrass remnants are considered a weed).

There are several options for the Xeriscape gardener who wants to try seeding the lawn, while still dealing with the weeds *and* keeping the watering down. One is to sow the grass seed anytime, knowing that it won't germinate until conditions are just right, which may take several weeks or months. This saves water, but birds *may* eat the seeds, and weeds will still grow.

Another alternative is to allow the weeds to grow along with the grass the first year (this actually makes sense because the weeds provide shade and protection for grass seedlings, which cuts down on watering). Bob Vilotti used this method to start his backyard fescue lawn in Denver. The second year he applied a pre-emergent herbicide to the lawn in early spring and knocked out the weeds before they had a chance to get started. The result was a thick stand of grass with little or no pain, and limited use of herbicide. A person who wanted to avoid the herbicide completely could use the same technique, realizing that he/she would have to commit to some serious hand-weeding in the second growing season to rid the lawn of weeds.

A third option is to get the weeds under control before starting the lawn. According to Warren Schultz, one of the best ways to get a new or improved lawn off to a good start is to reduce the weed population as much as possible before sodding or seeding. This will cut down as much as anything on the amount of time you have to spend maintaining the lawn later. (Realize, though, that it's not possible to eliminate all the weed seeds, some of which are said to be viable for scores of years. Typical soil contains about 5,000 weed seeds in the top six inches of soil per square foot. They may also be introduced when animal manures and imported top-soil are brought in.)

Ways to control weeds include several listed in the next section for getting rid of existing grass. The prairie garden section of the appropriate plant choice chapter has an in-depth discussion of the weed elimination process necessary to establishing a prairie reconstruction, which may take up to a year. (Soil sterilization is *never* recommended, of course, because beneficial soil organisms are killed as well as all the plants.)

Removing Existing Sod

A big dilemma for the prospective Xeriscape gardener renovating a landscape is finding a way to remove existing grass and replace it with a more drought-tolerant species or other ground cover. Several possibilities are suggested here for removing not only grass from an existing landscape, but also weed cover from a new site. No way is perfect, but knowing what you'll replace the grass with helps. For instance, the "easiest" way to get rid of existing lawn grass is to rent a sod cutter (or better yet, hire someone else to do it!) and remove the top layer of grass and roots. If you're planning to install native grasses that are adapted to poor soil, this method is just fine. If you want to put in a perennial bed, though, you'll want to retain as much of the nutrient value of the sod as you can. You can still use the same method, but save all the grass and attached dirt and compost it for later use in the garden. Here are some other methods.

Overseeding

Mow existing grass as short as possible. Rake new seed in thoroughly and water regularly for the first two weeks.

Advantages: Minimal labor. Some success if much-lower-water-requiring grass is overseeded because after initial seedling establishment, less frequent watering for the new grass will favor its survival over the old. May do better the second year.

Disadvantages: Doesn't work well. Increased water to start the seed encourages existing sod to start growing again. Not advised if changing from a cool- to a warm-season grass, because one will be dormant while the other is active, leading to a crazy-quilt effect of color.

Ripping Out I

Use a sod cutter, shovel, or sod spade (with a square, sharp edge) to cut roots at a depth of three to four inches. Give sod away, haul it away, or make it into a compost pile.

Advantages: Gets rid of most intense competition from existing grass roots and a thick layer of weed seeds.

Disadvantages: Backbreaking labor. Sod cutters are heavy and so is sod. In poor soil this method re-moves the most nutrient-rich soil layer (unless composted).

Ripping Out II

Same as above, except turn slabs of sod upside down in place and let them stay there till the grass is dead. Rototill or spade broken-up slabs into the soil along with soil amendments.

Advantages: Keeps nutrients in soil. May take shorter amount of time than tilling method described below. May be the best compromise.

Disadvantages: Still backbreaking. Weed seeds still present (but then they always will be, no matter what you do).

Tilling Up

Rototill area. Let sit four to six weeks to let grass and weeds resprout and dead grass/weeds decom-pose, then till area again. May have to repeat pro-cedure.

Advantages: Lets Rototiller do (most) of the work. Retains the nutrients and organic matter of the grass.

Disadvantages: Tiller may still be hard to handle. Ground is "under construction" for a long time.

Replacing with a Tough Ground Cover

Plant an aggressive ground cover such as juniper or purple-leaved wintercreeper in good-sized holes right in the grass. Mulch with three to four inches of wood chips or other mulch. Plants will eventually take over the grass. (Zoysiagrass in bluegrass is another example).

Advantages: Doesn't take chemicals or *too* much labor, just enough to dig the holes for the plants.

Disadvantages: Expensive if you have to buy all new plants. Might take one or two years to cover the grass.

Using Soil Solarization

Water the area to be redone deeply about a month before planting. Cover completely with clear plastic; anchor plastic with rocks or soil around edges. Leave until grass is dead (about one to two months).

Advantages: Grass and sprouting weeds are killed by intense heat under plastic. Easy technique.

Disadvantages: Doesn't seem to work well where nights are cool. Not enough heat generated to kill weeds. Plastic must be anchored or it will blow around.

Killing Grass with Herbicide

Follow directions for spraying area to be desodded, using "mild" herbicide such as glysophate. Wait two weeks, and either rake up the dead vegetation or till it under.

If you're preparing the ground for prairie grasses you may need to take a whole summer to eliminate the weeds in this way: During the rest of the growing season, weekly chase down and spray any green that appears with glysophate, especially about two weeks before the first frost when weeds are most actively absorbing nutrients (and herbicide) into their roots. If the problem appears to be fairly well handled by the end of the summer, then you can begin planting the following year. If you're still mixing up a large amount of the herbicide each week, then plan on spending another growing season on weed control.

Advantages: Little labor involved. Kills annual weeds as well.

Disadvantages: You may not want to use chemicals since they are stored in the tissues of woody ornamentals. Use of herbicide near existing trees and shrubs may damage them over the long run. Glysophate is not a harmless chemical.

Smothering with Mulch

Cover the area with a layer of newspapers several sheets thick. Overlap the pieces to avoid gaps. Do not use glossy color advertising pages because the ink is sometimes poisonous. Cover the newspapers with several inches of an organic mulch, such as shredded bark. (Gravel mulches will tear the newspaper and admit weeds too easily.) You can just leave the area alone to compost the grass till next year, or dig planting holes for flowers, trees, or shrubs.

Advantages: Extremely inexpensive and easy. (I tried this last year. Now instead of scrawny grass and compacted soil there is a thin black layer of compost from the newspaper and a thicker brown layer of decomposed grass and roots. Areas that were impenetrable with a shovel are now easy to turn over.)

Disadvantages: Newspaper must be well covered with mulch or it will be unsightly. Weeds can still come up through gaps or tears. (Don't try to spread out the newspapers while the wind is blowing, unless you like a lot of excitement!)

Last, but certainly not least, for the Xeriscape gardener most inclined to be economical with his/her time is the simple method of just leaving the grass there. Before you expend the energy to remove it, make sure it's not filling some important function for which grass is best suited. Then devote your time to renovating the grass itself for improved water thriftiness by aerating, overseeding, and/or fertilizing (or *not* fertilizing) and being a better-informed "irrigator" as explained in the irrigation chapter, or let it go to seed and become a grassy meadow.

When to Plant

The best time to plant a new lawn is when temperature and moisture are favorable for seed germination and for growth of seedlings or plugs, and when conditions are less favorable for weed growth. Most weeds germinate in the spring, languish in the summer heat, and sprout to a lesser extent in the fall. For seeding, sprigging, or plugging a new lawn,

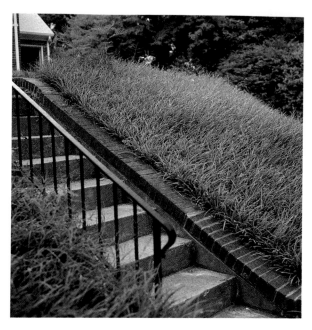

Several ground covers, including periwinkle (Vinca minor), *had been tried on this steep slope in Charlottesville, Virginia, but mondo grass* (Ophiopogon japonicus) *worked best. At the top of the slope a level patch of turfgrass is easy to maintain.*

you need six to eight weeks of favorable weather for the grass to become sufficiently established: for sodding, a month is needed.

For cool-season grasses, late summer to early fall is the recommended time to seed a turfgrass. Less water will be needed this way because cooler temperatures have slowed evaporation from the soil. You can lay sod anytime during the growing season, but you may use considerably more water if you do so midsummer. By laying sod in the spring you can sometimes take advantage of spring rains to eliminate some of the watering.

For warm-season grasses, late spring to early summer is said to be the best time for seeding because this is when soil temperatures are most favorable for germination. In the South some weeds germinate in the fall, making it hard to establish a seeded lawn at that time.

Preparing the Ground for a New Lawn

To get the most out of your lawn areas, several steps should be taken to prepare the ground for planting

regardless of the method of lawn establishment.

Preparing grade. If the surface grade is very uneven, remove and stockpile topsoil first, remove dead stumps and large rocks, and construct the subgrade, making sure the slope is evened out and large depressions are filled in.

For proper drainage a minimum of two percent slope is recommended (4.8-inch drop over twenty feet). The maximum slope should not exceed four to one, a one-foot drop in four feet. It's just barely possible to mow grass at a three-to-one slope (one foot drop in three feet), but let's face it—who wants to? Trying to maintain turfgrass at a three-to-one slope is one of the basic Xeriscape jokes. It appears in all the slide shows as an example of how not to do it, not only in the difficulty of mowing and the fact that it doesn't have much functional use, but also in the tremendous amounts of water needed to keep it green.

To put it more positively, a steep slope in a yard is just the place to do some creative Xeriscape landscaping with retaining walls or any of the wildflowers, wild grasses, or low-growing shrubs that don't mind growing on a slope. If you plant wild grasses, your kids can still slide down it if it snows.

Improving surface and subsurface drainage. Surface drainage is taken care of by ensuring a minimum slope to the turf as described. However, occasionally, the installation of drain tiles or dry wells is needed to correct a subsurface drainage problem brought about when poorly drained soils (usually high in clay) are present in a low spot with no outlet. (See any book on lawn establishment for details on how to install these.)

Adding soil amendments and cultivation. Cultivate the subgrade to a depth of eight inches. This will improve the water-absorbing capacity of clay soil so that when you are watering your lawn, less will run off. It's especially important to cultivate if there has been much compaction from construction traffic. Redistribute stockpiled topsoil, removing small rocks one to two inches in diameter in the top four inches (to allow for use of aerators or other equipment later), evenly spread any required or desired soil amendments over the top, and cultivate again to incorporate them into the soil.

In order to ensure even distribution of soil amendments, divide the quantity of amendment into two portions, then spread one-half beginning at one end of your yard and making passes back and forth. Start at the other end of your yard for the second half and make the passes perpendicular to the first set. This way, if you have miscalculated the rate at which you portion out the material, you won't end up with one section of your yard not having any of the amendments on it.

If you want to add hydro-gels to the lawn area, doing it before starting the grass is *much* easier than doing it later. You simply spread the material evenly over the soil with a fertilizer spreader and till it in with other soil amendments. Research still hasn't determined the optimum rates for hydro-gels in lawns, but a range of fifteen to thirty pounds per 1,000 square feet seems to give a lush lawn, with water savings of about thirty to fifty percent (at least in Colorado).

Like fertilizer, the only danger in using hydro-gels seems to be the problem of overdosing. In this case the lawn isn't "burned," it just gets a little squishy after a rain. This problem can be easily avoided by adding no more than five pounds per tilled inch per 1,000 square feet. For instance, if you want to use twenty-five pounds per 1,000, till it in at least five inches.

Soil pH

Most turfgrasses are adapted to a pH between 6.0 and 7.0, though there are exceptions. If a soil is too acidic for the lawn grass, its drought tolerance, as well as vigor, growth, and competitive ability, may decline. Soil becomes acidic as excessive rainfall or irrigation leaches calcium and magnesium below the root zone, because of the use of acidifying fertilizers such as ammonium sulfate, or because of irrigation with water high in sulfur. As a result, a soil whose acid pH has been adjusted to match the grass's tolerance level may become too acid again as a result of poor cultural practice. For that reason, you're better off choosing a grass whose pH requirements match the pH of your soil. However, if you've got your heart set on a grass whose pH preference requires your amending the soil, see page 39 for guidelines on changing soil pH.

Soil Fertility

Three primary nutrients may need to be added to the soil before establishing a new lawn. They are the same as those found in almost all commercial fertilizers—nitrogen, phosphorus, and potassium. Warren Schultz recommends two to three pounds of nitrogen, five to eight pounds of phosphorus, and one to two pounds of potassium per 1,000 square feet as a good basic fertilizer for the establishment of a new seeded lawn. Natural sources of phosphorus include bonemeal, rock phosphate, fish emulsion, sludge, bloodmeal, and cottonseed meal. Sources of potassium include greensand (glauconite), wood ashes, granite dust, tobacco waste, dried sheep manure, millet, and buckwheat straw.

These recommended rates assume that you'll be seeding with a traditional lawn grass rather than a native grass such as blue grama grass or buffalograss. If you're planning to use one of these grasses, please see the prairie garden section in the appropriate plant choice chapter. In some instances you may wish to add little or no fertilizer. Rick Brune, a native grass expert in Colorado, points out that in the alkaline soils of the semiarid West phosphorus is so immobile that many of our yards "probably still contain enough phosphorus to be mined." Potassium deficiencies are rare and, in the case of blue grama grass, the grass actually responds negatively to nitrogen.

For establishing a lawn, then, the best procedure is to use the information provided by a professional soil test for correcting soil fertility and pH, and making modifications as needed. Again, seek the advice of a local county extension agent. (Some communities have become heavily involved in ensuring that soil be amended proeprly before starting a lawn by requiring a permit to sod, issued only after the home landscaper has shown proof of purchase of the required soil amendments. In this way they are trying to take precautions so that the irrigation water used on a new lawn will have a better chance of being used efficiently for plant growth.)

Establishing the final grade. Various tools can be used to help in the final leveling and grading process, which ideally is done within twenty-four hours of planting. (Delay the process if the ground is very wet since this will destroy the soil's structure.) A wide steel rake, piece of chain link fence, or homemade leveling bar made of a heavy plank of wood with a pulling rope attached can be used to drag the area, smoothing out the grade. It's best to take some time with this step because it's difficult to alter the grade once the lawn is in. Low spots may cause puddling of water and high spots are more susceptible to scalping by mowers.

The goal is to create a soil base with a firm, granular (not dusty) texture, free of clods, rocks, and debris. After the ground is leveled it can be rolled to help firm it.

(If you will be sodding your lawn, leave the final grade about ¾ to one inch lower than if you are seeding, so that the sod will sit flush with driveways, sidewalks, and sprinklers.)

Seeding

The three essentials for the seeded lawn are soil moisture, soil preparation, and the amount and quality of seed. After spending considerable effort ridding your ground of as many existing weeds as you can, don't negate your work by purchasing cheap grass seed mixtures, which are more likely to contain weed seeds and unwelcome grass seeds such as annual bluegrass; it's important to avoid false economy on this point. Select high-quality seed from a reputable dealer.

Don't skimp on the amount of seed you buy, especially if you'll be raising bunch-type grasses that don't have the ability to spread and fill in open areas that sod-forming grasses do. A thin lawn takes more maintenance and provides more room for weeds to grow. Most grasses need about fifteen to twenty seeds per square inch to make a thick stand, given the fact that only eighty to ninety percent will germinate. The quantity of seed should be increased, too, by twenty-five to fifty percent if the seed is more than a year old, to make up for any decrease in germination rate.

Mixtures

Grass mixtures generally apply only to cool-season grasses since mixtures of the aggressive warm-season turfgrass tend to result in monocultures after only one or two growing seasons. Grass mixtures are usually sold on a percentage-of-weight basis. A mixture might be thirty-five percent perennial ryegrass, thirty-five percent creeping red fescue, and thirty percent Kentucky bluegrass. But because the number of seeds per pound varies tremendously, the actual percentages on a number-of-seeds basis will be different. The resulting mixture of grasses in the ground may vary substantially from what you had envisioned.

To determine the true ratio of each grass based on number of seeds per pound, multiply the number of seeds per pound for each grass by its ratio in the mixture.

Number of Seeds per Pound for Various Grasses

Bahiagrass	170,000
Bentgrass	8,000,000
Bermudagrass	2,000,000
Blue grama grass	725,000
Bluegrass	2,100,000
Buffalograss	40,000 (burs—uncleaned seeds)
	150,000 (cleaned seeds)
Centipedegrass	400,000
Red or chewings fescue	550,000
Tall fescue or perennial ryegrass	230,000

For the above mixture:
35% perennial ryegrass = (.35)(230,000) = 80,500 seeds
35% creeping red fescue = (.35)(2,100,000) = 735,000 seeds
30% Kentucky bluegrass = (.30)(550,000) = 165,000 seeds
TOTAL NUMBER OF SEEDS IN A POUND OF MIX: 980,500

Percentage of seeds/pound mix:
Perennial ryegrass   80,500/980,500 = 8.2%
Creeping red fescue   735,000/980,500 = 75%
Kentucky bluegrass   165,000/980,500 = 16.8%

The resulting grass mixture is quite different, although variances in germination will readjust the result again slightly. (Creeping red fescue has a germination rate of eighty-five percent compared to ninety to one hundred percent for the other two grasses.)

A grass seed listed as "certified" will be virtually one hundred percent pure seed. Most of the traditional lawn grasses from a reputable dealer will carry this label.

For seeding with native grasses, recommended rates may be given in terms of Pure Live Seed (PLS) rather than just bulk seed. This designation takes into account the purity of the seed and the germination rate of the variety. It's not always possible for seed companies to produce pure batches of native grass seed with absolutely no seeds of other grasses or plants present, nor any other nonseed materials, such as chaff. Using the PLS designation, buyers can figure out how much extra seed they'll need to purchase in order to allow for both the average purity and the average germination rate of the seed.

The poundage recommendations given in the individual grass entries represent PLS, and most seed companies will have calculated the PLS of their seed. If they haven't, you simply divide the number of pounds of PLS you need for your seeding area by the germination rate and the percent of purity to arrive at the number of pounds of seed you need to buy. For instance, to get one pound PLS of a grass that has forty percent purity and ninety percent germination (these values will be listed on the seed packaging):

$$\text{Number of pounds needed to buy} = \frac{1 \text{ pound PLS}/1{,}000 \text{ square feet}}{(.4)\,(.9)}$$
$$= 2.8 \text{ pounds}/1{,}000 \text{ square feet}$$

When you're ready to seed, divide the amount of seed for an area into two equal portions. Either by hand or using a drop seeder (this is better since it distributes more evenly and keeps the seed near the ground where the wind can't toss it around), spread the seed across the area, making back-and-forth passes. Spread the other half of the seed perpendicularly to the first half.

After seeding, firm the seeded area by tamping down with the back of a rake or rolling it lightly with a lawn roller. Mulching the seedbed conserves moisture, keeps rain from washing away the seed, and speeds germination by keeping the conditions more constant. Make sure the mulch is applied very thinly so that sunlight can get through, or else germination will not take place. You can mulch with weed-free straw (not hay, because it contains weed seeds). A sixty- to eighty-pound bale will mulch 1,000 square feet. Neither sand nor peat moss should be used because they can crust over and form a barrier that sheds water. Mulch paper is a relatively expensive but effective mulch. Make sure the mulch paper is securely fastened into the ground. Remove it when the grass is one inch high.

The soil should be kept moist but not saturated until the grass is two inches high. Don't allow the soil to dry out, even if it means sprinkling two or more times a day. Try to stay off the grass initially. Let it grow about an inch higher than it will be mowed before the first mowing. Keep the grass high throughout the first growing season.

Sprigging

For sprigging, individual plants, rhizomes, or stolons of grass are planted in channels four to twelve inches apart and allowed to fill in between. Each sprig planted includes a node and is capable of rooting and starting a new plant. Sprigs are purchased by the bushel or can be made by pulling sod apart into pieces. Make sure sprigs are kept shaded and slightly moist during planting. Soak the ground on the day before planting, then place the plants in small furrows, two to three inches long, at the appropriate distance (faster-growing grasses such as Bermudagrass and St. Augustinegrass are usually planted twelve inches apart, while slow-growing zoysiagrass is planted at six inches). Leave the greenest part sticking above the ground. Only plant as much at a time as you can keep moist.

After planting, roll lightly and irrigate. Keep weeds hoed till the grass fills in, which may take a few weeks for Bermudagrass and up to two years for zoysiagrass.

Plugging

Another less expensive alternative to sodding is plugging, in which small squares or circles of sod are set in the ground at regular intervals of a few inches to a foot apart and allowed to fill in over time. Plugging, like sprigging, is a vegetative method of producing a lawn, where the grass is grown from offshoots of existing plants rather than from seed. Vegetative methods are used when the seed is not yet available, or will not produce grass true to type.

After being planted in holes two to three inches deep, plugs are lightly rolled and kept moist until establishment. Zoysiagrass plugs set at one-foot intervals in an existing bluegrass lawn will take over in about four years and, as discussed earlier, plugs of buffalograss may be planted right into bluegrass previously killed with glysophate.

Sodding

It's best to buy sod that has been grown in soil that is not much finer than the soil in your yard. A soil grown on clay and laid over sandy soil will create an impermeable barrier where the two soils meet.

Thin sod roots more rapidly than thickly cut sod. Most grasses are cut with a 0.4- to 0.8-inch soil depth, with tall fescue, Bahiagrass, St. Augustinegrass, buffalograss, and blue grama sometimes cut deeper.

Try to have sod laid within twenty-four to sixty hours after being cut. This will minimize drying out and possible heating damage within the rolls or squares, which can occur if the internal temperature rises above 100 degrees Fahrenheit. Start unrolling the sod along a straight line such as a sidewalk, a line stretched between two stakes, or even a long board. Stagger the pieces like brickwork so they don't line up even with each other, but place them as close as possible together. Use a little topsoil in any cracks between the sod pieces. Water the sod thoroughly and keep evenly moist until the roots have grown into the soil (this usually takes two to three weeks of perhaps daily watering in the warmest part of the day). Do not walk on freshly laid and watered sod for ten days to two weeks. Mow sod after you have stopped watering for two or three days. Never mow wet grass!

Appropriate Plant Selection

ANOTHER Xeriscape landscaping fundamental that has undergone a change in focus is appropriate plant selection, formerly called low-water-demand plants. According to Doug Welsh, "Our judgment of 'low water demand' is very subjective. Except in turf species, research just doesn't exist." Because of the huge variety of plants and conditions it may never be possible to strongly define through research just which plants are "low water demand."

Furthermore, Welsh explains, "Every plant can be a Xeriscape plant. If the plant is adapted to the

Annuals and perennials shine in this Colorado flower bed, photographed in early October. Featured are garden chrysanthemums (Chrysanthemum × morifolium), *white alyssum* (Lobularia maritima), *blanket flower* (Gaillardia grandiflora), *and flowering kale* (Brassica oleracea).

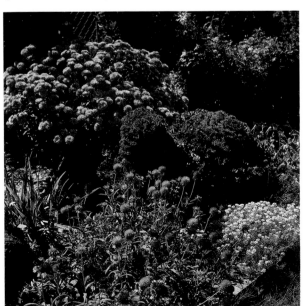

region in terms of heat, cold, soil, etc., and thus appropriate, then it can fit into a Xeriscape landscape." For now, the best judgment of plant water requirements will be the conventional wisdom of amateur and professional gardeners.

Your objective should be to carefully match the moisture requirements of plants to the best microclimate available for them in your landscape. A moisture-loving perennial, for instance, could still find a home in a dry-climate Xeriscape landscape if given some shade, protection from wind, moisture-retentive soil amendments, and drip irrigation if needed.

Again, it depends on what you want out of your Xeriscape garden. If you want to use some of the water-efficiency suggestions in this book in order to include favorite plants in your landscape, whether they are adapted to your normal rainfall pattern or not, you can. If you want to craft a no-water, or very low-water, Xeriscape landscape, you'll try harder to select the plants that survive and thrive with the normal amount of available precipitation in your area.

For some people plant selection is the most exciting and rewarding part of Xeriscape gardening. We may come to love the long-term vision and practicality of our plan or the elegance of our design, but few of us can fail to warm to the task of choosing plants. It's where we can be most creative and expressive. It's where we come to appreciate the diversity of plant species in our region and the intricacies of plant, insect, and wildlife interdependence. We see that complexity in the landscape, besides being more intriguing, brings benefits such as providing habitat for a greater variety of creatures.

In chapter 4 we looked at practical turf areas, and which species to use where lawn grass is appropriate. In this chapter we look at selecting plants other than turf, with details on how to choose, install, and/or propagate them.

In selecting plants, keep in mind one of the fundamental truths about Xeriscape gardening: You can water your plants to your heart's delight. If you don't drown them, they may flower more, they may be a little more fiercely green, and they may grow a little or a *lot* larger this year. *Or* you can do your best to choose the right plants, give them appropriate homes, and never water them after they're established. They may flower indifferently, they may have a subdued rather than brilliant green color, they may not grow an inch this year, but they *won't die!*

Having said that, we must immediately point out one of the equally important truths about creating any landscape, Xeriscape type or otherwise. All new plants in the landscape, whether started from seed or transplants, undergo a period of establishment during which *they need a sufficient quantity of water.* If rainfall doesn't provide it, then we must. We don't leave new plants to fend for themselves any more than we expect young children to tough it out on their own.

Thus you may be startled to see your water consumption actually increase the first year if you have introduced a large number of new plants into the landscape. Don't despair, though, for in the second year you should see a marked decrease in water consumption for trees and shrubs, and in the third year you should be able to eliminate any additional watering. With drought-tolerant perennials the period of establishment is shorter, and with appropriate annuals it's a matter of weeks.

With many water-thirsty species, however, we will likely be tied to watering as long as we want the plant to live.

General Characteristics of Drought-Tolerant Plants

Many drought-tolerant species have characteristics in common that have to do with how they adapt to and survive drought. You might keep these "habits" in mind when choosing plants for your Xeriscape garden. Most water-efficient or drought-tolerant plants will have one or more of them.

1. One rule of thumb (though not an ironclad one) is that the larger the leaf size, the more water the plant needs (and the easier it will scorch in the sun).

2. Grayish, fuzzy, or finely divided foliage usually means the plant is drought tolerant.

3. Plants with a low-growing habit may be drought tolerant. They hug the ground to stay out of drying winds.

4. Herbs and certain other plants with a scent, such as *Eucalyptus* and *Lavandula* (lavender) species, produce aromatic oils that prevent the plants from drying out.

For low-maintenance gardens, select slow-growing perennials or shrubs because they need little pruning and attention and they don't outgrow their spaces quickly. Also avoid any plants listed in plant botanies as having negative qualities such as "hard-to-establish, susceptible to disease and pests, needs frequent division, short-lived, needs staking."

If you've seen plants you'd like to include, but don't know their names, take photos of them and bring them to plant nurseries or send them to the nearest botanic garden for help in identification.

Natives Versus Nonnatives

The most obvious place to start looking for plants for Xeriscape landscaping is in native plants—plants that thrive in your region on the amount of rainfall given to them by nature. Native plants have the added advantage of being adapted to the general soil profile of the area. They need less fertilizer because they get needed nutrients from the native soil. They are usually more resistant to pests and diseases, so fewer pesticides are required to prevent those problems.

Native plants will usually withstand any record-breaking extremes of weather, especially long cold spells, which may kill nonnative plants. Droughts may come only every few years to a region, and the conditions in between may vary from flooding to optimum moisture to dry. Natives are adapted to almost all of these seasonal variations.

Where hot spells are commonplace, native plants have often developed adaptive mechanisms, such as deep root systems, leaves coated with protective waxes, and the secretion of substances that retard evaporation. These plants may have leaves coated with tiny hairs that reduce evaporation and give a grayish green cast to their foliage, or they may exhibit one or more of the other mechanisms mentioned here or in the introductory chapter.

Southwest native plant specialist Judith Phillips strongly recommends that prospective Xeriscape gardeners in any part of the country spend considerable time studying not only which plants grow easily in the wild near your home, but also where and with what other plants. Do they grow in wide open areas or in a well-sheltered spot? Do they grow along stream banks or on rocky hillsides? Are they found only where the soil has been undisturbed for centuries or spring up prolifically as sunflowers do where the soil is recently disturbed, as in road cuts? Do they prefer sunny, south-facing slopes or cooler, moister, north-facing slopes? Do they grow in groups, as isolated plants, or with a particular other species?

She emphasizes the practicality in this. If your goal is a self-sustaining landscape, it's especially important to choose plants with soil and exposure requirements similar to those of your site. The plant that can thrive on natural rainfall, as well as be tolerant of drought, is less likely to weaken and be susceptible to diseases and pests.

Grouping plants that grow together in the wild gives them a better chance to assist each other in the same ways they do in the wild, whether it be by providing shade for protection, increasing humidity, or moderating temperature fluctuations. This will reduce the nursing that *you* have to do to help plants along.

By using native plants you will very likely provide food or cover for native birds, and thus, in a small way, help preserve the habitat for more diverse species. This helps reverse the trend, endemic to typical suburban housing developments, of eliminating a complex habitat and replacing it with a monotonous and foreign one.

Some people assume that the flowers of native plant species aren't as vividly colored as those of more familiar garden favorites. However, careful study of natives anywhere in the country will reveal

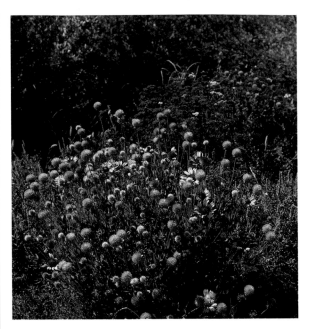

A late fall view of the tallgrass prairie reconstruction at the Denver Botanic Garden echoes the lavish growth that once blanketed much of the Midwest.

an array of brilliantly hued flowers and foliage enough to satisfy even the most avowed color lover.

However, keep in mind that because soil and microclimates can vary so significantly in a small area, a plant that is native to one side of a rock may be unable to survive on the other side. You can find out only through experimentation.

Nonnatives

The point was made to me repeatedly across the country that Xeriscape plants should *not* be equated with native plants. I was fervently asked to reassure prospective Xeriscape gardeners that if they don't favor native species or if native plants aren't available, many beautiful nonnative plants work well with Xeriscape landscaping, particularly those adapted to periods of drought and/or poor soil. Species native to the Mediterranean area, China, Australia, and New Zealand are often successful in American Xeriscape gardens.

Also, many adapted nonnative plants were introduced so long ago that it's hard to say what's native and what isn't. Crape myrtles are beloved from Texas to Virginia. Brought over originally from

China in 1747, they make an excellent choice for Xeriscape gardens. They feature not only drought tolerance but also astonishingly lavish flowers, ranging in color from white to hot pink, disease resistance (in the new cultivars), and the ability to thrive untended.

On the flip side, the following considerations should be part of your decision making when selecting native plants or determining whether to use them:

1. Suitability. The plant must be native to the specific area or environment you want to use it in. A plant native to creek bottom areas will not thrive on dry, rocky slopes.

2. Availability. *Some* natives are hard to grow under nursery conditions, and digging plants up from the wild is the fastest way to endanger them. Fortunately, the number of native plant nurseries is on the rise.

3. When using natives, make sure you group them with other plants with similar horticultural needs, not only in terms of water requirements, but soil nutrition and texture, too.

4. Natives may be just too "wild and woolly" for your taste. You may not like the untamed look or coarse features some of them have. Keep in mind, though, that they may look untamed because they *are* untamed, as well as untended, and if placed in your landscape and given the same care you give other plants, they may take on more ornamental qualities.

Invasiveness

"Invasiveness" is a term that crops up with some regularity in Xeriscape landscaping, particularly because some of the most drought-tolerant species are pretty tough plants. Their toughness is one of the reasons they survive drought. But problems can occur when certain plants "escape cultivation." Removed from their original environment, along with the attendant pests, diseases, and competition from other nearby species, to a more hospitable one (that is, one with more rainfall or irrigation and less competition), these plants start to take over. Russian olive is an unfortunate example of this. Because the seeds are delicious to birds, they are spread far and wide in the droppings. they have escaped cultiva-

tion in Minnesota and other parts of the Midwest, crowding out native species and even taking over pastureland.

For the most part the problem is more serious in areas of the country where rainfall is higher, especially in the East and Midwest. But it can happen anywhere, even in your own yard. The best advice for avoiding this problem is to keep potentially invasive species confined to areas surrounded by pavement or some other physical barrier. This doesn't completely solve the problem, however, because, as in the case of the Russian olive, the species may be propagated by other "agents."

For those who don't want to contribute to the problem in the larger environment, either stick to native species *for your area* or do some research about what's known of the invasive potential of exotic species. (An exotic can be any plant that is native to another place, even some other part of the United States.) Bonnie Harper-Lore, program coordinator for the Midwest Regional Office of the National Wildflower Research Center, suggests checking with regional offices of the Nature Conservancy (a group of nonprofit organizations that buy up undisturbed land around the country in order to preserve habitat), which seem to be particularly in tune with this type of problem. A partial list of invasive species that have become a problem in different areas of the United States appears here.

This list was assembled from several sources. Where known, the chief type of plant community where it is troublesome is noted. Some of these plants are obvious weeds that you wouldn't be choosing for a landscape anyway, but others appear on plant lists in the Appendix for areas of the country where they aren't considered invasive. You may decide you don't want to include plants in your landscape that are invasive anywhere in the country to avoid accidentally contributing to the problem. The same may be true of those plants whose exact trouble areas are not yet known.

Plant community where invasive
  F = forest
  P = prairie, glade, or savannah
  W = wetland

Botanical Name	Common Name(s)	Plant Community	Where Troublesome
Acacia melanoxylon and many other *Acacia* species			Southwest
Ailanthus altissima	Tree-of-heaven	F, P	Eastern U.S.
Albizia julibrissin	Mimosa	P	
Bamboo			Many parts of the country
Bellis perennis	English daisy		Northwest
Berberis thunbergii	Japanese barberry		Northeast, Midwest
Bromus inermis	Smooth brome, Hungarian brome	P	Midwest
Carduus nutans	Musk thistle	P	All U.S.
Casuarina equisetifolia	She-oak, ironwood		Gulf states
Celastrus orbiculatus	Leafy spurge, Oriental bittersweet	P	Northeast, Midwest
Chrysanthemum leucanthemum	Oxeye daisy		Northwest
Cichorium intybus	Chicory		Many parts of the country
Cirsium arvense	Canada thistle	P, W	All U.S.
Coronilla varia	Crown vetch	P	Midwest
Cortaderia jubata	Pampas grass		Southwest
Cynodon dactylon	Common Bermudagrass		Southwest, Gulf states
Cytisus scoparius	Scotch broom		Northwest, most species invasive in Southwest
Daucus carota	Queen Anne's lace	P	
Digitalis purpurea	Foxglove		Northwest
Dipsacus sylvestris	Wild teasel	P	
Elaeagnus angustifolia	Russian olive	P	Midwest
E. umbellata	Autumn olive	F, P	Midwest
Equisetum hyemale	Horsetail		Many parts of the country
Eucalyptus spp. (many)			Southwest
Euonymus alata	Winged wahoo, Winged euonymus	F	
E. fortunei		F	
Euphorbia esula	Leafy spurge	P	
Festuca elatior	Tall fescue	P	
Galium verum	Yellow bedstraw		Northeast, Midwest
Glechoma hederacea	Ground ivy		Northwest
Hedera helix	English ivy		Southwest, Northwest
Hypericum calycinum	Aaron's beard, St.-John's-wort		Northwest
Ipomoea spp. (most species)	Morning glory		Many parts of the country
Juniperus virginiana	Eastern red cedar	P	
Lantana hybrids			Gulf states
Lespedeza cuneata	Sericea lespedeza	P	
Ligustrum vulgare	Privet	F	Eastern U.S.
Lonicera japonica	Japanese honeysuckle	F, P	Northeast, Midwest
L. maackii	Amur honeysuckle	F, P	
L. tatarica	Tatarian honeysuckle	F, P	Eastern U.S.
Lysimachia vulgaris	Garden loosestrife	W	

Botanical Name	Common Name(s)	Plant Community	Where Troublesome
Lythrum salicaria	Purple loosestrife	W	Northeast, Midwest
Maclura pomifera	Osage orange	F, P	
Melaleuca quinquenervia	Punk tree, Cajeput tree		Gulf states
Melilotus alba	White sweet clover	P	Midwest
M. officinalis	Yellow sweet clover	P	
Myriophyllum brasiliense	Water-feather	W	
Nasturtium officinale	Watercress	W	Many parts of the country
Pastinaca sativa	Wild parsnip	P	
Paulownia tomentosa	Princess tree	F	
Pennisetum setaceum	Fountain grass		Southwest
Phalaris arundinacea	Reed canary grass	P, W	Midwest
Phragmites communis	Reed	W	
Pinus nigra	Austrian pine	P	
P. sylvestris	Scotch pine	P	
P. thunbergii	Japanese black pine	P	
Poa compressa	Canada bluegrass	P	
P. pratensis	Kentucky bluegrass	P	
Polygonum cuspidatum	Japanese knotweed	P, W	Many parts of the country
Populus alba	White poplar	P	
Portulaca oleracea	Purslane		Many parts of the country
Potamogeton crispus	Pondweed	W	
Pteridium aquilinum	Bracken fern		Northwest
Pueraria lobata	Kudzu vine	F	Southeast
Rhamnus cathartica	Common buckthorn	F, P	Midwest
R. frangula	Alder buckthorn	W	
Robinia pseudoacacia	Black locust	F, P	Midwest
Rosa multiflora	Multiflora rose	F, P	Northeast, Midwest
Rubus procerus	Himalayan blackberry		Southwest, Northwest
Schinus terebinthifolius	Brazilian pepper tree		Gulf states
Solidago canadensis	Goldenrod		Northwest
Sorghum halepense	Johnson grass	P	
Tamarix gallica	Tamarisk	W	Western U.S.
Typha angustifolia	Narrow-leaved cattail	W	
T. latifolia	Cattail		Northwest
Ulmus procera	English elm	P	
U. pumila	Dwarf elm	P	
Verbascum thapsus	Common mullein	P	
Viburnum opulus	Guelder rose	F	
Vinca major	Large periwinkle	F	Eastern U.S., Northwest
V. minor	Common periwinkle	F	Eastern U.S.

Plant Communities

Plants live together in communities, the nature of which is strongly dependent on the topography, orientation toward the sun, microclimate of the immediate area, and soil. The *dominant plants* of each community are also dependent on these conditions. In eastern forests, for instance, the high amounts of rainfall are favorable to the extremely large trees, some as high as 150 feet, which are (or once were, until interference from humans) the dominant plants in the region. They tower over the forest floor, creating shade and intercepting some rainfall, which, in turn, affects the development of the *understory*, or *subdominant* layer, of shrubs and smaller trees.

By contrast, the Midwest and Great Plains receive substantially less rainfall, not enough to support massive trees, which gives prairie grasses the opportunity to dominate the vast, sunny regions.

Within these two extremes there will be much crossover. The south-facing slope in the forest will have open patches of meadow where the trees have lost the fight for dominance because too much moisture evaporates from that side of the hill. In the grassland a north-facing hill will not lose as much moisture in the shade, thus giving shrubs and trees a foothold.

After taking the time to understand the localities in which various types of plants thrive and interact with each other, it begins to dawn on us where the plants we want in our landscape should be sited. We see that it makes sense not to plant grass under a very shady tree because we know that where grasses are most successful they don't have to contend with shade. By the same token, plunking a tree down in the middle of the lawn keeps it from doing its best because it has to compete with the grass for water and nutrients. (Grass should be planted no closer than eighteen inches from a tree, according to one expert, and if you can give it the width of the tree's branch spread both will do better.)

Trees and shrubs that can endure blazing sun and other extremes of weather can provide protection for some of the more tender perennials and shrubs. Sections of your house, fences, and walls can all provide unexpected microclimates. A south-facing flower bed protected by an L-shaped house may still have petunias blooming at Thanksgiving, even in cold, wind-battered Wyoming. (Mine did.)

Trying to mesh this "naturalistic" side of planning with the more "practical" concerns presented in the planning and design chapter may seem an overwhelming task at first. It's not, really, because such a wide variety of plants can be used for Xeriscape landscaping, and because naturalistic planning is really very practical, too. It will pay long-term dividends in terms of water and maintenance saved. It takes observation and thought, but eventually it all falls into place.

In choosing plants we also consider their ability to withstand cold. Zone maps in seed and plant catalogs refer to this criterion in the form of the United States Department of Agriculture (USDA) Plant Hardiness Zone Map (see page 137). These zones tie together areas where minimum annual temperatures are consistent. (They do not give reference to soil type, rainfall, or summer heat.) One is advised not to use plants that haven't traditionally been able to survive the lowest temperature in the zone. However, Panayoti Kelaidis, alpine plant specialist at the Denver Botanic Garden, feels that cold hardiness with respect to perennials has been over-emphasized. In Denver and other parts of the country he's visited, he has seen the smaller plants, particularly the more drought-tolerant ones, survive in much colder areas than they're "supposed to."

In Xeriscape gardening we also look for plants that can survive the minimum amount of precipitation a region can expect. A plant that can survive both drought and extremes of weather ranks among the truly tough.

This is where Xeriscape gardening becomes fascinating. It's a challenge to reproduce the conditions in which a plant can thrive, but it's also exhilarating to see a plant perform far beyond its expected limits.

Two rosebushes grow in my backyard on the west side of a fence downhill from the lawn. They've not been fed, watered except by runoff from the grass, or pruned beyond cutting off a few blooms in four summers, and they've endured bitter cold spells without being mulched. Yet each year they produce beautiful blooms on schedule.

The exciting results of a few years of experimentation with drought tolerance in plants seem to indicate that many, many more plants are drought tolerant than was previously believed. Often they have just never been given the chance to show what they can do, because gardeners are so addicted to watering.

You might like to experiment with plants, to see what they will endure, before you begin watering. You may break new ground for Xeriscape gardening. You might want to limit these trials to smaller, less expensive plants, and be more conservative with costly trees and shrubs. Here it is especially important to consult reliable local sources of plant information who may have many years of experience with how local conditions of climate affect plants. Be prepared to accept that some plants may be pushed beyond their limits and may die. It happens in nature, too.

SOME OUTSTANDING PLANT GROUPS FOR XERISCAPE GARDENING

What follows is a discussion of several categories of low-water-demand plants. My purpose here is not to reinvent the wheel—that is, to give exhaustive directions for how to grow perennials, wildflowers, ornamental grasses, etc., since dozens and dozens of excellent books provide that kind of detailed, basic information. Instead, I've tried to answer my own questions about how to incorporate some of these low-water-using plant groups into a Xeriscape design, give some rudimentary information about how to raise them, and bring out any points wherein the raising of them for Xeriscape gardening differs from the traditional advice.

Ornamental Grasses

Ornamental grasses are a natural for Xeriscape gardens because they not only require little water (if well chosen for the site) but also little maintenance. They need no deadheading (removal of spent flowers to promote continued bloom) or mowing; they are very pest- and disease-free; and too much fertilizer causes them to grow too quickly, spread in search of nutrients, and die out in the middle. They accommodate a wide range of soil and climatic conditions.

Grasses are one of the most successful plant families in the world. There are grasses in nearly every environment, from hard-baked desert to soggy marshes, from the tropics to the polar regions, from the seashore to the highest snow-covered mountains.

There are over 10,000 named species of grasses in the world, and except for ones that are commonly considered weedy invaders of turfgrass, many of them, when viewed individually, make lovely ornamental grasses. This is where appreciation of

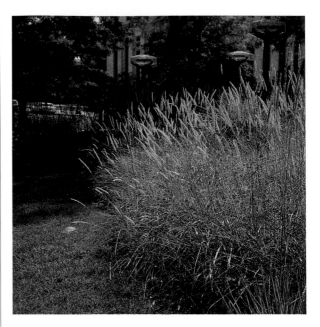

Despite the delicacy of individual Pennisetum incomptum *plants massed here, they lend a solid architectural element to this design. (Design: Oehme, van Sweden & Associates)*

native species comes into play. The grasses that have flourished unnoticed and neglected in abandoned areas, roadsides, and waste places might look elegant sorted and massed in your landscape. And their seeds are free and easy to gather.

In general, species from the family Gramineae (true grasses) will be most drought tolerant, or will be found in the driest regions of the world. Their needs are simple—just fertile, well-drained soil in an open, sunny location. Bamboos and the grasslike plants in the *Carex* (sedges) and *Juncus* (true rushes) genera, in that order, need progressively more moisture in the soil. The *Luzula* genus (woodrushes) is more adaptable, tolerating wet feet next to a stream and some drought if established in rich soil under trees.

Annual grasses are grown from seed each year. Seeds can be started indoors or out and will take three to four weeks to germinate. Plant thickly for a good stand when starting outdoors. It's important to mark the area planted with annual grasses because their seedlings may be indistinguishable from the weeds that will crop up, too, and you don't want to risk pulling them up by mistake. Seeds may be broadcast or planted in shallow rows drilled in a crisscross pattern. Cover them very lightly with soil or fine sand and give them temporary protection to prevent them from being eaten by birds. Chicken wire or black thread stretched across the bed between stakes may be protection enough.

Thin the seedlings when they are one to two inches tall. The spacing depends on the ultimate height of the plants; grasses up to two feet tall might be spaced at six inches and taller ones up to twelve inches. At the end of the season gather seeds from some of the plants for the next year's planting. None of the ornamental grasses are hybrids, so they will grow consistently from year to year. Store these seeds and any others you have in a cool, dry place such as the refrigerator.

Perennial grasses are slow-growing. They may take five to seven years to achieve maturity if you start them from seeds, and two to three years if you buy nursery-grown plants that have been propagated by division, which they usually are. When planning, keep in mind the ultimate size of the plant because it may be considerably larger than the plant you start with.

Most perennial grasses prefer full sun and fertile, well-drained soil. Plant grasses in early rather than late spring so they will have more moisture to help them get started. If you're planting grasses for a massed effect, plant them roughly the same distance apart that they grow in height. If you want the entire form of a plant to show, give them about twice as much room.

Prune larger perennial grasses in early spring before new growth begins to within six inches of the ground. Divide clumps if they begin to look dead in the center and replant the pieces to give them more room, or give extra pieces away.

A list of popular ornamental grasses appears in the Appendix, grouped into dry, average, and moist soil categories, with some grasses appearing in more than one group. Local experts may be able to suggest dozens more possibilities, along with advice on locating seeds and/or plants.

Perennials and Annuals

One of the delightful surprises of the Xeriscape experience is that flower beds can be incorporated into any Xeriscape design. With the right soil preparation and an understanding of water needs, they can be water-efficient, needing far less water per square foot than highly maintained turf.

Wilbur Davis, whose early Texas Xeriscape landscape is discussed in the section on Texas, has a simple and satisfying philosophy: "If part of my lawn starts giving me trouble, I just turn it into a flower bed."

If ornamental grasses are the darling of the landscape design world right now, perennials are the darling of the flower gardening world. Praised for their toughness, tenacity, refined beauty, and dependability, perennials are revered and loved by gardeners everywhere, especially those who aspire to elegance. On the other hand, try to talk perennials to an annuals fan and you may get: "Oh yes, per*enni*als. They take forever to cre-e-e-p across the landscape.

The good news is that there's no real need for this *versus* because both annuals and perennials have their place in a Xeriscape garden. Annuals are often well able to withstand the extremes of heat and drought that can occur in a summer, while

A mixed planting of yellow flag iris (Iris pseudacorus), *cornflowers* (Centaurea cyanus), *and* Astilbe thunbergii *makes a striking visual composition at the National Arboretum in Washington, D.C.*

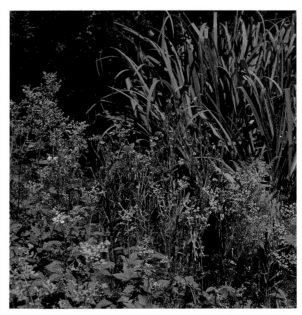

research at Colorado State University indicates that many perennials are as able to live without supplemental watering in their second year and beyond as trees and shrubs.

Both have an endless variety of flower and foliage colors and textures from which to choose, especially when you include native plants, and there are flowers for every condition of soil moisture, from desert-dry to boggy. Until recent years perennials have had the edge when it came to availability of more unusual species in bedding plants, but growers seem to be responding to public interest by propagating a wider variety of annuals.

The annuals listed in the Appendix are divided into cool- and warm-season species. Cool-season annuals grow fastest in the cooler weather of spring, fall, or winter (in subtropical climates), while warm-season annuals need summer heat to flower and thrive. In temperate climates, plant cool-season annuals as early in the spring as possible; the warm-season annuals should be planted later. In mild climates, plant cool-season annuals in the fall for winter flowering and warm-season annuals in spring.

Bulbs
·······

Spring-flowering bulbs are drought evaders and thus make good plants for Xeriscape gardens. In general, if conditions get too tough for them, not only in terms of drought, but also heat, they will shut down (go dormant) and survive. Some species of iris, especially bearded iris, are very popular for Xeriscape designs in many climates, particularly the Rocky Mountains and Great Plains.

(To keep the stand of flowers from one bulb increasing each year, make sure the bulb has adequate moisture and sunlight during its time of ripening, that period between flowering and when the leaves yellow and die down. During this time the bulb is storing food for next year's growth, and it's very important not to cut off the leaves while they're still green.)

Early spring bulbs such as crocuses, grape hyacinths, and daffodils can be scattered through lawns (called naturalizing) for a striking effect, as long as the plants will have ripened and the foliage

died down before it's time to start mowing the grass. This works especially well in conjunction with warm-season grasses such as buffalograss that don't green up till late spring. The flowers are set off by the gold color of the grass and the leaves give the lawn some spring greenery, so the lawn isn't in such strong contrast to the already green cool-season lawns that may surround it.

Planting

Annuals may survive in relatively poor soil, but for perennials, soil preparation is the single most important factor in getting them off to a good start, in part because they will be in place several years and it's difficult to improve the soil under existing plants, and in part because few perennials do well in heavy, poorly drained or unaerated soils. In addition to adding goodly quantities of nutrients, the efforts of double digging will pay off with more handsome plants the first year.

Double digging is accomplished by digging a trench one spade deep and about a foot wide at one end of your bed. The soil is put into a wheelbarrow, or carried one shovelful at a time, to the other end of the bed and deposited there. Back at the trench, spread any soil amendments you plan to use (at a rate to cover just the trench area) in the trench and mix it into the soil to another spade's depth. Spread the soil amendment over the next foot-wide area, and mix it in while also turning the soil over to rest in the previous trench, now just one spade deep again. Continue this process till you get to the far end of the bed. The soil first dug out at the other end of the bed becomes the top layer of the trench at this end.

This process takes a lot of work, especially if your soil is hard to break up, but perennial plants will achieve about twice the size the first year that they ordinarily would. Note: With all this digging in your future, you may want to invest in a narrow, pointed spade if you have particularly rocky soil, even little rocks.

When I'm planting a small area of flowers, I mix hydrated, water-absorbing polymer over the bed and till it in with the organic material. For flower beds a good rate to put in is one and a half quarts (hydrated) per square foot, tilled in six inches deep.

This is equivalent to three teaspoons dry crystals per square foot, or one dry pound (two and a half cups) per hundred square feet. Each plant also gets a handful of hydrated polymer mixed with the immediate backfill. This gives the plants a ready water supply and makes it less critical to keep watering regularly the first few days. For larger beds the dry polymer can be broadcast and incorporated.

Watering

When planting, either water the plants gently and thoroughly after setting them in place, or fill each planting hole with water and let it drain, then set in the seedling or plant and water a little extra for the sides. If the seedlings don't have much soil attached to them at planting time, check two or three times a day to make sure they haven't wilted during the first three days. After that, stick a finger into the soil up to the big knuckle every few days to check for soil moisture. If it's dry that far down, apply an inch of water (approximately two-thirds of a gallon per square foot) and don't water again till it's dry again. This will take into account rain doing some of your watering, and will let the soil moisture, not the calendar, dictate the watering frequency.

After the first three weeks or so you can check less often unless there's a particularly hot, dry spell, and in most parts of the country (all but perhaps the most arid sections) you can pretty much discontinue watering after midsummer.

The Colorado State University Horticulture Department did a revealing study with several annual flower species on the effects of watering on flowering and plant size. The test group received no additional watering above normal rainfall after the midpoint of the growing season (mid-July). The area receives only seven to ten inches of rainfall during the growing season, with the highest amount in May (our summer showers tend to be brief and intense). The group that was watered regularly showed increased plant size and flowering, but only an average of ten percent above that of the unwatered group.

I gave all my flowers the acid test last summer, watering them only a couple of times after the end of June. My yard is fairly protected from drying winds but gets a full measure of sun, and the only plants that ever even drooped mildly were the red annual salvias. The rest—blue salvia, cleome, celosia, nierembergia, cosmos, portulaca, stocks, linaria (all annuals) and purple coneflower, coreopsis, rudbeckia, variegated thyme, hardy ice plant, chrysanthemum, santolina, chocolate flower, pinks, and achillea (all perennials)—did fine.

Wildflowers
....

America is rediscovering wildflowers as a carefree alternative to traditional bedding plants. Wildflowers are ideal where a more natural, less formal appearance is desired. They also can provide season-long color with sometimes little or no additional water and maintenance than normally required for more formal gardens. A proper mix of wildflowers will provide peak flowering from April to frost. There are over 6,000 species of wildflowers in the United States. Like grasses, there are wildflowers for every region and for every conceivable combination of soil and climate.

Wildflowers are given star billing at the Brandywine Conservatory in Pennsylvania; all the medians in the parking and entrance area are packed with dozens of species so that something is in bloom throughout the growing season. Spike gayfeather (Liatris spicata) *is shown here.*

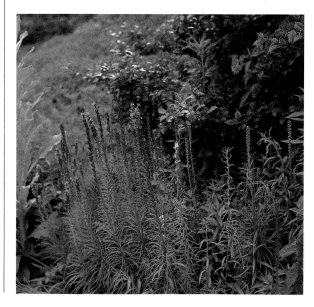

In some areas of the country where rainfall is ample, certain wildflowers grow so prolifically that they are considered "weeds." (The polite term is "escaped cultivation." Having seen poppy mallow—*Callirhoe involucrata*—(also called wine cups) plants trailing around my grandparents' hardscrabble Kansas farm on many childhood vacations, it never occurred to me to use them in a landscape until I saw them looking lovely in the Xeriscape demonstration garden at the Wichita (Kansas) Botanica. They're drought tolerant, make a good ground cover, and have beautiful flute-shaped flowers, similar to those of morning glories, in a stylish magenta shade.

For Xeriscape gardening, give those sturdy, familiar wildflowers a second look, for they are often the ones that demonstrate superior survivability and drought resistance. And don't reject a particular wildflower just because you've seen it around too often to suit you. Take time to consider its good qualities with respect to lower water use and maintenance, and look at its bloom from a different perspective.

Remember also that the untended, straggly wildflower growing by the road may have little resemblance to the propagated plant of the same species you raise in your yard, cared for and carefully situated. Properly managed and confined, wildflowers can lend charm to any landscape.

The reality for most wildflower gardeners is that the species they long to grow are the rarer or more temperamental (in terms of establishing them) types. The demand for native wildflowers has risen so much that unscrupulous growers are digging up plants from the wild to sell, in some cases collecting them to the point of near-extinction. The National Wildflower Research Center (NWRC) in Austin, Texas, explains that while most native plants that are available commercially are propagated, some, such as the pink lady's slipper (*Cypripedium acaule*), have never been successfully propagated on a commercial scale. All of those being commercially sold are wild-collected. An estimated 100,000 of these plants were wild-collected and sold in a recent year by one supplier, despite the sad fact that this species rarely survives being transplanted.

When buying native plants the NWRC suggests that you make sure the nursery you buy from propagates their own plants and doesn't dig them from the wild. Some claim to have nursery-grown stock, but may have dug them from the wild and potted them for a short time before selling them.

Ask questions about how the plants were propagated. If the nursery can't tell you how, then they were probably wild-collected. Retail outlets should also be held accountable for the plants they sell, and if *they* can't tell you how the plants were raised, find a more reputable source. (For $2 and a self-addressed, stamped envelope you can obtain a list of sources for propagated native plants in your area from the Wildflower Center Clearinghouse (NWRC, 2600 FM 973 North, Austin, TX 78725-4201). The Wildflower Center also provides lists of recommended native species for each state.

Wildflower Culture

Most popular woodland flowers prefer a very light soil, and particularly dislike compacted roots. This makes sense when you examine their native soil—hundreds of years of leaf mulch and loosely packed ground litter (leaves and dead flowers plus twigs and branches). Add to that decaying animal matter such as droppings and occasional carcasses of forest animals. The result is almost pure humus, what we strive to re-create with our compost piles. When we consider that common garden soil may have only five percent or less organic matter, we begin to see what we're up against. Fortunately, most forest wildflower roots are not particularly deep, usually no more than twelve inches, so you can overexcavate the soil for a wildflower bed if you have particularly inhospitable soil.

Humus-rich soil is almost constantly moist because of its tremendous capacity to store water. Woodland soil holds up to ten times its weight in water, while ordinary garden soil may hold only fifteen to thirty percent of its weight. To grow any kind of woodland wildflower, even those of the Rocky Mountains, you will have to re-create this environment.

You may want to make some leaf mold as described in the soil improvements chapter and use as much as possible when developing soil pockets

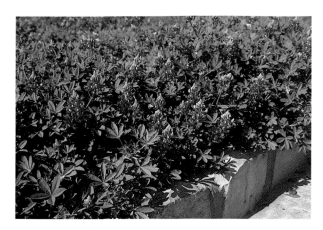

Wildflowers are a natural for Xeriscape gardens, whether used in a prairie garden or as a flowering annual, as is the Texas bluebonnet (Lupinus texensis) *in this photo. (Photo: Doug Welsh)*

for woodland flowers. Another possibility is to incorporate a higher than normal rate of hydro-gel (see page 44) to the area where the wildflowers will be grown.

Wildflowers that grow in meadows and fields will generally grow in more "average" garden soil. The soils in these environments are lighter than the very heavy soils of semiarid lands and poorer than the humus-rich soils of woodlands. Many of the species native to these soils, such as purple coneflowers (*Echinacea purpurea*), sunflowers (*Helianthus* spp.), gaillardias, gayfeather (*Liatris* spp.) and salvias are common garden favorites.

Alpine flowers thrive in rocky soil because in their native environment smaller soil particles are washed downhill by rainfall and snowmelt. To succeed with alpine flowers you need an extremely gravelly soil with a small amount of humus of a depth sufficient to meet the needs of those deeply rooting plants while allowing for drainage below the roots. A planting could be as deep as twelve to twenty-four inches. Free-standing berms are often constructed as a home for alpine wildflowers to ensure proper drainage, and because it's easier to build a berm than to excavate a deep soil area.

Planning a Wildflower Garden

If your site is overgrown with existing trees and shrubs and you want to create a wild woodland garden, you may want to keep selected mature trees and remove weak or diseased ones and seedlings that will crowd the flowers. Retain some groupings of underbrush for a naturalized layered effect.

Since wildflowers like loose soil, try not to step on the ground after you've prepared it. If your wildflower beds are wide enough that you can't reach all the flowers from the edge in order to tend them, create a path with stepping-stones or small gravel set among the plants so they're always visible, to let you and your visitors know where it's safe to step.

Choose a site that receives at least six hours of sunlight a day and a minimum of foot traffic. Ultimately a large wildflower area is more effective than a small one, but you may want to start small and spread the establishment of a large wildflower garden over several years. It's easy to underestimate how much weeding will be necessary. *Remember, you will no longer be able to use broadleaf "weed controls" in your yard because they will have disastrous consequences for your wildflowers.*

If your wildflower bed will be located next to a lawn area and you live in a part of the country where soil is acid, so that you must regularly put lime on the lawn to keep its soil neutral, you may want to install a nine-inch-wide edging set so the top is flush with the ground to keep the alkalizing lime from harming the wildflowers.

Obtaining Plants

Because some wildflowers may take several years to flower and produce seed, it's best to consult a wildflower gardening encyclopedia as to the best species or form to buy, and whether it grows best from seed, cultivated nursery plants, or by division of established rootstock.

Your best bet is to buy nursery-grown plants because they are likely to be tougher and more tolerant of transplanting than plants found in the wild. Unfortunately, the number of varieties available may be limited.

If the wild plants you've chosen are amenable to transplanting, it is okay to move them from a friend's property or from a property that is going to be cleared and built on. Always obtain permission before collecting plants. It's considered unethical to take plants from the wild under any other circumstances, and in some states it's illegal unless you have a native plant handler's permit.

You can also propagate your own plants from seed, division of rootstock, or cuttings. This is inexpensive and gives you the widest choice of plants, but it is time-consuming and requires specialized knowledge or study about each plant species that you are propagating.

Planting a Wildflower "Meadow"

In nature most wildflower meadows include more grasses than flowers, but you may want a swath of wildflowers only, similar to a cultivated flower garden, but more random and natural-looking. Fastest results are obtained by plugging individual plants into cleared ground. A dense mat of wildflowers, known as wildflower sod, is available commercially in the West. It gives instant color, flowering the first year, but is expensive for large-scale plantings. Experience has shown that after the second growing season one or two of the fifteen or more species originally present in the wildflower sod come to dominate the planting, with the rest being crowded out. This may be okay for you. If you want long-term variety, though, a better use for the wildflower sod might be to separate the plants and set them out individually with six to twelve inches in between (vary the spacing for a more natural look). This gives the less aggressive species a better chance to establish themselves and survive competition from the dominant plants.

The same phenomenon results from many commercially available "wildflower mixes." They often include annual wildflower species to give blooms the first year while the perennial species are becoming established. The annual species may or may not reseed themselves, depending on how much competition they get from aggressive perennials or the ever-present weeds. (In one experiment at the Denver Botanic Garden a few years ago, an area was actually fumigated—to kill *everything*, including weed seeds—then planted with a supposedly weed-free "wildflower mix." The resulting wildflower meadow still had generous quantities of weeds in it, suggesting that it's virtually impossible to keep weed seeds out of mixes—or even seeds of individual species, for that matter.)

Wildflower mixes often include species that may or may not be native to your area. This is not the worst thing in the world that can happen. The intent is usually to create a colorful palette of easy-to-grow wildflowers (some of the most popular species in wildflower mixes are practically "gardener-proof"—*anyone* can grow them) and to give quick, if not always permanent, results. However, if you want a true native mix of wildflowers, research what grows in your area and purchase seeds of individual species from a reputable seed firm. Try to select a minimum of five perennial and five annual species.

Rick Brune, who writes and lectures from personal experience on the establishment of prairie gardens (his explanation of how to re-create a prairie garden appears in the next section), gives this "recipe" for starting wildflowers from seed. He has tried many different methods and has found this to be the best:

1. Clear the ground with a sod cutter (assuming it previously had turf), water, and wait for the remaining rhizomes to sprout. Dig them up as they appear. This process may take three to four weeks. Hoe or dig up weeds that appear.

2. Unless your soil is exceptionally poor, don't add organic soil amendments as many wildflowers

A small, sloping front yard is partly filled with wildflowers in this Colorado garden (which also appears on the cover), giving visitors a warm welcome.

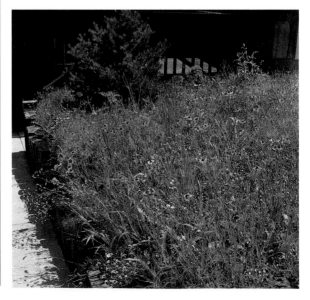

are adapted to poor soil. Don't till the ground unless it's very compacted as this will increase weed germination.

3. Rake random furrows in the soil no more than ½ inch deep. Either broadcast the wildflower seed mix (which is rather wasteful and contributes to the crowding-out process) or lightly scatter seeds of individual species in groups spread randomly over the area, with some overlap. This will give the less aggressive species a slightly better chance to establish themselves in colonies. (You may also want to select species from the list in the Appendix that are not among the more dominant ones.)

4. Cover the seeds with a thin layer of soil (¼ to ½ inch) and tamp lightly with the back of a rake. For fastest germination and establishment, water gently once or twice a day if it doesn't rain for two to three weeks. (Germination takes ten to twenty days.)

An alternative to the first step is to kill the grass with glysophate in midsummer and leave it to rot over the winter. The dead vegetation can be tilled into the soil in the spring. You can supposedly plant in a sprayed area just two weeks after applying the herbicide, but small-print warnings about many species that can't be planted in the area for six to twelve months indicate that there may be other species, including wildflowers, that would be sensitive to the chemical.

Tom Cramer of Wildseed, Inc. (Eagle Lake, Texas), recommends another method.

1. Mow existing vegetation as close to the ground as possible.

2. Rake and remove clippings (the drawback to this is that it removes the nutrients that are in the clippings, too). Rake or hoe shallowly (½ inch maximum).

3. Mix seed with a carrier such as potting soil or sand (four parts inert material to one part seed) to help distribute the seed evenly, and broadcast the mix over the area.

4. Rake lightly to promote good seed-soil contact.

5. Water if it doesn't rain.

Cramer recommends planting in the autumn in the southern and western parts of the country. Seeds will sprout and establish plants before going dormant. Warm-season grasses are winding down their growing season, so they will provide less competition, and seasonal rains often occur at this time. The plants will reemerge in early spring and be six inches high before the warm-season grass starts to grow.

In northern and northeastern parts of the country bitterly cold winter is too damaging to the new seedlings, so early spring planting is recommended. Cramer cautions that this overseeding method won't work in grasses that grow during the winter, such as fescue and annual ryegrass. Since Kentucky bluegrass follows much the same growing pattern as fescue and ryegrass, it may be that the method described earlier will be more successful for establishing wildflowers where bluegrass has grown.

Realize that patience is necessary no matter what method you use. The seeds may wash away if it rains heavily, or may be eaten by birds. (If you have a slope, build dikes of small rocks across the slope, removing them later after the flowers are somewhat established, or put down plastic netting designed to prevent erosion.) The perennial wildflowers will probably not flower the first year. Count on it taking up to three years for your wildflower garden to be

Wildflower gardens take many forms. In this October scene both the gaillardia (Gaillardia grandiflora) *and yarrow* (Achillea spp.) *have gone to seed, yet still have a dramatic, colorful presence.*

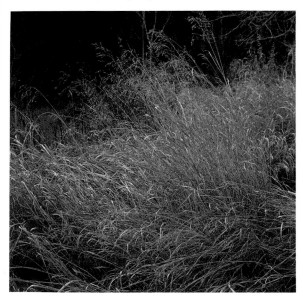

well established and effective. A short list of popular wildflowers appears in the Appendix.

Prairie Gardens
....

Growing up in the West, seeing only the grazed-over desiccation of the former prairie and grassland, and never being particularly inspired by photographs of reconstructed prairie, which fail to do them justice, I was unprepared for the lushness and splendor of the reconstructed tallgrass, midgrass, and shortgrass prairies at the Denver Botanic Garden that I saw on a recent Indian summer visit.

The "understory" grasses were thick on the ground, and the taller grasses ranged over them in an endless weaving of delicate gold silhouettes. In ten seconds I came to see why devotees of prairie gardens labor patiently, sometimes for years, to re-create this scene.

Prairies are mixtures of grasses and wildflowers in varying ratios, but usually about sixty to ninety percent grasses. They once covered thousands of square miles of the central United States, blanket-ing the ground in what truly must have been a blaze of glory. We can try to approximate how they might have looked, though we can never really replicate the vegetative history represented by this very stable and complex ecosystem.

Once established, which may take three years or more, prairie gardens are model Xeriscape landscapes; they are drought tolerant, low maintenance, and require no watering, fertilizing, or mowing. They are an ideal way to take advantage of a full-sun environment (this is what they prefer) and to attract birds and butterflies. Native grasses grow naturally on soils moderately low in nitrogen and potassium. They often tolerate soils high in clay and slow to drain. Since prairies are found in climates that get lots of winter precipitation, but not as much in summer, they can usually be maintained without supplemental irrigation.

Although there are twenty-five different kinds of prairies that developed with the advance and retreat of each ice age, they are grouped into three main categories. Tallgrass prairies covered the eastern part of the American grasslands, where higher rainfall amounts supported larger plants, some as high

Real prairie may have up to fifteen flowering plants in a square yard, but you don't realize it because they don't all bloom at once. This peaceful scene is from the shortgrass prairie reconstruction at the Denver Botanic Garden. In bloom are Indian paintbrush (Castilleja integra), *gaillardia* (Gaillardia grandiflora), *and prairie coneflower* (Ratibida columnifera). *The small shrub is rabbitbrush* (Chrysothamnus nauseosus).

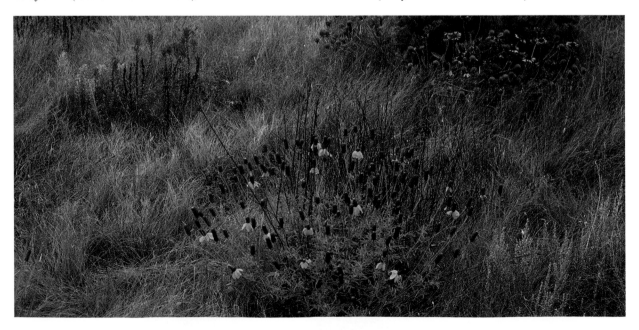

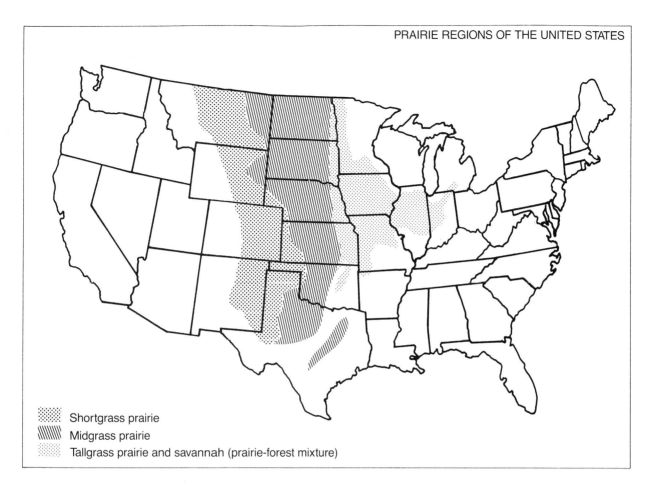

PRAIRIE REGIONS OF THE UNITED STATES

Shortgrass prairie
Midgrass prairie
Tallgrass prairie and savannah (prairie-forest mixture)

as eight to nine feet. Typical dominant species included big bluestem (*Andropogon gerardii*), Indiangrass (*Sorghastrum nutans*), and switch grass (*Panicum virgatum*). Re-creating a tallgrass prairie may include seeding or setting out individual plants at intervals. Weeds will probably grow in the spaces between the plants for several years until the grasses become tall enough to shade them out.

Farther west were midgrass prairies dominated by grasses about knee-high such as needle-and-thread (*Stipa comata*), little bluestem (*Schizachyrium scoparium*), and western wheatgrass (*Agropyron smithii*). Midgrass prairies contain large quantities of needle grasses, which have sharp seeds that lie on the ground from mid-July to about mid-August until they have burrowed into the ground, making it difficult to walk barefoot through the grass. This may make those species less desirable for home use unless you don't plan to walk on the grass anyway. One is also cautioned that the species *Stipa virigila* reseeds rather aggressively

and may end up dominating your small prairie garden.

There is debate over whether shortgrass prairie is really a climax prairie or simply the result of overgrazing, but in any case a blue grama grass (*Bouteloua gracilis*)–buffalograss (*Buchloe dactyloides*) prairie is fairly simple to re-create because of seed availability and the ability of the grasses to form a dense cover.

Weed Ordinances

Many communities have weed ordinances that prohibit grasses from being grown at greater than twelve, eight, or sometimes even six inches tall. These were originally designed to protect citizens from the health hazards and inconvenience of having "weed-seed factories" in the form of neglected properties within established neighborhoods.

Although a weed ordinance can't be used to force someone else's aesthetic standard on you, the government *does* have the right to make sure your property is not a fire or health hazard. With a tallgrass prairie, especially, it's important to protect your property and your neighbors' properties from fire. This can be done easily by keeping a mowed swath between your garden and house as well as around the perimeter of your property. Noxious plants like ragweed and poison ivy should be pulled out, as should European weeds like dandelions and chicory that may spread to neighbors' yards.

If neighbors object to your efforts to re-create a grass prairie, you may have to go to court to explain that your yard is indeed well cared for and that you feel your grasses and prairie wildflowers are far less of a hazard than the barrage of chemicals poured on a typical lawn.

In the Midwest the use of prairie in the landscape is becoming more accepted. Several cities have amended their ordinances to allow for "naturalistic plantings." You may save yourself some trouble by confining your prairie-raising project to your backyard. Unless you live in a particularly rustic neighborhood, it *is* fairly tricky to find a way to blend a whole yard of prairie grasses into the surroundings. One option is to confine the prairie to a large, curv-

ing central bed outlined smartly with gravel or bark, and surrounded to the edge of the property with either more of the same or a continuation of the turfgrass common to the neighborhood. You could also limit yourself to a more understandable swath of wildflowers in the front yard, or let the prairie fill in a small space with a built-in boundary such as an area cut off by the approach sidewalk, or an island planting bed.

Stand Establishment

This plain-spoken technical term simply means the successful establishment of a good stand of whatever you're trying to raise, be it native grass, wildflowers, or a crop. In this section are several suggestions for stand establishment of prairie gardens, especially a shortgrass prairie.

Rick Brune says that the single most important factor in successful prairie gardening is weed control FIRST! If you don't take that step, you'll have an ongoing and perhaps overwhelming battle trying to establish prairie grasses and wildflowers in the midst of the more aggressive weeds. The number of weeds you have in the existing ground cover governs the technique for starting the garden.

Method 1: Few weeds present. If you have a fairly weed-free sod, except for a few dandelions, you can rent a sod cutter and remove the sod, which has the advantage of removing many of the weed seeds as well. Since buffalograss and blue grama grass are adapted to poor soil, the fact that you are also removing the richest layer of humus is not a large concern.

Be sure to remove all rhizomes (runners) of bluegrass or quackgrass in the remaining soil. If you are not sure they are all out, water and wait two weeks, digging out any grasses that sprout. Then rototill and plant. Buffalograss and blue grama grass like lumpy soil for establishment, so the only further soil preparation is leveling the seedbed. Brune doesn't add any organic soil amendments when establishing a native grass stand because, though organic amendments might help the plants become established faster, they then tend not to be as durable and long-lived. Organic amendments also encourage weed growth. The addition of fertilizers is *not* recommended. Blue grama grass reacts nega-

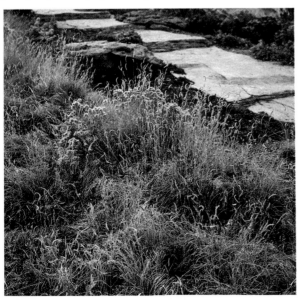

Blue grama grass (Bouteloua gracilis) *still hits a striking note in mid-November at the Denver Botanic Gardens. A prairie garden is effectively set off (and viewed from) a pathway of slate, pebbles, or other material.*

tively to nitrogen, and phosphorus and potassium deficiencies are rare in most soils.

You can plant wildflower seedlings started indoors (more cost-effective than broadcasting seeds) at the same time as you sow the grass seed if you have a fairly weed-free base. To give them a head start on competition from the grass, lay out six-inch cardboard circles or bottoms of tin cans where you will plant the flowers and plant the grass seed around them. The advantage of planting wildflowers with the grass seed is that it gives you a blooming prairie sooner and everything can be watered together. The disadvantage is that the only option for weed control will be hand-weeding because the herbicides such as glysophate that target broad-leaved weeds will kill the wildflowers.

Either spread wildflowers randomly for a natural look or group them in clumps for patches of color. Real prairies may have up to fifteen flowering plants per square yard, but it's hard to realize that because they're not all in bloom at once. With a large prairie project you may not be able to manage more than about four plants per square yard, though more can be added later by digging a six-inch-wide and six-inch-deep planting hole through the grass sod for each plant.

You can plant prairie grass seeds in fall or spring. With fall planting the seeds will germinate at the earliest possible time in the spring, but may be eaten by birds or washed away in the meantime. Furthermore, cool-season weeds will probably germinate before the warm-season grasses.

Brune has found planting between May 1 and mid-June to be most successful. Later than that and the heat and drought of the summer may kill many of the seedlings. The planting time might vary depending on your location, so check with your County Extension Service. Spring planting gives you one more chance at weed control.

Buffalograss is planted ½ to ¾ inch deep. Brune recommends making furrows about an inch deep and six to twelve inches apart. Broadcast the seed and rake it in across the furrows. This way more of the seed is buried deeper than if you just raked it in. Blue grama grass can be broadcast over the area just seeded with buffalograss and raked in, too.

Blue grama is usually more abundant than buffalograss in a shortgrass prairie, a typical ratio being about six to one. Blue grama seed is much lighter than buffalograss seed, so a pound contains many more seeds. Planting half a pound of blue grama and one pound of buffalograss gives a ratio of eighteen to one, which is close enough for this purpose, and produces a turf thick enough to crowd out weeds the second year, if not the first.

Buy blue-green buffalograss seeds because they are treated to reduce germination time from up to three years to seven to ten days.

Other shortgrass prairie species such as side oats grama may be overseeded for variety, but it's not necessary. After completing the seeding, rent a roller and roll the entire seedbed. Planting wildflowers is done after rolling and before watering. It's okay to walk on the newly seeded area; just try not to disturb the seedbed except where you plant.

After several years of following the traditional technique of sprouting wildflower seeds in soilless medium, then transplanting them to another container before finally transplanting them outdoors, it occurred to Brune that the second step might be unnecessary since most of the plants in question are adapted to a short growing season and tough conditions. He now transplants many prairie wildflowers directly into the ground in the seedling stage and has very good success. This method would probably work for wildflower gardens as well.

Establishing a good cover of prairie grasses requires as much watering as a bluegrass lawn. They must be kept constantly moist for the first three weeks, which may mean watering several times a day if it's windy and hot. After that watering can be reduced to every two to three days, tapering to one deep watering once a week the first year. Avoid producing drought stress in the plants, as evidenced by wilting, rolling leaves, or a gray appearance in the plant. From the second year, you should be able to eliminate watering, or at most water two to three times a year.

Method 2: Heavy weeds. If you have a heavy or unknown weed problem, go through several cycles of watering to germinate seeds after removing the sod, then hoe to control the weeds and get some indication of the severity of the problem. If it looks hopeless, you might consider spraying glysophate to kill the bluegrass and annual weeds, and damage the bindweed and thistle (see page 67).

If you don't want to use the broadcast herbicide method, you can either plan on doing a tremendous amount of hand-weeding until the prairie grasses fill in, or till the ground every two to three weeks as new weed crops appear during the growing season. Soil solarization (see page 67) did not work well in Denver when Brune tried the technique; because of the cool nights, not enough heat was generated to kill the seeds, but it may work in other parts of the country where nights stay warmer.

Bindweed (*Convolvulus arvensis*) and thistle (*Cirsium arvense* and *C. vulgare*) are very difficult to eradicate. Hand-pulling bindweed is said to stimulate it to further growth, and thistle will grow back if only a tiny amount of root is left in. You may have to resort to spot-killing these pests, but even if you only want to hand-weed make sure you don't let them overrun your planting area.

You may want to plant grass seed the second year (after your year of weed control) and wait another year to plant wildflowers. This leaves the option open for spraying for weeds during the grass-growing year, if your problem is severe. The main disadvantage is that then you will have to water the wildflowers individually when you plant them, and help them compete for light and nutrients by keeping runners from the grass out of their planting areas.

Proceed with seeding, rolling, and watering grass seed as described and add the wildflowers the following spring.

Seeds of some prairie grasses and flowers have a fairly low germination rate. They have evolved many protective mechanisms to ensure that their seeds won't germinate until conditions are just right. In some cases seeds must be helped to germinate by scarifying them (rubbing them with rough sandpaper to create cracks whereby moisture can get in and induce germination) and cold-stratifying (simulating the cold dormancy period most perennials need to go through to germinate by storing the seeds in the refrigerator for several weeks or months).

A partial list of prairie grasses for landscaping (see the Appendix) was adapted from an Iowa State University Extension Service publication. It includes grasses from each of the three main prairie types.

Ground Covers

Ground covers are a mainstay of Xeriscape landscapes because they fulfill many of the functions of grass except wearability. They can duplicate the lush, green feeling of lawn grasses for those who love the "sea of green" look, without the high-maintenance and watering costs, and they can be used in many places where lawn grasses are impractical. Suitable places for ground covers include narrow strips between sidewalks or structures and steep slopes where mowing is difficult; hot, dry exposures; and dense shade under trees and behind buildings.

A well-chosen ground cover will provide cooling for adjacent buildings, have year-round color, spread by itself, have a compact growth habit, be dense enough to keep out weeds, be (generally) low maintenance, and have a dense, fibrous root system (valuable for erosion control). Evergreen ground covers need the least amount of maintenance. Ground covers provide a variety of texture and colors, and can serve as transition between lawn

Ground covers don't just cover the ground with a practical living mulch that cools the air around it without high water use; they can be exciting, *too, as are lamb's ears* (Stachys byzantina) *and* Artemisia ludoviciana *'Silver Mound' at the Cornell Xeriscape Demonstration Garden.*

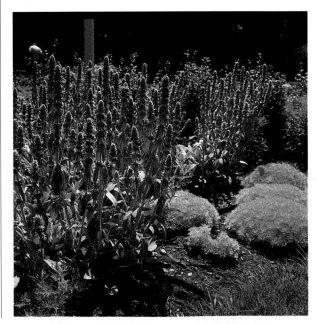

areas and shrub or flower borders. They make an excellent replacement for areas previously covered with gravel.

Most drought-tolerant ground covers will do best in full sun, though some will do better in partial shade. Ground covers specific to different regions of the country are included in the regional plant lists in Part 2. A short list of drought-tolerant ground covers for areas throughout the United States appears in the Appendix.

Planting Ground Covers

Walkways of concrete or stepping-stones should be planned and installed before planting ground covers if heavy foot traffic is expected. Most ground covers will not survive being walked on. You'll want to loosen and improve the soil for ground covers as much as you can, with two exceptions:

• If the ground is definitely sloping, try to disturb the native soil as little as possible to minimize erosion.
• If the area is infested with perennial weeds, tilling will actually help propagate them. In this case, leave the soil alone and treat individual weeds with glysophate, or spray the whole area if the number of weeds is overwhelming.

Normally, the soil should be generously improved before planting. Most ground covers spread by off-shoots or runners, and they'll be more apt to fill in quickly where the soil has good aeration, organic matter, and drainage. Heavy clay soils should be improved extensively throughout the bed or over-excavated, as they are not suitable even for ground covers that can survive in poor soils.

It's important to control as much of the weed cover as possible before planting, especially perennial weeds. Annual weeds can be hoed out, pulled out, or chemically controlled. Glysophate controls most weeds, but it's best to use it sparingly, perhaps saving it for only the most intractable weeds such as bindweed.

Incorporate at least three cubic yards of shredded bark, compost, or well-rotted manure into each 1,000 square feet of area. (A three-way mix of one-third compost or bark, one-third aged manure, and one-third topsoil can be incorporated at up to nine

yards per 1,000 square feet, as indicated in the soil improvements chapter.) This is a suitable place to incorporate hydro-gels as well since they help to improve drainage. Use ten to fifteen pounds per 1,000 square feet tilled in at least nine inches deep. After soil amendments have been incorporated, water the area and fill in any low spots that may occur.

The spacing between plants varies tremendously, depending on species, from six inches to ten feet. It's best to study books that discuss ground covers in detail to determine the spacing as well as the best plant suited for the location you want it in, or discuss the matter with local nursery growers.

Plant ground covers when they will have the longest time to establish themselves before unfavorable weather sets in. In cold winter climates plant early in the spring. In mild winter climates plant in the fall. Avoid planting in summer, because ground covers will be stressed by heat and will need close attention on watering.

When setting out the plants, treat them as trees and shrubs (see following). Dig holes just to the depth of the root ball, letting larger plants actually sit on a plateau with a little trench around them. If the plants are being installed on a slope, give each one its own little terrace with a watering basin (slightly depressed trench) behind the plant. Backfill around the plant.

Groundcover areas are good candidates for drip or underground irrigation systems. The regular spacing of the plants lends itself well to tailoring the systems to water just the plants without a lot of waste. The watering needs of ground covers vary tremendously as with every other type of planting in a Xeriscape garden, so use the type of plant, type of soil, amount of rainfall, and amount of shade as guidelines. To avoid overwatering, use the "knuckle method" described on page 83.

Trees and Shrubs
....

Trees and shrubs are vital to Xeriscape landscapes because they provide not only drama, seasonal color, and architectural interest, but also one of the key water-saving devices, shade. The temperature under a shade tree may be as much as ten to fifteen

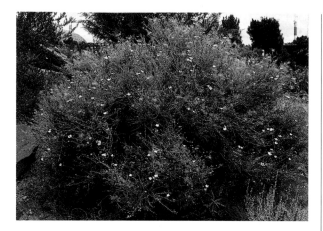

Apache plume (Fallugia paradoxa) *is one of the most drought-tolerant native shrubs, and it gives a summer-long show with starlight blooms and feathery pink seed heads.*

degrees cooler than in the open, and that cuts down on evaporation from surface plants. Trees and shrubs (as well as fences) also act as wind barriers, reducing evaporation not only from the plants themselves, but also from the top layer of soil. Many plants that will grow only in moist soil if in full sun will survive in dry shade.

Because of their extensive root systems, trees and shrubs are among the lowest users of applied water, especially native or adapted species. The roots of one large tree may actually take more water from the soil than an equal area of grass, but tree roots are so efficient at tapping groundwater sources or moist subsoil that in much of the nation they rarely need irrigation after establishment. Many trees and shrubs will survive one or two droughty seasons or will get by with less than the ideal amount of water; they will just grow less.

Of course, the same cautions apply to trees and shrubs as to other types of plants about watering during establishment, which may take up to three growing seasons. It's best to plant trees and shrubs in areas that are separate from irrigated lawn areas, for several seasons. Some lawn grasses will not tolerate shade and will only fare indifferently if placed under a tree. Bumping a tree with a lawn mower can seriously damage a tree. If the lawn grass requires frequent irrigation, it may encourage the tree or shrub to grow shallow roots under the grass which

will compete with the grass. And, as with wildflowers, if the tree likes acid soil and the grass needs neutral soil, putting the two close together may cause them both to suffer.

Putting shade-tolerant, low-water grasses, flowers, or shrubs near trees may be more successful. Especially in sandy soil this tactic helps fully utilize the water applied, since the root systems of these plants grow to different depths. Water not used by the shallower-rooted plants drains on down to the deeper-rooted ones. Recent research indicates that many trees have much wider, shallower root systems than was previously believed, so before you plan to interplant heavily around trees, find out how their roots grow. It may be simpler just to give them lots of room and plan to situate the massed beds elsewhere.

If the soil is extremely heavy, it may be necessary to plant all trees and shrubs on berms (mounds) of well-drained, loamy soil brought into the site, but avoid planting trees on turfed berms. When trees are planted on other slopes or berms, try to build in permanent saucerlike depressions around them to catch water.

Size of Plants

It's tempting to try to make room in your budget for the largest trees or shrubs you can afford, in order to see a satisfying instant change in your landscape. This is okay, but please be aware that the larger the plant at transplant time, in general the longer it will be before the tree or shrub recovers from the process and begins growing again.

Tree expert Dr. Carl Whitcomb has found that when the caliper (diameter) of a tree trunk gets larger than about three inches, the tree generally has so many twig and leaf cells to support above ground that transplanting it at that size leaves it in shock for years. The tree expends all its energy rebuilding roots to support that topgrowth again. Meanwhile, he says, a one- or two-inch-caliper tree transplanted at the same time may catch up to or even surpass the larger tree in size after just a few years.

Also, slow-growing plants such as *some* oaks (not all) will tolerate very little change, so transplant them when small.

When to Plant

Early spring is the best time to plant trees and shrubs where winters are cold, as soon as the ground can be worked, or as they say in Colorado, "as soon as you can jackhammer through the ground." It's best to avoid disturbing a plant that has recently broken bud and is producing new, soft growth. Balled-and-burlapped stock (see following) should be planted either before bud-break or after new growth has hardened (early summer), not during soft-growth stage.

Container-grown stock can usually be planted all summer, but it's still best to avoid planting when the new growth is soft. For evergreens, it's safe to plant when a pine candle (new growth at branch tip) can be broken off; this means new growth has hardened off. In cold winter climates there is greater risk of losing a plant transplanted in the fall, but if planting at that time is necessary, mulch with a layer of about five inches of wood chips to prevent early freezing of soil. New root growth generally ceases when the soil temperature goes below forty degrees, and mulching can delay this a little longer. You want to give the tree or shrub about a month to take hold before the soil temperature gets that cool. Check with local experts as to the latest time to plant for your area.

In very mild climates trees and shrubs may never experience true dormancy, but they have a "resting" stage midwinter. Fall planting is recommended, since the roots of newly planted trees and shrubs will continue to grow all winter in non-frozen soil. The established root system is then ready for spring shoot growth.

Planting Trees and Shrubs

Trees and shrubs are usually purchased bare root, balled-and-burlapped (B-and-B), or container-grown.

Bareroot plants are dug from the field when dormant; the roots are cleaned, trimmed, and kept moist for transport. These plants are usually the least expensive to purchase. In the past bare root-stock has been available only for small deciduous trees and shrubs because they have the longest dormancy period. Dormancy for evergreens is shorter, and they generally don't tolerate having their roots exposed for any period of time. A few nurseries are starting to carry very large bareroot stock, some as large as twenty feet tall. Dave and Linda Rock of Picadilly Nursery in Brighton, Colorado, have gone to this method because they find it makes for an easier transplant than if the same size plant is B-and-B or container-grown. One Colorado gardener who planted several trees this way reported that they had a few leaves the first year after their April planting, and had normal foliage cover by the second year.

Bareroot stock is usually available only in early spring. In some cases, if the roots have dried out, they can be soaked to restore moisture and will survive, but most bareroot stock will die if the roots dry out.

Balled-and-burlapped plants have been dug from the field with a ball of soil attached, and wrapped in burlap to keep the root ball intact. Because they are dug in the field, part of the root system is often lost (up to 98 percent), and it may take the plant awhile to recover from transplanting and begin growing.

Container-grown stock is raised in plastic or fiber pots. The root stystem is complete within the pot, so there is no loss of roots. However, if the plant is large the roots may have become coiled in the pot and may eventually girdle (encircle) the tree, thereby killing it by damaging the inner bark that carries water and nutrients up the tree.

Keep the soil or roots of newly purchased plants moist and keep the plants in the shade until planting. Bare roots can be kept moist by keeping the roots sealed in a plastic bag, wrapping them in moist peat moss, or dipping them in a slurry solution of finely ground hydro-gel, which clings to the roots.

The planting hole should be dug at least twice the diameter of the root ball or root mass. Some experts recommend that you dig the hole as much as five times the diameter of the root ball or mass. Wide holes, only as deep as the rootball, are now recommended rather than deeper ones in response to the research that has shown root growth to be more shallow and lateral (sideways). And, as recommended in the soil improvements chapter, *don't* add organic matter to the planting hole unless you

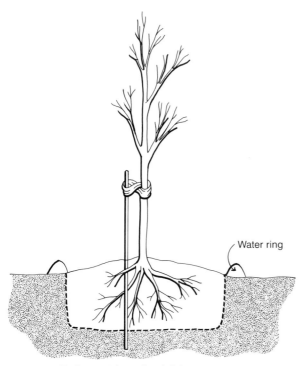

For bareroot plants, dig a hole large
enough to permit the roots to be spread
out without crowding or curving around the
walls of the hole.

can mix in enough to supply the plant's root zone at least three years. For a silver maple, for instance, this would be a six- to eight-foot-diameter circle amended twelve to eighteen inches deep.

For most people, though, this is more work than they can face, so if you're doing it yourself, the next best alternative is to loosen the soil through that area as much as possible and skip the organic amendments.

When Dr. Whitcomb retired from the university, he set up a tree propagation business. He has since made an interesting discovery. He's found that with a wide variety of species, if he lowers the pH of the soil medium he plants them in to about 5.0 (fairly acid), they have much increased root growth and topgrowth.

For the experimentally minded Xeriscape gardener, Dr. Whitcomb offers this suggestion: Go ahead and amend the soil around tree transplants with granular elemental sulfur (an acidifying amendment) by mixing it into the planting hole at a rate of about four pounds per hundred square feet. This can be done for existing trees, too. Just sprinkle it on the ground and water it in. The sulfur takes

a long time to assimilate into the soil, so wait six months, and if you still don't note any improvement in the plant, make another application, gradually lowering the pH.

To plant bareroot stock, prune off broken, damaged, or diseased roots and hold the plant as you backfill the soil so it will be at the same ground level as it was in the nursery before. A color difference on the stem will indicate what this level is.

Balled-and-burlapped trees and shrubs should be planted on an undisturbed base with the top of the ball even with the surrounding ground level (for sandy or average soils) and two to four inches above the ground for heavy soils that don't drain well. If the top is set below ground level, soil may settle around the base of the trunk, covering it up, or water may collect around the roots, causing root suffocation. A small berm, or water ring, may be constructed around the edge of the planting hole to hold water.

Remove all wires, ropes, or twine as well as pins or nails that may have been used to hold the root ball together before backfilling the hole. Cutting the burlap or removing it from the top will help the roots grow out more quickly.

Hydro-gels can be incorporated into the backfill as you plant, at the rate of two dry ounces (⅓ cup) or two gallons hydrated per cubic foot of backfill (not counting the rootball volume, if any). This will help reduce transplant shock and the chance of the soil drying out too much during establishment.

For container-grown stock, remove paper pots as well as plastic ones before installing the plant in a wide, shallow hole as described here. Place the plant on an undisturbed base dug about two to four inches shallower than the soil mass to allow for settling. You want the base of the trunk to end up at ground level after settling, not below it.

If container-grown plants have pot-bound roots at the bottom of the root mass, cut through any roots that circle more than halfway around the pot, as these are in danger of growing all the way around and girdling the trunk. Backfill and water in well. Allow water to settle the soil; don't tamp the backfill.

Mulching with wood chips, bark chunks, or similar material after planting reduces the need for frequent watering and competition by the turfgrasses for nutrients and water. Bonnie Lee Appleton, au-

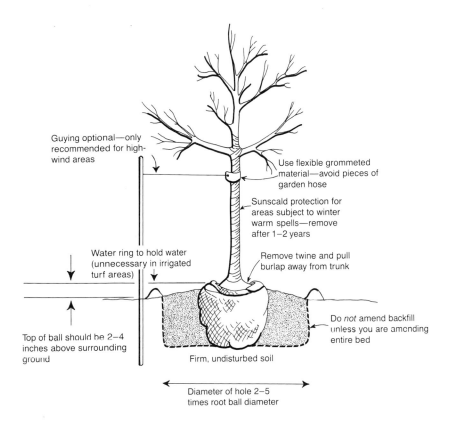

Guying optional—only recommended for high-wind areas

Use flexible grommeted material—avoid pieces of garden hose

Sunscald protection for areas subject to winter warm spells—remove after 1–2 years

Water ring to hold water (unnecessary in irrigated turf areas)

Remove twine and pull burlap away from trunk

Do *not* amend backfill unless you are amending entire bed

Top of ball should be 2–4 inches above surrounding ground

Firm, undisturbed soil

Diameter of hole 2–5 times root ball diameter

Planting a balled-and-burlapped tree or shrub. (For container stock, use the same procedure, first removing the plant from the container.)

thor of *Landscape Rejuvenation* (Pownal, Vt.: Storey Communications, Inc., 1988), recommends layering the mulch no more than two to three inches, in order not to smother roots or create a soggy environment. This recommendation applies to humid climates; in drier areas you can mulch up to five inches deep. A landscape fabric weed barrier may be used to keep weed growth down, but never use solid polyethylene sheet plastics, as these will exclude air and water exchange to roots, which can kill the plant.

It was formerly recommended that no fertilizer be added to the planting hole to avoid "burning" the roots, but this applies only to fast-acting inorganic fertilizers. Organic fertilizers or slow-release inorganic fertilizers may be added to the backfill to provide a source of nutrition for the roots once they start growing again.

Recommended pruning of newly planted trees and shrubs has undergone a change, too. You used to be advised to cut back about twenty-five percent of the topgrowth to compensate for root loss during transplanting. However, the latest advice from experts favors pruning only damaged or broken branches and saving more extensive shaping for the following growing season. By leaving all the leaves possible, you give the plant a chance to generate more food, and overcome transplant shock sooner.

Staking

New research evidence seems to show that unstaked trees develop thicker trunks with the additional movement they experience. If your trees are planted in a protected area, follow this advice, and stake only trees on which the crown is disproportionately large for the root ball, or which may blow over in their planting holes because of being in an exposed location.

Some landscape architects/contractors specify staking new trees from three sides, not just one or two, to keep wind from wiggling the root ball. Make sure there is a little give in the staking or the thickness of the trunk won't increase below the guying. The best choice for staking is wide strips of a strong, soft material such as indoor-outdoor carpet or the webbed strapping used in backpacks, attached to the guying wires via grommets. Wire through pieces of garden hose is no longer recommended because it may cause girdling injury. Guying should be below the midpoint of the tree.

Sunscald Protection

Young transplanted trees may experience an injury known as sunscald due to excessive heat on the tree's trunk and branches. Sunscald occurs more commonly in trees planted on the south sides of buildings, when the absorption of sunlight causes the surface temperature of the trees to rise. The cells in the bark may become active and thus be subject to injury when the temperature drops again at night.

To protect against this, it may be advisable to wrap the trunk with a commercial crepe wrap, starting at the base of the tree and overlapping as you go up. Wrap as far as the lowest branch, securing the top with a single staple or small tack. Remove the wrap during the spring and summer to prevent it from harboring diseases and insects, and use it only for one or two growing seasons.

Watering to Establish Trees and Shrubs

Shallow watering leads to shallow roots, which defeats the purpose of a Xeriscape planting. An easy way to gauge how long it takes to deep-water roots is to water the plant for a measured amount of time, let it soak in for a couple of hours, and then dig a hole six to ten inches deep (outside the range of the newly planted root ball). If the soil is wet at the bottom of the hole, then water that amount of time at the next watering interval.

Dr. Jim Feucht, with the Colorado State University Cooperative Extension Service, recommends a more precise watering method to maximize water-use efficiency and the development of deep root systems. He advises watering with a soil needle (root feeder) attached to the hose. The area to be watered is from about one foot outside the dripline (below the extremities of the branches) halfway back toward the trunk. Insert the soil needle twelve to eighteen inches deep, let the water run thirty to sixty sec-

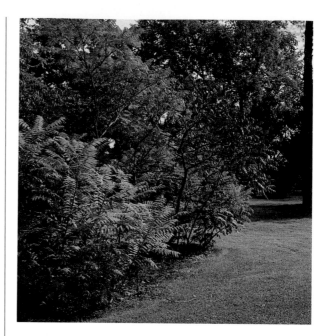

*Sumacs (*Rhus *spp.) are native to much of the United States. In the East they tower up to fifty feet; in Colorado they usually reach only moderate to tall shrub height (eight to twenty feet). Extremely drought tolerant, they also give a brilliant red show in the fall. Sumacs are best planted in clumps or groves as they tend to be thinly foliaged at the bottom.*

onds, then move the needle six to eight inches away, and repeat. Move in a zigzag pattern around the tree to water all feeder roots. After the circle is completed, repeat the procedure with the needle angled slightly away from the tree. Large balled-and-burlapped trees can be watered right in the root ball, though you must reduce the water pressure when watering in the root ball or in the backfill. This type of watering is very time-consuming, but it eliminates the oxygen starvation that can result from flood-watering, and will help your tree become established and grow faster.

Watering frequency of new transplants depends on soil moisture at the root zone, not the calendar. Take time initially to establish on average how long it takes the soil to dry out to that ten-inch depth. Dig down a few days after transplanting, and water again only if the soil is powdery or crumbles when squeezed. Take cool weather and precipitation into account when determining a rough schedule for watering. It may be about once or twice a week for a month or so, then you can slowly spread the interval out a little unless the tree shows signs of drought stress (primarily leaf wilting). During the second growing season roughly double the interval for watering, and by the third, you should be able to discontinue additional watering above precipitation if you haven't already.

Using Hydro-gels in Tree Planting

For many applications the use of hydro-gels is still experimental, but one area where it really shines and has proved consistently beneficial, at least in the western, more arid parts of the country, is in tree planting and transplanting. Several million seedlings are planted with hydro-gel each year through the Colorado and other state forest services, using the "survival technique." The bareroot seedlings are dipped in a slurry solution of a fine grind of the hydro-gel, and all seedlings, whether bare root or container-grown, get a handful (cup to a pint) of the hydrated crystals mixed in with the backfill. This small amount of hydro-gel seems to give the seedlings enough of a water supply to help get them through the crucial first year of establishment.

In July 1989 seventeen Joshua trees in Utah (some of which may be fifty to two hundred years old) had to be transplanted to make way for a highway project. Thirty years before, the same trees and over forty others were moved for the same reason. At that time the transplanting was done under ideal conditions, in cool weather, in October. Despite the careful procedure thirty of the sixty trees died. This time there wasn't time to wait for better weather and the trees had to be moved in July, when the temperature soared to 108 degrees Fahrenheit.

The trees were lifted with a tree spade, all of the exposed roots were brushed with the bareroot dip solution, and hydrated crystals were mixed in the planting holes. Two years later all seventeen Joshua trees are still alive.

Vines

Vines are one of the most underrated category of landscape plants. They can be very useful for Xeriscape landscapes because of their ability to provide shade when grown on arbors and trellises, and to add a welcome note of lushness to the landscape.

Some vines such as Hall's honeysuckle (*Lonicera japonica* 'Halliana')—use only in semiarid to arid climates, where it's not invasive—can double as a ground cover, anchoring soil and providing greenery in deep shade where grass doesn't thrive. They can provide cooling shade for plants as well as living areas, not only patios and decks, but also interior rooms. A vine-covered wall is several degrees cooler than a blank wall.

A simple frame with wide spaces can be constructed and anchored in the ground about a foot away from a south- or west-facing window. A vine growing up this frame will absorb heat in the summer that would ordinarily reflect into the room, yet will not substantially block the light.

Because all the growing energy of vines goes into producing foliage rather than supporting themselves, they can fill a vertical space quickly while using a minimum amount of space on the ground, sometimes as little as one square foot. They often possess not only luxuriant foliage but also beautiful flowers, and sometimes provide brilliant fall color. They can serve to mask eyesores such as an unattractive view, a chain link fence, or a stark concrete wall.

Vines need support and well-drained, well-prepared soil in the planting hole. Plant vines about six inches away from the wall or support and maintain a three-inch space between the vine and wall; vines do better when there is air circulating around them. Use a three-inch layer of mulch over the roots to keep them cool, especially in summer. The best location for vines is where their roots can be kept cool (either by shade or mulching), but their leaves can drape over into the sunshine. If roots must be in the sun, place a large rock or mulch over them to keep them cool. Water vines well when young and keep weak or dead wood pruned out. Wisteria and other large vigorous species need moderate to severe pruning nearly every season to avoid the vines taking over trees and damaging shutters and wooden structures. Grapevines need pruning in order to bear fruit. Remember the old saying about vines: "The first year they sleep, the second year they creep, and the third year they leap." Be prepared.

Vegetable and Herb Gardens

Vegetable gardens in general are a good choice for Xeriscape landscapes for the simple reason that they are not usually hooked up to the "pour-it-on" lawn sprinkler system. Instead, hand-watering or any of the various drip irrigation systems are the norm. Some crops are harmed by overhead watering because it wets the leaves, which can attract undesirable insects or lead to disease.

"Edible landscaping" has been championed by author Rosalind Creasy in recent years. Citing the decorative nature of many garden crops, especially leafy vegetables, she recommends blending them with ornamental landscaping in containers, flower borders, and massed beds. On the flip side, several

Raised bed gardens put the plants within easier reach and provide architectural interest as well. (The lawn shown here is irrigated with belowground drip irrigation.) (Design: Thomas L. Stephens)

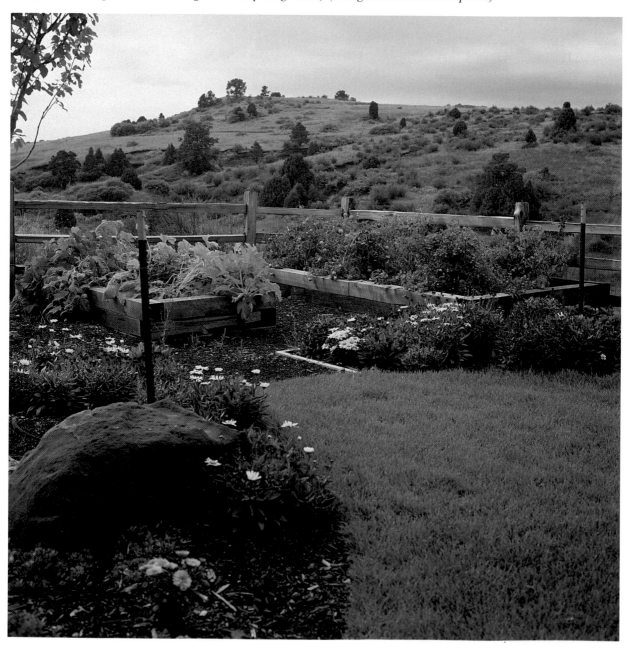

traditional garden flowers, such as nasturtiums (*Tropaeolum majus*), cottage pinks (*Dianthus caryophyllus*), and daylilies (*Hemerocallis* spp.), are edible and drought tolerant, too.

In any vegetable garden where the soil is poor, it's a good idea to improve it as much as possible and continue improving it every year because, unlike some flowers that may give you more flowers with poorer soil and herbs that may produce more of the flavor you want in poor rather than rich soil, vegetable crops are very clear on the fact that they need good nutritious soil if you want them to produce lots of vegetables. So for vegetable gardens, go ahead and incorporate organic soil amendments at the maximum rate recommended for your area.

Vegetable garden crops also need to have frequent watering at specific times during their fruiting cycle, but not, interestingly enough, throughout the whole cycle. If you pay attention to their needs during these critical times, you should be able to be a little more lax during other parts of the plants' cycle.

Critical Moisture-Sensitive Period

VEGETABLE	PERIOD
Asparagus	Need consistent watering
Beans	Pollination and pod formation
Beets	Need consistent watering
Broccoli	Early in season to prevent buttoning (extremely small heads) and during head formation and enlargement
Brussels sprouts	Need consistent watering
Cabbage	Head formation and enlargement
Carrots	Uniform watering till three-quarters final size. Reduce watering to prevent splitting.
Cauliflower	Early in the season to prevent buttoning (extremely small heads) and during head development
Celery	Need consistent watering
Chinese cabbage	Need consistent watering
Collard greens	Need consistent watering

VEGETABLE	PERIOD
Corn	Tasseling through silking and ear filling
Cucumbers	Need consistent watering
Eggplant	Flowering through harvest
Kale	Need consistent watering
Lettuce	Leaf lettuce: throughout growing season
	Head lettuce: during head development
Okra	Need consistent watering
Onions	Bulb enlargement. Stop watering when tops fall.
Peas	Flowering and pod filling
Peppers	Flowering to harvest
Potatoes	After initial tuber formation
Pumpkins	Need consistent, high watering
Radishes	Need consistent watering
Spinach	Need consistent, low watering
Squash, summer and winter	Bud development and flowering
Tomatoes	Blossom set through fruit enlargement
Turnips	Beginning of root development through root enlargement

Author Mel Bartholomew's "square foot gardening" method is an example of a conservation-minded way to look at vegetable gardening because it saves many resources (not the least of which is your time) as well as water. In *Square Foot Gardening* (Emmaus, Pa., Rodale Press, 1981), he says that the traditional way of dropping hundreds of seeds out in a long, straight row is more suited to big-time agriculture than weekend home gardeners. Instead, he advocates setting the seeds out at their ultimate spacing, giving each a little well of sand to start in so there is less chance of damping off. The beds are misted daily or more often if needed to keep them moist till the seeds sprout, then they are mulched to conserve moisture. After that they are watered weekly or twice weekly according to their needs, using Bartholomew's favorite precision watering vessel, an empty two-cup cottage cheese container.

The watering schedule is based on what we want from the plant, whether it be the roots, fruits, or seeds. All root, leaf, and head crops need a steady, even supply of moisture because they have shallow root systems. They will produce larger vegetables with sufficient moisture. They should be watered about twice a week for average soil after sprouting and being mulched. Examples include:

Beets	Lettuce
Broccoli	Radishes
Cabbage	Spinach
Carrots	Swiss chard
Cauliflower	Turnips

When we want the fruit or seed of a crop, it's better to water less frequently to encourage these deep-rooted plants to develop good root systems. Some suggest that when a plant undergoes drought stress, it begins to flower and set seed in an attempt to complete its life cycle before it dies. If we give this type too steady a water supply, it tends to produce lots of leaves and not much fruit. They include:

Beans	Melons
Corn	Peppers
Cucumbers	Squash
Eggplant	Tomatoes

Other factors influence watering frequency. If the soil is sandy rather than average, you'll need to water more often, but with less water. If it is clayey, it will hold moisture longer and you will water less often to avoid overdoing it. If the garden is subjected to a lot of drying wind, make adjustments in the watering schedule. Seedlings and new transplants may need watering more frequently to get started.

When planting seeds or transplanting plants, always try to place them in a slight saucer-shaped depression to help catch water and prevent runoff. You can also form little trenches linking the seedlings so that the overflow from the watering of one plant will run to the next one.

Herbs

Many herbs are very drought tolerant. Many are native to the Mediterranean coast, where they thrive in conditions of poor soil, good drainage, and usually full sun. In hot sun many herbs generate their essential oils that in some way protect the plants from drying out. If overwatered or fertilized they will produce little oil, but sometimes lavish growth.

Well-drained soil is essential for most herbs, so if this isn't what you have on your lot you might consider raised-bed or container gardening. Most herbs need about a foot of well-drained soil.

Some herbs can be used as landscape plants. Rosemary is an old favorite perennial herb that is welcome as a small shrub in most gardens. Herbs can also be mixed decoratively through the vegetable garden, or used to form a design of their own.

The following list of basic herbs will grow in or require moist soil to thrive:

Angelica	Mints
Basil	Sweet bay
Chervil	Sweet marjoram
Comfrey	Summer savory
French sorrel	Watercress
Leeks	Winter cress
Lovage	

These herbs will tolerate dry soil:

Aloe vera	Garlic
Anise	Hyssop
Borage	Lavender
Caraway	Parsley
Chamomile	Rosemary
Chicory	Sage (all)
Chives	Shallots
Coltsfoot	Tarragon
Coriander	Thyme (all)
Cumin	Top onion
Dill	Winter savory
Fennel	Wormwood
Fenugreek	

Efficient Irrigation:

Making Every Drop Count

LANDSCAPE irrigation is used to supplement rainfall only when necessary to promote plant health and vigor. If water conservation is your goal in landscaping your property, then thinking through your watering "policy" is of first importance. You may decide that you wish to do little or no watering after your Xeriscape landscape has become established. In this case you'll carefully match the plants you select with the existing soil and site conditions (that is, climate, rainfall, heat, cold) or else you'll improve your soil to provide for enhanced water-retaining capability. This option is easiest for people who live in areas that receive forty inches of rainfall or more each year, but is quite do-able even for areas receiving less.

If you've done a good job with the other Xeriscape guidelines, the only sacrifice you might need to make is in the quality (that is, lush greenness) of

Three Xeriscape principles show up in this photo: the use of mulch to reduce soil moisture loss, efficient irrigation with a drip system, and appropriate plant selection—blue plumbago (Plumbago auriculata) *is an excellent Xeriscape plant choice for the South. (Photo: Doug Welsh)*

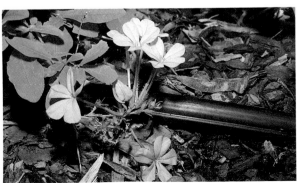

your turfgrass or drought-sensitive plants, but even they can be adequately maintained with a little spot-watering during prolonged drought.

A second option, suitable for areas receiving roughly twenty to forty inches of precipitation a year, is to plan to irrigate regularly only the highly visible, highly used, and/or drought-sensitive areas of the landscape. Unless you make big mistakes and select plants that need much more moisture than you receive naturally, most trees, shrubs, ground covers, and many flowers can usually thrive without additional watering in these areas.

If you live in an area that receives less than twenty inches annually, chances are you'll have to plan on doing some additional watering of most turfgrass and other plants to keep them in good condition.

When people think of irrigation, they often automatically think "irrigation system" (or sprinkler system). But for the well-informed Xeriscape gardener, this shouldn't be the first and only choice. In fact, for much of the eastern United States irrigation systems in home landscapes are the exception rather than the rule. People simply drag out the hose when needed to revive parched grass. In more arid climates, having an automatic system in place saves lots of time, water (if properly used), and often plants. Even there, though, if you keep areas that must be irrigated to a minimum, you may be able to do without an automatic irrigation system.

Probably most of us will decide whether or not to include an automatic system based on one of these personal reasons. However, if you've decided you want one, first take a look at your site's opportunities for water harvesting. If you can capture every drop of water your site receives by way of the various methods described here, you may be able to decrease the size of the system you will need.

DO YOU NEED AN IRRIGATION SYSTEM?

Reasons to Include One

1. A well-designed system delivers water very efficiently when used correctly.

2. Your turf area is large enough that it would be difficult to manually water without a great deal of moving around of hoses and sprinklers.

3. You travel a great deal during the "drought season" (whenever that is for your area) and might lose a turf area or planting bed if it isn't watered in your absence.

4. You've installed a lot of new plants in your landscape and don't want to take the time to hand-water them until they're established (which may take two or three seasons). One option for this situation is to put in a temporary irrigation system, the least expensive and efficient one you can, knowing it will come out later.

5. It's extremely important to you to have a lush green lawn as much of the year as possible.

6. Your site has a lot of grade changes, which makes manual irrigation difficult.

7. You live in a part of the country where the climate is so hot and dry that if a plant was accidentally left unwatered for a few days it might die.

Reasons to Forgo One

1. Your turf area is small or nonexistent. Most people can deal with manually watering 800 to 1,000 square feet of turf without much problem.

2. You live in a part of the country that gets ample rainfall to keep your turfgrass alive and are willing to tolerate a higher degree of drought dormancy (browning) in your lawn. You realize, too, that your ornamental plants will grow more slowly if they're not watered regularly. (This may be okay.)

3. You want to save a lot of money.

4. You don't want to bother with the maintenance of an irrigation system, prefer to remain as low-tech as possible, or want to make the least impact on the environment as possible (that is, use one or two hoses, sprinklers, and accessories, rather than several hundred feet of pipe and all the appurtenances of an automatic system).

WATER HARVESTING

A 1,000-square-foot roof will generate 150 gallons of water during a ¼-inch rain. Rather than letting it run off the site, you can "harvest" the water that Mother Nature provides you free, via rainfall and snowfall, and use it in your Xeriscape landscape. The following are a few simple methods for water harvesting.

1. Use slightly depressed median strips in between driveways and walks to save runoff from rain, snowmelt, and irrigation.

2. If you are building a new driveway and walk system, you should design the surfaces to slope into turfgrass areas, planting beds, holding ponds, or cisterns.

3. On steeply sloping sites, use terraces to slow down and collect the runoff.

4. Provide small depressions at the bottom of slopes to catch runoff.

5. Avoid directing runoff from your neighbor's yards into your flower beds and lawn since you can't control their use of chemicals, such as "weed-and-feed."

Downspout collection. Extend the existing downspouts from your roof gutters into the ground with a manufactured plastic adapter attached to the metal downspout pipe and a four-inch-diameter solid pipe. The solid pipe should extend a minimum of five to eight feet away from the house or building.

At the end of the solid pipe, change to a slotted drainage pipe to allow the water to percolate into the planting bed soil. Usually the pipe can be laid in a trench that is approximately twelve inches deep and ten inches wide, with the pipe surrounded by coarse gravel. The trench should slope at a minimum grade of two percent, or ¼ inch per foot away from the house. The gravel is then covered with a layer of porous landscape fabric that allows water to flow through the fabric, but stops fine particles of soil from filtering into the gravel. The voids in the gravel become small reservoirs for water and allow it to percolate into the surrounding soil gradually.

It is best that all such underground drainage pipes eventually open up to daylight at some point on the site to prevent water from backing up and/

YOUR ROOF CAN HARVEST WATER FOR YOUR LANDSCAPE

To calculate the amount of water your home's roof can harvest, use this formula:

$$\frac{\text{amount of rainfall (in inches)} \times \text{area of roof (in square feet)}}{\text{area to receive the water (in square feet)}} = \begin{array}{l}\text{inches of water} \\ \text{harvested for the} \\ \text{landscape area}\end{array}$$

For example,

$$\frac{1 \text{ inch rain} \times 500 \text{ square feet of roof}}{1{,}000 \text{ square feet of landscape}} = {}^{1}\!/_{2} \text{ inch of harvested water}$$

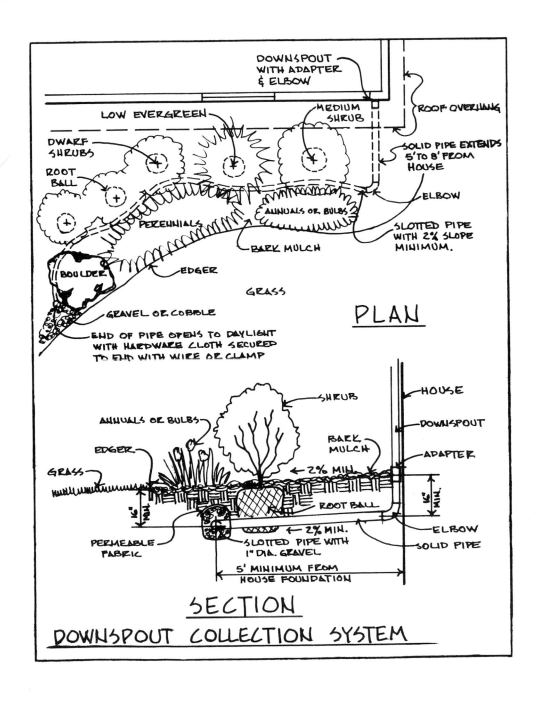

DOWNSPOUT COLLECTION SYSTEM

or freezing in the pipe and causing damage to the house and roof. When the pipe comes to the surface, it should be capped at the end with a piece of hardware cloth or screen wire. This will prevent small rodents from using the pipe as a home and clogging it with nesting materials. Clamp or wire the cloth onto the end of the pipe so that it can be removed easily for regular cleaning if debris accumulates.

This downspout collector can snake through the planting beds. Often with native or naturalized plants, this is the only source of water necessary after the plants have become established. Similar manufactured French drain materials can be used instead of the pipe.

Cobblestone runoffs. Instead of the unattractive solid concrete splash blocks at downspouts, try using a shallow swale with three- to six-inch-diameter cobblestones extending to the edge of the

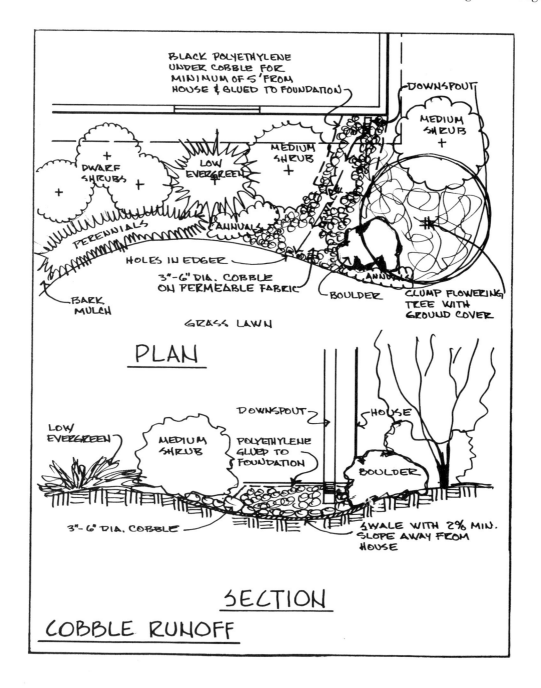

PLAN

SECTION

COBBLE RUNOFF

planting bed and lawn or turf area. The cobblestones should be placed on a solid black plastic or Visqueen sheet for the first five to eight feet away from the house or building.

Beyond the five to eight feet, you can use the porous landscape fabric or nothing at all. This will allow the water to percolate into the mulch and soil of the planting, flower beds, or lawn. Cobblestones rather than smaller gravel are used because they stay in place during heavy rains or periods of rapid snowmelt.

Collection basins, ponds, and cisterns. If there are large areas of solid surfaces, such as roofs, driveways, parking areas, patios, or game areas, that would contribute excessive amounts of runoff water during heavy rains or snowmelt, consider installing a collection basin, pond, and/or cistern for holding the water. Such collection basins and ponds should be lined with either hard-packed clay, concrete, or nonporous vinyl liners to prevent the water from percolating into the soil. A small galvanized horse trough can also serve as a tiny pool/collector.

Cisterns can be relatively small in diameter (two to five feet) and can be concrete or metal pipes normally used as drainage culverts under roads and driveways. These pipes can be installed vertically underground and can have solid or open bottoms.

All solid and slotted drainpipes should end in a collection basin, pond, or cistern. A pump with a filtration system or gravity flow siphons can be used to remove the water for use in your landscape. Adequate overflow provisions should be included in any collection system to prevent possible damage from flooding.

After using every water-harvesting method you can think of to utilize your free water, you're now ready to consider irrigation methods.

NO SPRINKLER SYSTEM

If you've decided you can easily maintain your landscape without the use of an automatic irrigation system, you will be using hand-held hoses and portable sprinklers during the establishment of your plants and for irrigating drought-sensitive plants during dry spells. The equipment is available at nearly every hardware store and nursery and garden center, and includes hoses, sprinklers, quick-couple devices for joining hoses instantly, and automatic shutoff timers that can be attached at the spigot to prevent overwatering.

Research by the Rodale Institute several years ago on sixteen different sprinklers representing five broad categories found that for uniformity, efficiency, and range (distance) of coverage, the impulse- or impact-type sprinklers were the best. Inexpensive revolving sprinklers (with revolving arms that move by water pressure), as well as fixed sprinklers that shoot water through a pattern of holes in their tops, gave the least uniform coverage, often leaking and/or distributing most of the water near the sprinkler. Oscillating sprinklers cover a square area, but often deposit too much water at the ends of their oscillations, where they pause to reverse direction. In addition, though oscillating sprinklers may be great for children to play in, throwing water high in the air increases evaporation and wind drift losses. Traveling sprinklers (the ones that look like little tractors) have revolving arms and move across the lawn for better distribution and efficiency.

When buying a sprinkler, pick one with a low precipitation rate (the information should be on the package) if you have clay soil, and a high rate for sandy soils (to get the job done quickly). Also, the bigger the drops produced by the sprinkler, the less the water loss through evaporation; this is why the impulse sprinkler is so efficient. Uniformity is important to prevent puddling or dry spots. Try not to put the sprinkler in the same place each time you water. Efficiency and convenience can also be added to portable sprinklers by using the new automatic timers. These relatively inexpensive devices connect to the spigot and hose, and can turn the sprinkler on and off.

The efficiency of manual methods of irrigation varies, depending on the knowledge the person operating the sprinklers has about the actual water requirements of the landscape; efficiency can run from as low as ten to as high as eighty percent. (For information on the watering needs of different types of plants other than turf, see the specific sections in the appropriate plant selection chapter.)

NEW AUTOMATIC IRRIGATION SYSTEM

If you've decided you want to install an automatic irrigation system, you will be using an automated sprinkler irrigation and/or drip, low-volume irrigation. With an automated system, a wide variety of piping, sprinkler heads, drip equipment, and controllers allows the homeowner to apply measured amounts of water in a very precise way. This method can achieve seventy to eighty percent efficiency.

There is no "standard" irrigation system, and a well-designed system may include several different types of equipment, such as pop-up and fixed-riser sprinklers, bubblers, drip emitters, microsprinklers, and soaker hoses. Knowing the basic types of equipment is essential in designing an irrigation system, and is also helpful for the non-do-it-yourselfer in communicating with professional irrigators when getting designs and job estimates. Most homeowners should leave the irrigation design to the professionals. Installation, however, is do-able for many folks.

Pop-up and fixed-riser sprinklers are ideal for watering lawn areas and low-growing ground covers and shrubs. These days sprinkler heads, whether mounted in pop-ups or fixed risers, are available in several types, such as spray heads, impulse and stream rotors. Spray heads offer perhaps the most flexibility and efficiency in small home landscapes,

Some people prefer pop-up spray emitters of microjets to drip irrigation for the convenience of being able to see the emitter working and to spray water over a larger area. (Photo: Doug Welsh)

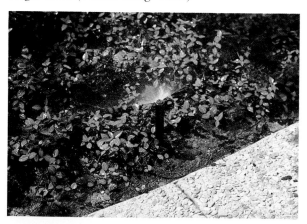

while expansive lawn areas are probably best irrigated with impulse or stream rotors. The latter throw a larger stream of water which is less likely to evaporate or be blown by wind. Different sprinklers operate at different water pressures, so it is important to determine the water pressure of your water supply during the planning process (see page 20).

Bubblers are used primarily to flood irrigate planters, newly planted trees and shrubs, and parking lot medians (because it's almost impossible to irrigate medians with spray heads without overspraying and wasting lots of water). Bubblers are designed to deliver a lot of water in a short period of time, so if they're left on too long they can waste water. Be sure to include some containment method around the area (such as a small berm) to keep the water where you want it.

A sprinkler system can be manual, or it can be automated with an irrigation controller, the brains of the system. The controller directs the watering cycles by activating valves at various stations throughout the system. Within a home landscape, there may be four or five stations. A variety of controllers are available ranging from $100 to $500, depending on the features included (that is, solid state versus mechanical programming capacity).

Drip Irrigation

The watering equipment that offers the greatest potential for water conservation is drip irrigation, often called low-volume irrigation. Drip irrigation is the controlled, slow application of water to the soil. Water flows at low pressure through plastic pipes or hose laid along each row or grouping of plants. The water oozes out into the soil through emitters, or pre-punched holes.

Drip irrigation can be used in flower and shrub beds, vegetable gardens, and home fruit orchards. It is not commonly used in irrigating lawns; however, this use is on the upswing.

Many benefits of drip irrigation have been documented, the primary being an increase in plant health and performance. This is achieved through its ability to maintain a more constant soil moisture level. In other watering methods, there tend to be

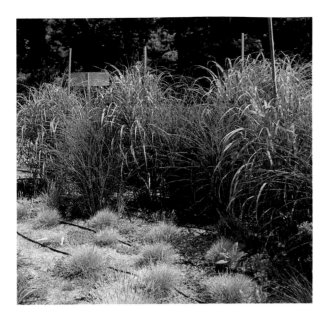

Miscanthus sinensis *'Variegatus' and blue fescue* (Festuca ovina *var.* glauca) *with drip irrigation lines in place. An emitter can be installed at each plant for precise metering out of water. Later the lines will be covered with organic mulch.*

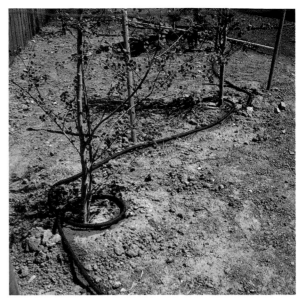

Drip irrigation being installed around small trees.

extreme fluctuations, resulting in plants experiencing a "flood to dust" cycle.

From an insect and disease standpoint, drip irrigation increases plant health by eliminating the splashing up of water on the plant foliage by sprinklers. Drier foliage means fewer pest problems. Drip also increases irrigation efficiency by placing the water directly on the soil, reducing any chance for water loss by evaporation or wind drift.

The major problems experienced with drip are damage by chewing rodents and clogging by sand, silt, or calcium deposits. These can be managed with filters and self-cleaning emitters.

There are many drip irrigation products on the market today, including button emitters, drip tapes, and pressure-compensating emitters. You can either design the system yourself or have a professional irrigation designer do it. With a little coaching, installation is relatively simple.

In addition to drip-type emitters, there are a variety of other low-volume irrigation devices called microsprinklers. These miniature sprinklers operate at reduced pressure, yet function like a sprinkler. The result is a little spitting or spraying

sprinkler that achieves the benefits of drip, plus the sprinkler wets a larger area of soil and you can see it working. One complaint often heard by drip owners is, "I can't see if it is working without getting down on my hands and knees." If seeing the water come out of the irrigation system is reassuring to you, microsprinklers may be your best choice. The only disadvantages are that the microsprinklers wet the foliage and may not wet the soil evenly because of plants blocking or disrupting the sprinkler pattern.

One other low-volume irrigation device is the soaker hose or porous pipe. This type includes the rejuvenated canvas soaker hose that Grandma used and the new porous rubber hoses now on the market. Both types offer irrigation efficiency primarily as a temporary, portable watering device.

For low-volume irrigation systems to operate properly, both a filter and a pressure regulator are recommended. Impurities in the water are a primary enemy of low-volume irrigation, and can be eliminated by inexpensive filters. The pressure regulator is designed to reduce the water pressure coming from the main water source (that is, hose bib or water line) to acceptable levels for low-volume irrigation, around 10 to 30 pounds per square inch (psi).

Existing Automated Irrigation Systems

If you have an existing irrigation system and want to evaluate its performance or plan to make changes in it, you or a professional irrigator should perform an irrigation water audit on the system. An irrigation water audit determines the system's working efficiency. Hydraulic data of the system, such as the system's pressure, precipitation or flow rate, and the sprinkler distribution uniformity, plus the soil's infiltration rate, are collected. With this information, adjustments or design changes can be made to ensure the efficient operation of the system. Remember, though, this efficiency measurement is only for the mechanical operations of the system. Total efficiency of the system—a comparison of the amount of water put out by the system and the amount of water that is actually absorbed and held by the soil—requires efficient performance of the irrigation system and proper management of the system by you.

One way large amounts of water are wasted is by irrigating too frequently and for too long a time. Also, the water applied by sprinkler systems is too often lost before it reaches the ground because of evaporation; runoff that can cause erosion of the soil; overspraying on sidewalks, driveways, and fences; and deep percolation through the soil below the plant's root system.

A water audit can determine and pinpoint these inefficiencies and provide you with the information needed to modify an existing system and correct inefficient operating procedures. It can also be used to design an efficient irrigation system from the beginning. With a thorough water audit, you or your professional irrigator can develop an irrigation schedule custom designed for your Xeriscape landscape.

Modification of an existing sprinkler system to a full or partial drip system is relatively easy if you know the design of your existing system and the basics of drip irrigation. You cannot just remove a sprinkler head and install a drip emitter in its place. It is best to convert an entire zone with a separate valve for the areas covered with the drip irrigation to allow for the precise control of the amount of water applied. It is also important to have a controller that can be programmed to allow for different frequencies of watering for drip versus sprinkler irrigation.

There are a number of adapter units that can be inserted in the place of a sprinkler head that have small diameter tubes (spaghetti tubes) and emitters that can be run to individual plants. The key to converting sprinkler irrigation to drip is reducing the existing water pressure to the proper level required for drip and low-volume irrigation equipment. Many of the adapter units available have pressure-regulating capabilities.

Care should be taken when retrofitting an existing system to make sure that all components are compatible and the system will function properly. If you feel that your knowledge of irrigation is not quite up to the task, contact a professional irrigator for help.

Irrigation System Maintenance

A perfectly designed and installed irrigation system can be ruined without routine maintenance. Many factors can affect the efficient performance of an irrigation system, including vandalism, traffic, electrical problems, landscape equipment damage, debris in the water system, freezing weather, mineral deposits, wearing out of equipment, and defective materials or workmanship.

During a regular maintenance check (once a month), turn each zone on and inspect each sprinkler head within the zone for proper pop-up and seating (return to ready position), nozzle obstructions, and correct spray throw. Usually, only minor adjustments are necessary to correct any of these problems. Trim the grass around each sprinkler head regularly.

Any malfunctioning valves or controller problems will show up when you check the system zone by zone. If the water pressure is too high for the system, the nozzles create fog or mist instead of water drops. The mist is easily windblown and the landscape may start to show drought stress. In the summer this problem may become apparent in as short a time as a week or two, but if your system is operated through the winter, the problem may go undetected.

The plants may not suffer as much, but water will be wasted. To correct this situation, adjust the sprinkler head according to the manufacturer's instructions.

Too little water pressure shortens the throw distance of the water from the nozzle, leaving a pattern of green circles in the lawn. This will also become evident more quickly in hot weather. Correct by changing the nozzle size in the sprinkler head.

Slow leaks can occur in any irrigation system. Higher than usual water bills may be the first sign of a slow leak. Areas in the landscape may also appear more lush than their surroundings. An irrigation specialist should be called in to find the leak with a leak detector.

To ensure that you know exactly how much water you are using with your irrigation system, you should install a water meter and record on a regular basis (at least once each month at approximately the same time) the volume of water your system has consumed. By charting the flow of water through your system, you will be able to know exactly how much you have saved in water and money by applying the Xeriscape fundamentals to your project.

IRRIGATION MANAGEMENT

For much of the nation, the key to conserving water in the landscape is to irrigate properly. You can design and install the most elaborate and efficient irrigation system available, yet through poor management waste huge amounts of water. Drip irrigation equipment, for example, does not save water unless the operator manages the system properly. The point is that irrigation systems and equipment don't save water, people do. Realize, too, that our lawns have a drinking problem and we are the cause. People make the decisions on when and how to irrigate. It is our responsibility to do it correctly.

To water properly, it helps to be able to think like a plant. Asking a plant whether it is thirsty gets little response; therefore, you must be able to read the minds of your plants. Be a clairvoyant of the plant world.

Why Do Plants Need Water?

Here are some basics of how plants use water and where they get it. Water provides four primary functions in the plant. First, water helps inflate the plant, which keeps it standing up and growing. When a plant wilts, it's telling you that there is not enough water in the plant to keep the cells inflated, or turgid, for plant growth and health.

Water is used in photosynthesis, a sugar-making process that converts energy from the sun, plus water and oxygen, into food for the plant. Water is also the blood of the plant and aids in the circulation of food, nutrients, and hormones throughout the plant.

And finally, water helps cool the plant through transpiration, a perplexing process in the plant. Transpiration, the evaporation of water from the plant's leaves, cools the plant leaves on a hot day and is the driving force in "sucking" water out of the soil into the roots. However, transpiration has a wasteful side in that large amounts of water can be lost each day through transpiration with no visible benefit to the plant. On a hot summer day in the South, a pecan tree can transpire 120 gallons of water every day. The challenge in irrigation is to provide enough water for the plant health without applying luxuriant amounts that may simply be lost to transpiration.

The rate of transpiration by a plant is directly affected by the soil moisture level and the weather. As soil dries, transpiration slows, since it becomes increasingly difficult for the plant to suck water from the soil. Transpiration increases as temperature and light intensity increase. This is why summer, the hottest and brightest time of year, causes plant water-use rates to peak. Increases in wind speed also increase water use. Recognizing these factors in plant water use will help you decide when to water.

How Do Water, Soil, and Plants Relate?

The soil is the primary source of water for landscape plants. The soil serves as the reservoir, or "bank account," of water for the plant. As discussed in the soils chapter, each soil type can hold a specific amount of water. The strategy in irrigation management is to keep the bank account at acceptable levels for the plant to withdraw water, and to refill that bank account completely at every watering.

Soil is also a reservoir for oxygen, which is needed by the plant in order to take up water. If oxygen is forced out of the soil by flooding (water fills all available spaces in the soil), then most plants can't take up water. This phenomenon explains how plants can wilt when they are overwatered. It also explains the often used answer to questions about plant problems, "You're watering too much or too little."

How Do Plants Respond to a Lack of Water?

When plants experience a lack of water in the soil, several responses can occur. The most common sign of drought stress is wilting. However, plants also show other signs, including leaf rolling, color changes, leaf burning, and loss of leaves.

Most of the turfgrasses show stress by wilting, as indicated when your footprints are seen after a walk across the lawn. The turfgrasses with wider leaves (for example, St. Augustinegrass) will roll their leaves lengthwise in an attempt to reduce the leaf area and water loss. Lawn grasses often show a dullness versus the shiny green of a healthy plant.

Many tender flowers and shrubs will show these signs and/or a burning of the leaf edges or margins. The crispy margins occur when less than adequate supplies of water are flowing through the plant. Some plants in the landscape will also drop leaves during drought stress. The plant is simply attempting to lighten the demand for water and increasing its ability to survive drought. A prime example of this plant response is seen in ocotillo (*Fouquieria splendens*), a desert plant.

Philosophy for Efficient Irrigation

The philosophy for irrigating the landscape centers on meeting the water requirements of each plant without waste. Actual water requirements vary with the species, as evident by their natural environments (for example, desert plants versus rain forest plants). However, most plants are considered opportunistic, and will use excess water through wasteful transpiration and lush growth. By zoning plants according to water requirements as described in the planning and design chapter (page 22), you can concentrate on watering groups of plants instead of individual plant types.

Irrigation should enhance the plant's natural ability to obtain water. By watering deeply to fill the bank account of soil moisture at each irrigation, the plant is encouraged to have as deep a root system as possible. Remember, though, that soil types will also affect the depth of rooting. Clay restricts root growth more than sand; therefore, any given plant will usually have a deeper root system in sand than clay.

One of the simplest ways to reduce water waste, yet one that's often ignored, is not to irrigate during the daytime. The sun can evaporate as much as fifty percent of the water sprayed by sprinklers before it hits the ground. Irrigation should take place between dusk and about ten in the morning, with the optimum time being between 3 and 6 a.m. At this time irrigation avoids evaporation by the sun, plants dry out as the sun comes up and avoid potential disease problems, and watering is completed before in-house water use begins with bathing. If you do not have an automatic system and don't want to wake up before the chickens, please do your watering between dusk and bedtime. The concern for disease epidemics caused by watering at night is blown out of proportion in my judgment. If disease occurs, there are ways to control it.

Similar to time of day, season of the year greatly affects how you manage your watering. Whether you irrigate your landscape with a manual or automatic system, changes in the frequency and amount of irrigation should be made at least *monthly!*

Determining exactly when to irrigate a newly planted landscape may initially be a matter of trial and error. Watering during the establishment period is completely different from watering an older, established landscape. The best method is to start with a weekly watering and increase or decrease frequency as necessary based on observing the plants.

Allowing irrigation water to run off a landscape is a terrible waste. The rate at which a soil will absorb water is called the infiltration rate. If the irrigation system applies water (called the precipitation rate) faster than the infiltration rate, then runoff will occur. The following table shows the infiltration rates for selected soils:

Light, sandy soils	½ to ¾ inch per hour
Medium-textured clay or loam	¼ to ½ inch per hour
Heavy-textured clay	1/10 to ¼ inch per hour

To determine the precipitation rate of your sprinkler system, place three to five straight-sided containers (for example, tuna cans) in a line from a sprinkler out as far as the spray pattern extends. Turn the sprinkler on for a half hour. Then measure the amount of water (in inches) in each can, total the amounts, and divide by the number of cans to obtain an average. This number multiplied by two will give you a precipitation rate in inches per hour. Use this rate to gauge how long to irrigate to get one inch on the landscape.

As a rule, one inch of water is enough to penetrate the soil to a depth of one foot for sand and six inches for clay. Try to apply one inch of water at each irrigation for turfgrass, ground covers, and annual and perennial flowers. Deeper watering is recommended for shrubs and trees, since their root systems are usually deeper. An open, slow-running hose is probably the best equipment for this job.

On a heavy clay soil (which has a low infiltration rate), a one-inch irrigation will most likely cause runoff unless you multicycle your irrigation. This means irrigating a landscape area until just before runoff, stopping the irrigation in that spot, and irrigating another area. Then come back to the initial area and irrigate again after an hour or so to allow the previous watering to soak down into the soil. Keep cycling until one inch is applied. This multicycling of irrigation can be performed whether you use an automatic system or hose-end sprinklers.

Scheduling Irrigation

The answer to the age-old question "How long and when do I water?" is often very complex. Usually it is determined by whim, by old habits, or "by the seat of your pants." Now that you are thinking like a plant and have the basic philosophy of irrigation, here are six methods of scheduling irrigation (first described by Bill Pogue, Irrometer Company, Riverside, California).

"Set It and Forget It"

This method came with the advent of the automatic irrigation system. Although this system is the easiest and most convenient, it is the most wasteful because it does not take into account the ever-changing needs of the plant.

Much of the water waste in automatic irrigation systems occurs when people set their systems to water for the midsummer heat as soon as they turn them on in the spring, and never change them.

Remember that environmental conditions are the primary factors affecting plant water needs. Cloudy skies in the summer can reduce water use by half compared to clear blue skies.

Also, as a general rule, plants are capable of withstanding moderate drought more easily than too much moisture. For this reason it is important to let the soil become fairly dry between thorough waterings. If you "set it and forget it," this drying-out process may not have a chance to happen, so you're reducing your plant's health.

Plant Appearance

Sometimes a plant wilts on a hot day because moisture is evaporating from the leaves faster than the roots can supply it. If there is enough soil moisture, the plant absorbs water in the evening to firm up the stems and leaves. However, when the leaves remain wilted the following morning, watering is recommended. Wilting for a short time does not harm the plant, but over a prolonged period it can cause permanent damage. If turfgrass is showing drought stress, you have twenty-four to forty-eight hours to water it before damage occurs. See page 112 for other signs of stress from lack of water.

The Calendar

By now you should know why this is not a good method for scheduling watering. However, the reality for many of us living with voluntary or enforced watering restrictions is that this is unavoidable. If you can water only every three or four days, then missing a chance to water may be damaging, so people try not to miss a day, which in turn develops plants that have poor drought endurance and need regular watering!

The only solution is to do whatever you can by way of cultural practices to help your plants go longer between waterings (not to mention *your* letting them go longer), and try to help local water authorities find other ways to deal with temporary water shortages.

"Feel Method"

Probably the oldest and simplest method of measuring the soil moisture content is to squeeze a little bit of soil between your thumb and index finger. Crude and unscientific as this method might seem, it can give the experienced home gardener a quick field check. A soil sample can be obtained by a shovel, soil sampling tube, or soil auger.

Much of the value of the feel method is gained by your experience of how plants react to different levels of soil moisture without being damaged. Remember that in order to encourage deeper root growth you will want to take your soil sample near the bottom of the root zone. You may or may not want to go to the trouble of digging a hole in your lawn every week or so and will arrive at rough watering intervals that work for you. With a soil sampling tube the damage is minimal.

Moisture-Sensing Method

To increase the efficiency of either the sprinkler- or drip-type irrigation system, it is a good idea to use any one of the available and proven soil moisture and rainfall sensor devices. If you have an automatic system, you can use moisture sensors to override the wasteful watering practices of conventional timer controllers. The technology has been available since the early 1950s, but only recently have there been both products and management information geared toward the home landscape.

Rain shutoff sensors. This is one of the easiest ways to improve an existing automatic irrigation system. The rain shutoff unit is mounted where it is exposed to the open sky and will not be filled up by leaves or other debris. When the rainwater in the collection pan or cup reaches as much as ¼ inch deep, it turns off the entire system. The normal watering schedule resumes when the pan dries. These units cost $15 to $50 and are being used more and more to prevent watering during rain.

Soil moisture sensors. The main advantage of soil moisture sensors is that they can eliminate much of the irrigation management decisions. These devices indicate the soil moisture available to the plant and reduce the need for knowledge of the site-specific variables of soil type, microclimates, root/plant activity level and water-use rate, and root depth.

The main types of soil moisture sensing devices are tensiometers and gypsum blocks. They offer scientific measurements of soil moisture status, which is an indirect measurement of plant water use and need. As plants dry the soil through water uptake, the instruments read the soil dryness level and indicate the irrigation needs of the plants.

Cost and maintenance are important considerations in choosing a soil moisture sensor. Regardless of the type of sensor, it is best to install more than one sensor in most home landscapes to account for differences in microclimates and plant water-use zones. Tensiometers range in price from $35 to $50 in sizes suitable for home landscapes. Concerns have arisen, though, about their long-term maintenance, although great efforts are being made to develop a maintenance-free device.

Gypsum blocks are relatively inexpensive ($5 to $10 each), but the meter required to read the blocks may cost $200 to $300. The accuracy of the blocks will change over time, and each block may last about two years before needing to be replaced.

Advances in soil-sensing technology are developing rapidly in response to concern for water conservation. Computerized controllers for collecting and interpreting sensor-collected data are increasing the automation and efficiency of irrigation systems. Switching-type sensors, which are wired into valve circuitry of an automated irrigation system, operate like a soil moisture "thermostat" for the system. Some of the newest sensors look like metal tongue depressors that are stuck into the soil, read soil moisture levels, and communicate with the controller. There is great hope that these devices will be more maintenance-free, "user friendly," and cost-effective.

With any of the soil moisture sensors, a level of soil moisture must be selected by the irrigator as a trigger to begin irrigation. This will be a higher moisture level for water-loving plants and a lower level for the drought-tolerant ones. Once a moisture level has been selected, the system nearly runs itself. Further accuracy in scheduling can be achieved by combining this method with weather data, seasonal changes, additional equipment, and experience.

Although this method of scheduling seems fully automated, there is still need for regular maintenance. The sensors and other components should be inspected periodically (every four to eight weeks). Avoid being misled by claims that anything is "maintenance-free."

Moisture Balance Method

The moisture balance method combines knowledge of both soil moisture holding capabilities and estimates of plant water use. The goal is to balance incoming and outgoing soil moisture.

Evapotranspiration (ET) includes both evaporation from the soil and transpiration from the plant. The sun, wind, and plants themselves are constantly making withdrawals from the bank account of soil moisture. Each soil type holds a different amount of water available to plants. Sandy soil may hold only one-third as much as clay soil.

SOIL TEXTURE		READILY AVAILABLE MOISTURE/FOOT
Light, sandy	coarse sand	0.7 inch
	fine sand	0.9 inch
Medium, loamy	fine sandy loam	1.5 inches
	silt loam	1.9 inches
Heavy, clay	clay loam	2.1 inches
	clay	2.0 inches

For shallow-rooted plants, such as turf and annual flowers, their main root mass is only in the top foot of soil. Deeper-rooted plants, such as trees, shrubs, and ground covers, may have roots throughout the top twelve to thirty-six inches of soil. When using the moisture balance method, you need only consider the soil depth of plant roots to avoid overwatering and wasting water that flows down beyond the roots.

For instance, a clay soil holds two inches of moisture per foot of soil. For a turf area, be concerned only with the top foot; therefore, two inches of water are available to the plant. With a shrub having roots two feet in depth, there would be a total of four inches of available water.

University research indicates that it is best to irrigate when fifty percent of the soil moisture reserve is used up by ET to avoid plant stress. For the turf area with shallow roots, this means that irrigation should be applied when one inch of water has been lost to ET. For example, the daily ET rate for Dallas, Texas, in July is estimated at slightly over ¼ inch of ET lost per day. This means that a turf area in Dallas in a clay soil should be irrigated every four days to maintain the soil moisture level above fifty percent. And at that watering, one inch of water should be applied to bring the soil moisture back to capacity. By contrast, during March the turf area should be irrigated only every seven days because of the reduction in ET.

As a further contrast, the shrub area with a two-foot root zone in the same location in August should be irrigated only every seven or eight days. These irrigation frequencies must be adjusted when rainfall occurs, and the soil moisture level should be monitored, at least by feel, to determine if insufficient or excess irrigation is being applied.

Evapotranspiration data for your town can be obtained through the National Weather Service, your Cooperative Extension Service, or in the publication *Rainfall-Evapotranspiration Data, United States and Canada* (The Toro Company, Riverside, Calif., 1966). Keep in mind, though, that the ET estimates may be based on the most popular local turfgrass. Its water-use rate may or may not be indicative of other turfgrasses (especially native grasses), shrubs, and ground covers. You will need to judge whether your plants are using less water or more.

The moisture balance method, although not perfect, is useful for knowing when and how much to irrigate plants of various types on different soil types. The accuracy of this method can be increased by utilizing site-specific ET measurements, rainfall data, and/or soil moisture sensors.

Your experience and management skills still play the most important role in conserving water in the landscape. And don't lose sight of the fact that in a Xeriscape landscape, the whole idea is to eliminate unnecessary watering.

Irrigation, whatever the method used, is an important part of keeping Xeriscape projects looking their best in many parts of the country. Some landscape projects do not have irrigation systems, and the homeowner simply harvests the water Mother Nature furnishes, waters by hand only as needed, or allows the plants to survive on their own with no supplemental watering.

Even though irrigation is sometimes necessary, we must remember that the technology for irrigating anything other than agricultural crops has been prevalent for only about fifty years. Before that time some landscapes were very beautiful with only minimal supplemental water. Our culture has created the need for lush green grass at a very high cost in water use regardless of natural precipitation.

To keep our landscapes lush and green in areas of the country where rainfall won't support that, we must understand the new technologies that will assist us in doing so at a minimal cost to the environment by conserving and using water wisely. In addition, there should be much more study and research into how, exactly, to irrigate as efficiently as possible and to reuse and recycle treated wastewater, another byproduct of our current civilization and lifestyle. Some municipalities are reusing treated wastewater from processing plants on golf courses, open spaces, and parks. And some communities have tried to implement this use of "gray water" in new subdivisions, with mixed success. There are decided advantages and disadvantages to using recycled water, but we must continue to research and develop new techniques that will allow us to reuse this most precious resource, water, to its fullest extent.

Mulching

A TEST made in the spring of 1988 at the University of California/Irvine compared moisture savings and soil temperature reduction under several mulching materials:

• peat moss, costing 30 cents/square foot for each two-inch layer
• commercial compost, at 18 cents/square foot for each two-inch layer
• shredded fir bark, costing 6 cents/square foot for each two-inch layer.

The materials were compared at depths of one, two, and four inches. Those that did best in preventing moisture loss proved to be the fir bark at two inches and four inches. The soil beneath all three was ten degrees cooler one inch below soil line than the unmulched controls. In another experiment a three-inch layer of mulch reduced soil temperatures as much as ten degrees as far down as eight inches below the surface. Unmulched soil reached temperatures as high as 100 to 108 degrees Fahrenheit in the top few inches, high enough to kill roots.

These tests point out what gardeners have known for millennia. Mulching, the sixth Xeriscape principle, is a very good thing. In fact, with a few cautions, there's almost nothing bad to say about mulching.

Reducing soil temperature is one way mulching preserves moisture. It also reduces exposure to wind, which can pull moisture up and out of the soil through evaporation. One study showed that a two-inch layer of leaf litter reduced evaporation forty-five to sixty-five percent, depending on the type of leaf. (Pine needles did the best.)

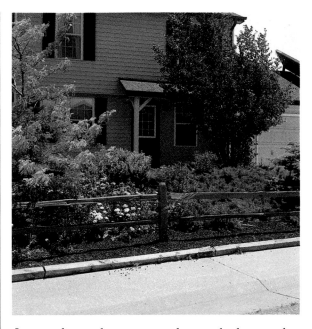

Lava rock was chosen to complement the house color and to set off the plants in this nonturf Xeriscape garden. Plants include quaking aspen (Populus tremuloides), junipers (Juniperus spp.), sweet William (Dianthus barbatus), garden tiger lilies (Lilium spp.), and honey locust (Gleditsia triacanthos).

Interestingly enough, what makes the best mulch for water conservation may or may not be the one that looks the best, is the least expensive, or reduces heat alone. A mulch should do the following:

Limit reflectivity. Bare sand or clay soil develops a very light reflective surface during the hot summer months which bounces the heat and light of the sun back onto plants, adjacent surfaces and buildings, and to the atmosphere. Mulch provides a darker and more fragmented surface that cuts down on the reflectivity and cools the area around plant stems and leaves. As a result, less water is often evaporated out of the soil and plants.

Curtail heat. The soil surface is cooled when mulch is used, so less water is evaporated from the heated soil. It helps seal in the moisture around the root zone by protecting them from extremes of heat and cold. (Winter protection is a big part of the function of mulch. It regulates the temperature of the soil around the roots, preventing freeze damage, frost heave, and too-early emergence of spring bulbs.)

Hold and build the soil. By insulating against freezing and thawing, mulch prevents cracks from forming in the soil surface. By retaining moisture in the root zone, mulch encourages root growth that stabilizes the soil. It allows water to move in an orderly way into the root zone. Organic mulch eventually breaks down and improves the quality and water-holding capacity of the soil near the surface.

Prevent weeds. By blocking out sunlight, mulch helps prevent weed seeds from germinating and competing with landscape plants for available soil moisture. In gardens it's safer to mulch to control weeds than to cultivate (break off or dig them out with a hoe) because the roots of the garden plants are left undisturbed.

Keep water in the root zone. Water is retained in the upper layers of the soil where most annuals, perennials, and ground covers draw their moisture since mulch reduces evaporation and transpiration.

Control erosion. Mulch softens the impact of falling rainwater and slows it down so it can soak into the soil before running off. It also prevents soil from being disturbed or washed away from around plants.

Reduce maintenance. No water is needed to maintain mulch, compared to any type of plant cover, either to sustain the plants or to water in fertilizers, for instance. Periodic weeding and occasional replacement are all that's needed for the maintenance of mulch areas.

Uses no water as a groundcover planting would. Whether turf, ground cover, or other plant material, all plant soil coverings are growing and using water out of the soil. Mulch doesn't use water and seals it in, making it available for nearby plants.

Mulches fulfill many functions in Xeriscape gardens. In addition to all their water-conserving qualities, they serve to separate water-use zones when used under shrub and tree plantings. As discussed in the tree and shrub section of the appropriate plant selection chapter, there are many reasons for keeping these plantings separate from turf, and mulch provides a nonwater-using soil covering for those areas. Mulch can be used as attractive ground coverings for utility areas or other areas where turf is deemed nonfunctional.

Of course, entire landscapes covered with mulch are unattractive, but when combined with water-conserving vegetation and a well-designed hardscape, they are effective and attractive.

Mulches can be an important design feature when used as an accent for turf. Many organic materials such as shredded bark, compost, and leaf mold are dark brown in color and provide a background color for flowers and plant materials. In general, organic mulches lend a naturalistic, informal note, while inorganic mulches such as gravel are often used for more formal designs.

Some potential problems with mulching that must be considered when selecting a mulch and mulching depth include:

The hazard of fire. especially with dried pine needles, straw, and evergreen boughs. Locate mulch beds with flammable mulches away from wooden walls and fences.

Nitrogen deficiency. Extremely fresh organic mulching materials such as sawdust, grass clippings, straw, nut and grain hulls, manure, and chipper waste may draw nitrogen out of the soil as the material breaks down and cause a temporary deficiency in the soil. (Yellowing of the lowest plant leaves is a sign of this.) This problem can be prevented by adding nitrogen in the form of ammonium sulfate, calcium nitrate, or nitrate of soda (one tablespoonful per bushel of material) once or twice each growing season, or three pounds actual nitrogen (slow-release fertilizers such as ureaform are best) per cubic yard of material. Use whatever form of nitrogen is recommended by your local extension agent.

Salt. Partially composted mulches such as mushroom compost and manure can have a high level of salts that can damage plants. Rather than applying them in the spring, use them in fall so winter rains and snowmelt can wash out the salts.

Rodent and pest problems. Some organic mulches encourage insect pests such as slugs, snails, sowbugs, and earwigs by creating a dark, moist environment. Rodents may tunnel under a thick layer of mulch, especially straw, leaves, and corncobs. When these mulches are used, they should not be placed closer than six inches from the base of woody plants. When they are placed too close, rodents living in the mulch will chew the bark of the plants, girdling and killing them.

Overmulching. Too thick a layer of mulch may reduce the penetration of oxygen and water into the soil, which may kill shallow-rooted plants. In humid parts of the country, roots may grow along the soil surface under a layer of mulch that's too thick (over two inches) because they are able to take moisture from the air. They are then at risk during drought periods.

Undermulching. If weed control is a primary consideration and you live in a part of the country not subject to the humidity problem just discussed, you may want to consider that ultraviolet light has been shown to penetrate as much as four inches into bark or similar-density mulching materials. To prevent sunlight from encouraging weeds to grow, layer your mulch four to six inches deep, *or* use a three-inch mulch layer over a weed-barrier fabric.

Depth of Mulch

The guidelines for mulch depth given in the following table are general. You may want to increase or decrease the depth depending on local climatic conditions. Just remember that going too thin usually leads to weed problems. A rule of thumb suggests using a one- to two-inch layer for a mulch with mostly ½-inch particles, and using thicker layers for larger particles.

One cubic yard of mulch (twenty-seven cubic feet) covers:

80 square feet	when four inches deep
100 square feet	when three inches deep
160 square feet	when two inches deep
325 square feet	when one inch deep

It takes three cubic yards to cover 1,000 square feet one inch thick, and two cubic feet to cover

eight square feet three inches deep. To figure out the number of bags or cubic yards of mulch you'll need, multiply the area by the desired depth of mulch expressed in feet, then divide that amount by the number of cubic feet in the bag, or cubic yard (twenty-seven cubic feet). For example:

900 square feet at a 3-inch mulch depth:
$$900 \times {}^3/_{12} = 225 \text{ cubic feet}$$
225 cubic feet/3 cubic feet per bag $= 75$ bags
OR
225 cubic feet/27 cubic feet per yard $= 8$ cubic yards (rounded off)

Time to Mulch

The best time to mulch for water conservation is in late spring, after the soil has absorbed water from spring rains but before summer heat starts to pull the moisture back out. Mulches to enhance appearance and control weeds may be applied at any time. Those applied to protect fall transplants from freezing should be put in place soon after transplanting. This helps keep the temperature of the soil warmer longer for better root growth. If the mulch is to be used to prevent early spring emergence of bulbs or to reduce frost heave, it should be applied after the ground has frozen (usually after the second or third freeze of the fall). Pull the mulch back in spring from emerging plants, especially perennials, when danger of hard frost is past.

MULCHING MATERIALS

The advantages and disadvantages, especially with respect to water conservation, of numerous mulching materials are discussed here. Mulches are either organic or inorganic. Inorganic mulches are man-made or created from inorganic natural sources, while organic mulches come from plant and animal sources, as waste material, trimmings, or decaying leaves. They are part of the life-death-decay-life cycle that occurs in nature, so they must all be understood to be temporary, to different degrees.

They will all break down eventually, whether in one year or less, or over several years depending on the mulch and the climate, so they need to be periodically replenished. In the process of their breaking down, organic mulching materials enrich the soil. If a primary aim is to improve the soil, choose an organic mulch. Earthworms will assist by incorporating some of the mulching material into the top layer of the soil.

Organic Mulches

The most appropriate mulch for each plant is the leaf and twig litter from the plant itself; pine trees do best with pine needle mulch, deciduous trees and shrubs utilize nutrients from their own leaves. You can take a cue from nature by not raking up the dead leaves from all the shrubs and trees but letting them mulch themselves. This is especially beneficial over the winter when leaf layers provide some insulation for the roots. If you can't bear not to be spic-and-span, at least wait till spring to do the cleaning, then compost the leaves.

Shredded bark mulch serves as a design element, linking planting beds and stairway. Zinnias (Zinnia spp.), marigolds (Tagetes spp.), and a rosebush are still in bloom in this October photo.

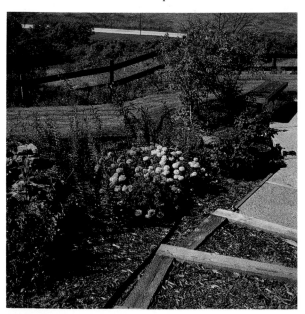

MATERIAL	RECOMMENDED DEPTH
Shredded bark	3–4″

Advantages: Binds the soil, lets water in and holds it in the soil well. Builds the moisture-holding capacity of soil. Pieces tend to knit together, making the mulch sturdier and less prone to wash away than chunk bark or wood chips. Slow to break down because of the lignin (plant carbohydrate that decomposes slowly) in it.

Disadvantages: Expensive. May compact over time. Can be unsightly and ineffective if applied in too thin a layer.

Wood chips	3–4″

Advantages: Let water in effectively. Keep some in the mulch layer, but allow little out. Cool and seal the soil. Keep down weeds. Improve the water-holding capacity of the soil. Many sizes available but largest and smallest should be avoided.

Disadvantages: Break down and disintegrate in a year or two, depending on the source of wood and type. Small sizes break down quickly and will require the addition of nitrogen to replenish what they initially take from the soil as they decay.

Chunk bark	4–6″

Advantages: Coarse texture. Large size lets more water in but doesn't hold it in as well as finer-textured materials. Can be long-lasting. Recent research has shown it to have superior weed control capability compared to shredded bark. (Bird netting can be put over it to keep it in place.)

Disadvantages: May blow around in windy areas, or wash away on slopes. Fairly expensive. Not always available, except regionally. Breaks down slowly, so doesn't add to soil texture and nutrients.

Chipper debris	3–4″

Advantages: A mixture of shredded bark, wood chips, and leaves available from tree-trimming operations, often free for asking and hauling from city or private tree crews. (Look in the White or Blue Pages for municipal arborist or parks department, or in the Yellow Pages for private companies.) Some cities are recycling Christmas trees this way. Lets

MATERIAL	RECOMMENDED DEPTH

water in effectively. Adds humus as it breaks down. (Avoid chipper waste from eucalyptus trees. It may retard plant growth.)

Disadvantages: Mixture of materials may lead to uneven appearance. May create nitrogen deficiency in soil as it breaks down. In spring add half of the nitrogen fertilizer dose recommended on page 118. I use chipper debris and find it gives a very rustic appearance, which is usually okay for the effect I want especially at the extremities of the landscape. However, very delicate plants are hard to discern against the mottled surface. Mulch around small plants with a higher-quality, more even-looking material.

Sawdust and wood shavings   1–3″

Advantages: Available and comparatively inexpensive in many areas. Decompose, adding humus to the soil. Easily applied and give favorable appearance. Free of most weed seeds and diseases. Help water-holding capacity of the soil as they disintegrate.

Disadvantages: Increase soil acidity. This may be favorable for some plants, but toxic to others. Should be weathered for one or more years before being applied. Injury may occur to many plants if applied too heavily because the sawdust holds a great deal of water itself, increasing its weight. Not all of the water reaches the soil. They can form a barrier that compacts in time. Break down rapidly, blow in the wind when dry. Nitrogen must be added to the soil or to the sawdust (see page 118) to avoid nitrogen depletion. Burn easily and are hard to extinguish.

Pine needles   2–3″

Advantages: Easily applied and give favorable appearance. Available and cheap in many areas. Increase water-holding capacity of the soil. Loose, light, but help bind soil. Let in a lot of water, hold little itself, and let some water be transpired back out. Decompose, adding humus to the soil and increasing soil acidity, which helps acid-loving plants such as pines, azaleas, rhododendrons, camellias, and blueberries.

MATERIAL	RECOMMENDED DEPTH

Disadvantages: Not always available. Settle and form a water-impervious mat. Last a short time.

Evergreen boughs   2–4″

Advantages: Available and comparatively inexpensive in many areas. Easy to handle; quickly applied and easily removed.

Disadvantages: Fire hazard when dry. Should not be applied adjacent to buildings. Make great homes for mice and other small rodents.

Lawn clippings   1″ at a time

Advantages: Experts say it's better to leave the clippings on the lawn unless they've become matted, but if you don't remove your clippings you undoubtedly have some die-hard neighbors who've gathered theirs. Dry out the clippings in thin layers on plastic or pavement for a day to prevent the anaerobic decomposition of fresh grass, which can lead to slime, smell, and flies. Readily available. Let some water in, hold little, and inhibit transpiration. Best used in small areas. One caution: Don't put weed-and-feed treated grass clippings on your vegetable garden or wildflower plantings.

Disadvantages: May contain weed seeds. Heat up and create offensive odor if not dried first. Correct for nitrogen deficiency as directed on page 118.

Sphagnum peat moss   1–3″

Advantages: Improves physical conditions of most soils. Source of fertility that is slowly available to plants. Greatly increases the water-holding capacity of the soil. Holds water in the soil very effectively, and holds a great deal of water itself. Easy to handle and adds to the appearance of the soil. Often increases the soil acidity, which is generally advantageous.

Disadvantages: Not always available and often rather expensive. Impervious to water when dry. May blow in windy sites. May not let water in when it is wet. Cannot easily be used on slopes because it erodes; best used in small confined areas. Breaks down rapidly.

MATERIAL   RECOMMENDED DEPTH

Bog or sedge peats   1–3″

Advantages: Much less expensive where regionally or locally available. Hold water, but also let water in effectively. May not drift as much as sphagnum peat when dry. Usually lower in organic matter than sphagnum. Can be bought in bulk.

Disadvantages: Not always weed-free. Not as uniform or predictable as sphagnum. Not ecologically sound, because mountain sedge peats in Colorado, for instance, are mined from 10,000-year-old meadows, so one ancient ecosystem is being decimated in favor of another. Break down rapidly.

Straw from wheat, oats, barley,   4–6″
or rye (not hay—too many weed seeds)

Advantages: Generally available and comparatively inexpensive. Decomposes slowly, adding humus to the soil. Easily lets water in, cools the soil, and holds some water in the soil, though not as well as some other mulches. Good for temporary cover, gardens, and grass seeding.

Disadvantages: Often rather unsightly. May blow and scatter. Will mat down. Harbors insects, diseases, weed seeds, and rodents. Some danger from fire when dry, so should not be applied next to buildings. Needs addition of nitrogen (see page 118).

Leaves/leaf mold   2–4″

Advantages: Lets some water in and keeps it in. Holds the soil. Readily available at little or no cost, but should be partially rotted before being applied. Improves the water-holding capacity of the soil. One of the best mulching materials for trees, woody perennials, and wildflowers. Shredded leaves are more compact and easier to use.

Disadvantages: Leaves, when used exclusively, frequently pack too heavily when applied over tender herbaceous perennials and may be injurious. Harbor insects, diseases, weed seeds, and rodents. Nitrogen needs to be added (see page 118). Matting may lead to runoff of water. Can be a fire hazard. Dries and blows. Unshredded leaves are difficult to handle.

MATERIAL   RECOMMENDED DEPTH

Partially decomposed compost   2–4″

Advantages: Can be made from garden and kitchen waste. Readily available. Costs little other than labor and storage. An excellent method of incorporating organic matter into the soil and improving water-holding capacity. Is average at letting water in. Holds some water itself, but is excellent at holding it in the soil. Before spreading, sift to remove all large, uncomposted pieces.

Disadvantages: Needs to be stored and aged on or near the site. Is unsightly and bulky during storage. Takes time to collect and compost. May have weed seeds.

Strawy manure   2–4″

Advantages: Acts as a low-level fertilizer and improves the water-holding capacity of the soil. Will be incorporated into the soil and have to be renewed each year. A good soil builder, adds humus, and contains available plant food.

Disadvantages: Source of supply may be limited. May contain high levels of salt. Harbors insects, disease, and weed seeds. Unsightly, objectionable to apply, and may "burn" plants because of high ammonia content unless heat-treated or aged. Decomposes rapidly; should be replenished frequently.

Tobacco stems   2–3″

Advantages: Available in limited areas. May aid in the control of many insects and repel rodents. Add fertility and humus to the soil.

Disadvantages: May have offensive odor if not cured (weathered). Carrier of certain diseases (tobacco mosaic) that may affect some plants, such as tomatoes.

Ground or crushed corncobs   2–3″

Advantages: Generally available at comparatively low costs. They should be finely ground. Decompose very slowly. Easily applied, and give favorable appearance. Greatly increase water-holding capacity of the soil.

MATERIAL   RECOMMENDED DEPTH

Disadvantages: Attract rodents, especially when first applied. Soil nitrogen is less available, so supplementing may be needed (see page 118).

**Spent hops; oat, peanut,   2–3″
buckwheat, and cottonseed hulls; pecan shells;
mushroom compost; cocoa bean and rice hulls**

Advantages: Regionally available mulching materials that are attractive, easy to handle, and effective in letting water into the soil and holding little themselves. Can be low-level fertilizers, adding humus to the soil. Some are excellent soil conditioners. Comparatively inexpensive in limited areas. Decompose slowly. Greatly increase the water-holding capacity of the soil. May be available for the hauling of it.

Disadvantages: Available in limited areas. Cost, if any, depends on transportation expense. May change the soil chemistry. May need to be ground or processed before use. Soil nitrogen is less available, so supplementing may be needed (see page 118). Rice hulls may blow around; to prevent this, cover them with a thin layer of a heavier material.

Newspaper   1″ or less

Advantages: Available and cheap. Easily applied. Lay down six to eight sheets thick and immediately weigh down with a light covering of soil or sand, wetting to hold it in place. Keeps some water in, controls erosion, and can be incorporated into the soil as it weathers. May be used in small areas as a temporary mulch.

Disadvantages: Decomposes rather rapidly. Lets little water in. Unsightly and may dry out and blow away if not covered.

Snow

Advantages: Sometimes called "the poor man's mulch," an excellent insulator against cold and drying winds. Nature's best mulching material. Keeps plants in dormancy during midwinter warm spells.

Disadvantages: Sometimes objectionable, depending on the circumstances. Usually not available in the South!

Inorganic Mulches

Inorganic mulches consist generally of sheet plastic, woven fabric, or any of several types of rock. Sheet plastic is fairly inexpensive while woven fabric is quite expensive. In both cases these mulches are usually covered with some other mulching material for a more attractive appearance. What we really think of when it comes to inorganic mulches is rock, whether crushed stone, river rock, gravel, etc.

It would be tempting to try to oversimplify in commenting on the amount of energy (as in fossil fuel) it takes to bring rock mulch to your yard—the price is an indication of how much it takes—but it's not quite that easy. It undoubtedly takes lots of energy to mine, possibly crush, and transport rock products; it also takes energy to grind up wood products or other organic mulches and transport them. In addition, rock mulches last for several years, while organic amendments must be renewed every year in many cases. Between the two options it's hard to say which takes more energy.

However, there is one cost involved in using rock mulches that is inescapable: the fact that every rock used is being irrevocably moved from one environment to another, with no chance for regeneration. With river rock, for instance, you should realize that natural areas such as stream beds, shorelines, and mountains are being plundered to make decorative landscapes.

Rock mulches, though they can be very striking and decorative, are not perfect. They usually let through all the water they receive, but they can also exclude air and water from the roots of trees and shrubs. They're long-lasting, but hard to clean. They'll block weeds *if* installed thickly enough, but they bounce tremendous amounts of heat and light back to adjacent plants, people, and homes.

(On the other hand, rock mulches are a better choice for alpine wildflowers. These plants are adapted to very poor soil and little moisture, and may actually die if mulched with a more moisture-retentive bark-type mulch.)

MATERIAL	RECOMMENDED DEPTH

Plastic film   **3—10 mm**

Advantages: Holds water in very effectively. Controls weeds unless holes are punched to allow water in. Easy to transport, thin, light.

Disadvantages: Must be covered or masked with other materials. Heat that develops under the plastic can injure plant roots. Lack of air and oxygen exchange is very hard on nearby plants. Doesn't work well on slopes because whatever material is used to cover it slides off. Labor-intensive to install. Increases danger of creating "zero-scape" or "ugly-scape."

Woven fabrics   **3—10 mm**

Advantages: Used to exclude weeds. Often combined with organic mulches for a more natural appearance.

Disadvantages: Expensive. Labor-intensive to install.

Gravel, river rock   **1—3″**

Advantages: Lets water in very well, holds none itself, and keeps water in the soil. Lasts a long time, comes in a variety of sizes and colors, and doesn't break down.

Disadvantages: Expensive. Must be mined from natural areas. Can be pushed down into the soil. Doesn't help water-holding capacity of the soil. Unsightly if used in large areas. Tends to slide or be washed down slopes. Hard to keep clean under

MATERIAL	RECOMMENDED DEPTH

pines and other fine-needled leaved trees. Will not prevent growth of some weedy grasses unless combined with plastic or weed-barrier fabric.

Crushed stone   **1—3″**

Advantages: Lets all moisture into the soil, keeps none itself, and keeps moisture in the root zone. Many colors available.

Disadvantages: Expensive. Can be be very reflective if too white. May change the soil chemistry when it breaks down. Will not prevent growth of some weedy grasses unless combined with plastic or weed barrier fabric.

Pumice   **2—3″**

Advantages: Holds some water in the pores of the rock, but allows much of the water into the soil. Lightest and most porous of the inorganic mulches. Available in a variety of colors.

Disadvantages: Breaks down in a few years, but does not integrate into the soil to improve its water-holding capacity. Only regionally available. Will not prevent growth of some weedy grasses without being combined with plastic or weed-barrier fabric.

Decomposed granite   **2—3″**

Advantages: Long-lasting. Lets water in and holds it in the soil. Holds some water itself. Very dense mulch that excludes weeds. Many colors possible.

Disadvantages: Only regionally available. Disintegrates over several years.

Appropriate Maintenance

MAINTENANCE in Xeriscape landscaping, as in any landscaping, basically includes five tasks: weeding, feeding, pruning (this includes mowing), pest control, and watering. These tasks are interrelated, with watering being the key task. You'll have less of both weeding and pruning if you can keep the watering to a minimum. Overwatering contributes to the presence of insects and diseases, and excessive feeding (which must usually be watered in) may lead to more weeding and pruning. One of Xeriscape landscaping's truisms is the higher the water requirement of a landscape, the higher the maintenance needs will be.

Much of the maintenance you may detest can be avoided by thorough planning and design, appropriate installation techniques, and timely observation of the condition of grasses, plants, planting bed conditions, and irrigation system components.

Early in my teaching career I found William Morwood's little paperback book, *The Lazy Gardener's Garden Book* (New York: Tower Books, 1970), and have taken many of its helpful and humorous bits of information to heart. Some of his information is dated, but the general idea is not to let the maintenance of your landscape become such a demanding and "work"-oriented task.

If you hate weeding, then make sure your mulched areas have a thick-enough layer of mulch (three to five inches), or include the use of weed-barrier fabric beneath the mulch (not a good idea in annual and perennial flower beds or in ground-cover areas, for reasons I will elaborate on later), and learn what it takes to maintain a thick, healthy stand of turf to keep out weeds in your lawn. Plant flowers, annuals and perennials, and ground covers close enough together so that they will compete with and shade out weeds.

If you dislike pruning, select plants that are dwarf varieties, that will grow slowly, or that can be left to assume their natural form and shape. *Always* give your plants enough room away from walls and other structures, utilities, paving surfaces, and each other so they will mature to fulfill the purpose you intended in your design and won't outgrow their space.

If you don't like to mow, plan to install low-maintenance ground covers, use slow-growing native grasses, budget and design practical hardscape areas, or use only minimal lawn areas.

If fertilizing is not your bag, you could learn environmentally safe feeding methods (*Jerry Baker's Flowering Garden*, New York: Collier Books, 1990, has several recipes for homemade plant food formulas), or you could just not worry about it too much and let the plants grow using the nutrients available in the well-prepared soil you have provided. Except for lawn grasses, many plants will survive and look great without supplemental feeding. This is especially true if you've designed primarily with native or hardy adapted plants.

If pest control is a concern, don't overwater. Also design your Xeriscape landscape to include a wide variety of plants, and try to use plants and pools or basins of water to attract wildlife and birds to your landscape. You should try to create an environment that will encourage a variety of creatures (including beneficial insects) to visit, and possibly live in, your yard; that will help create an ecological balance of prey and predators that will more nearly duplicate the natural "web of life" John Storer talks about in his excellent little book by the same name.

If watering is not your idea of fun, then make sure you know your soil type and follow the guidelines in the chapter on soil improvements for keeping watering to a minimum. In many parts of the country you should have a "sense of humus" about your soil, since much of it lacks organic matter that is always helpful in absorbing and retaining water. Most of the suggestions in the previous sections of this book are designed to get you to the place where you have a beautiful landscape that doesn't require much watering or, for that matter, much of the other maintenance chores, except for doing regular seasonal cleanup, checking and adjusting the irrigation system (if you have one), and adding mulch to planting bed areas to control weeds.

Observation and Planning

After you have successfully planned and designed your project, installed it properly using the best techniques for soil preparation and an efficient irrigation system (if you choose), and selected and planted low-water-demand plants, you are ready for the task that will take up your time for the life of your project, the oft-dreaded word "maintenance."

The first and very important step in a good maintenance program is the timely and thorough observation of the conditions you have created or enhanced in your Xeriscape landscape. There is no substitute for physically being in your landscape on a regular basis and carefully checking on the conditions of your plants. Now this doesn't mean you need to live in the landscape, but that you should at least be there regularly, a minimum of once a week during the growing season, and become familiar with the general health of your plants and lawn.

You should be aware of the general appearance of the plants and lawn, and whether they are showing signs of stress from lack of water, disease and insect infestations, competition from weeds, shortages of nutrients in the soil, or other problems that may have resulted from any severe weather conditions that occurred since your last visit.

Be alert for signs of disease and insect damage such as holes in leaves or deposits of larvae inside curled leaves. By early detection, you may prevent the need for massive use of chemicals to rid your landscape of these problems.

Weed infestations are easily controlled. With a few minutes of each day spent pulling the most

recent invaders, you will prevent the later back-breaking job of a major weed war, either by hand-weeding or applying chemicals.

If leaves turn yellow or a pale green, you might have a lack of nutrients in the soil; an application of liquid fertilizer may be necessary as a foliar or deep root feeding to restore vigor to the plant.

It is a good idea to record what you see either in a brief journal or notebook format, or you may photograph or videotape the conditions for comparisons during the planning and preparation for maintenance during the year. This is where an accurate as-built drawing of the final results of your Xeriscape landscape will help you to recognize and record changes in your project. You can use it to locate specific elements that will need special attention and record the results for future planning.

Thoroughness, attention to details, and good planning will help you keep on top of the maintenance conditions, and will allow you to make timely judgments and decisions to enhance the success and enjoyment of your Xeriscape project. Neglect and haphazard scheduling of regular maintenance tasks will lead to short- and long-term problems that will compound with time and cause you more problems and grief than is necessary. So try to keep on top of the situation and be in control rather than have to put out "fires" as difficulties and problems with your plants and lawn arise.

WEED CONTROL

One of the most disconcerting situations that occurs when you have tried to apply all of the Xeriscape fundamentals, especially when you have used large planting bed areas of flowers and ground covers, is that you are often confronted with numerous weeds during the first year of your project. This frequently occurs when you have incorporated soil amendments, such as manure or topsoil, that carry a high level of weed seeds, or when you have rototilled the existing soil without removing the weeds first. Or you may have overwatered the plants and lawns during the establishment period or had an excess of natural rainfall, both creating excellent growing conditions for weeds as well as your new plants.

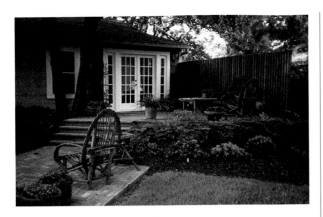

Doug Welsh's first Xeriscape garden (San Antonio, Texas) featured a wood deck and interlocking pavers, drip irrigation, exciting drought-tolerant plants, a functional turf area, mulched beds, and, of course, appropriate maintenance. (Design: Terry Lewis/John Troy, San Antonio, Texas. Photo: W. A. Adams)

The best thing to do if this occurs is to pull the weeds, rake the planting bed areas regularly to stir up the mulch material, thereby disturbing the germinating and growing conditions for the weeds, and add more mulch to prevent further weed growth.

Pulling the weeds is the best way if you have a heavy infestation, and the earlier the better, even though as a certified "lazy gardener" I hate the idea of crawling around on the ground and snatching these new growing creatures from their snug locations. I have often thought that we should allow the weeds to grow and take over an area since they seem to do so well in spite of all our efforts to control them.

Using any one of the many fabric-type weed barriers under organic or inorganic mulches is often recommended as a way to control weeds. In theory, this seems like a good idea, but in practice I have found several problems. First, when used in flower beds or groundcover areas the weed-barrier material is often cut so many times to allow for the planting of flowers that it becomes as useless as a holey raincoat. In addition, when used in groundcover areas it will often not allow the spread of the plants, restricting the growth of runners and spreading roots.

Second, when using weed-barrier materials in combination with organic mulch you will have a buildup of decomposed mulch forming a composted soil that will grow weeds on top of the fabric while still restricting the growth of weeds through it. In a period of less than four years in my own planting bed areas, I removed the fabric material because I found that the weeds flourished in the compost where the barrier was left intact and that we had shredded the fabric in areas where we had planted the many beautiful perennials and ground covers that were intended to reduce the amount of watering we had been doing in our typical bluegrass lawn.

When you use weed-barrier materials under inorganic mulch, such as rocks and gravel, you will also create a barrier for fine particles of dust and dirt that are not allowed to wash through the gravel and into the soil layer beyond. This again creates a great growing environment for the many weed seeds that are also spread by the wind and water and that fall into the spaces between the rocks and gravel, promoting growth on top of the barrier material. Usually a hosing down or a vigorous raking of the mulched areas will help in the removal of weed seeds. The earlier you do this, the better off you will be. Nip the little rascals in the bud by stirring up their happy home with a rake. Don't be bashful at this point, since early action with a rake and a hoe will keep you from stooping to their level and pulling them once they have gotten a firm hold in your soil or mulch area.

FEEDING AND FERTILIZING

Feeding new plants often is discouraged since doing so may cause burning and other damage to tender roots and leaves. But if you have planted ground cover in a bed area and mulched with an organic material, you may have set up a condition that will retard the establishment of the plants. Fresh organic mulch often requires a high level of nitrogen in the initial stages of the decomposition process at the same time the new plants need the same nitrogen for vigorous leaf and root growth during the establishment process.

The best recommendation, then, is to apply a liquid or slow-release granular fertilizer with a relatively high nitrogen content that will help balance the nitrogen supply to the plants during the early establishment period. Sometimes only one application of fertilizer is required, but you must observe the situation carefully and be prepared to do additional feedings as necessary. Usually after the first growing season an aggressive ground cover will fill in completely and discourage further weed growth. On occasion, however, the timid and less aggressive ground covers such as *Mahonia repens* (Oregon grape holly) will require additional feedings to promote quick covering in a planting bed area.

Feeding a lawn is another matter entirely. Because turfgrasses use up the nitrogen supply in the soil more rapidly than most other plants, it is often essential to fertilize the lawn on a regular basis. In addition, one of the best ways to prevent weed problems is to have a healthy and well-fed lawn.

You should not apply fertilizer arbitrarily, but rather take soil samples as explained in the planning and design and soil improvement chapters. Find out the exact conditions of your soil and add only the required nutrients and elements that will produce the healthy lawn and plants you want. All too often we, both homeowners and professional turf managers, will purchase the latest or best fertilizer, according to the sales and promotions at our local garden supplier, and not be sure of what our plants and grasses really need. We often force-feed our lawns simply because it seems the thing to do. Don't let all the media commercials make you buy something because it looks good. Use only those products that your lawn really needs and that will be good for the total environment.

PRUNING AND MOWING

The control of growth by pruning and mowing is a never-ending battle in the maintenance war. By nature, the physical act of pruning actually encourages more vigorous growth; the more you prune and mow, the more you will have to keep doing it. Allowing plants to attain their natural growth habit actually provides a more pleasing appearance and considerably reduces the amount of pruning you will have to do.

It is best to know the rate of growth and mature size of a plant when selecting it for a specific purpose and location in your project, and to allow for the maximum space for it to mature and fill in, rather than to overplant an area and have to "harvest" from

it by pruning and removing overgrown plant materials. The tendency, however, by both the homeowner and the professional designer is to overplant for immediate effect. To do so is to ask for future problems during the maintenance process.

It is often very difficult to settle for fewer plants and a relatively stark appearance during the early years of a project, however; most projects will have a more finished appearance after three to four years, and will cost less in the initial installation and during the long-range maintenance.

Mowing is the most dreaded word in the "lazy gardener's" vocabulary. Most turf-type grasses in the vast majority of lawns in this country are mowed more often than necessary, usually because that seems to be the thing to do. By mowing less frequently, you allow the grass plants to mature and to provide a healthier defense to the many diseases and insects that seem ready to devour them during times of stress caused by drought, overwatering, or other excesses that the unknowing (but well-meaning) homeowner perpetrates on them.

Unless you are going to play a sport such as golf, baseball, or croquet on your grass, where a true and consistent path of the ball is important, it is not necessary to mow the grass extremely short or on a regular schedule. I have found that allowing bluegrass to reach a height of at least three to three and one-half inches and only mowing off approximately one-third at any one time is best for the grass and does not put it in a stress condition. Bermudagrass and other lawn grasses have their own requirements (see the individual entries in the turf chapter), but the best suggestion is to mow only as often as is absolutely necessary for the health of the grass and the general neatness of your property. Mowing less often, and thus letting grass grow taller, also results in the taller grass acting as a living mulch, shading the soil surface, reducing loss of soil moisture by evaporation, and encouraging a deeper root system.

Another important recommendation is to mow only with a sharp mower blade, whether rotary- or reel-type, to avoid damaging the grass leaves and causing stress that will invite attack by diseases or pests. It is recommended that you sharpen the blade of a rotary-type mower at least after every other mowing, not just once a year or never, as is so often the case. Sharp tools of any type will help do a better and cleaner maintenance job.

Another way to reduce the mowing, watering, and feeding of a lawn is to use shorter-growing grasses such as dwarf fescue, buffalograss, and blue grama. They can provide an alternative to bluegrass and other turfgrasses and meet many of the homeowner's needs for a lawn, while requiring considerably less maintenance. One of my clients/students installed a combination of buffalograss and blue grama sod over a year ago, watered it only three times after the first month of establishment, and mowed it only three times during a typical Colorado summer. He and his wife liked the thought of less water and mowing so much that they installed the same mix of native sod in their backyard this past spring and are looking forward to reducing their maintenance requirements even more. In addition, native grasses have a more natural appearance, and can be walked or played on.

PEST CONTROL

The more diverse the landscape environment, the less likely is the possibility of a major disaster from an attack of disease or insects. By having a mono-culture (only one type of plant growing), which is what most of our lawns are, we promote the like-lihood of inviting not only one grass-gnawing crea-ture or disease, but also all its relatives and kin, to feast on our lawns if we neglect some of the simple maintenance requirements and put the grass in a stress condition.

Here, again, a healthy lawn is a happy lawn, so the best way to control pests is to eliminate the conditions that promote and allow their existence. By providing the essentials for good growth, such as good soil, adequate light, and only necessary watering, we can provide the environment that will aid in good health and relieve stress in our lawns, thereby reducing the possibility of attack by the many diverse diseases and insects that are lurking to feed on our lawns.

However, if you get an infestation of some pesky creature, then use only the best preparations rec-ommended by your landscape nursery or garden center expert and very carefully follow the direc-tions on the label. Do not be indiscriminate in their application since to do so may cause an imbalance in the environment by eliminating the good or ben-eficial creatures along with the problems.

The better answer, of course, is to try to correct the underlying problem, probably a soil deficiency or watering problem or poor plant selection, which may be more costly in the short run but much more efficient and better for the environment, both in your immediate landscape and in the world. Be careful and be wise, not foolish. This is the only world we have and we had better take good care of it now, not later when we have damaged it beyond repair.

WATERING YOUR LAWN AND IRRIGATION SYSTEM MAINTENANCE

As stated in the chapter on efficient irrigation, over-watering is a fact of life in many of the irrigated lawns in this country. The best way to control the amount of water applied is to install a moisture sensor controlled system. It monitors the available moisture in the soil that is needed for good plant growth, and then applies only the amount that is necessary to replenish the amount lost from eva-potranspiration (ET).

Whether or not you have an irrigation system, you must be observant of the water needs of the landscape. To water just because it is your day on the restricted or ET schedule is sheer folly. Seek out the ET rate for your local area and use that information to help you determine the amount of water you need to apply. Never go for more than a month without checking the watering times and du-rations on an "automatic" controller.

One of the best ways to know when your lawn is in stress from lack of water is to walk over it; if footprints remain (because the grass did not spring back) it is stressed. Often, especially with bluegrass or St. Augustinegrass, the leaves turn blue or gray-green, and sometimes begin to curl slightly to re-duce the leaf surface and the transpiration rate. It is best to water just before this condition occurs. By being observant, you can soon learn when your lawn is approaching this stage, and apply the amount of water necessary to relieve the stress. Care should be taken not to apply more water at any time than your soil can absorb, so you don't create an excess that will run off into the street or onto your neighbor's lawn.

A regular inspection of your irrigation system will also alert you to conditions that will require repair or modification of the system or the way you operate it. Most sprinkler heads and drip emitter devices can clog up from dirt or roots, and can cause malfunctions that will waste large amounts of water if you are not alert to the situation.

With drip systems you will usually have some type of filter to remove small particles in the water before it reaches the microscopic openings in the emitters or porous pipe. You should check and clean or replace these filters on a regular basis.

Always have enough spare parts on hand to correct any condition that occurs, or have the phone number of your irrigation system installer or maintenance person handy so you can call him/her when you see or suspect a problem. Early attention to a problem often will save lots of money and water.

Often we get hung up on having our lawns and landscapes conform to a specific system of mowing, watering, fertilizing, and spraying, when all of this work and chemical application is not essential to achieving an attractive landscape. Probably one of the best reasons for Xeriscape landscaping, in my opinion, is that it reduces the amount of maintenance time and money and the damage to the natural environment from the overuse of chemicals and water, and allows us to do something that is more fun, relaxing, and enjoyable with our "leisure" time.

It was from Anna Thurston, landscape architect and water conservation specialist for Aurora, Colorado, that I first heard the expression, "Xeriscape landscaping is really just good gardening practice." That really put Xeriscape gardening into perspective for me—how it's primarily a matter of putting to use all the information about good cultural practices and plant selection with respect to microclimate. We've learned a lot in the last few years that has altered some of those practices, especially with respect to soil improvement and overfertilization of lawns, but the knowledge has always been there, available from the plants, if only we'd pay attention. But that's

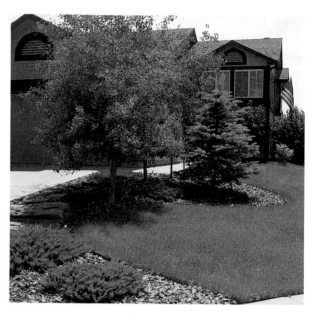

A simple Xeriscape design—easy to maintain, and doubly pleasing because it is meticulously maintained.

the whole point of gardening, learning by paying attention to the plants.

Still a young concept, Xeriscape landscaping has much growing, changing, and refining to do. The plant lists in this book will undoubtedly change over time as we learn more about the limits of plants' drought tolerance, and the danger of introducing plants wholesale from different climates and environments. It's always exciting, though, because it's a win-win situation for everyone.

Maintenance is an important part of Xeriscape gardening. If people have a bad picture of Xeriscape landscaping, it's often related to the fact that they've seen a weed-riddled gravel expanse "zero-scape" at some time and have decided that's what a Xeriscape landscape is. If for no other reason than to promote Xeriscape gradening's good name, please take good care of your Xeriscape garden.

When all is said and done, it may just be that the truly essential issue in "water conservation through creative landscaping" lies in what we do with the watering side of maintenance—whether we rush out on schedule and turn on that tap (or even worse, let the automatic timer make all our watering decisions for us), or elect to just sit tight. You have masses of information here to help make that second choice possible. The rest is up to you.

P·A·R·T T·W·O

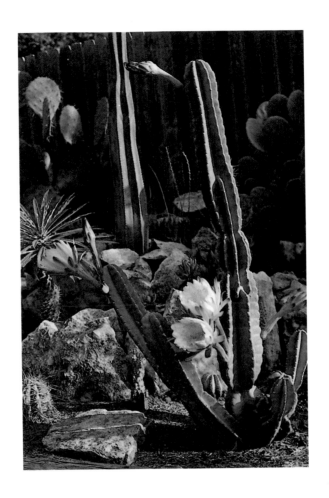

The Plants

Xeriscape Plants for the American Garden

MY PRINCIPAL aim with this book has been to show Xeriscape gardening devotees, skeptics, and complete neophytes that a well-planned Xeriscape design is compelling and beautiful, despite its "restriction" of limiting water use. I have tried to convey that it's an ecological approach, the ideal Xeriscape landscape being closely related to the ecological region of the country in which we each live. The Xeriscape principles are the same no matter where one lives; only the plant lists change.

Realizing that Xeriscape gardening is very much a regional experience, I have tried to provide a starting point for choosing plants in eleven broad regions of the country. However, the more I delved into the subject, the more I realized how difficult a task it is to address adequately in one book because there are so many other variables to consider in trying to determine whether a certain plant will be drought tolerant—soil nutrition and structure, orientation toward the sun, protection from wind, etc., all have their impact on the plant's success or failure there.

I set out to define a no-nonsense set of Xeriscape plant regions in order to rescue myself and my readers from the sea of indecision we founder in about plant choices. I even rounded up a map of the United States complete with all county boundaries, so you could locate *exactly* which region you are in. I planned to take into consideration soil, weather, and elevation, and to delineate those lines boldly and without vacillation.

Of course I was floored by the size and diversity of this huge land. It absolutely refused to fit itself into fifteen or so distinct regions. I learned that the West generally has alkaline and heavy clay soils, and that the East, in part because higher rainfall

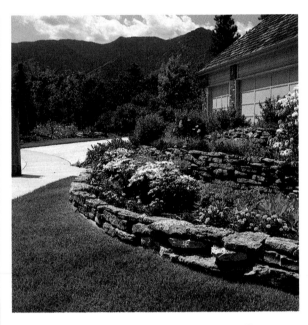

This Colorado Springs yard effectively handles an inconvenient slope with a dazzling display of drought-tolerant flowers that are efficiently watered with drip irrigation. A minimal turf area serves as an accent to the rock wall. (Design: John Genz)

amounts leach out certain chemicals, has generally acid soils, ranging from sand to rich loam to heavy Georgia gumbo clay. Aside from that there's no way to characterize a region's soil type. More than 14,000 different soils are classified in the United States, and topsoil may vary from the most cumbersome clay to pure sand within a few square miles.

Differences in elevation, terrain, and climate can cause striking differences in vegetation over a very short distance. Seaside plants in the twenty- to sixty-mile-wide coastal plain along the East Coast may not be found where the terrain turns to the gently rolling hills of the Piedmont. In turn, Piedmont plants will differ from those of the Appalachians farther inland. All three plant communities may occur in one state, as in Virginia or the Carolinas. Even when defining regions as broadly as possible, there are still three or four distinct plant communities in Texas and California, and the vegetation of north Florida is different from that of south Florida.

On the other hand, the vegetation doesn't change abruptly. There is extensive overlap not only within a region but across several states as well. A few adaptable plants will appear on drought-tolerant lists for nearly every part of the country.

So I must mark my Xeriscape plant regions with very dashed lines, if any. The general regions I arrived at vary in size and are based roughly on a

map called Ecological Research Areas in the 1975 *United States Atlas*, produced by the United States Geological Survey, with modifications to reflect more specific information on plant communities, cold hardiness, and available moisture.

The largest region covers the Great Plains (grassland), Rocky Mountains, and Great Basin (cold desert). This is due in part to the fact that most of that region is semiarid and experiences the same harsh extremes of weather, and in part to the fact that there is so much overlap in the Xeriscape plant lists available for each region that it seemed unnecessary to further subdivide them.

On the other hand, there is a separate list for central Florida (a relatively minute area), in part because an extensive and interesting list had been developed by the Southwest Florida Water Man-

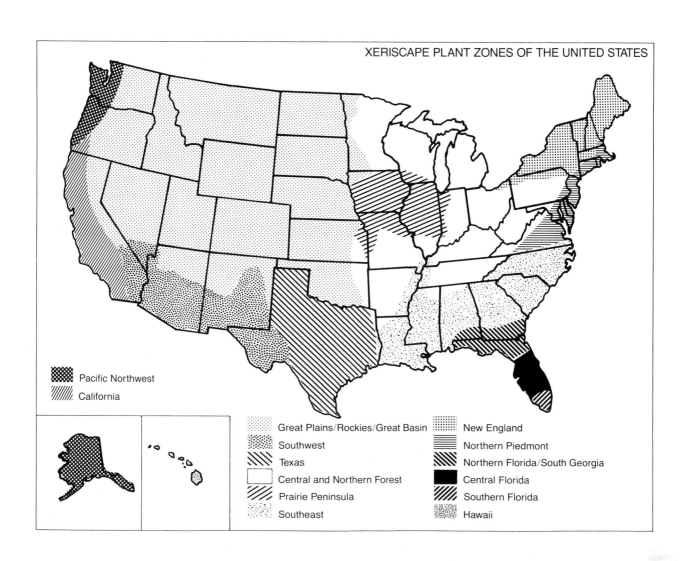

XERISCAPE PLANT ZONES OF THE UNITED STATES

Pacific Northwest
California
Great Plains/Rockies/Great Basin
Southwest
Texas
Central and Northern Forest
Prairie Peninsula
Southeast
New England
Northern Piedmont
Northern Florida/South Georgia
Central Florida
Southern Florida
Hawaii

agement District for the area, and in part because central Florida covers most of the Southeast's Hardiness Zone 9.

The plant lists for each region were developed using a number of sources, including the National Wildflower Research Center (which publishes a list of recommended species for a variety of habitats, both wet and dry, for each state), dozens of reference texts on each of the different kinds of plants, and recommendations from specialists.

Wherever possible, published lists from extension agencies or local entities concerned with Xeriscape landscaping were used to form all or part of the lists. Those agencies are noted where used.

Using the Regional Plant Lists

Begin by locating on the map the region of the country where you live:

• Look closely at where you live in relation to the general region. If your home's elevation and exposure are very close to the region's in general, you may choose from the Xeriscape plant lists for that region fairly confidently. If, however, you live in a discontinuous area, such as a low valley tucked into a mountainous region, or on the leeward side of a mountain in the middle of the desert, you can look as well at the plant lists associated with the next warmer or wetter areas, respectively.

• The zone lists are set up to indicate which plants have roughly the same water needs in a region. The Natural Rainfall or Very-Low-Water-Use Zones would require the least added water. After an establishment period ranging from a few weeks (for annual flowers) to three years (for some trees and shrubs), they should be able to survive without additional watering. Plants listed in these zones also generally do better, or can survive, in dry soil.

Plants that are listed in the Occasional Watering (or Low-Water-Use) and Regular Watering (or Moderate-Water-Use) Zones will need progressively more soil moisture in order to thrive. These designations also indicate that the plant prefers average or moist soil, respectively. In some instances, a plant appears in a "Moderate" zone, not because it needs copious amounts of water, but because it will

tolerate poor drainage, or because it lives happily with wet feet next to a stream or pond. Many of these will also survive in drier conditions, and there are probably many more plants that are adaptable in this way.

• The zones of the regional lists may be looked at and used two different ways. One of the best ways to use water and effort efficiently is to group plants together that have similar watering needs. It's pointless, for instance, to select sagebrush and cactus for their water-conserving properties, then plant them right next to an aspen, a plant that prefers moist soil. You'll drive yourself crazy trying to make sure the aspen gets enough water while not overwatering the drier-preferring plants. In fact, you may kill one or the other of them.

If you are designing a new Xeriscape landscape, you can use the lists to plan a watering "zone" in your landscape based on the plants within one group, or as a check to make sure you are not grouping together in one part of your yard plants that have very different water needs. (The planning and design chapter of this book discusses zoning.)

Another way to use the lists is to address the microclimates within an existing landscape. In many instances, some areas of your yard will be drier or moister than others. A hollow or small swale may become evident as you do your site survey, or you may have decided to continue having an area of turf that must be irrigated regularly. Then you *want* to know which plants like moister soil, so you can place *them*, rather than plants that will suffer from too much moisture, where additional water will naturally be present, either in the hollow or swale or adjacent to the turf. Similarly, you can get ideas for which plants will grow in the sunny, drier sections of your existing landscape.

• For some regions the plant lists are broken down into three water-use zones, in others there are two groups, and in a few instances only one list is included. This has to do partially with the nature of the available soil moisture for each part of the country and its variability within the region.

In Appalachia (part of the Central Eastern Forest), for instance, the demand for irrigation water rarely exceeds the supply, even in years of lower than average rainfall. In addition, the terrain of the region leads to ample moisture being fairly uni-

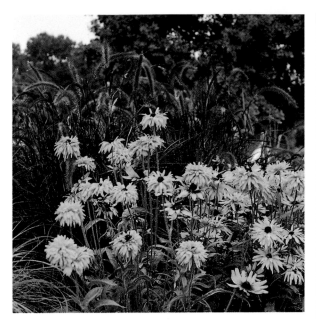

This combination of black-eyed Susans (Rudbeckia hirta) *and purple fountain grass* (Pennisetum setaceum) *has become a classic in Xeriscape gardens across the nation.* (Photo: Doug Welsh)

formly distributed. There are no deserts or significantly drier zones in that part of the country, so the list includes just two zones to be used in the Xeriscape concept of zoning as explained here.

In the Rocky Mountains and Great Plains states, however, precipitation zones include ecological areas ranging from desert (receiving zero to ten inches of precipitation a year) to high plains (averaging ten to eighteen inches a year) to mountainous areas that may get as much as thirty inches of precipitation a year. As a result, I have three zones for the region to reflect some of that variability.

The number of zones within each region may also reflect the shortage or abundance of information about plants' water needs. This has in part to do with how long Xeriscape landscaping has been a topic of interest in that area, and in part with the fact that so many thousands of different plants grow that it's unlikely there will ever be definitive information about just how much drought every plant can tolerate.

• Many of the trees and shrubs appearing on our lists, especially from the eastern part of the country, are native species. In some instances, the plants may have characteristics such as low disease re-

sistance or untidy habits of dropping fruit that make them less desirable as landscape plants. Often a variety may have been cultivated to improve on the native species. Here is where it's helpful to get local information as to suitable substitutes or varieties.

• I have tried to be consistent in providing information about as many different types of plants as possible for each region. However, trying to include all the annuals, perennials, vines, and ornamental grasses that adventurous American gardeners raise in every part of the country became an overwhelming task.

As a result, I decided to create overall lists of annuals, perennials, grasses, etc., for the whole country according to whether they prefer dry, average, or moist soil. Those lists are found in the Appendix, and they include some of the most popular, best-known, or most commmercially available cultivated species and hybrids.

You will also find listings of those categories of plants in each regional list. However, there they will tend to include more wildflowers, uncommon plants, or plants that have been specifically recommended for Xeriscape gardens in that part of the country. There may be some overlap.

• In all lists the botanical name is given first, then one or more common names. Although common names are usually more fun, I chose to make the listing this way in deference to the national nature of the book. A plant may have a dozen or more common names, depending on what part of the country you live in, and a common name may refer to two completely different plants in different regions. Thus, the scientific nomenclature is used for consistency to ensure that we're all talking about the same plant. (Unfortunately, botanical names change over the years, too, but much more slowly.)

Use these lists as a starting point for suggested plants, then gather additional information to help narrow your choices and complete your design with assistance from successful Xeriscape gardeners and local or regional experts such as botanic garden horticulturists, teachers of classes in gardening and Xeriscape landscaping, nursery growers, propagators, and county extension agents.

Books on local plants and gardening are another good source of information. There is even a small, but growing number of regional plant books that directly address the concerns of drought-tolerant plants or low-water gardening. Basic plant encyclopedias can be consulted for information on soil and nutrient requirements, shade tolerance, time and color of bloom, texture of foliage, etc., though you may have to search diligently for information on soil moisture and water needs. (I did!)

I can't emphasize enough how important it is to seek additional local information in designing your Xeriscape garden. The people you consult will likely have many years of cumulative experience about which plants work within your local area with respect to soils, cold hardiness, longevity, availability, and what they have observed about plants' water needs. Judith Phillips, native-plant propagator in Albuquerque, New Mexico, emphasizes the need for *extremely* local information. She remarked that she was struck recently about how differently she and another grower in Santa Fe, just sixty miles north, at the edge of the Sangre de Cristo Mountains, regarded the water needs of several plants.

The U.S. Department of Agriculture released a new hardiness zone map in the spring of 1990. However, most plant references used in preparing the lists in this book are based on the old zone maps. To avoid confusion, the old zone map is shown here until such time as the plant references are updated. Note that for the two largest regions (Great Plains/Rockies/Great Basin and Central and Eastern Forests), hardiness has been indicated for all of the appropriate plants, since the regions cover so many different hardiness zones. This has been done for the New England list as well, because cold hardiness is often more of a factor than drought tolerance. **On all the other lists you can assume that any plant listed is hardy throughout the area, *unless* it is otherwise indicated in the zone column of the list. If just one zone is listed, that is the coldest zone in which the plant is still hardy.**

You should regard these lists as a starting point, from which you may add or subtract plants, depending on what you find out locally.

One of my most rewarding experiences in searching out plant lists was learning that there are many favorite Xeriscape plants and many plants in general that will survive and thrive in a wide variety of climates and rainfall regions. Santolina, or lavender cotton, a gray-green foliage plant with masses

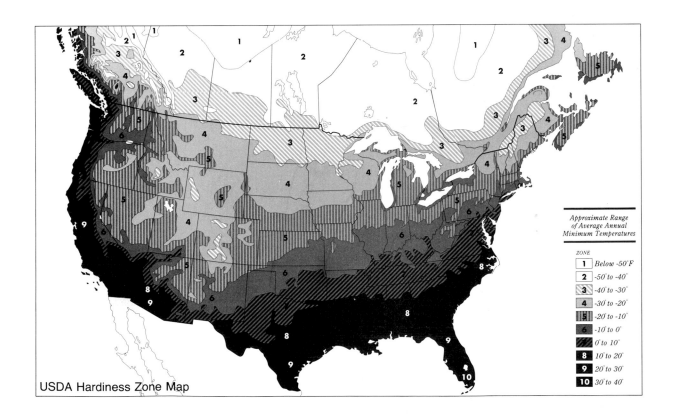

USDA Hardiness Zone Map

Approximate Range of Average Annual Minimum Temperatures

ZONE
1 Below -50°F
2 -50° to -40°
3 -40° to -30°
4 -30° to -20°
5 -20° to -10°
6 -10° to 0°
7 0° to 10°
8 10° to 20°
9 20° to 30°
10 30° to 40°

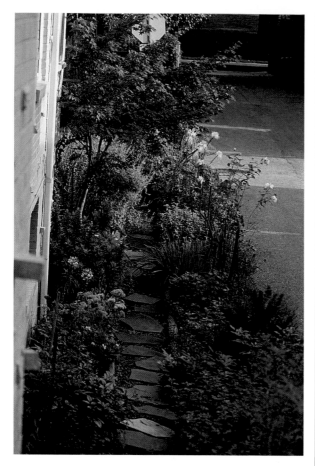

A slate path provides not only access to the back of this Washington, D.C., townhouse, but a way to view this charming, old-fashioned garden as well.

of bright yellow buttonlike flowers, lives happily with a little drip irrigation in Albuquerque as well as on its own in Washington, D.C., enduring a twenty- to thirty-inch difference in precipitation totals.

Many other plants will survive wide variations of temperature, soils, and weather. Even cold hardiness has some flexibility if a potentially tender plant is installed in a location shielded from prevailing winter winds.

I have tried to include plants native to each region, giving consideration to availability of plant materials. One of the frustrations faced by early Xeriscape landscaping enthusiasts was the lag time for propagation in nurseries. Eager to try native plants, they often found few to purchase. In some cases native plants are slow or difficult to germinate, then slow-growing to reach marketable size.

The industry is making some progress in catching up with the demand for xeric plants. You can be part of the process of making native and xeric plants more available by "encouraging" your local nursery growers with frequent requests for specific plants— nursery growers need to know we're serious about Xeriscape gardening before they invest time and money in growing plants.

I offer these lists, again, as a starting point, and hope they will generate some experimentation and results that will confirm or alter them for greater accuracy in future editions. I welcome your input.

Xeriscape Plants for New England

BLESSED with abundant and fairly evenly dispersed rainfall (thirty to fifty inches per year), New England has long been the model for traditional landscapes—lush green lawns, stately trees, English-style perennial borders. For most of the year this type of landscaping is well matched to its environment, but there is a two-month period in the summer when dry spells can occur, and landscape plants conditioned by the climate to a steady input of moisture show drought stress. Dr. Don Rakow of Cornell University sees stress in some trees even after ten days without any significant moisture.

People may water their lawns from April to September to maintain a lush green lawn, though irrigation is rarely necessary for maintaining woody plants. Dr. Rakow feels turfgrass in the New England area may be overwatered when put under automatic irrigation, and trees often get overwatered when they are part of a landscape that's watered regularly. Here the Xeriscape concept of zoning might be well employed, particularly separating turf areas from trees, not only to meet their individual watering needs but to separate the soil pH as well. Lawn grasses generally fare better with neutral pH (6.0 to 7.0) while many native New England trees will prefer acid soil. Selecting one of the new turf-type tall fescues rather than Kentucky bluegrass for lawns will also reduce some of the disparity in water needs.

The urban conditions of the many large cities in the Northeast give rise to "heat islands" that worsen drought stress on street trees. Faced with that situation people must either select the most drought-tolerant species or plan on regular irrigation of street trees.

The concept of Xeriscape landscaping was introduced in the New England area only in the late 1980s. Because of the high rainfall the region experiences, the idea seemed to have no bearing, in part because it was assumed that Xeriscape landscaping in New England meant using the same plants as in a Xeriscape-style landscape in Arizona. But Xeriscape gardening is definitely regional. In New England (as in every other part of the country) a strong accent must be made on appropriate plant selection—those suited to New England's generally moister environment, and able to withstand the summer dry season.

Interest in water conservation is definitely on the upswing in the Northeast. In recent years the squeeze has been put on water supply systems in some areas there partly because of increased watering in the summer, but compounded by a large influx of new residents. Water rates, especially in urban

Plant breeders have taken some wildflowers and enhanced their use in the landscape, as with blue salvia (Salvia farinacea *'Victoria Blue'*), *seen with its domesticated cousin, annual red salvia* (S. splendens). *(Photo: Doug Welsh)*

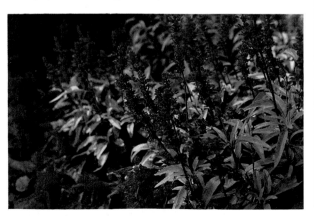

areas, have risen substantially, giving people a reason to take a second look at water-conserving landscaping.

Rakow points out that an additional reason for selecting drought-tolerant species and using other fundamental Xeriscape design concepts is that it reduces the stress trees experience which may weaken them and make them more susceptible to disease.

At the eastern Massachusetts nursery he operates, Dr. Jeff Licht has done considerable research into what plants do well in the Northeast, using water-efficient landscaping as the criterion. He has found that with a few exceptions, such as asters, phlox, potentilla, and silene, the mesic plants did better at adapting to drier conditions than the xeric plants used out West did at adapting to the moister situation of the Northeast.

As usual, natives shine when it comes to adapting to what the weather brings, but Licht found that many natives of Far East Asia and Eastern Europe did well at his location, too. For drought tolerance he recommends choosing narrow- rather than wide-leaved plants; those with waxy, hairy, or gray-colored leaves; and spring bloomers (they avoid drought damage by going into early dormancy).

He recommends adding organic matter to the soil to improve drainage and air circulation, and thus reduce the fungal activity common in high rainfall areas that can lead to plant disease. He also cautions against the excessive use of fertilizer, noting that plants can't utilize surplus soil nutrients during drought and late in the growing season, and this may lead to problems for the plants.

Although Ruth Dyckman didn't plan her upstate New York yard as a Xeriscape garden, it has the lushness one could expect from Xeriscape landscaping in that setting. The showcase is the large island bed of flowers in front of her house full of perennials that are easily able to withstand dry spells. It features bee balm (*Monarda didyma*), a popular New England native wildflower, hostas nestled in the midst of tall flowers that give them shade, *Achillea ptarmica* 'The Pearl', sunflowers, tulips, daffodils, grape hyacinths, snowdrops, and daylilies.

Dyckman says she waters only five or six times during the summer when there is a long dry spell.

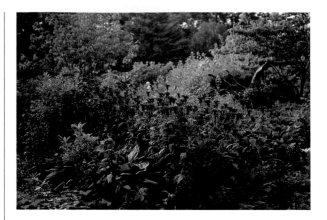

A portion of Ruth Dyckman's upstate New York garden features bee balm (Monarda didyma) *and hostas. The island bed of flowers is the showcase of her extensive, yet water-thrifty garden.*

Her gardening is limited more by the cold winter weather than by lack of moisture.

Manny Shemin, founder of Shemin Nurseries, speaks of the "monolithic" look common in many of New England's forests. A very appropriate Xeriscape theme for New England might duplicate this theme—a rock garden designed around large rocks and featuring woodland plants and wildflowers. This is especially suitable if you've been "blessed" with a collection of boulders brought in by the glaciers, or have rocky soil. Native wildflowers (many of which are listed in the plant list that follows) make an excellent foil for large or small rocks. Many New England wildflowers are acid-loving, but if you want to try some that prefer alkaline soil, you can replace the existing soil with pockets of appropriate soil mix. This is made easier by the fact that woodland wildflowers generally have roots less than one foot deep. (See pages 83–88 for more information on wildflowers.)

The Xeriscape plant list for New England is relatively short compared to some of the others. Location in Hardiness Zones 3, 4, and 5 limits the number of species in the area, and invasive plants have been removed. As with other areas of temperate climate (that is, those having cyclic weather, from warm summers to cold winters), the plant list can be expanded by using the lists in the Appendix for specific categories of drought-tolerant plants/situations. Just remember to pay attention to the Hardiness Zone designations.

Xeriscape Plants for New England
Natural Rainfall Zone

BOTANICAL NAME	COMMON NAME(S)	HEIGHT	ZONES
DECIDUOUS TREES			
Acer tataricum	Tatarian maple	30'	4
Amelanchier arborea	Downy serviceberry	10–40'	3–9
Betula papyrifera	Paper birch	50–75'	2
(susceptible to birch borer)			
B. populifolia	Gray birch	35–50'	4
(more resistant to birch borer)			
*Carya cordiformis***	Bitternut hickory	90'	4
C. ovata	Shagbark hickory	75–100'	4
C. tomentosa	Mockernut hickory	90'	5
Catalpa speciosa	Northern catalpa	40–60'	4–8
Crataegus crusgalli	Cockspur hawthorn	20–35'	4
C. mollis	Downy hawthorn	35–50'	3
C. phaenopyrum	Washington hawthorn	20–35'	5
C. pruinosa	Frosted hawthorn	10–20'	3
C. punctata	Dotted hawthorn	20–35'	4
C. viridus 'Winter King'		30'	5–7
(Note: Many hawthorns are susceptible to pests)			
Malus spp.	Flowering crab apple	50'	2
Ostrya virginiana	American hophornbeam	35–50'	4
Phellodendron amurense	Amur cork tree	30'	3
Prunus pensylvanica (short-lived)	Wild red cherry, Pin cherry	20–35'	2
Ptelea trifoliata	Common hop tree	20–35'	5
Quercus alba	White oak	75–100'	4
Q. coccinea	Scarlet oak	60–100'	4
Q. ellipsoidalis	Northern pin oak	50–75'	4
Q. montana	Chestnut oak	50–75'	5
Q. muehlenbergii	Chinkapin oak	35–50'	4
Q. rubra	Red oak	40–100'	3
*Q. velutina**	Black oak	75–100'	4
Syringa reticulata, syn.	Japanese tree lilac	30'	4
S. amurensis var. *japonica*			
Tilia cordata	Littleleaf linden, Basswood	75'	3–8
*Ulmus americana****	American elm	75–100'	2
(Susceptible to many diseases—including Dutch elm disease—and pests)			
EVERGREEN TREES			
Abies concolor	White fir	75–100'	4
A. veitchii	Veitch fir	75'	3
Picea abies	Norway spruce	150'	2
P. glauca	White spruce	40–90'	2
Pinus aristata	Bristlecone pine	8–45'	5
P. banksiana	Jack pine	50–75'	2
P. cembra	Swiss stone pine	75'	2
P. resinosa	Red pine	75–100'	2
P. rigida	Pitch pine	50–75'	5

Natural Rainfall Zone

BOTANICAL NAME	COMMON NAME(S)	HEIGHT	ZONES
DECIDUOUS SHRUBS			
Buddleia alternifolia	Alternate leaf butterfly bush	15′	6–8
Caragana spp.	Peashrub	4–18′	2
Colutea arborescens	Bladder senna	12′	5
Comptonia peregrina	Sweetfern	3–6′	2–5
Gaylussacia baccata	Huckleberry	2′	5–6
Hypericum kalmianum	Kalm's St. Johnswort	3′	4
Kolkwitzia amabilis	Beautybush	10′	4
Ligustrum spp.	Privet	9–15′	3
Malus sargentii	Sargent crab apple	6′	5
Philadelphus spp.	Mock orange	3–9′	4
*Rhododendron roseum***	Rose rhododendron	9′	3
Rosa caroliniana	Carolina rose	3′	4
R. hugonis	Father Hugo rose	7′	5
Salix humilis	Prairie willow	6–12′	3
Sambucus canadensis	American alder	6–12′	3
Shepherdia canadensis	Russet buffaloberry	6–9′	2
Stephanandra incisa 'Crispa'		2′	5
*Vaccinium angustifolium**	Lowbush blueberry	3′	2
Viburnum carlesii 'Compacta'	Korean spice viburnum	5′	4
V. rafinesquianum	Rafinesque viburnum	3–6′	3
EVERGREEN SHRUBS			
Rhododendron carolinianum	Carolina rhododendron	6′	5
GROUND COVERS			
Euphorbia corollata	Spurge	3′	4
Sedum acre	Goldmoss sedum	2″	4–9
S. ternatum	Mountain sedum	3–6″	3
S. × 'Vera Jameson'	Stonecrop	2–4″	4
PERENNIALS (all are hardy to at least Zone 3)			
Armeria caespitosa	Thrift	9″	
Aslepias speciosa	Showy milkweed	2–4′	
Aster linearifolius	Savory-leaved aster	12–18″	
A. novi-belgii	New York aster	3–4′	
Baptisia tinctoria	Yellow false indigo	2–3′	
Geranium robertianum	Herb Robert	1–2′	
Geum triflorum	Prairie smoke	6–12″	
Grindelia robusta	Shore grindelia	2–4′	
Hepatica acutiloba	Sharp-lobed hepatica	8″	
H. americana	Round-lobed hepatica	6″	
Lilium philadelphicum	Wood lily	2–3′	
Lupinus perennis	Wild lupine	15″	
Oenothera hookeri (biennial)	Hooker evening primrose	3–6′	

BOTANICAL NAME	COMMON NAME(S)	HEIGHT	ZONES
PERENNIALS cont'd			
Oxalis violacea	Violet wood sorrel	4–6″	
Penstemon digitalis	White penstemon	3′	
Thalictrum dioicum	Early meadow rue	8–30″	
T. polycarpum	Sierra meadow rue	16–40″	
Verbascum olympicum	Mullein	6′	
Veronica incana	Woolly speedwell	12–18″	
Viola canadensis	Canada violet	12–18″	
V. papilionacea	Blue violet, Butterfly violet	6–12″	
V. pedata	Bird's-foot violet	2–6″	
V. pedunculata	California violet	6–24″	
VINES			
Celastrus scandens	American bittersweet	35′	2
Clematis verticillaris	Rock clematis	3–20′	2
C. virginiana	Virginsbower	10–20′	3
Lonicera dioica	Limber honeysuckle	9′	2
Parthenocissus quinquefolia	Virginia creeper, Woodbine	35′	2
Vitis riparia	Riverbank grape	20–35′	2

Occasional Watering Zone

BOTANICAL NAME	COMMON NAME(S)	HEIGHT	ZONES
DECIDUOUS TREES			
Acer pensylvanicum	Striped maple	35–50′	3
A. rubrum	Red maple	100′	3
A. saccharinum	Silver maple	100′	3–9
*A. saccharum***	Sugar maple	75–100′	3–8
A. s. var. *nigrum*	Black maple	75–100′	3
*A. spicatum**	Mountain maple	20–35′	2
*Betula lenta**	Sweet birch	50–75′	3
B. pendula	European birch	60′	2
(Note: Many birches are susceptible to borers. Drought stress increases susceptibility.)			
Carpinus caroliniana	Hornbeam	35–50′	2
Cercis canadensis	Redbud/Judas tree	20–35′	5–8
*Fagus grandifolia***	American beech	75–100′	3
Fraxinus americana	White ash	60–120′	3–9
*Juglans cinerea****	Butternut	50–75′	3
*J. nigra****	Eastern black walnut	150′	4
Nyssa sylvatica	Black gum, Black tupelo	50–75′	5–9
Platanus occidentalis	American plane tree	75–100′	4
Populus alba	White poplar	90′	3
P. deltoides	Eastern cottonwood, Eastern poplar	75–150′	3
P. tremuloides	Quaking aspen	35–50′	2
Sorbus alnifolia	Korean mountain ash	45′	4–7

(This species most resistant to borers that often kill other mountain ashes)

Occasional Watering Zone

BOTANICAL NAME	COMMON NAME(S)	HEIGHT	ZONES
EVERGREEN TREES			
Ilex opaca	American holly	45'	5
Picea glauca	White spruce	50–75'	2
Pinus strobus	White pine	100–150'	2
DECIDUOUS SHRUBS			
Amelanchier canadensis	Shadblow serviceberry	24'	3
A. laevis	Allegheny serviceberry	36'	4
Cornus amomum	Silky dogwood	9'	5
C. mas	Cornelian cherry	24'	4
Corylus cornuta	Beaked filbert	6–12'	3
Dirca palustris	Atlantic leatherwood	3–6'	3
Hamamelis virginiana	Witch hazel	15'	4
Sambucus pubens	Scarlet elder	6–12'	3
*Viburnum acerifolium**	Mapleleaf viburnum	3–6'	3
*V. alnifolium****	Hobblebush viburnum	6–12'	3
*V. cassinoides****	Witherod viburnum	3–8'	3–6
V. corymbosum	Highbush blueberry	6–12'	4
*V. dentatum****	Arrowwood viburnum	6–12'	3
V. trilobum	American cranberry bush	6–12'	2
EVERGREEN SHRUBS			
*Kalmia latifolia**	Mountain laurel kalmia	12–20'	5
*Taxus canadensis***	Canada yew	3–6'	2
GROUND COVERS			
Convallaria majalis	Lily-of-the-valley	6–8"	3–9
*Galax aphylla**		4–6" (foliage), 12–18" (flowers)	5–6
*Gaultheria procumbens**	Winterberry, Checkerberry wintergreen	2–6"	2
Lotus corniculatus	Birdsfoot trefoil	2–4"	5
Mitchella repens	Partridgeberry	2–4"	2
Vinca minor	Periwinkle	3–6"	5–9
PERENNIALS (all are hardy to at least Zone 3)			
Actaea alba	White baneberry	18–24"	
Aletris farinosa	Star grass	18–24"	
Anemone canadensis	Meadow anemone	2'	
A. deltoides	Threeleaf anemone	6–12"	
Aquilegia chrysantha	Golden columbine	4'	
A. formosa	Sitka columbine	12–40"	
Asarum shuttleworthii	Mottled wild ginger	4–12"	
A. virginicum	Heartleaf	4–12"	
Bergenia purpurascens	Saxifrage	1'	
Campanula americana	Tall bellflower	7'	

BOTANICAL NAME	COMMON NAME(S)	HEIGHT	ZONES
PERENNIALS cont'd			
Chimaphila maculata	Striped pipsissewa	3–12″	
C. umbellata	Common pipsissewa	3–12″	
Chrysopsis falcata	Yellow aster	4–16″	
Claytonia caroliniana	Spring beauty	8″	
C. virginica	Spring beauty	4–6″	
Coptis groenlandica	Common goldthread	4–6″	
C. trifolia	Alaska goldthread	4–6″	
Desmodium canadense	Tick trefoil	3–6″	
Disporum lanuginosum	Hairy fairy bells	16–30″	
D. trachycarpum	Wartberry fairy bells	1–2′	
Epilobium angustifolium	Fireweed	2–8′	
Gentiana andrewsii	Andrew's gentian	1–3′	
G. crinita (biennial)	Fringed gentian	1–2′	
Geum macrophyllum	Largeleaf geum	1–3′	
Goodyera pubescens	Downy rattlesnake plantain	6–18″	
G. tesselata	Checkered rattlesnake plantain	1′	
Helenium bigelovii	Bigelow sneezeweed	1–3′	
Helianthus decapetalus	Golden thin-leaved sunflower	2–5′	
H. tuberosus	Jerusalem artichoke	5–10′	
Houstonia caerulea	Bluet	2–8″	
Hydrastis canadensis	Golden seal	6–24″	
Jeffersonia diphylla	American twinleaf	10″	
Lilium canadense	Canada lily	2–6′	
L. pardalinum	Leopard lily	1–7′	
L. superbum	Turk's-cap lily	3–8′	
Mitella diphylla	Miterwort	1–2′	
Oxalis acetosella	Common wood sorrel	3–5″	
Podophyllum peltatum	Common mayapple	12–18″	
Polygonatum commutatum	Great Solomon's seal	2–6′	
Rudbeckia laciniata	Cutleaf coneflower	9′	
Sisyrinchium angustifolium	Common blue-eyed grass	4–20″	
S. bellum	Western blue-eyed grass	2′	
S. californicum	Golden-eyed grass	16″	
Streptopus roseus	Rosy twisted stalk	1–2′	
Tradescantia virginiana	Virginia spiderwort	1–2′	
Uvularia perfoliata	Wood merrybells	1–2′	
U. sessilifolia	Little merrybells	8″	
Viola blanda	Sweet white violet	2–4″	
VINES			
Wisteria sinensis 'Purpurea'	Purple wisteria	40′	

*Best in acid soil.

**Demands cool moist soil.

***Not often planted, but preserve if on-site.

Xeriscape Plants for the Northern Piedmont

THE EASTERN foothills of the Appalachian Mountains are known as the Piedmont. This area extends in a wide band from Massachusetts to Georgia. Many of the plants that grow in this region of oak, hickory, and pine forests and moderate upland topography will grow throughout, because of the similarity of rainfall (forty to fifty inches a year) and temperatures (most of it falls into USDA Hardiness Zones 5, 6, and 7). Yet there are some differences in the plant lists for the northern and southern Piedmont areas, so I elected to make an arbitrary and not completely clear-cut break between North and South Carolina, lumping the southern Piedmont area in with the Southeast.

The need for Xeriscape gardening has become acute in some areas of the northern Piedmont in recent years, in part because of changes in demographics. Jeff Featherstone of the Delaware River Basin Commission says the residential water demand doubles in the summer. This situation has been exacerbated in recent years by the fact that many people are moving out of the city into the suburbs, especially around Philadelphia, and taking up gardening and landscaping as a hobby. The area he helps manage is only 13,000 square miles, but it contains 25 million people, and the three main rivers that supply the region have all had lower levels in recent years because of drought.

Elizabeth Brabec, a landscape architect in Washington, D.C., uses her own yard to test plants and design strategies for Xeriscape gardening. When she and her husband bought this fifty-six-year-old home several years ago it had six old oaks and several thirty-five-year-old azaleas in the middle of the sunny side of the front yard and nothing else but tired grass stretching the long distance from the street to the porch. They moved the azaleas to shadier locations on the north side of the yard so they wouldn't need so much watering and added a few more drought-tolerant species such as cherry laurel (*Prunus laurocerasus*) and pyracantha, and perennials.

The northern Piedmont area is fortunate in having considerable rainfall as well as enough cold weather for perennial flowers to go through the period of dormancy they need. Brabec has had good luck with most of the perennials and shrubs she has tried, including artemisia, lychnis, aucuba, and blue spirea. She notes that plants for Xeriscape landscapes in the northern Piedmont need to be not only drought tolerant for dry July and August, but also able to withstand waterlogged soils in spring and fall, so they must be very durable.

The northern Piedmont is one area of the country where mulch should not be installed more than two inches deep because the humidity and high rainfall

In the Northeast, Xeriscape landscapes are often filled with beautiful evergreen conifers, with different growth habits and foliage colors. This garden is in Philadelphia. (Photo: Doug Welsh)

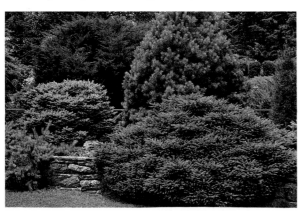

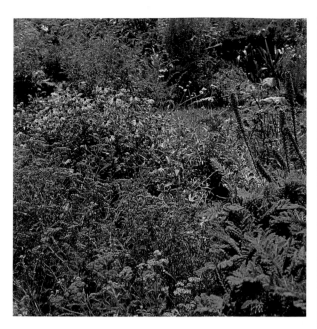

This perennial garden in downtown Washington, D.C., features many drought-tolerant flowers. Shown here are yellow coneflowers (Ratibida columnifera), *spike* gayfeather (Liatris spicata), *and* Achillea millefolium 'Summer Pastels'.

can cause the roots to grow shallow, sometimes right on top of the ground if the mulch is too deep. This makes it harder for the plants to survive drought. Brabec also recommends that decorative white rock mulch be avoided because it reflects too much light and heat in the winter, causing plants to come out of dormancy and sometimes scalding bark.

One of the first in-depth regional brochures on Xeriscape gardening for the East Coast, entitled "Save Water, Save Maintenance, Save Money," was initially produced in 1989 by the Anne Arundel County (Maryland) Department of Utilities. It was used as one of the references for the plant list in this chapter. Individual copies of this full-color brochure, which includes more information on individual plants, can be obtained by writing that department at 7409 Baltimore-Annapolis Boulevard, Glen Burnie, MD 31061 (phone: 301-760-7740).

Xeriscape gardening has an enthusiastic booster in Richard Weir, the county extension agent for Cornell, who helped design and install an extensive Xeriscape demonstration garden on Long Island through the university. Long Island, which is com-

pletely dependent on in-place aquifers, has suffered from the drawing down of the aquifers during drought periods in recent years. This has resulted in increased salinization and pollution, and an increased cost of water treatment to the consumer. In 1990 water cost an average of $6 per 1,000 gallons on Long Island, roughly twice that of upstate New York. Nonetheless, many of the vacation homes on Long Island, some less than a block from the beach, duplicate the typical tree-and-turf landscapes of upstate New York. The demonstration garden has been in place since 1988, so the plants, some of which are suitable for seaside gardens as well as New England gardens, have had a chance to mature nicely. Weir hopes to show how colorful Xeriscape landscapes on Long Island can be and still alleviate some of the problems associated with high-water-using landscapes.

Coastal areas of the northern Piedmont may have extremely sandy soil, as well as high amounts of salt in the soil and air. The southern third of New Jersey features an ecological community known as the Pine Barrens. The dominant plant for this community is the pitch pine (*Pinus rigida*), which is a pioneer plant that moves in after an area has been burned. To propagate naturally, the cones of the pitch pine must be burned open. Grasses are sparse to nonexistent in the excessively sandy soil. Instead, the ground may be covered with any of several beautiful, drought-tolerant ground covers such as bearberry (*Arctostaphylos uva-ursi*), wintergreen/New Jersey tea (*Gaultheria procumbens*), lowbush blueberry (*Vaccinium angustifolium*), and beach heather (*Hudsonia* spp.). (Beach heather is impossible to transplant, so it is found only in natural areas.)

Because of the sandy soils, turfgrasses in beach and pine barrens areas can't be maintained without constant inputs of water and fertilizers. Home landscapers are encouraged to find alternatives to turf.

In order to preserve this natural community all new landscaping in the area comes under the jurisdiction of the Pinelands Commission, which requires that native plants be used. Dr. Bruce Hamilton, professor of landscape architecture at Rutgers University in New Jersey, helped establish two seaside Xeriscape demonstration gardens in Cape May, New Jersey, which feature many of the plants adapted to both sandy and salty soil. (Another demonstration garden of inland plants has been developed at Rutgers University.)

Dr. Hamilton and Dr. Theodore Shelton coauthored a brochure entitled "Landscaping for Water Conservation: A Guide for New Jersey," which features several color photographs of appropriate plants. (Single copies may be ordered by writing the Rutgers Cooperative Extension Service in your county if you live in New Jersey, or the New Jersey Department of Environmental Protection, Division of Water Resources, Office of Water Conservation, CN029, Trenton, NJ 08625.)

This brochure offers the intriguing suggestion that dedicated native plant buffs might let a portion of their properties be turned over to nature for the ultimate in low-water landscaping. You can then watch a succession of plants take hold over the years, starting with annual weeds, followed by perennials and grasses, such as little bluestem grass (*Schizachyrium scoparium*), poverty grass (*Danthonia spicata*), daisies (various species), black-eyed Susan (*Rudbeckia hirta*), Queen Anne's lace (*Daucus carota* var. *carota*), goldenrod (*Solidago* spp.), and New England aster (*Aster novae-angliae*). Next, native trees and shrubs such as gray dogwood (*Cornus racemosa*), bayberry (*Myrica pensylvanica*), sumacs (*Rhus* spp.), red cedars (*Juniperus virginiana*), pin oaks (*Quercus palustris*), red maple (*Acer rubrum*), and green ash (*Fraxinus pennsylvanica*) will appear.

Remove the worst alien invaders as soon as they

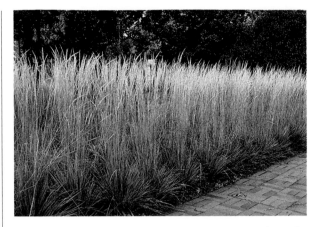

Calamagrostis acutiflora var. stricta *strikes a formal note at the National Arboretum in Washington, D.C. (Photo: Doug Welsh)*

appear, especially Hall's honeysuckle (*Lonicera japonica* 'Halliana'), which kills anything it twines on, and multiflora rose (*Rosa multiflora*). Others that may be considered pests include Norway maple (*Acer platanoides*), tree-of-heaven (*Ailanthus altissima*), and white mulberry (*Morus alba*).

Rainfall amounts are similar throughout the northern Piedmont region, and many of the plants suitable for seashore plantings will be similar all the way to the northern edge of this area. If you live inland, take care that the plants you select are within your cold-hardiness range. A special section on drought- and salt-tolerant plants is in the Appendix. Look for those within your hardiness zone.

Xeriscape Plants for the Northern Piedmont
Natural Rainfall Zone

BOTANICAL NAME	COMMON NAME(S)	HEIGHT	ZONES
DECIDUOUS TREES			
See Natural Rainfall Zone for New England, page 141, plus:			
Acer campestre	Hedge maple	25'	5–6
Castanea mollissima	Chinese chestnut	40–60'	
Catalpa bignonioides	Southern catalpa	30–40'	
Cladrastis lutea	American yellowwood	50'	
Cotinus coggygria	Smoke tree	10–15'	
Diospyros virginiana	Persimmon	75'	

BOTANICAL NAME	COMMON NAME(S)	HEIGHT	ZONES
DECIDIOUS TREES cont'd			
Elaeagnus angustifolia	Russian olive	12–15′	
Fraxinus quadrangulata	Blue ash	50–70′	
Liriodendron tulipifera	Tulip tree	80–120′	
Malus baccata mandschurica 'Midwest'	'Midwest' Manchurian crab apple	50′	
Platanus acerifolia	London plane tree	100′	
Pyrus calleryana	Bradford pear	30–50′	
Quercus borealis	Red oak	75′	
*Q. imbricaria**	Shingle oak, Laurel oak	75′	
*Q. stellata**	Post oak	40–50′	
*Tilia americana**	American linden	90′	
Zelkova serrata	Japanese zelkova	50–80′	

EVERGREEN TREES
See Natural Rainfall Zone for New England, page 141, plus:

Pinus flexilis	Limber pine	30–50′	
P. nigra	Austrian pine	30–50′	
P. thunbergii	Japanese black pine	20–80′	

DECIDUOUS SHRUBS

Aronia arbutifolia	Red chokeberry	9′	
Baccharis halimifolia		6–12′	
Chaenomeles spp.	Flowering quince	7′	
Cystisus scoparius	Scotch broom	4–9′	7
*Gaylussacia baccata**	Box huckleberry	2′	5–6
Hibiscus syriacus	Rose of Sharon	5–15′	
Jasminum nudiflorum	Winter jasmine	4–6′	7
Malus sargentii 'Roselow'		6′	5
Prunus cistena	Purpleleaf sand cherry	8–10′	
Rhododendron calendulaceum	Flame azalea	9′	
Spiraea × *bumalda*	Bumald spirea	3′	
S. japonica	Japanese spirea	4–6′	

EVERGREEN SHRUBS

Buxus microphylla	Littleleaf box	6′	
Hypericum kalmianum	Kalm St.-John's-wort	2–3′	
Ilex cornuta	Chinese holly	8–15′	
Juniperus excelsa	Spiny Greek juniper	10–15′	
Ligustrum japonicum	Japanese privet	6–12′	7
L. sinense	Chinese privet	10–15′	
Nandina domestica		6–8′	7

GROUND COVERS
See Natural Rainfall Zone for New England, page 142, plus:

Epigaea repens	Trailing arbutus	3–6″	
Fragaria vesca	Wild strawberry	6–8″	
F. virginiana	Virginia strawberry	3–6″	
Hedera helix	English ivy	6″	

Natural Rainfall Zone

BOTANICAL NAME	COMMON NAME(S)	HEIGHT	ZONES

PERENNIALS

See Natural Rainfall Zone for New England, pages 142–43, plus:

BOTANICAL NAME	COMMON NAME(S)	HEIGHT	ZONES
Aster ptarmicoides	White aster	30″	
Campanula divaricata	Allegheny bellflower	3′	
Coreopsis maritima	Pacific coreopsis	1–3′	
Eupatorium coelestinum	Mistflower	6′	
Hypoxis hirsuta	Yellow star grass	6–12″	
Liatris pycnostachya	Kansas gayfeather	4–5′	
L. scariosa	Tall gayfeather	2–4′	
Polygonatum biflorum	Small Solomon's seal	1–3′	
Saxifraga virginiensis	Virginia saxifrage	12–18″	
Silene caroliniana	Wild pink	8–12″	
Xanthorhiza simplicissima	Yellowroot	3–6′	
Xerophyllum asphodeloides	Turkey-beard beargrass	5′	

ANNUALS

BOTANICAL NAME	COMMON NAME(S)	HEIGHT	ZONES
Dimorphotheca aurantiaca	African daisy	6–12″	
Helipterum manglesii	Everlasting flower, Immortelle	1–2′	
Mirabilis multiflora	Four-o'clock	18–36′	

VINES

BOTANICAL NAME	COMMON NAME(S)	HEIGHT	ZONES
Campsis radicans	Trumpet creeper	30′	
Parthenocissus quinquefolia	Virginia creeper, Woodbine	35′	

*Not often planted, but preserve if on-site.

Occasional Watering Zone

BOTANICAL NAME	COMMON NAME(S)	HEIGHT	ZONES

DECIDUOUS TREES

See Occasional Watering Zone for New England, page 143, plus:

BOTANICAL NAME	COMMON NAME(S)	HEIGHT	ZONES
Amelanchier arborea	Downy serviceberry	20–30′	
A. canadensis	Shadblow serviceberry	60′	
*Asimina triloba**	Pawpaw	15–30′	
Betula nigra	River birch	90′	
Celtis laevigata	Sugarberry	30′	
Chionanthus virginicus	Fringe tree	15–30′	
Halesia carolina	Silverbell	30′	
H. monticola	Silverbell	30′	
Liquidambar styraciflua	Sweet gum	50′	
Magnolia grandiflora	Bull bay, Southern magnolia	80′	7
*M. macrophylla**	Bigleaf magnolia	50′	
*M. tripetala**	Umbrella tree	45′	

BOTANICAL NAME	COMMON NAME(S)	HEIGHT	ZONES

DECIDUOUS TREES cont'd

*Populus grandidentata**	Largetooth aspen	50–75'	
Quercus palustris	Pin oak	75'	
Sassafras albidum		30–60'	
Sorbus americana (susceptible to borers)	American mountain ash	35'	

DECIDUOUS SHRUBS

See Occasional Watering Zone for New England, page 144, plus:

Calycanthus floridus	Carolina allspice	4–8'	
Clethra alnifolia	Summer sweet	6'	
*Cornus alternifolia** (shallow-rooted)	Pagoda dogwood	24'	
C. sericea, syn. *C. stolonifera*	Red-osier dogwood	6'	
E. atropurpurea	Wahoo	6'	
Fothergilla spp.*	Witch alder	3–6'	
Ribes hirtellum	Wild gooseberry	3'	
Xanthorhiza simplicissima	Yellowroot	3'	

EVERGREEN SHRUBS

Aucuba japonica	Japanese aucuba	4–15'	
Pieris floribunda	Mountain andromeda	3–6'	
Rhododendron maximum	Great laurel, Rosebay rhododendron	6–20'	

PERENNIALS

Anemonella thalictroides	Rue anemone	8"	
Aquilegia chrysantha	Golden columbine	4'	
A. formosa	Sitka columbine	12–40"	
Aruncus sylvester	Goatsbeard	7'	
Chelone glabra	White turtlehead	6'	
Cimicifuga americana	American bugbane	5'	
Dicentra canadensis	Squirrel corn	6–10"	
Erythronium albidum	White fawn lily	1'	
E. americanum	Common fawn lily, Trout lily	1'	
E. grandiflorum	Lamb's-tongue fawn lily	1'	
E. montanum	Avalanche lily	18"	
E. revolutum	Mahogany fawn lily	1'	
Eupatorium perfoliatum	Boneset	3'	
E. purpureum	Bluestem	3'	
E. rugosum	White snakeroot	2–4'	
Melanthium virginicum	Bunchflower	30–72"	
Panax quinquefolius	American ginseng	6–18"	
Sanguinaria canadensis	Bloodroot	8"	
Spiranthes cernua	Ladies' tresses	16"	
Tiarella cordifolia	Allegheny foam flower	1'	
Trillium spp.		6–24"	

*Not often planted, but preserve if on-site.

Xeriscape Plants for the Southeast

XERISCAPE landscaping has found an enthusiastic home in the Southeast with the help of many far-thinking individuals. Dr. Philip Karr of the Cobb-Marietta Water Authority says, "In twenty years the population of the north metro Atlanta area is expected to double. We're just trying to plan ahead for that, and Xeriscape landscaping is part of the plan." Atlanta is already feeling the pinch, despite the fact that the average rainfall in the region is high (forty-nine inches) and usually adequate to supply the population. "The water is there, in reservoirs," says Fox McCarthy, who promotes Xeriscape landscaping with nearly matchless zeal on behalf of Cobb-Marietta. "It's just that the delivery systems haven't been able to keep pace with the population growth in some areas." The result in 1990 was a confusing, frustrating, and often changing array of watering restrictions in some districts.

Post Properties, a developer and manager of apartment and business communities, has long been a leading promoter of Xeriscape gardening in the public sector, even before it was a concept with a name. Post simply called it low-maintenance landscaping, or good business sense. In building their communities, they invest in lavish landscaping with beautiful, drought-tolerant plants, creating environments in which people love to live and work.

Says Todd Tibbitts of Post Landscape, an offshoot of the development company, "We irrigate about ten percent of our properties, concentrating the irrigation on the most visible, public areas, such as entrances, parkway medians, and the areas around the leasing offices. Hose bibs are scattered throughout the other areas such as flower beds in case we need to do some spot watering of [drought-] stressed areas. We use zoysiagrass on irrigated areas only and where there is some shade. We use hybrid Bermudagrass on irrigated and nonirrigated areas in full sun.

"Oddly enough, Xeriscape landscaping is really a return to the way things were in the Atlanta area twenty years or more ago. There used to be no irrigating of landscapes at all. People stayed with native plants and other tried-and-true dependables that could survive without additional watering. The

Bright annuals create a warm welcome at a commercial property entrance in Atlanta. These high impact areas are often irrigated, while more remote areas are nonirrigated. The company has saved thousands of gallons annually with such targeted watering policies. Pictured here are periwinkle (Catharanthus roseus), Coleus spp., and tall verbena (Verbena bonariensis). Summer-flowering cannas (Canna indica) are in the background. (Design: Post Landscape)

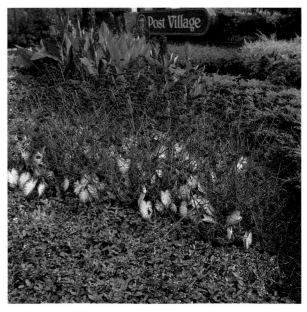

interest in the colorful, water-thirsty exotics has been more recent, leading to the use of irrigation."

Post tries to use a balanced canvas of plants, including some of the old favorites as well as newer drought-tolerant strains. They grow much of their own stock and often "design on the ground," says Andy Hull, also of Post. "We do a lot of mass plantings with low-maintenance ground covers." He reports that the use of Xeriscape plantings saves the company thousands of gallons of water yearly. A partial list of the plants in Post landscapes was used to help develop the list here. Hull cautions, however, that *any* "list" of drought-tolerant plants should not be taken as a complete list of the only ones that will work. "There are hundreds of other plants available in Georgia nurseries that would work just fine in a Xeriscape garden. The key is to site them right, and keep them grouped with other plants having the same water needs." Gary Wade, extension horticulturist with the University of Georgia, echoes that thought: "Many native plants and most of the introduced species you find at nurseries and garden centers in Georgia can survive long periods of limited water availability once they are established."

Bermudagrass is the turfgrass of choice for drought tolerance in the Southeast. Common Bermudagrass resists drought better and improved strains withstand cold better without turning brown. Zoysiagrass is also drought tolerant, though not quite as resilient to cold. One minus for common Bermudagrass is that its root system is invasive if not confined and it's very difficult to eradicate; zoysiagrass is slower growing. Other warm-season grasses may go dormant or brown out during drought if not watered, but will green up when water is again available.

In a brochure available from South Carolina's Clemson University ("Xeriscape: Landscape Water Conservation in the Southeast") mowing heights of three to three and a half inches are suggested for cool-season grasses like fescues, one inch for Bermudagrass, and one and a half inches for centipedegrass.

The Southeast includes very diverse soil conditions, ranging from red clay to sandy, alluvial coastal plain soils. However, Brian Smith, with Clemson's Extension Service, reports that temper-

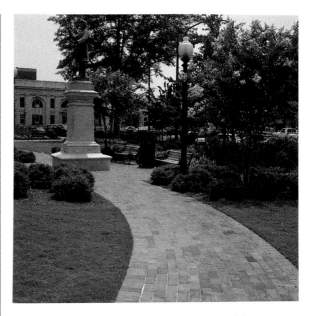

A classically designed city center park in Marietta, Georgia, is actually a model Xeriscape landscape featuring many drought-tolerant, yet formal plants that thrive in the Southeast, such as crape myrtle (Lagerstroemia indica), yaupon holly (Ilex vomitoria), celosia, creeping lilyturf (Liriope spicata), and zoysiagrass. (Design: Post Landscape)

ature affects plant selection more than soils. "Rhododendrons, for instance, aren't grown in southern South Carolina because of temperature. It's just too hot here."

The University of Georgia Extension Service has also published a lengthy booklet on Xeriscape gardening for Georgia. One highlight from this publication points out the importance of shade in southeastern Xeriscape landscapes: one mature oak can dissipate as much heat as four heavy-duty home air conditioners running twenty-four hours a day. This evaporative effect cools the surrounding environment and reduces water loss from nearby plants. Many established landscapes have an abundance of shade, and a balance must be struck between the energy and water savings provided by numerous trees, and the lack of air flow over lawn grasses if a landscape becomes overgrown; good air circulation is important in the prevention of disease in grasses in humid climates.

An important reversal of typical Xeriscape gardening advice is recommended for southeastern landscapes. We are often advised to place the high-

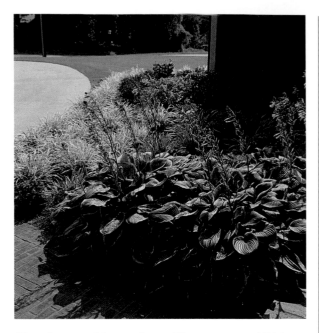

*Though green foliage plants (*Hosta *spp. and* Liriope spicata*) predominate in this composition, the overall effect is kept lively with pink accent flowers. The zoysiagrass lawn is watered in this Atlanta landscape, but the entrance garden survives on natural rainfall.*

water-use plant zones near the entry or otherwise close to the building where the most visual impact will be gained for the amount of water used. The Clemson brochure notes, however, that moisture and mildew damage to houses in the Southeast caused by landscaping is substantial, according to recent studies. In this region (and in other high-humidity, high-moisture areas) it would be strongly advisable to plan low-water-use zones adjacent to houses and buildings to alleviate mildew and moisture problems. In addition, dense shrubs should not be planted near the building foundation; this would block vents originally installed to allow good air circulation under the building floor.

SOUTHEAST GEORGIA/NORTHERN FLORIDA

An area that includes northern Florida and southeast Georgia is classified as part of the Southeast because the climate, soils, and flora are "more sim-

ilar to those of the Southeast than of southern and central Florida," according to Gary Knox, extension specialist at the University of Florida.

The experimental station near Tallahassee out of which he works researches varieties of crape myrtle, testing for colors, resistance to disease, etc. The station is right off a twenty-five-mile stretch of state highway all along which crape myrtles planted forty years ago by north Florida nursery growers and left completely untended for most of those years are still thriving, a tribute to the toughness and beauty of the species.

Knox reports that there isn't much concern for landscape water conservation in north Florida, in part because rainfall is almost always adequate. However, people still water lawns, sometimes too often and too shallowly. Knox recommends that site conditions be taken fully into account when planning a landscape, and he emphasizes appropriate plant selection when talking with people about Xeriscape gardening.

"Many people in north Florida raise annuals for flower color. Perennials usually need more of a cold spell, so they don't grow well here. Vincas, begonias, and impatiens are favorite warm-season annuals, and pansies and snapdragons are often grown over the winter."

Because of the high rainfall rate in the Southeast, the plant lists contain only one category, drought-tolerant plants. Other species would work for a Xeriscape design, too, especially if their native habitat were subject to the same two-month dry season that most southeastern landscapes experience—that is, they don't grow normally along a stream or in a bog. The list was compiled from the Clemson and University of Georgia brochures, with additional plants suggested by Post Landscape, and the second list was provided by the University of Florida Extension Service.

If you have sandy soil or a seashore setting, consult the list of seashore plants in the Appendix, choosing those within your cold-hardiness zone.

Though 1991 brought the opposite problem, five of the driest years on record in the Southeast occurred in the 1980s. The wise southeastern Xeriscape gardener will choose plants that can endure more than normal drought as well as some wetter years.

Xeriscape Plants for the Southeast
Natural Rainfall or Occasional Watering Zone

BOTANICAL NAME	COMMON NAME(S)	HEIGHT	ZONES
DECIDUOUS TREES			
Acer buergeranum	Trident maple	20'	
A. floridanum	Florida maple, Southern sugar maple	20–50'	
A. rubrum 'October Glory', 'Red Sunset'		25–50'	
A. saccharum 'Legacy'		40–80'	
Albizia julibrissin	Mimosa	36'	
Alnus glutinosa	Black alder	80'	
Betula nigra		90'	
Carpinus betulus	European pyramidal hornbeam	50'	
C. caroliniana	American hornbeam	36'	
Carya illinoinensis	Pecan	150'	
Catalpa bignonioides	Southern catalpa	30–40'	
Celtis laevigata	Sugar hackberry	90'	
Cercis canadensis		25–30'	
C. chinensis		40'	
C. reniformis		40'	
Chionanthus virginicus	Fringe tree	10–20'	
Cornus kousa	Chinese dogwood	21'	
Cotinus coggygria	Smoke tree	25'	
C. obovatus	American smoke tree	30'	
Crataegus spp.	Hawthorn	15–25'	
Fraxinus americana	White ash	60–120'	
Ginkgo biloba		125'	
Halesia carolina	Silver bell	20–30'	
Koelreuteria bipinnata	Chinese flame tree	60'	
Lagerstroemia indica		20–30'	
Liquidambar styraciflua	Sweet gum	75'	
Liriodendron tulipifera	Tulip poplar	75–150'	
Magnolia × *loebneri*		50'	
M. × *soulangiana*		25'	
M. × *stellata*		20'	
Malus baccata		50'	
M. floribunda	Japanese flowering crab apple	30'	
M. sieboldii var. *zumi*		25'	
Metasequoia glyptostroboides	Dawn redwood	125'+	
Oxydendrum arboreum	Sourwood	30–40'	
Pistacia chinensis	Chinese pistachio	60'	
Populus spp.	Poplar	50–150'	
Prunus × 'Mt. Fuji'	Mt. Fuji cherry	20–35'	
P. × 'Okame'	Okame cherry	24'	
P. subhirtella	Autumn cherry	30'	
P. s. 'Pendula'	Weeping cherry	30'	
P. × *yedoensis*	Yoshino cherry	48'	
Pyrus calleryana 'Bradford'	Bradford pear	30'	
Quercus acutissima	Sawtooth oak	35–45'	
Q. coccinea	Scarlet oak	75'	
Q. falcata	Southern red oak	70–80'	

Xeriscape Plants for the Southeast
Natural Rainfall or Occasional Watering Zone

BOTANICAL NAME	COMMON NAME(S)	HEIGHT	ZONES
DECIDIOUS TREES cont'd			
Quercus nigra	Water oak	80–90'	
Q. palustris	Pin oak	70–80'	
Q. phellos	Willow oak	80–100'	
Q. robur	English oak	75–150'	
Sapium sebiferum	Chinese tallow	40'	
Sophora japonica	Japanese pagoda tree, Chinese scholar tree	75'	
Taxodium distichum	Bald cypress	150'	
Ulmus alata	Winged elm	20–70'	
U. carpinifolia	Smoothleaf elm	90'	
Zelkova serrata	Japanese zelkova	90'	
EVERGREEN TREES			
Cedrus deodara	Deodar cedar	150'	7–8
Cryptomeria japonica	Cryptomeria cypress	150'	
Cupressocyparis leylandii	Leyland cypress	100'	
Eriobotrya japonica	Loquat	10–20'	
Ilex latifolia	Lusterleaf holly	60'	7
I. opaca	American holly	50'	
I. vomitoria	Weeping yaupon	12–20'	
Ligustrum recurvifolium	Tree-form ligustrum	10–15'	7
Magnolia grandiflora		80'	7–9
Pinus elliottii	Slash pine	80–100'	
P. strobus	White pine	80–100'	
P. taeda	Loblolly pine	80–100'	
P. thunbergiana	Japanese black pine	90'	
Prunus caroliniana	Carolina laurel cherry	15–30'	
Quercus spp.	Oak	30–150'	
Sabal palmetto	Cabbage palm	60'	
Trachycarpus fortunei	Windmill palm	30'	
DECIDUOUS SHRUBS			
Abelia grandiflora 'Prostrata'		1–3'	
Berberis thunbergii var. atropurpurea 'Rose Glow'		1–3'	
Callicarpa americana	Beautyberry, French mulberry	5–8'	7
C. dichotoma	Purple beautyberry	6'	
Chaenomeles lagenaria, syn. *Cydonia japonica*	Flowering quince	5–8'	
C. speciosa		6'	
Chimonanthus praecox	Wintersweet	8'	7
Cytisus scoparius	Scotch broom	6'	
Euonymus alata 'Campacta'		4'	
Exochorda racemosa	Common pearlbush	15'	
Forsythia × *intermedia*	Border forsythia	9'	
F. × *suspensa*	Weeping forsythia	9'	
Hamamelis vernalis	Witch hazel	10'	

BOTANICAL NAME	COMMON NAME(S)	HEIGHT	ZONES
DECIDUOUS SHRUBS cont'd			
Hydrangea paniculata	Peegee hydrangea	25'	
H. quercifolia	Oakleaf hydrangea	6'	
Ilex decidua	Possumhaw holly	30'	
Itea virginica	Virginia sweetspire	3–9'	
Kerria japonica	Single-flower kerria	4–6'	
Kolkwitzia amabilis	Beautybush	10'	
Ligustrum × vicaryi	Golden privet	12'	
Punica granatum	Pomegranate	15'	7–8
Rhododendron 'Austrinum'		10'	
Rosa carolina	Carolina rose	3'	
R. laevigata	Cherokee rose	15'	7
R. 'Nearly Wild'		1–3'	
Salvia greggii (semideciduous)	Gregg salvia, Autumn or Cherry sage	2–3'	
Spiraea × bumalda 'Anthony Waterer'		2'	
S. nipponica		7'	
Viburnum × juddii		8'	
V. lantana		15'	
V. macrocephalum	Chinese snowball	12'	
V. × 'Mohawk', *×* 'Cayuga'		9'	
V. plicatum var. *tomentosum*		9'	
EVERGREEN SHRUBS			
Aucuba japonica	Aucuba	6–8'	7
A. j. 'Nana'	Dwarf aucuba	3–4'	7
Berberis julianae	Wintergreen barberry	5–6'	
B. j. 'Nana'	Dwarf wintergreen barberry	1–3'	
B. verruculosa	Warty barberry	6'	6–8
Buxus microphylla	Japanese boxwood	6'	
B. m. var. *japonica*	Japanese boxwood	3–4'	
B. sempervirens	Common boxwood	5–8'	
Camellia japonica		8–10'	7
C. sasanqua	Sasanqua camellia	8–10'	7
Chamaecyparis obtusa 'Nana Gracilis'	Dwarf Hinoki cypress	4'	
Cleyera japonica	Japanese cleyera	8–10'	
Elaeagnus macrophylla		9'	
E. pungens	Thorny elaeagnus	12'	7
Fatsia japonica	Japanese aralia	10–12'	8
Gardenia jasminoides	Cape jasmine	2–5'	8–9
G. radicans	Creeping gardenia	1–4'	
Ilex × attenuata		8–10'	
I. cornuta	Chinese holly	8–15'	7
I. c. 'Burfordii'		8–12'	7
I. c. 'Burfordii Nana' (dwarf)		5–6'	
I. c. 'Rotunda' (dwarf)		3–4'	7
I. crenata		3–4'	

Xeriscape Plants for the Southeast
Natural Rainfall or Occasional Watering Zone

BOTANICAL NAME	COMMON NAME(S)	HEIGHT	ZONES
EVERGREEN SHRUBS cont'd			
Ilex crenata 'Green Lustre'		1–3'	
I. c. 'Helleri'		2–3'	
I. c. 'Hetzii'		4–5'	
I. glabra 'Compacta' (dwarf)		5'	
I. vomitoria	Yaupon holly	8–12'	7
I. v. 'Nana'	Dwarf yaupon holly	3–4'	7
I. v. 'Schellings'		1–3'	
Illicium parviflorum	Anise	6–8'	
Jasminum nudiflorum	Winter jasmine	4–5'	7
Juniperus divaurica 'Expansa'	Parson's juniper	1–2'	
Kalmia latifolia	Mountain laurel	5–8'	
Leucothoe populifolia	Florida leucothoe	12'	
Ligustrum japonicum	Japanese privet	7–10'	7
L. sinense 'Variegatum'	Variegated Chinese privet	12'	7
L. × *vicaryi*	Golden privet	10–12'	
Loropetalum chinense		6–12'	7
Mahonia bealei	Leatherleaf mahonia	6–7'	
Myrica cerifera	Wax myrtle	8–10'	
Nandina domestica and dwarf cvs.	Heavenly bamboo	6–8'	7
Osmanthus × *fortunei*	Fortune's osmanthus	8–10'	7–8
O. heterophyllus	Holly osmanthus	15–20'	7
Photinia × *fraseri*	Fraser photinia	10–12'	7
P. glabra	Japanese photinia	6–10'	7
Pinus densiflora	Dwarf Japanese red pine	1–3'	
Pittosporum tobira	Japanese pittosporum	8–10'	8
P. t. 'Wheeler's Dwarf'	Dwarf pittosporum	3–4'	8
Podocarpus macrophyllus	Southern yew	8–12'	8
Pyracantha coccinea var. lalandei		6–9'	6–7
P. koidzumii	Formosa firethorn	10–12'	8
Raphiolepsis indica	Indian hawthorn	2–4'	8
R. umbellata	Yedda hawthorn	4–6'	8
Rhododendron 'Glenn Dale'		3–5'	
R. 'Kurume'		3–4'	
R. 'Silver Sword'		1–3'	
Sabal etonia	Scrub palmetto	3–4'	
Ternstroemia gymnanthera	Cleyera	30'	
Viburnum 'Eskimo'		1–3'	
V. × *pragense*	Pragense viburnum	10'	
Yucca aloifolia	Spanish bayonet	4–10'	
Y. glauca 'Pendula'	Weeping yucca	6–8'	
Y. gloriosa	Spanish dagger	10'	

BOTANICAL NAME	COMMON NAME(S)	HEIGHT	ZONES
GROUND COVERS			
Ajuga reptans 'Bronze Beauty', 'Burgundy Glow'		8–10"	
Cephalotaxus harringtonia 'Drupacea'	Spreading yew	18–24"	
C. 'Prostrata'	Spreading yew	18–24"	
Cotoneaster salicifolius	Willowleaf cotoneaster	12–18"	
Dianthus spp.		6–12"	
Euonymus fortunei var. *colorata* (considered invasive in some areas)	Wintercreeper euonymus	6–18"	
E. f. var. *kewensis*	Kewensis	2"	
Hedera canariensis	Algerian ivy	6–8"	
H. helix	English ivy	6–12"	
Liriope muscari 'Big Blue'		8–15"	
Lonicera pileata	Box honeysuckle	4'	
Ophiopogon japonicus	Mondo grass	5–6"	
Rosa pimpinellifolia	Petite pink Scotch rose	2–3"	
Sarcococca hookerana var. *humilis*	Himalayan sarcococca	18"	
Trachelospermum asiaticum	Asiatic jasmine	4–6"	
Vinca minor	Periwinkle	5–6"	
PERENNIALS			
Digitalis purpurea	Foxglove	2–6'	
Echinacea angustifolia	Purple coneflower	3–5'	
Liatris scariosa	Gayfeather	2–6'	
Solidago altissima	Goldenrod	1–5'	
Verbena canadensis	Clump verbena	6"	
V. tenuisecta	Moss verbena	6"	
VINES			
Akebia quinata	Fiveleaf akebia	30–40'	
Clematis armandii	Evergreen clematis	15'	
C. henryi		30'	
C. paniculata	Sweet autumn clematis	30'	
Cocculus laurifolius	Snail seed	15'	
× *Fatshedera lizei*	Tree ivy	8'	
Ficus pumila	Creeping fig	40'	
Gelsemium sempervirens	Carolina jessamine	10–20'	
Lonicera × *heckrottii*	Goldflame honeysuckle	12'	
Trachelospermum asiaticum	Yellow star jasmine	15'	
Wisteria floribunda	Japanese wisteria	24'	

Xeriscape Plants in North Florida/Southeast Georgia

BOTANICAL NAME	COMMON NAME(S)	HEIGHT
DECIDUOUS TREES		
Acacia spp.		20–60'
Citrus spp.		10–30'
Maclura pomifera	Osage orange	60'
Morus spp.		30–80'
Parkinsonia aculeata	Jerusalem thorn	20–30'
Prunus angustifolia	Chickasaw plum	16'
P. cerasifera	Cherry plum	25'
Ptelea trifoliata	Hop tree	20–35'
Quercus incana	Bluejack oak	25'
Q. laevis	Turkey oak	20–50'
Q. prinus	Chestnut oak	90'
Q. shumardii	Shumard oak	40–125'
Q. stellata	Post oak	40–50'
Q. velutina	Black oak	50–90'
Sapindus saponaria	Soapberry	35–45'
EVERGREEN TREES		
Cinnamomum camphora	Camphor tree	40–50'
Cupressus spp.		20–60'
Evodia spp.		10–30'
Ficus spp.		40–80'
Juniperus silicicola	Southern red cedar	25–30'
Persea spp.	Bay	30–60'
Pinus clausa	Sand pine	60–80'
Platycladus arborvitae	Oriental arborvitae	40'
Quercus ilex	Holly oak	60'
Q. laurifolia (semievergreen)	Laurel oak	60'
Q. suber	Cork oak	60'
Q. virginiana	Live oak	60'
Ziziphus spp.	Jujube	25–40'
PALMS		
Butia capitata	Pindo palm	10–20'
Chamaerops humilis	European fan palm	6–12'
Cycas revoluta	Sago palm	10'
Phoenix spp.	Date palm	25–90'
Rhapidophyllum hystrix	Needle palm	6'
Rhapis excelsa	Lady palm	6–8'
Sabal minor	Dwarf palmetto	5–7'
Serenoa repens	Saw palmetto	8'
Washingtonia filifera	California fan palm, Desert fan palm	40–60'
W. robusta	Mexican fan palm, Washington palm	50–80'
DECIDUOUS SHRUBS		
Cassia spp.	Senna	2–25'
Cytisus spp.	Broom	8"–6'
Erythrina herbacea	Coral vine	20–30'
Rhamnus spp.	Buckthorn, Indian cherry	10–20'
Vaccinium spp.	Blueberry, Sparkleberry	1–12'

BOTANICAL NAME	COMMON NAME(S)	HEIGHT
EVERGREEN SHRUBS		
Acacia spp.		3–20'
Agave spp.	Century plant	2–5'
Artemisia spp.	Sage, Sagebrush	1–10'
Baccharis halimifolia	Eastern baccharis, Groundsel bush, Saltbush	8'
Callistemon spp.	Bottlebrush	8–15'
Ceratiola ericoides	Rosemary	4–5'
Cereus peruvianus	Hedge cactus	10'
Cotoneaster spp.		2–12'
Eugenia spp.	Stoppers	8–10'
Feijoa sellowiana	Pineapple guava	14'
Ficus spp.	Fig	10–12'
Fortunella japonica	Kumquat	12–15'
Genista spp.	Broom, Woadwaxen	2–10'
Ilex glabra	Gallberry	9'
Lespedeza spp.	Bush clover	1–10'
Leucophyllum frutescens	Texas sage	5–6'
Lyonia ferruginea	Rusty lyonia	10–20'
Myrtus communis	Myrtle	15'
Nerium oleander	Oleander	12–15'
Opuntia ficus-indica	Indian fig, Prickly pear	18'
Punica granatum	Pomegranate	10–15'
Rosmarinus officinalis	Rosemary	2–4'
Ruscus aculeatus	Buther's-broom	3'
Sesbania punicea	Rattle box	6'
Severinia buxifolia	Boxthorn	3–4'
GROUND COVERS		
Asparagus densiflorus 'Sprengeri'	Asparagus fern	12–18"
Ficus pumila	Creeping fig	10–12"
Helianthemum nummularium	Sun rose	6–8"
Helianthus debilis	Beach sunflower	1–2'
Hemerocallis spp.	Daylily	1–3'
Ipomoea spp.	Morning glory	4–12"
Ruellia brittoniana	Mexican bluebell	18–24"
Sesuvium portulacastrum	Sea purslane	12–18"
Tetrapanax papyriferus	Rice-paper plant	1–2'
Tulbaghia violacea	Society garlic	1'
Zamia floridana	Coontie	1–3'
VINES		
Bignonia capreolata	Crossvine	60'
Clematis drummondii	Drummond clematis	Varies
C. texensis	Texas clematis	6'
Lycium spp.	Matrimony vine, Christmasberry	6–12'
Macfadyena unguis-cati	Cat's-claw vine	25–30'
Vitis spp.	Grape	Varies

Xeriscape Plants for Central and Southern Florida

EVEN THOUGH Florida experiences an average of fifty-five inches of rainfall per year, the fact that the dry season occurs in winter when Florida's population doubles or triples with tourists and winter residents puts a severe strain on its freshwater supplies. The drawing down of aquifers to supply water for all these people sometimes causes salt water to intrude into the groundwater. When salt water starts to show up in a well's water, it must sometimes be capped and retired from use. Although Florida has high humidity, it also has high solar radiation and a fairly steady wind at fifteen miles per hour. The result is that the evapotranspiration rate equals the rainfall rate, and the demand for domestic water threatens to outstrip water supplies. Although the national average demand for water is 140 gallons per capita per day (gpcd), in southern Florida the average is 200 gpcd, and may range as high as 1,000.

Bruce Adams, former president of the National Xeriscape Council, now water conservation coordinator for the South Florida Water Management District (SFWMD), has been instrumental in getting legislation passed in 1991 in Florida that directly addresses the issue of Xeriscape landscaping. Among other things, the new laws define Xeriscape landscaping, provide for a five-year phase-in plan for all state properties and highways (including interstates) to be changed to Xeriscape designs, and require any new sprinkler system installed to include a rain-sensing shutoff device. Adams is very pleased with this progress, noting that Florida is the first state to enact legislation that includes Xeriscape landscaping and the seven principles as being part of what "a landscape architect can and shall do."

Three of the five water management districts in Florida have passed daytime watering bans, and all

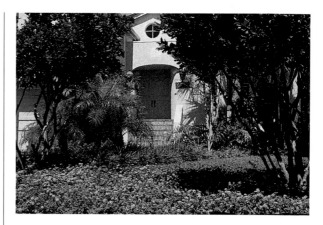

Florida Xeriscape gardeners have a rich palette of Xeriscape plants from which to choose. This model Xeriscape design features Lantana camara, *pygmy date palm* (Phoenix roebelenii), *mondo grass* (Ophiopogon japonicus), Ligustrum japonicum, *and* 'Floratam' St. Augustinegrass.

local governments are being strongly encouraged to publicize Xeriscape landscaping and provide information on how it can be achieved.

Obviously, considerable effort is being made to promote Xeriscape concepts in southern Florida, and to showcase the value of using native plants adapted to the cycle of winter drought and summer flooding experienced by the region. There is even building code legislation requiring that native plants growing on a proposed site be kept, to the greatest degree possible, and removed only by permit.

However, prospective Xeriscape gardeners are assured that many exotic (and noninvasive) species are also adapted to this type of landscaping. Pat Dailey, who teaches classes in Xeriscape landscaping, says she tries to promote the idea that "all plants [in southern and central Florida] are Xeriscape plants. We just have to put them in their proper place." She's talking specifically about the concept of zoning within a landscape, locating plants in a microclimate in your yard that will serve their water or dry soil needs.

From the following lists, it's evident that a very broad spectrum of plants is available for Xeriscape designs. (The lists feature plants commonly used and available through the nursery trade, not rare, hard-to-find species.) Part of the excitement of Xeriscape gardening for south and central Florida, Dailey says, is that there's such a rich palette of plants in use. "From Orlando south, you can grow things that can't be grown anywhere else in the continental United States." Drought-tolerant plants from Australia, New Zealand, Southeast Asia, and South Africa are common, including avocadoes, mangoes from India, and many other exotic fruits.

The term "perennials" takes on a different meaning in this part of the country. Most traditional perennial flowers grown elsewhere don't thrive in south/central Florida, in part because they need a below-freezing period each year in which to undergo dormancy, and in part because fungus is a problem. A few perennials such as gaillardia, butterfly weed (*Asclepias tuberosa*), and firebrush (*Hamelia patens*) will survive. The plant lists that follow may include some perennials that also appear on the overall lists of perennials on pages 282–91. In this part of the country it isn't possible to generalize and assume that all the plants on the overall list can be raised, so the ones that *can* are listed.

Dailey says "perennials" are usually not pulled out separately in plant lists, but are included in other lists as flowering color (usually present year-round). For instance, daylilies (*Hemerocallis* spp.), a Xeriscape favorite in nearly every part of the country, and rain lilies (*Zephyranthes* spp.) are used as ground cover in Florida because they spread so exuberantly. Bougainvillea is used as both a vine and a bush. Coleus is used as an accent plant. Many of the trees and shrubs on the list are deciduous in other parts of the country, but evergreen in Florida.

People often plant warm-season annuals such as marigolds over the hot, humid summer and cool-season annuals such as salvia over the winter. (See the overall list of annuals in the Appendix for other ideas.) Incorporating generous quantities of organic

matter or appropriate amounts of hydro-gels in Florida's predominantly sandy soils can cut down substantially on the need to water annuals.

Because the climate is subtropical, with the abundant heat and moisture required by many tropical plants, some introduced plants and a few native plants have a tendency to become invasive when removed from their normal habitat. Care must be used in selecting these often extremely drought-tolerant and rugged survivors in areas where they might escape cultivation. They should be used only in median strips or other areas where they will be carefully confined. The species that are prone to invasiveness are noted in the plant list.

The SFWMD's "Xeriscape Plant Guide II" issues a warning against the following species as being particularly invasive:

Bischofia javanica	Bishopwood (in southern areas)
Casuarina spp.	Australian pine
Melaleuca quinquenervia	Punk tree, Swamp tea tree
Schinus terebinthifolius	Brazilian pepper tree

They warn, too, that the following plants should not be planted near sidewalks or sewer lines because they have large, aggressive root systems:

Enterolobium cyclocarpum	Ear tree
Ficus benjamina	Weeping fig
F. retusa 'Nitida'	Laurel fig

As Xeriscape gardeners, it's important for us to be aware of new knowledge about invasiveness, to make sure that the landscapes we plan will not threaten nearby natural plant communities. One source for this type of information is the County Cooperative Extension Service.

For southern and central Florida the lowest-water-using lawn grasses are Bahiagrass, Bermudagrass, and zoysiagrass. Moderately drought-tolerant grasses include St. Augustinegrass and centipedegrass. Carpetgrass is an "oasis" plant, requiring regular watering.

Mulching with organic materials that degrade slowly and help enrich the soil is recommended. Mulch should be applied at a three-inch depth, but should be kept pulled away from stems and trunks to avoid rotting. Citrus trees should not be mulched, because they are extremely susceptible to trunk and root rot.

The plant lists are divided into three zones. The "natural" or "very drought tolerant" zone includes plants that will survive on natural rainfall after establishment. The "moderate drought tolerance" zone plants will require supplemental irrigation during extreme dry periods to maintain an attractive appearance. The "oasis" zone plants will need frequent watering. An oasis plant may become drought tolerant if adapted to shade, and may survive without watering if the soil is poorly drained. In many cases the "oasis" plants are called that because of their native habitat, which may be a swamp, a stream bank, or an area subject to frequent flooding. Plants with high salt tolerance are noted.

These lists have been taken directly from the extensive brochures available from the South and Southwest Florida Water Management districts. If you live in this region it would be very worthwhile to obtain copies of them because they include other useful and interesting information about the plants. The brochure from the Southwest District even notes the habitats for the native plants in the list, such as "Beach/Strand—sand and shell soil, dry, salty, windy" or "scrub—deep acid soils, extremely well drained," etc., for the Xeriscape gardener interested in creating a consistent habitat, or matching soils and conditions as closely as possible. You can get the brochures by writing to Planning Department, Southwest Florida Water Management District, 2379 Broad Street, Brooksville, FL 34609-6899. The phone number is (904) 796-7211, or call toll free at 800-423-1476. You can also write to the South Florida Water Management District, P.O. Box 24680, West Palm Beach, FL 33416-4680. Their water conservation line is 800-662-8876.

The St. Johns River Water Management District in north Florida will very soon publish a plant list as well. Write to them at P.O. Box 1429, Highway 100 West, Palatka, FL 32177.

Xeriscape Plants for Central Florida

This plant list was prepared for an area extending roughly fifty miles north, east, and south of Tampa, Florida. At the northern end the minimum temperature may go as low as 18 degrees Fahrenheit, while at the southern end and along the coast it may stay as high as 34 degrees. The plants on the list are all hardy to the 18-degree temperature, except where noted. Those with the notation "not SF" are not suitable for southern Florida.

Natural Rainfall Zone

BOTANICAL NAME	COMMON NAME(S)	MATURE HEIGHT	MINIMUM TEMPERATURE (FAHRENHEIT)
DECIDUOUS TREES			
Carya illinoinensis	Pecan	100'	
Celtis spp.	Hackberry, Sugarberry	60–80'	
Chorisia speciosa	Floss-silk tree	50'	26°
Crataegus spp.	Hawthorn	15–30'	
Dalbergia sissoo	Indian rosewood	45'	26°
Gleditsia triacanthos (not SF)	Honey locust	60–90'	
Jacaranda acutifolia	Jacaranda	50'	26°
*Koelreuteria elegans***	Goldenrain tree, Golden shower tree	55'	
Lagerstroemia indica	Crape myrtle	20'	
Liquidambar styraciflua	Sweet gum	85'	
Parkinsonia aculeata	Jerusalem thorn	25'	

BOTANICAL NAME	COMMON NAME(S)	MATURE HEIGHT	MINIMUM TEMPERATURE (FAHRENHEIT)
DECIDUOUS TREES cont'd			
Peltophorum dubium	Yellow poinciana	50′	22°
Pistacia spp. (not SF)	Pistachio	30–40′	
Prunus angustifolia (not SF)	Chickasaw plum	25′	
Ptelea trifoliata (not SF)	Hop tree	15′	
Quercus chapmanii	Chapman oak	30–45′	
Q. incana	Bluejack oak	20–30′	
Q. laevis	Turkey oak	40–50′	
Q. macrocarpa	Burr oak	50–140′	
Q. nigra	Water oak	75′	
Q. prinus (not SF)	Chestnut oak	40–100′	
Q. shumardii	Shumard oak	85′	
Q. stellata (not SF)	Post oak	15–65′	
Q. velutina (not SF)	Black oak	60–90′	
Rhus spp. (not SF)	Sumac	8–30′	
Sapindus spp.	Soapberry	35–45′	
*Sapium sebiferum**	Chinese tallow tree	40′	
Sophora spp. (not SF)	Japanese pagoda tree	15–75′	
Tamarix spp.	Tamarisk	10–30′	
Ulmus alata	Winged elm	50′	
U. americana var. *floridana* (not SF)	Florida elm	60′	
Zelkova serrata (not SF)		60–80′	
EVERGREEN TREES			
*Araucaria heterophylla***	Norfolk Island pine	50′	22°
Brassaia actinophylla	Schefflera	40′	22′
Cedrus spp.	Cedar	30–50′	
Cinnamomum camphora	Camphor tree	60′	
Coccoloba diversifolia	Pigeon plum	70′	30°
*Cupressus sempervirens***	Italian cypress	50′	
Cycas circinalis	Queen sago	20′	26°
Eriobotrya japonica	Loquat	20′	
Erythrina crista-galli	Coral tree, Cockspur coral tree	15–25′	
Eucalyptus spp.	Gum tree	60′	22°
Eugenia spp.	Stoppers	20′	
Ilex × *attenuata* (not SF)	American holly	50′	
I. opaca	American holly	20–50′	
I. vomitoria	Yaupon holly	25′	
Juniperus silicicola	Southern red cedar	40′	
Macadamia integrifolia	Macadamia nut	30′	
Magnolia virginiana (not SF)	Sweet bay	75′	
Mangifera indica	Mango	50′	34°
*Melia azedarach**	Chinaberry tree	60′	
Persea borbonia	Red bay	50′	
Pinus clausa	Sand pine	60′	
P. elliottii	Slash pine	80′	
P. palustris	Longleaf pine	100′	

Xeriscape Plants for Central Florida
Natural Rainfall Zone

BOTANICAL NAME	COMMON NAME(S)	MATURE HEIGHT	MINIMUM TEMPERATURE (FAHRENHEIT)
EVERGREEN TREES cont'd			
Pinus taeda	Loblolly pine	80'	
*Platycladus orientalis***	Oriental arborvitae	15–20'	
*Podocarpus macrophyllus***		40'	
Pongamia pinnata (not SF)	Pongam	40'	34°
Pyracantha coccinea	Firethorn	20'	
Quercus myrsinifolia	Myrtle oak	10–25'	
Q. palustris	Pin oak	60–100'	
Q. suber (not SF)	Cork oak	60'	
Q. virginiana	Live oak	70'	
Tamarindus indica	Tamarind	50'	30°
Ulmus parvifolia	Weeping elm, American elm	40'	
PALMS			
Arecastrum romanzoffianum	Queen palm	40'	
Butia capitata	Butia palm, Pindo palm	20'	
*Caryota mitis***	Fishtail palm	25'	
Chamaedorea microspadix (needs deep shade)	Bamboo palm	10'	
*Chamaerops humilis***	European fan palm	10'	
Cycas revoluta	Sago palm	10'	
Livistona chinensis	Chinese fan palm	20'	
Phoenix canariensis	Canary Island date palm	60'	
P. reclinata	Senegal date palm	35'	
Rhapidophyllum hystrix	Needle palm	6'	
Sabal minor	Dwarf palmetto	5–7'	
S. palmetto	Cabbage palm	60'	
Serenoa repens	Saw palmetto	8'	
Trachycarpus fortunei	Windmill palm	20'	
Washingtonia filifera	Desert fan palm	40–60'	
W. robusta	Washington palm	60'	
DECIDUOUS SHRUB			
Lagerstroemia indica 'Nana'	Dwarf crape myrtle	6'	
EVERGREEN SHRUBS			
Abelia × *grandiflora***	Glossy abelia	6'	
Allamanda neriifolia	Bush allamanda	5'	22°
Baccharis halimifolia	Groundsel, Saltbush	8'	
Befaria recemosa	Tarflower	5'	
Buxus microphylla var. *japonica***	Japanese boxwood	4'	
Callicarpa americana	Beautyberry	8'	
Carissa spp.	Natal plum	4'	26°
Coccoloba uvifera	Sea grape	18'	30°
Cycas revoluta	King sago	6'	

BOTANICAL NAME	COMMON NAME(S)	MATURE HEIGHT	MINIMUM TEMPERATURE (FAHRENHEIT)
EVERGREEN SHRUBS cont'd			
Elaeagnus pungens	Silverthorn	18'	
Euphorbia pulcherrima*	Poinsettia	12'	22°
Feijoa sellowiana**	Pineapple guava	14'	
Ilex cornuta**	Chinese holly	10'	
I. glabra**	Gallberry	9'	
I. vomitoria		3'	
Ixora coccinea**		7'	26°
Jasminum mesnyi**	Primrose jasmine	5'	
J. nitidum**	Shining jasmine	5'	22°
Leucophyllum frutescens	Texas sage	5'	
Lyonia lucida	Tetterbush	8'	
Murraya paniculata**	Orange jasmine	12'	22°
Myrica cerifera	Wax myrtle	12–15'	
Nandina domestica	Heavenly bamboo	6'	
Nerium oleander	Oleander	12'	
Platycladus orientalis**	Oriental arborvitae	25'	
Plumbago auriculata**		4'	22°
Raphiolepis indica	Indian hawthorn	5'	
Russelia equisetiformis	Firecracker plant	4'	30°
Schefflera arboricola**	Dwarf schefflera	8'	26°
Ternstroemia gymnanthera (not SF)	Cleyera	15'	
Yucca aloifolia	Spanish bayonet	20'	
GROUND COVERS			
Asparagus densiflorus	Asparagus fern	1'	
Aspidistra elatior	Cast iron plant	2'	
Borrichia frutescens	Sea oxeye daisy	2'	
Catharanthus roseus	Periwinkle	1'	
Dietes bicolor	African iris	2'	
Helianthus debilis	Beach sunflower	1'	
Hemerocallis spp.	Daylily	2'	
Hippeastrum spp.	Amaryllis	2'	
Hymenocallis spp.	Spider lily	2'	22°
Kalanchoe spp.		1'	26°
Lantana montevidensis	Weeping lantana	1'	26°
(Do not use where pets might eat the plant—causes kidney problems)			
Piloblephis rigida (not SF)	Pennyroyal	1'	22°
Rhoeo spathacea 'Nana'	Dwarf oyster plant	8"	26°
Setcreasea spp.	Purple queen	1'	26°
Tulbaghia violacea**	Society garlic	1'	
Wedelia trilobata*		1'	26°
Zamia pumila	Coontie	3'	
PERENNIALS			
Aletris lutea	Yellow colic root	2–3'	
Asclepias tuberosa	Butterfly bush	1'–3'	
Baptisia lanceolata	Pineland baptisia	3'	

Xeriscape Plants for Central Florida
Natural Rainfall Zone

BOTANICAL NAME	COMMON NAME(S)	MATURE HEIGHT	MINIMUM TEMPERATURE (FAHRENHEIT)
PERENNIALS cont'd			
Ipomopsis rubra	Standing cypress	6'	
Liatris tenuifolia	Dense blazing star	3'	
Phlox nivalis	Creeping phlox	6'	
ANNUALS			
Gaillardia pulchella		1–2'	
Helianthus debilis	Beach sunflower	6'	
Monarda punctata	Horsemint	3'	
(can also be biennial or perennial)			
Rudbeckia hirta (biennial)	Black-eyed Susan	1–3'	
Salvia coccinea	Tropical sage	30"	
VINES			
Antigonon leptopus	Coral vine	40'	26°
Bougainvillea spp.		Varies	26°
Clerodendrum thomsoniae	Bleedingheart vine	8'	22°
Ipomoea stolonifera	Beach morning glory	Varies	26°
Tecomaria capensis	Cape honeysuckle	6'	26°

*Considered a noxious weed in some areas.
**May need occasional watering in southern Florida, especially in sandy soil.

Occasional Watering Zone

BOTANICAL NAME	COMMON NAME(S)	MATURE HEIGHT	MINIMUM TEMPERATURE (FAHRENHEIT)
DECIDUOUS TREES			
*Acer rubrum***	Red maple	40'	
A. saccharum	Florida maple	30'	
Bauhinia variegata	Orchid tree	25'	26°
Bursera simaruba	Gumbo-limbo	60'	22°
Carya glabra	Pignut hickory	60'	
Cercis canadensis	Redbud, Judas tree	30'	
Chionanthus virginicus	Fringe tree	25'	
Chrysalidocarpus lutescens	Areca palm	20'	
Delonix regia	Royal poinciana	35'	30°
Diospyros kaki	Oriental persimmon	20'	
*Ilex decidua**	Deciduous holly	25'	
Liriodendron tulipifera	Tulip tree	110'	

BOTANICAL NAME	COMMON NAME(S)	MATURE HEIGHT	MINIMUM TEMPERATURE (FAHRENHEIT)
DECIDUOUS TREES cont'd			
Magnolia soulangiana	Saucer magnolia	25′	
Morus spp.	Mulberry	30–45′	
Platanus occidentalis	Sycamore	100′	
*Sapium sebiferum**	Chinese tallow tree	45′	
Tabebuia chrysotricha		40′	
Taxodium distichum	Bald cypress	100′	
EVERGREEN TREES			
Callistemon rigidus	Upright bottlebrush	25′	
C. viminalis	Weeping bottlebrush	20′	26°
Citrus spp.		20′	30°
Conocarpus erectus	Buttonwood	40′	34°
Ficus nitida	Rubber tree	50′	26°
Ligustrum japonicum		15′	
L. lucidum	Glossy privet	30′	
Magnolia grandiflora (not SF)	Southern magnolia	50′	
Persea americana	Avocado	40′	22°
*Prunus caroliniana**	Cherry laurel	30–40′	
Psidium guajava/****	Guava	30′	
Quercus ilex	Holly oak	60′	
Ravenala madagascariensis	Traveler's tree	25′	34°
Vaccinium arboreum	Sparkleberry	20′	
Vitex trifolia (not SF)	Chaste tree	20′	22°
Ziziphus spp.	Jujube	30–40′	
PALMS			
Acoelorrhaphe wrightii	Paurotis palm	30′	22°
Chrysalidocarpus lutescens	Areca palm	20′	30°
Phoenix roebelenii	Pygmy date palm	10′	26°
Rhapidophyllum hystrix	Needle palm	6′	
Rhapis excelsa	Lady palm	10′	
DECIDUOUS SHRUB			
*Ficus carica**	Edible fig	10′	
EVERGREEN SHRUBS			
Agave americana	Century plant	4′	22°
Ardisia crenata	Coral ardisia	6′	
Aucuba japonica	Japanese aucuba	5′	
Bambusa spp.	Bamboo	Varies	
Calliandra haematocephala	Powderpuff	15′	30°
*Calycanthus floridus** (not SF)	Sweet shrub	8′	
Camellia japonica	Camellia	25′	
*C. sasanqua***	Sasanqua camellia	15′	
Codiaeum variegatum	Croton	10′	26°
Dizygotheca elegantissima	False aralia	10′	30°
Eugenia uniflora	Surinam cherry	15′	26°

Xeriscape Plants for Central Florida
Occasional Watering Zone

BOTANICAL NAME	COMMON NAME(S)	MATURE HEIGHT	MINIMUM TEMPERATURE (FAHRENHEIT)
EVERGREEN SHRUBS cont'd			
Fatsia japonica		3′	
Galphimia glauca	Thryallis	6′	
Gamolepis chrysanthemoides	Bush daisy, African daisy	2′	26°
Gardenia jasminoides	Gardenia	8′	
Halesia diptera (not SF)	Silverbell	20′	
Hibiscus syriacus (not SF)	Rose of Sharon	10′	
Hypericum spp.	St.-John's-wort, Aaron's beard	3′	
Ilex crenata 'Compacta' (not SF)	Dwarf Japanese holly	4′	
Illicium floridanum	Florida anise	20′	
Jasminum multiflorum	Downy jasmine	5′	26°
Ligustrum sinense		4–6′	
Magnolia stellata (not SF)	Star magnolia	8′	
Mahonia bealei (not SF)	Leatherleaf mahonia	8′	
M. lomariifolia	Chinese holly grape	6′	
Michelia figo (not SF)	Banana shrub	12′	
Philodendron selloum		8′	26°
Photinia × fraseri	Red tip	12′	
Pittosporum tobira		10′	
Psidium littorale	Strawberry guava, Cattley guava	14′	22°
Rhododendron spp.		8′	
Strelitzia nicolai	White bird-of-paradise	20′	
S. reginae	Bird-of-paradise	4′	22°
Viburnum obovatum	Walter viburnum	10′	
V. odoratissimum	Sweet viburnum	10′	
V. suspensum	Sandankwa viburnum	8′	
GROUND COVERS			
Aechmea spp.	Urn plant	2′	26°
Agapanthus africanus		2′	
Begonia spp.		1′	
Billbergia spp.		2′	26°
Caladium × hortulanum	Fancy-leaved caladium	2′	
Convolvulus 'Blue Daze'		6″	26°
Cuphea hyssopifolia	False heather	1′	26°
Cyrtomium falcatum	Holly fern	2′	
Gerbera jamesonii	Gerbera daisy	1′	
Liriope muscari	Lilyturf	8″	
Mitchella repens	Partridgeberry	3″	
Nandina domestica 'Nana'	Dwarf nandina	8″	26°
Neoregelia spp.		1′	22°
Nephrolepis exaltata	Sword fern	2′	
Ophiopogon japonicus	Mondo grass	8″	
Portulaca spp.	Moss rose, Rose moss	6″	22°
Ruellia caroliniensis		1′	
Rumohra adiantiformis	Leatherleaf fern	3′	

BOTANICAL NAME	COMMON NAME(S)	MATURE HEIGHT	MINIMUM TEMPERATURE (FAHRENHEIT)
GROUND COVERS cont'd			
Sisyrinchium spp.	Blue-eyed grass	1'	
Spathiphyllum spp.	Peace lily	2'	30°
Trachelospermum asiaticum	Dwarf Confederate jasmine	8"	
PERENNIALS			
Aletris farinosa	Colic root, Star grass	3'	
Aster dumosus	Aster	3'	
Rhexia alifanus	Tall meadow beauty	2'	
VINES			
Allamanda cathartica	Yellow allamanda	50'	22°
Campsis radicans	Trumpet vine	30'	
*Epipremnum aureum**	Pothos	40'	26°
Ficus pumila	Creeping fig	40'	
*Hedera canariensis**	Algerian ivy	30'	
H. helix (not SF)	English ivy	90'	
Ipomoea pes-caprae	Railroad vine	60'	22°
Lonicera sempervirens	Coral honeysuckle	50'	
Pyrostegia venusta	Flame vine	6'	22°
Trachelospermum jasminoides	Confederate jasmine	30'	

*Considered a noxious weed in some areas.
**May need occasional watering in southern Florida, especially in sandy soil.

Regular Watering Zone

BOTANICAL NAME	COMMON NAME(S)	MATURE HEIGHT	MINIMUM TEMPERATURE (FAHRENHEIT)
DECIDUOUS TREES			
Acer palmatum	Japanese maple	20'	
Betula nigra	River birch	75'	
Cornus florida	Dogwood	30'	
Nyssa sylvatica var. *biflora*	Black gum	80'	
Salix babylonica	Weeping willow	40'	
S. caroliniana	Coastal plain willow	40'	
Taxodium ascendens	Pond cypress	70'	
EVERGREEN TREES			
Gordonia lasianthus	Loblolly bay	70'	
Ilex cassine	Dahoon holly	40'	

Xeriscape Plants for Central Florida
Regular Watering Zone

BOTANICAL NAME	COMMON NAME(S)	MATURE HEIGHT	MINIMUM TEMPERATURE (FAHRENHEIT)
DECIDUOUS SHRUBS			
*Cephalanthus occidentalis**	Buttonbush	20'	
Hibiscus coccineus	Swamp hibiscus	6'	22°
H. rosa-sinensis		10'	26°
GROUND COVERS			
Canna flaccida	Yellow canna	2'	
Crinum americanum	String lily, Swamp lily	2'	
Cryptanthus spp.	Earth stars	3"	26°
Guzmania spp.		1"	26°
Impatiens spp.		1'	26°
Iris hexagona	Blue flag	2'	
Osmunda regalis	Royal fern	4'	
Saururus cernuus	Lizard's tail	2'	
Vriesea spp.		2'	26°
PERENNIALS			
Coreopsis gladiata	Tickseed	3'	
Lobelia cardinalis	Cardinal flower	3–6'	

*Considered a noxious weed in some areas.

Sources: Southwest Florida Water Management District, "Plant Guide," Brooksville, Florida. University of Florida Cooperative Extension Service, "Drought Tolerant Plants for North and Central Florida," Circ. 807, Gainesville, Florida. National Wildflower Research Institute, "Recommended Wildflowers for Florida," Austin Texas.

Xeriscape Plants for Southern Florida
Natural Rainfall Zone

See Natural Rainfall Zone for Central Florida, pages 164–68, plus:

BOTANICAL NAME	COMMON NAME(S)	HEIGHT
DECIDUOUS TREES		
Albizia julibrissin	Mimosa	30–40'
A. lebbeck	Mother-in-law's tongue	50–80'
Bauhinia spp.	Orchid tree	20–30'
Bursera simaruba	Gumbo-limbo	40–60'
Carya floridana	Scrub hickory	20–70'
C. glabra	Pignut hickory	80–120'
Cassia fistula	Golden shower tree	30–40'
Ceiba pentandra	Silk cotton tree	50–80'
Celtis laevigata	Sugarberry	40–60'
Cercis canadensis	Redbud, Judas tree	20–30'

BOTANICAL NAME	COMMON NAME(S)	HEIGHT
DECIDUOUS TREES cont'd		
Clusia rosea	Pitch apple	25–30'
Coccoloba pubescens	Bigleaf sea grape	60–80'
Cochlospermum vitifolium	Buttercup tree	30–40'
Delonix regia	Royal poinciana	25–40'
Diospyros virginiana	Persimmon	30–45'
Harpullia arborea	Tulipwood	30–50'
Jacaranda mimosifolia		40–50'
Lagerstroemia speciosa	Queen's crape myrtle	15–25'
Lysiloma bahamensis	Wild tamarind	40–50'
L. latisiliqua	Sabacu	20–30'
Morus rubra	Red mulberry	30–35'
Pachira aquatica	Guiana chestnut	25–30'
Plumeria rubra	Frangipani	15–25'
Pongamia pinnata	Pongam	30–40'
Sapindus saponaria	Soapberry	35–45'
Tabebuia caraiba	Silver trumpet tree	20–30'
T. chrysotricha	Golden tabebuia	35–50'
T. heterophylla	Pink trumpet tree	15–30'
T. impetiginosa	Purple tabebuia	15–20'
T. umbellata		15'
Taxodium distichum	Bald cypress	60–100'
Terminalia catappa	Tropical almond	20–45'
Thespesia populnea	Seaside mahoe	35–45'
EVERGREEN TREES		
Acacia auriculiformis	Earleaf acacia	40–50'
A. farnesiana	Sweet acacia	10–12'
Beaucarnea recurvata	Ponytail	15–25'
Bucida buceras	Black olive	40–50'
B. spinosa	Spiny black olive	15–20'
Citharexylum fruticosum	Fiddlewood	25–30'
Citrus spp.		10–30'
Conocarpus erectus	Buttonwood	30–50'
Cordia sebestena	Geiger tree	20–25'
Dracaena draco	Dragon tree	40–60'
Drypetes diversifolia	Milkbark	30–40'
D. lateriflora	Guiana plum	20–30'
Enallagma latifolia	Black calabash	30–45'
*Ficus aurea**	Strangler fig	40–50'
F. citrifolia	Shortleaf fig	40–50'
*F. elastica**	Indian rubber tree	40–60'
F. lyrata	Fiddleleaf fig	40–50'
F. religiosa	Sacred fig	50–80'
Grevillea banksii	Bank's grevillea	15–20'
Guaiacum sanctum	Lignumvitae	10–30'
Guapira discolor	Blolly	35–50'
Gymnanthes lucida	Crabwood	15–30'
Hypelate trifoliata	White ironwood	30–40'

Xeriscape Plants for Southern Florida
Natural Rainfall Zone

BOTANICAL NAME	COMMON NAME(S)	HEIGHT
EVERGREEN TREES cont'd		
*Hibiscus tilaceus**	Mahoe	30–45'
Krugiodendron ferreum	Black ironwood	20–30'
Magnolia grandiflora	Southern magnolia	60–100'
Manilkara roxburghiana	Mimusops	15–25'
Mastichodendron foetidissimum	Mastic	45–70'
Melicoccus bijugatus	Spanish lime	40–50'
Millettia ovalifolia		20–35'
Moringa oleifera	Horseradish tree	20–25'
Murraya paniculata	Orange jasmine	10–20'
Noronhia emarginata	Madagascar olive	40–50'
Ochrosia elliptica		10–20'
Pinus elliottii var. *densa*	South Florida slash pine	80–100'
Piscidia piscipula	Jamaican dogwood	35–50'
Pittosporum ferrugineum	Rusty pittosporum	40–60'
Quercus laurifolia	Laurel oak	60–100'
Q. nigra	Water oak	60–100'
Reynosia septentrionalis	Darling plum	20–30'
Simarouba glauca	Paradise tree	35–50'
Spathodea campanulata	African tulip tree	40–60'
Swietenia mahogani	Mahogany	35–60'
Syzygium cumini	Jambolan plum	50–100'
S. jambos	Rose apple	20–30'
Tecoma stans	Yellow elder	10–20'
Ximenia americana	Tallowwood plum	20–25'
Yucca elephantipes	Spineless yucca	20–30'
PALMS		
Acrocomia totai	GruGru palm	25–35'
Archontophoenix alexandrae	Alexandra palm	40–45'
Arikuryroba schizophylla	Arikury palm	10–15'
Bismarckia nobilis	Bismarck palm	30–60'
Chrysalidocarpus lutescens	Areca palm	20–30'
Coccothrinax argentata	Silver palm	10–20'
Cocos nucifera	Coconut palm	60–100'
Heterospathe elata	Sagisi palm	30–45'
Latania loddigesii	Blue latan palm	20–50'
Licuala grandis	Licuala palm	10'
Phoenix dactylifera	Date palm	60–90'
P. rupicola	Cliff date palm	25–30'
P. sylvestris	Wild date palm	40–60'
Pritchardia spp.	Prichardia palm	10–25'
*Pseudophoenix sargentii***	Buccaneer palm	10–15'
Ptychosperma elegans	Solitaire palm	15–25'
P. macarthurii	Macarthur palm	20–30'
Roystonea regia	Cuban royal palm	50–70'
Thrinax morrisii	Key thatch palm	15–30'

BOTANICAL NAME	COMMON NAME(S)	HEIGHT
PALMS cont'd		
*T. parviflora***	Thatch palm	15–25'
*T. radiata***	Florida thatch palm	15–30'
Veitchia merrillii	Manila palm	10–25'
V. montgomeryana	Montgomery's palm	25–40'
V. winin	Winin palm	40–65'
DECIDUOUS SHRUBS		
Capparis cynophallophora	Jamaican caper	8–10'
Erythrina herbacea	Cardinal-spear	20–30'
EVERGREEN SHRUBS		
Acacia cyanophylla	Orange wattle	14–18'
Agave attenuata	Century plant	2–5'
Angadenia berterii	Pineland allamanda	2–4'
Asparagus spp.	Asparagus fern	2–6'
Bauhinia punctata	Red bauhinia	3–10'
Beaucarnea recurvata	Ponytail	5–15'
Borrichia arborescens	Silver sea oxeye	2–4'
Bougainvillea spp.		6–12'
Bucida spinosa	Spiny black olive	6–15'
Byrsonima cuneata	Locustberry	15–20'
Cassia clusifolia	Seven-year apple	5–10'
Ceratiola ericoides	Rosemary	4–5'
Chiococca alba	Snowberry	6–9'
Codiaeum variegatum	Croton	4–6'
Colubrina arborescens	Coffee colubrina	15–20'
Conocarpus erectus 'Sericeus'	Silver buttonwood	15–20'
Conradina grandiflora		3–4'
Cordyline terminalis	Ti plant	3–6'
Cryptostegia grandiflora	Palay rubber vine	6–8'
Cycas circinalis	Queen sago	6–12'
Dalbergia ecastophyllum	Coin vine	6–9'
Dioon spp.**	Dioon cycad	3–7'
Dodonaea viscosa	Varnish leaf	5–7'
Dracaena marginata	Red-edged dracaena	8–12'
D. reflexa	Reflexed dracaena	6–12'
D. sanderana	Ribbon plant	3–5'
Elaeagnus philippinensis	Lingaro	8–10'
Enallagma latifolia	Black calabash	20–30'
Eugenia spp.	Stoppers	8–10'
Euphorbia milii	Crown-of-thorns	1–2'
E. tirucalli	Pencil tree	10–20'
Fortunella japonica	Kumquat	12–15'
Hamelia patens	Scarletbush, Firebush	5–6'
Jacquinia keyensis	Joewood	15–20'
Jatropha integerrima	Peregrina	5–7'
J. multifida	Coral plant	12–15'
Lantana camara	Common lantana	4–6'

Xeriscape Plants for Southern Florida
Natural Rainfall Zone

BOTANICAL NAME	COMMON NAME(S)	HEIGHT
EVERGREEN SHRUBS cont'd		
Lantana involucrata	Wild sage	3–4'
L. montevidensis	Trailing lantana	2'
Ligustrum japonicum	Japanese privet	6–8'
Lycium carolinianum	Christmas berry	6–8"
Lyonia ferruginea	Rusty lyonia	10–20'
Malpighia glabra	Barbados cherry	6–10'
Maytenus undatas	Maytenus	4–10'
Myrsine guianensis	Rapanea	15–20'
Ochrosia parviflora	Kopsia	8–10'
Pandanus veitchii	Veitch screw pine	12–15'
Pedilanthus tithymaloides	Devil's-backbone	2–4'
Pithecellobium guadalupense	Blackbead	15–20'
P. unguis-cati	Cat's claw	15–20'
Podocarpus macrophyllus	Yew podocarpus	8–12'
Polyscias spp.	Aralia	3–10'
Savia bahamensis	Maidenbush	8–10'
Scaevola plumieri	Inkberry	1–6'
S. taccada	Beach naupaka	5–6'
Severinia buxifolia	Boxthorn	3–4'
Suriana maritima	Bay cedar	15–20'
Synadenium grantii	African milkbush	6–8'
Tournefortia gnaphalodes	Sea lavender	4–6'
Triphasia trifolia	Limeberry	2–15'
Turnera ulmifolia	Yellow alder	2–3'
Vaccinium myrsinites	Shiny blueberry	1–2'
Westringia rosmariniformis	Victorian rosemary	4–6'
Yucca elephantipes	Spineless yucca	15–20'
Zamia spp.**	Cardboard palm	2–3'
GROUND COVERS		
Aloe spp.		1'
Bauhinia punctata (vinelike)	Red bauhinia	4–8'
Borrichia arborescens	Silver sea oxeye	2–4'
Bougainvillea spectabilis (vinelike)		6–8'
Canavalia maritima	Beach bean	6–12"
Carissa macrocarpa	Dwarf carissa	12–18"
Chiococca pinetorum	Pineland snowberry	2–3'
Ernodea littoralis	Golden creeper	1–3'
*Ficus montana**	Oakleaf fig	2–3'
*F. pumila**	Creeping fig	10–12"
F. sagittata	Trailing fig	10–12"
*Ipomoea pes-caprae**	Railroad vine	4–6"
Ipomoea spp.*	Morning glory	6–12"
Lantana depressa	Dwarf lantana	8"
Licania michauxii	Gopher aapple	3–12"
*Lippia nodiflora**	Matchweed	3"
Liriope muscari	Lilyturf	1'

BOTANICAL NAME	COMMON NAME(S)	HEIGHT
GROUND COVERS cont'd		
Liriope spicata	Creeping lilyturf	6–18″
*Okenia hypogaea***	Beach peanut	6″
Peperomia obtusifolia		18–20″
Ruellia brittoniana	Mexican bluebell	18–24″
Serenoa repens	Saw palmetto	4–8′
Sesuvium portulacastrum	Sea purslane	12–18″
Trilobus terrestris	Puncture vine	1′
*Uniola paniculata**	Sea oats	3–6′
Urechites lutea	Wild allamanda	1–2′
*Zamia floridana***	Coontie	1–3′
PERENNIALS		
Achillea millefolium	Yarrow	2′
Anemone canadensis	Meadow anemone	2′
Aralia nudicaulis	Wild sarsaparilla	1′
Arenaria lateriflora	Sandwort	8″
Artemisia stellerana	Dusty miller, Beach wormwood	42″
Asclepias lanceolata	Red milkweed	4′
Aster linearifolius	Linear-leaved aster	12–18″
Euthamia tenuifolia	Flat-topped goldenrod	1–3′
Hedyotis caerulea	Bluet	7″
Hypericum perforatum	St.-Peter's-wort	2′
Hypoxis hirsuta	Yellow star grass	6–12″
Leucanthemum vulgare	Ox-eye daisy	3′
Liatris graminifolia	Blazing star	4′
Lilium philadelphicum	Wood lily	2–3′
Lupinus perennis	Lupine	15″
Oenothera fruticosa	Sundrops	1–2′
O. humifusa	Dunes evening primrose	12–20″
Opuntia humifusa	Prickly-pear cactus	1′
Oxalis stricta	Yellow wood sorrel	2′
Potentilla argentea	Silvery cinquefoil	18″
P. recta	Rough-fruited cinquefoil	1–2′
Rhexia nashii	Meadow beauty	1–3′
Saponaria officinalis	Soapwort, Bouncing bet	1–3′
Scutellaria integrifolia	Common skullcap	1–2′
Sisyrinchium albidum	Blue-eyed grass	6–18″
Smilacina stellata	False Solomon's seal	2′
Solidago rugosa	Rough-leaved goldenrod	6′
Trientalis borealis	Starflower	9″
Trifolium hybridum	Alsike clover	2′
Viola pedata	Bird's-foot violet	2–6″
ANNUALS		
Geranium carolinianum	Carolina cranesbill	2′
Heterotheca subaxillaris	Camphorweed	3′
Lepidium virginicum	Peppergrass, Pepperwort	2′
Linaria canadensis	Toadflax	42″
Matricaria maritima	Scentless chamomile	6″

Xeriscape Plants for Southern Florida
Natural Rainfall Zone

BOTANICAL NAME	COMMON NAME(S)	HEIGHT
ANNUALS cont'd		
Portulaca oleracea	Common purslane	3–5"
Salvia coccinea	Scarlet sage	30"
Triodanis perfoliata	Venus'-looking-glass	3'
VINES		
Asparagus falcatus	Sicklethorn vine	40'
Campsis radicans*	Trumpet vine	30'
Cissus incisa	Marine ivy	30'
Crypotostegia madagascariensis	Madagascar rubber vine	Varies
Ficus pumila*	Creeping fig	40'
Parthenocissus quinquefolia*	Virginia creeper	35'
Pseudocalymma alliaceum	Garlic vine	20–30'
Pyrotesgia ignea*	Flame vine	6'

*Invasive plant.
**Protected—no part of the plant may be gathered from the wild.

Occasional Watering

See Occasional Watering Zone for Central Florida, pages 168–71, plus:

BOTANICAL NAME	COMMON NAME(S)	HEIGHT
DECIDUOUS TREES		
Annona reticulata	Custard apple	20–25'
Bombax ceiba	Red silk-cotton tree	50–75'
Butea frondosa	Flame-of-the-forest	35–40'
Cassia javanica	Pink-and-white shower	40–50'
Colvillea racemosa	Colville's glory	40–50'
Dillenia indica	Hondapara	30–45'
Enterolobium cyclocarpum	Ear tree	80–100'
Fraxinus pennsylvanica	Green ash	40–60'
Hura crepitans	Sandbox tree	40–60'
Pseudobombax ellipticum	Shavingbrush tree	20–30'
Sterculia foetida	Bangar nut	50–80'
Ulmus americana	American elm	80–100'
EVERGREEN TREES		
Annona squamosa	Sweetsop	15–20'
Araucaria bidwillii	Bunya-bunya tree	60–70'
Ardisia escallonioides	Marlberry	15–25'
Averrhoa carambola	Carambola	15–30'

BOTANICAL NAME	COMMON NAME(S)	HEIGHT
EVERGREEN TREES cont'd		
Bixa orellana	Annatto	10–30'
Bulnesia arborea		30–40'
Caesalpinia granadillo	Bridalveil tree	30–40'
Calophyllum inophyllum	Mastwood	30–45'
Cananga odorata	Ylang-ylang	30–40'
Cassia siamea	Kassod tree	35–40'
C. surattensis	Glaucus cassia	10–20'
Cecropia palmata	Snakewood	40–50'
*Cupaniopsis anacardiopsis**	Carrotwood	30–40'
Diospyros digyna	Black sapote	30–40'
Euphoria longan	Longan	30–40'
Exostema caribaeum	Princewood	20–25'
Ficus rubiginosa	Rusty fig	15–20'
Grevillea robusta	Silk oak	45–60'
Ilex cassine	Dahoon holly	25–40'
Kigelia pinnata	Sausage tree	40–45'
*Leucaena leucoscephala**	Lead tree	20–30'
Ligustrum japonicum	Japanese privet	10–15'
Litchi chinensis	Lychee	30–40'
Muntingia calabura	Capulin	20–30'
Myrciaria cauliflora	Jaboticaba	10–25'
Nectandra coriacea	Lancewood	30–40'
*Pithecellobium dulce**	Manila tamarind	30–40'
Podocarpus gracilior	Weeping podocarpus	15–35'
P. nagi	Nai podocarpus	20–40'
Pouteria campechiana	Eggfruit	20–25'
Prunus caroliniana	Cherry laurel	30–40'
Ravenala madagascariensis	Traveler's tree	20–30'
Stenocarpus sinuatus	Firewheel tree	35–45'
Trevesia palmata	Snowflake tree	15–20'
DECIDUOUS SHRUBS		
Caesalpinia pulcherrima	Dwarf poinciana	8–10'
Forestiera segregata	Florida privet	10–15'
Ilex ambigua	Ambigua holly	15–20'
Vitex agnus-castus	Chaste tree	10–15'
V. trifolia		10–12'
EVERGREEN SHRUBS		
Amyris elemifera	Torchwood	12–16'
Anthurium salviniae	Bird's-nest anthurium	4–5'
Ardisia escallonioides	Marlberry	12–15'
Bixa orellana	Annatto	15–20'
*Breynia disticha**	Snowbush	5–6'
Brunfelsia americana	Lady-of-the-night	4–6'
B. australis	Yesterday-today-and-tomorrow	6–8'
Buddleia officinalis	Butterfly bush	10–20'
Bumelia reclinata	Slender buckthorn	20–30'
Callistemon spp.	Bottlebrush	8–15'

Xeriscape Plants for Southern Florida
Occasional Watering

BOTANICAL NAME	COMMON NAME(S)	HEIGHT
EVERGREEN SHRUBS cont'd		
Carissa macrocarpa	Dwarf carissa	1–3'
Cassia alata	Candlebush	6–10'
C. bahamensis	Bahama cassia	10–15'
C. bicapsularis		10–12'
C. surattensis	Bush cassia	5–15'
Cestrum nocturnum	Night-blooming jessamine	10–12'
Chrysobalanus icaco	Cocoplum	6–8'
Citronella mitis	Calamondin orage	8–10'
*Clerodendrum paniculatum**	Pagoda flower	6'
*C. speciosissimum**	Java glorybower	6–8'
Cocculus laurifolius	Snail seed	12–15'
Cuphea hyssopifolia	False heather	1–2'
Dracaena deremensis		8–10'
D. fragrans	Corn plant	8–10'
D. surculosa	Gold-dust dracaena	3–6'
Euphorbia leucocephala	Pascuita	6–8'
Flacourtia indica	Governor's plum	15–20'
Galphimia gracilis	Thryallis	4–6'
Hamamelis virginiana	Witch hazel	15–20'
Homocladium platycladum	Ribbon bush	3–4'
Illicium anisatum	Anise tree	20'
Jasminum humile	Yellow jasmine	15'
J. volubile	Wax jasmine	2–3'
Loropetalum chinense		10–12'
Malpighia coccigera	Singapore holly	2–3'
Maytenus phyllanthoides	Florida mayten	4–8'
Myrciaria cauliflora	Jaboticaba	10–12'
Philodendron williamsii		4–6'
Photinia glabra	Redleaf photinia	8–10'
Podocarpus gracilior	Weeping podocarpus	10–25'
Psychotria nervosa	Wild coffee	4–6'
Punica granatum	Pomegranate	10–15'
Pyracantha coccinea	Red firethorn	8–12'
Randia aculeata	White indigo berry	6–10'
Rhodomyrtus tomentosa	Downy myrtle	8–10'
Serissa foetida		2–3'
Sophora tomentosa	Necklace pod	6–10'
Syzygium paniculatum	Brush cherry	12–15'
Tecoma stans	Yellow elder	10–12'
Tecomaria capensis	Cape honeysuckle	6–8'
Tetrapanax papyriferus	Rice-paper plant	8–10'
Thevetia peruviana	Yellow oleander	12–15'
Trevesia palmata	Tropical snowflake	8–12'

BOTANICAL NAME	COMMON NAME(S)	HEIGHT
PALMS		
Allagoptera arenaria	Seashore palm	5–6'
Chamaedorea elegans	Parlor palm	2–3'
C. seifrizii	Bamboo palm	6–8'
Dictyosperma album	Hurricane palm	25–40'
Hyophorbe lagenicaulis	Bottle palm	15–25'
Rhapidophyllum hystrix	Needle palm	3–5'
Roystonea elata	Florida royal palm	60–125'
GROUND COVERS		
Bromeliaceae family	Bromeliads	6–18"
Chlorophytum comosum	Spider plant	10–12"
Dichondra micrantha		1–3"
Evolvulus spp.	Blue daze	10–12"
Jasminum spp.		2–6'
Pilea microphylla	Artillery plant	1'
Pittosporum tobira 'Wheeleri'	Dwarf pittosporum	1–2'
VINES		
Allamanda violacea	Purple allamanda	10'
*Argyreia nervosa**	Woolly morning glory	Varies
Aristolochia elegans	Calico flower	20'
A. grandiflora	Pelican flower	15–20'
Beaumontia grandiflora	Herald's trumpet	10'
Clematis dioscoreifolia	Japanese clematis	15'
Monstera deliciosa	Ceriman	30'
Rhabdadenia biflora	Rubber vine	Varies
*Thunbergia grandiflora**	Bengal clock vine	6'

*Invasive plant.

Regular Watering Zone

BOTANICAL NAME	COMMON NAME(S)	HEIGHT
DECIDUOUS TREES		
Carpinus caroliniana	American hornbeam	25–35'
*Carya aquatica**	Water hickory	60–100'
Liriodendron tulipifera	Tulip tree	80–100'
Magnolia virginiana	Sweet bay	40–60'
Nyssa sylvatica	Black tupelo	50–80'
Platanus occidentalis	Sycamore	70–150'
Prunus persica	Peach	10–15'
EVERGREEN TREES		
*Avicennia germinans***	Black mangrove	20–30'
Gordonia lasianthus	Loblolly bay	30–40'
Laguncularia racemosa	White mangrove	40–60'
Ligustrum lucidum	Glossy privet	30–35'

Xeriscape Plants for Southern Florida
Regular Watering Zone

BOTANICAL NAME	COMMON NAME(S)	HEIGHT
EVERGREEN TREES cont'd		
*Rhizophora mangle***	Red mangrove	30–80'
*Salix caroliniana**	Coastal plain willow	20–30'
PALMS		
Carpentaria acuminata		35–45'
Chamaedorea cataractarum	Cat palm	4–6'
DECIDUOUS SHRUB		
Cephalanthus occidentalis	Buttonbush	15'
EVERGREEN SHRUBS		
Abutilon megapotamicum	Trailing abutilon	2–6'
Acalypha hispida	Chenille plant	5–6'
A. wilkesiana	Copperleaf	5–8'
Brugmansia x *candida*	Angel's trumpet	12–15'
Cleyera japonica		15–25'
Dombeya spp.	Tropical snowball	8–10'
Eranthemum pulchellum	Blue sage	4–6'
Eugenia brasiliensis	Grumichama	10–12'
Euphorbia cotinifolia	Red spurge	6–8'
E. pulcherrima	Poinsettia	6–8'
Evodia suaveolens var. *ridleyi*	Lacy-lady aralia	5–7'
Graptophyllum pictum	Caricature plant	4–6'
Holmskioldia sanguinea	Chinese hat plant	6–8'
Justica carnea	Flamingo plant	4–6'
J. spicigera	Mohintli	4–6'
Leea coccinea	West Indian holly	4–6'
Licuala spinosa	Spiny licuala	4–7'
Malvaviscus arboreus	Turk's-cap	6–8'
Medinilla magnifica		4–8'
Myrtus communis	True myrtle	8–10'
Odontonema strictum 'Variegatum'	Cardinal flower	3–6'
Pachystachys lutea	Golden shrimp plant	2–4'
Pseuderanthemum atropurpureum	Cafe con leche	4–6'
P. reticulatum		4–6'
Rhododendron hybrids	Azalea	2–6'
Sanchezia speciosa		5–6'
Synsepalum dulcificum	Miracle fruit	6–8'
Tabernaemontana divaricata	Crape jasmine	6–8'
Thunbergia erecta	Bush clock vine	4–6'
Tibouchina clavata		4–6'
T. urvilleana	Glorybush	8–12'
Viburnum suspensum	Sandankwa viburnum	6–8'

BOTANICAL NAME	COMMON NAME(S)	HEIGHT
GROUND COVERS		
Ajuga reptans*	Bugleweed	8–10″
Cyrtomium falcatum	Holly fern	1–2′
Dissotis rotundifolia	Spanish shawl	5–6″
Lantana montevidensis	Trailing lantana	18–24″
Nephrolepis spp.*	Sword fern	1–3′
Ruellia makoyana*	Monkey plant	8–12″
Rumohra adiantiformis	Leatherleaf fern	18–30″
Selaginella involvens	Erect selaginella	8–12″
S. uncinata	Blue selaginella	8–20″
Zephyranthes spp.	Rain lily	8–12″

*Invasive plant.
**Protected—no part of the plant may be gathered from the wild.

Xeriscape Plants for the Eastern and Northern Forests

THE Eastern Forest covers a broad area stretching from West Virginia southwest along the Appalachian Mountains, then west to eastern Texas, north into the Ozarks, and northeast again along the southern areas of Illinois, Indiana, and Ohio. This is the home of vast oak, hickory, and pine forests, dominant because the high rainfall rates support the trees. Receiving forty to fifty-six inches of precipitation each year, this region rarely experiences water shortages even in a "dry" year.

Because of this, Xeriscape gardening is not well known, nor is the need for it as critical as in other parts of the country. Yet David Draper, landscape designer and contractor in Nicholasville, Kentucky (near Lexington), reports that some people still water their lawns despite the fact that bluegrass is adapted so well to Kentucky that it's practically considered a native there. Draper promotes the Xeriscape spirit by emphasizing the energy savings that can be realized if landscape design is used to augment natural cooling and heating of houses and the energy cost of purifying the water that's poured on lawns. He uses native plants wherever possible in the landscapes he designs, especially locally grown plants. Draper has been using more perennials, native grasses, and ground covers recently, especially *Juniperus* spp., *Ajuga reptans* 'Bronze Beauty', *Euonymus fortunei* var. *coloratus*, and periwinkle (*Vinca minor*).

He also favors cypress mulch or rock. Because of the predominance of hardwood forests, mulches made from maple, oak, and sycamore trees are readily available.

Dr. Mary Witt, consumer horticulture specialist with the University of Kentucky, reports that the biggest problem faced by gardeners in the region is not drought, but late spring frosts. Extremes of temperature, both in winter and summer, wreak havoc on ornamental plants. "Basically, we get the worst of both southern and northern climates—weeds, weather, fungus, and diseases!" Many Xeriscape plants successful in other parts of the country such as hackberry (*Celtis occidentalis*), Virginia creeper (*Parthenocissus quinquefolia*), lavender cotton (*Santolina chamaecyparissus*), and black cherry (*Prunus serotina*) can't be used here because they are so invasive in the moist climate.

Dr. Witt has seen a refreshing trend in the last few years of more and more people being willing to just let their bluegrass and fescue lawns go brown (dormant) during the summer and not worry about it. "People are tired of having the problems associated with overmanaged lawns. Ten years ago, people routinely used lots of chemicals to keep perfectly manicured lawns." Now they skip the chemicals and the watering, too.

From a botanical standpoint, Eastern Forest gardeners are lucky; in terms of the number of different wildflowers and native trees and shrubs that grow in the region, this is one of the richest. The rather long list of suggested plants reflects this. The list includes low- and moderate-water-use plants. Although a list of plants requiring occasional watering might seem unnecessary (and perhaps ludicrous) in this high-rainfall region, it may still be put to use by Xeriscape gardeners faced with a very soggy area or poorly drained soil, such as some of the soils found in southern Illinois.

The Central Eastern Forest includes Hardiness Zones 6, 7, and 8. The plants in the list are all hardy to Zone 6, unless noted otherwise in individual entries. According to Draper, hardiness plays a big part in plant selection for this region. "In Cincinnati, many of our shrubs have winter problems, but most trees do fine as far north as Cleveland, with the exception of some of our evergreen trees. In Nashville, Tennessee, many of our borderline shrubs do well, especially during light winters." The famous southern magnolia (*Magnolia grandiflora*—Zone 7) simply won't make it in Zone 6 Kentucky, but usually will in Nashville.

NORTHERN FOREST XERISCAPE GARDENING

The Northern Forest covers the eastern half of Minnesota, most of Wisconsin, and all of Michigan. It is more similar to New England in terms of cold hardiness (ranging from Zone 3 to 5, with two pockets of Zone 2 in northern Minnesota) than the Eastern Forest, but its rainfall rate is significantly lower than both other areas (ranging from twenty-two to thirty-two inches).

Because of its forest "heritage," trees, shrubs, and woodland wildflowers do very well here. Many traditional perennials that thrive in cool weather, such as delphiniums (*Delphinium elatum*), bellflowers and harebells (*Campanula* spp.), peonies (*Paeonia* spp.), lupines (*Lupinus* spp.), and irises and other bulbs, shine in this environment. Summer precipitation is high enough to encourage exuberant growth.

Madison, Wisconsin (near the southern end of this area), has become a leader in the movement to allow tallgrass prairie restoration as part of accepted landscape options. It's located in an area that was originally a "mosaic" of tallgrass prairie interspersed with oak groves (known as oak savannah). In Madison, prairie restorations have become familiar enough that people are able to include this type of landscaping in their front yards without raising eyebrows. Several years of drought in the late 1980s were part of the spur for this movement.

The plant list for this region includes the hardiness zones for all trees and shrubs, since cold hardiness is so important here. Several native wildflowers are also included, if you'd like to try your hand at introducing a little habitat gardening into your Xeriscape landscape. Part of the pleasure of this type of gardening is that it often brings the side benefit (for some the main benefit) of drawing animals such as songbirds, squirrels, chipmunks, rabbits, and toads or small lizards. Additional information about appropriate native plants may be obtained from the National Wildflower Research Center—Midwest Branch, 725 Spring Hill Road, Wayzata, MN 55391; the Institute for Urban Wildlife, 10921 Trotting Ridge Way, Columbia, MD 21044, (301) 596-3311; or the National Wildlife Federation, 1400 16th Street, N.W., Washington, DC 20036. These last two organizations have programs for encouraging the establishment of "backyard habitats."

Although there's no shortage of water in southern Michigan, Mike Miller of Shemin Nurseries in Taylor, Michigan, promotes Xeriscape principles, especially drip irrigation, from a cost standpoint. Since the water isn't free, drip irrigation helps reduce the possibility of wasted water from overwatering. It also cuts down on the danger from "nonpoint source pollution" (the introduction of pollutants into waterways from many different sources, rather than one identifiable one, such as fertilizer and herbicide runoff from thousands of lawns), which is of major concern to many these days. In Mike's area, the water has a high iron content, so over time sidewalks as well as the bricks near the ground on houses become permanently stained red. Drip irrigation helps reduce this problem, too, he says.

Diane Hoagland of Sylvan Lake, Michigan, near Detroit, is a coordinator of the Master Gardener Program for her county. She has begun publicizing Xeriscape gardening by encouraging people to include native plants in their landscapes and to recycle organic material as much as possible on-site. Her home has many old oak trees, and she recycles the leaves into a mulch that helps acidify the soil for the many native acid-loving understory trees such as dogwoods (*Cornus* spp.) and azaleas (*Rhododendron* spp.) she has planted. For Diane, Xeriscape gardening is a way of saving energy. Although people wonder why she is promoting water conservation in an area of plentiful water, a recent move on the part of the small town she lives in to tie into Detroit's water system (which will double water rates) may increase the interest of her audience.

Xeriscape Plants for the Eastern and Northern Forests Natural Rainfall Zone

See Natural Rainfall Zone for New England, pages 141–43, plus:

BOTANICAL NAME	COMMON NAME(S)	HEIGHTS	ZONES
DECIDUOUS TREES			
Acer platanoides	Norway maple	90'	3–7
Aesculus glabra	Ohio buckeye	35–50'	4–8
A. hippocastanum	Horsechestnut	75'	3
A. octandra	Sweet buckeye	50–75'	4
Castanea mollissima	Chinese chestnut	60'	4
C. pumila	Allegheny chinquapin	30–50'	4
Catalpa speciosa	Northern catalpa	90'	4–8
Celtis laevigata	Sugar hackberry	90'	5–9
Chionanthus virginicus	Fringetree	8–30'	4
Cladrastis kentukea	Yellowwood	20–60'	4
Corylus colurna	Turkish filbert	75'	4
Diospyros virginiana	Common persimmon	75'	4
Euonymus atropurpurea	Eastern wahoo	20–35'	5
Fraxinus quadrangulata	Blue ash	50–75'	5
Malus coronaria	Wild crab apple	15–40'	4
Paulownia tomentosa	Royal paulownia	45'	5–9
Platanus × acerifolia	London planetree	100'	5
Ptelea trifoliata	Wafer ash, Hoptree	18'	4
Pyrus calleryana 'Bradford'	Bradford pear	30–50'	4–9
Quercus falcata	Southern red oak	50–100'	5
Q. imbricaria	Shingle oak	40–100'	5–8
Q. marilandica	Blackjack oak	35–50'	6
Q. prinus	Chestnut oak	90'	4
Q. shumardii	Shumard oak	50'	4
Q. stellata	Post oak	40–50'	5
Rhamnus caroliniana	Carolina buckthorn	10–40'	5
Sassafras albidum	Common sassafras	30–60'	4
Tilia americana	American linden	50–120'	3
T. platyphyllos	Bigleaf linden	120'	3
Ulmus rubra	Slippery elm	35–100'	2
Zelkova serrata	Japanese zelkova	50–80'	5–8
EVERGREEN TREES			
Pinus echinata	Shortleaf pine	70–100'	5
P. koraiensis	Korean pine	90'	3
P. nigra	Austrian pine	50–80'	4–8
P. ponderosa	Ponderosa pine	75–100'	5
P. sylvestris	Scots pine	70–100'	3–8
P. taeda	Loblolly pine	80–120'	7–9
P. virginiana	Virginia pine	45'	4
DECIDUOUS SHRUBS			
Amorpha fruticosa	Indigobush amorpha	12'	3
Ceanothus ovatus	Inland ceanothus	18'	4

BOTANICAL NAME	COMMON NAME(S)	HEIGHTS	ZONES
DECIDUOUS SHRUBS cont'd			
Cytisus scoparius	Scotch broom	4–9'	7–9
Deutzia gracilis	Slender deutzia	3'	4
Hibiscus syriacus	Rose-of-Sharon	5–15'	5
Hypericum prolificum	Shrubby St. Johnswort	3'	4
Ilex decidua	Possumhaw	12–20'	4
Jasminum nudiflorum	Winter jasmine	4–5'	7
Prunus × *cistena*	Purpleleaf sand cherry	8–10'	3
Ribes missouriense	Missouri gooseberry	3–6'	4
Robinia hispida (can be invasive)	Roseacacia locust	6–9'	4
Rosa setigera	Prairie rose	6–12'	4
Quercus prinoides	Dwarf chinquapin oak	12'	5
Spiraea spp.	Spirea	3–9'	Vary
Syringa chinensis 'Villosa'		12'	4
EVERGREEN SHRUB			
Ligustrum sinense	Chinese privet	20'	7
GROUND COVERS			
Ajuga reptans	Carpet bugle, Bugleweed	8–10"	4
Armeria maritima	Common thrift, Sea pink	6"	3
Ceratostigma plumbaginoides	Dwarf plumbago	6–12"	6
Chamaemelum nobile	Chamomile	12"	3
Epigaea repens	Trailing arbutus	6"	2
Epimedium spp.		12–15"	3–9
Fragaria chiloensis	Wild strawberry	6–12"	6
F. virginiana	Virginia strawberry	3–6"	5
Gaultheria procumbens	Winterberry, Checkerberry wintergreen	6"	4–9
Hedera helix	English ivy	6"	6
Liriope muscari	Lilyturf	18"	6
Nepeta faassenii	Catmint	12–18"	4 (West)
Polygonum capitatum	Knotweed	6"	Annual (reseeds itself)
PERENNIALS (all are hardy to at least Zone 3)			
Aster subspicatus		12–18"	
Bergenia purpurascens	Saxifrage	1'	
Campanula divaricata	Allegheny bellflower	3'	
Coreopsis maritima	Pacific coreopsis	1–3'	
Hypoxis hirsuta	Yellow star grass	6–12"	
Liatris pycnostachya	Kansas gayfeather	4–5'	
L. scariosa	Tall gayfeather	2–4'	
Oenothera fruticosa	Common sundrop	1–3'	
Penstemon canescens	Grey beardtongue	1–3'	
Polygonatum biflorum	Small Solomon's seal	1–3'	
Saxifraga virginiensis	Virginia saxifrage	12–18"	

(Flower is 12–18", leaves grow about 3" tall)

Xeriscape Plants for the Eastern and Northern Forests
Natural Rainfall Zone

BOTANICAL NAME	COMMON NAME(S)	HEIGHTS	ZONES
VINES			
Lonicera sempervirens	Coral honeysuckle	50'	4–8
Passiflora incarnata	Passion flower	20'	7
Smilax tamnoides	Bamboo greenbriar	20–35'	3–9
Vitis aestivalis	Summer grape, Pigeon grape	50'	5–9
V. labrusca	Fox grape, Plum grape	20–35'	5–8
FERNS			
Dennstaedtia punctilobula	Hayscented fern	20–32"	2–8

Occasional Watering Zone

See Occasional Watering Zone for New England, pages 143–45, plus:

BOTANICAL NAME	COMMON NAME(S)	HEIGHT	ZONES
DECIDUOUS TREES			
Alnus glutinosa	European black alder	75'	3
Asimina triloba	Pawpaw	15–30'	5
Betula nigra	River birch	90'	5
Cladrastis lutea	American yellowwood	50–75'	3
Halesia carolina	Carolina silverbell	30'	5
H. monticola	Mountain silverbell	90'	5
Liquidambar styraciflua	Sweet gum	50'	
Liriodendron tulipifera	Tulip tree, Tulip poplar, Yellow-poplar	80–120'	
Magnolia acuminata	Cucumber tree	60–100'	5
M. grandiflora	Bullbay, Southern magnolia	80'	7
M. macrophylla	Bigleaf magnolia	50'	
M. virginiana	Sweet bay magnolia	20–40'	
Morus rubra	Red mulberry	50'	
Oxydendrum arboreum	Sourwood, Sorrel tree	35–50'	6
Quercus palustris	Pin oak	75'	5
Q. phellos	Willow oak	50–100'	5
*Salix alba***	White willow	20–75'	3–9
*S. fragilis***	Crack willow	30–100'	
EVERGREEN TREES			
Rhododendron maximum	White rhododendron, Rosebay rhododendron	12–36'	
DECIDUOUS SHRUBS			
Aronia arbutifolia	Red chokeberry	9'	3
Callicarpa americana	American beautyberry	5–8'	7
Calycanthus floridus	Carolina allspice	6–12'	5

BOTANICAL NAME	COMMON NAME(S)	HEIGHT	ZONES
DECIDUOUS SHRUBS cont'd			
Cephalanthus occidentalis	Buttonbush	5–12'	4
Clethra alnifolia	Summer sweet	6'	4
Cornus rugosa	Roundleaf dogwood	6–12'	3
C. sericea, syn. *C. stolonifera*	Red-osier dogwood	6–12'	2
Euonymus americanus	Strawberry bush	6–12'	6
Fothergilla spp.	Witch-alder	3–6'	6
Hydrangea arborescens	Wild hydrangea	3–6'	4
Ilex verticillata	Winterberry	6–12'	3
Ligustrum amuense	Amur privet	15'	3
Lindera benzoin	Spicebush	6–12'	5
Rhododendron arborescens/**	Smooth azalea, Sweet azalea	12–20'	4
R. calendulaceum	Flame azalea	9'	5
R. peridymenoica var. *nudiflorum*	Pink Pinxter azalea	6'	
Salix discolor	Pussy willow	10–20'	3
Sambucus canadensis	Elderberry	6–12'	3
Spiraea × *bumalda*	Bumald spirea	2'	5
*Vaccinium corymbosum**	Highbush blueberry	3–10'	4
Viburnum rufidulum	Southern blackhaw	8–30'	5–6
V. trilobum	American cranberry bush	6–12'	2
Xanthorhiza simplicissima	Yellow-root	3'	5
EVERGREEN SHRUBS			
Aucuba japonica	Japanese aucuba	4–15'	7
Ilex glabra	Inkberry	6–12'	4
Leucothoe fontanesiana	Drooping leucothoe	2–6'	4
Nandina domestica		6–8'	7
Pieris floribunda	Mountain andromeda	3–6'	5
*Rhododendron carolinianum**	Carolina rhododendron	3–6'	5
*R. catawbiense**	Purple azalea, Catawba rhododendron	6'	4
R. maximum	Great laurel, Rosebay rhododendron	6–20'	3
GROUND COVERS			
Arenaria balearica	Corsican sandwort	2–4"	6
Cotula squalida	New Zealand brass buttons	2–4"	6
Erica carnea, syn. *E. herbacea*	Heath	16"	5–8
Galax urceolata		6–9"	3–8
Galium odoratum	Sweet woodruff	6–12"	5
Lysimachia nummularia	Moneywort, Creeping Jenny	2–4"	3
Mazus reptans		2"	4
Myosotis scorpioides	Forget-me-not	6–12"	4
Paxistima spp.		1–2'	5–9
Ranunculus repens 'Pleniflorus'	Creeping buttercup	1'	4–9
Sagina subulata	Irish moss, Scotch moss	1–2"	5
Sarcococca hookerana var. *humilis*		18"	6
Taxus baccata 'Repandens'	Spreading English yew	2'	6
*Vaccinium macrocarpon**	American cranberry	1–3'	3
V. vacillans	Late low blueberry	1'	3
*V. vitis-idaea minus**	Mountain cranberry	4–8"	3
Veronica prostrata, syn. *V. rupestris*	Speedwell	8"	6

Occasional Watering Zone

BOTANICAL NAME	COMMON NAME(S)	HEIGHT	ZONES
GROUND COVERS cont'd			
Veronica repens	Creeping speedwell	2–4″	6
Viola hederacea	Australian violet	6–8″	6
V. sororia, syn. *V. priceana*	Confederate violet	6–8″	6
PERENNIALS			
Anemonella thalictroides	Rue anemone	8″	
Arisaema dracontium	Green dragon	30″	
A. triphyllum	Jack-in-the-pulpit	30″	
Aruncus sylvester	Goatsbeard	7′	
Asclepias incarnata	Swamp milkweed	3′	
Chelone glabra	White turtlehead	6′	
Cimicifuga americana	American bugbane	5′	
Dicentra canadensis	Squirrel corn	6–10″	
D. cucullaria	Dutchman's breeches	10″	
D. eximia	Fringed bleeding heart	2′	
Erythronium albidum	White fawnlily	1′	
E. americanum	Common fawnlily, Trout lily	1′	
E. grandiflorum	Lamb's-tongue fawnlily	1′	
E. montanum	Avalanche lily	18″	
E. revolutum	Mahogany fawnlily	1′	3
Eupatorium fistulosum	Joe-pye weed	3–10′	4
E. perfoliatum	Boneset	3′	4
E. purpureum	Bluestem	3′	4
E. rugosum	White snakerooot	2–4′	4
Gillenia trifoliata	Bowman's root	3′	3
Helianthus angustifolia	Narrow-leaved sunflower	2–5′	3
Iris douglasiana	Douglas iris	6–30″	6
I. verna	Vernal iris	6″	4
I. versicolor	Blue flag iris	2–3′	6
Panax quinquefolius	American ginseng	6–18″	4
Penstemon canescens	Grey beardtongue	1–3′	5
P. digitalis	Beardtongue	3′	4
P. laevigatus	Smooth beardtongue	3′	5
Sanguinaria canadensis	Bloodroot	8″	4
Tiarella cordifolia	Allegheny foam flower	1′	3
VINES			
Menispermum canadense	Common moonseed	6–12′	2
Wisteria sinensis 'Purpurea'	Purple wisteria	40′	3
FERNS			
Adiantum pedatum	Maidenhair fern	10–20″	3–8
Athyrium felix-femina	Lady fern	3′	7
Dryopteris austiaca var. *spinulosa*	Spinulose shield fern	3′	3–8
D. marginalis	Marginal shield fern	15″	3–8
Matteuccia struthiopteris	Ostrich fern	3–5′	3–8
Osmunda cinnamomea	Cinnamon fern	2–5′	3–8

BOTANICAL NAME	COMMON NAME(S)	HEIGHT	ZONES
FERNS cont'd			
Osmunda claytoniana	Interrupted fern	2–5'	3–8
O. regalis	Royal fern	6'	3
Polystichum acrostichoides	Christmas fern	1–3'	3–8
P. munitum	Western swordfern	18–36"	7
Pteridium aquilinum	Bracken fern	1–3'	3

*Best in acid soil.
**Demands cool, moist soil.

Additional Xeriscape Plants for the Northern Forest
Natural Rainfall Zone

(A few additional shrubs and wildflowers are recommended for the Northern Forest.)

BOTANICAL NAME	COMMON NAME(S)	HEIGHT	ZONES
DECIDUOUS SHRUBS			
Prunus besseyi	Western sand cherry	6'	2
P. pumila	Sand cherry	6'	2
PERENNIALS (all are hardy to at least Zone 3)			
Anemone patens	American pasqueflower	1'	
Dodecatheon meadia	Common shooting-star	20"	
Eryngium yuccifolium	Rattlesnake-master	3'	
Geranium maculatum	Spotted geranium	2'	
Liatris aspera		6'	
Lithospermum canescens	Hoary puccoon	18"	
Penstemon grandiflorus (biennial)	Shell-leaf beardtongue	3'	
Petalostemum candidum	White prairie clover	30"	
P. purpureum	Purple prairie clover	3'	
Ratibida columnifera	Prairie coneflower	3'	
R. pinnata	Gray-headed coneflower	3'	
Rudbeckia laciniata	Cutleaf coneflower	9'	
Sisyrinchium campestre		20"	
Solidago nemoralis	Gray goldenrod	3'	

Xeriscape Plants for the Great Plains/Rockies/Great Basin

Xeriscape gardening in the Great Plains/Rockies/Great Basin is at once challenging and rewarding. It's challenging because we often experience hot, dry summers, fierce wind, and cold, dry winters. Spring weather can be wildly erratic, balmy for several days to entice plants to bud out, then freezing suddenly. Much of our precipitation occurs in spring and summer, but summer precipitation often comes in the form of intense rainstorms that can drain off quickly, rather than slow, soaking rains. With eight to fourteen inches of precipitation annually (up to thirty inches in the mountains), the western part of this region fits into the semiarid classification. Toward the eastern edge of the region the rainfall can range up to thirty-five inches per year, yet the extremes of climate are just as severe, and summer temperatures are enough higher that the additional rainfall is offset by the increased evapotranspiration.

On the other hand, Xeriscape gardening is rewarding here because we have such a wide plant palette. Everything from desert plants to prairie grasses to foothills and montane trees and shrubs can find a niche in the Mountain West. Much of the area was once grassland, so it's an ideal region for incorporating a prairie garden or other grassland adaptation into your Xeriscape design.

Because the climate is suited for it, a landscaping scheme including grass has a very high chance of success. Buffalograss and/or blue grama grass lawns can be successfully established, though some patience and weeding will be necessary the first two or three years till the grass fills in. Jim Knopf, Boulder landscape architect and author of a book on perennials for Xeriscape gardens in the Rockies (*The Xeriscape Flower Gardener*, Boulder, Co.: Johnson Publishing Co., 1991), recommends the use of turf-type tall fescues as the best alternative to bluegrass for a "bluegrass look-alike" lawn. Even bluegrass can be incorporated into a water-efficient landscape here without creating the need for excessive watering. (A strong understanding of proper watering practices and, in some cases, the use of water-absorbing polymers can help.)

The Great Plains/Rockies/Great Basin region is also a great place to grow perennial flowers. Cold winters give them the needed dormancy period, and the lack of humidity and general sogginess minimizes insect and disease problems. You can develop a splendid English-style perennial border using drought-tolerant perennials and have flower beds every bit as lavish and colorful as the originals. You'll probably even be using some of the same plants as in New England flower beds.

Very-low-water-using plants make a colorful hillside display at the Denver Botanic garden. Bigleaf sagebrush (Artemisia tridentata) *provides a background for pink* (Verbena tenera *var.* elegans) *and blue* (V. tenuisecta) *verbena.*

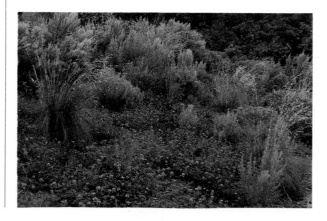

In the plant list that follows, the starred plants are ones that did well at Fort Collins, Colorado (Colorado State University), in a drought-tolerance test of several years' duration.

ROCKY MOUNTAINS

Anna Thurston, landscape architect and water conservation specialist for Aurora, Colorado, tries to emulate nature in her designs, using native plants wherever possible. She likes to use trees such as bur oak (*Quercus macrocarpa*) and northern catalpa (*Catalpa speciosa*), even though they require some maintenance in the fall; she feels that tasks which make us spend some time in the garden are helpful in keeping our link with nature. Her favorite Xeriscape plant is blue-mist spirea (*Caryopteris* x *clandonensis*).

Prairies, dry streambeds, rocky areas with boulders and native plants (rock gardens), and slices of coniferous forest are all found in the Rockies, and make great themes for Xeriscape gardens. In hotter areas try to keep the rocks (including gravel mulch) away from the house because they will tend to increase the interior temperatures of the house in the summer.

A "Rocky Mountain" look is very easy to achieve, even though the rainfall can get as high as thirty-two inches in the mountains. The mountain plants, conifers such as Rocky Mountain juniper (*Juniperus scopulorum*), ponderosa pine (*Pinus ponderosa*—be careful, it gets *very* large), bristlecone pine (*P. aristata*), and limber pine (*P. flexilis*), are adaptable to much lower amounts of precipitation, and favorites such as aspen (*Populus tremuloides*) and Rocky Mountain columbine (*Aquilegia caerulea*) which need extra moisture can be carefully sited for maximum water efficiency. There are, of course, dozens of other flowers and wildflowers that can help give the Rocky Mountain wildflower look.

Dale Greenwood, a Colorado amateur gardener, has found an unusual native plant he recommends for Xeriscape landscapes. It's a species of "true" blueberries (*Vaccinium scoparium*), which is native to the Colorado mountains where soil is acid. He says it not only forms a uniform low-maintenance

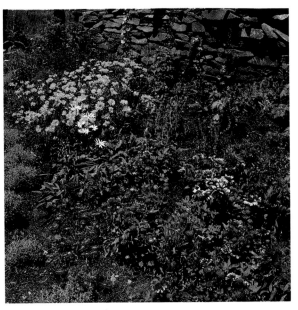

This northern New Mexico mountain flower bed features several of the perennials that do extremely well in the Rocky Mountain region. Clockwise from upper left: coreopsis (Coreopsis lanceolata), *Shasta daisy* (Chrysanthemum maximum), *delphinium* (Delphinium elatum), *gaillardia* (Gaillardia grandiflora), *hardy ice plant* (Delosperma cooperi), *and santolina* (Santolina chamaecyparissus). (Santolina and hardy ice plant are not reliably hardy in Zone 6 or below.)

ground cover about a foot high that will grow in either sun or shade, but it also produces some delicious berries, which are mistakenly called huckleberries. He also recommends *V. membranaceum* var. *ovalifolium*, a bush that grows about three feet tall and does best in a pH of 4.7 to 5.2, and *V. caespitosum*, which reaches about eighteen inches in height.

Recently while driving to the little town south of Denver where I work, I was much struck by how lush and very green the untended areas of the town and countryside looked despite our "low" rainfall rate of fourteen to sixteen inches per year. My boss, Dan Wofford, pointed out, "It doesn't matter. Look at all the summer monsoon rains we get." Something clicked for me at last. I always thought those monsoon rains (which usually last about ten minutes and come fairly regularly most evenings, just in time to rain out thousands of amateur softball games) were worthless, but I realized that they aren't. If you get nine or ten inches of precipitation during the growing season, spread out over the summer, and the plants are dormant during the rest of the year, then plants well adapted to this regime will thrive. It would be equivalent to two or three times as much rainfall in a warmer area where plants aren't dormant as long.

GREAT BASIN

I asked Dick Hildreth, director of the Red Butte Garden and Arboretum (Salt Lake City), what kind of plants grow in the desert there. He said, "Don't forget to say *cold* desert. *Please!*" Which is what they all say from the Great Basin, the area west of the Rocky Mountains to the mountains of eastern California. They're justifiably proud of how tough their plants are to be able to live there where the average annual precipitation can be as low as zero to seven inches annually and the temperature can be as bitterly cold as it gets in the Great Plains. The plants on the list look familiar because many of them are the same rugged, adaptable species I've found on Xeriscape plant lists from Georgia to the Northwest and from New England to north Texas.

Tom Stille, Reno, Nevada, landscape architect, helped develop a list of Xeriscape plants for his area that not only reflect varying levels of water needs, but also tie in with three large-scale natural plant communities near Reno. The "Sierra Nevada" community (which in nature receives the most rainfall—sixteen to sixty-four inches) includes representatives of the range of mountain conifers said to be the most diverse in the world. It also includes some of the largest conifers, such as sequoia (*Sequoiadendron giganteum*); *Pinus lambertiana*, the largest soft pine in the world; *Juniperus occidentalis*, the largest juniper; and *Calocedrus decurrens*, the largest incense cedar. The plant community also features deciduous trees and shrubs that grow along streams and lakes, such as serviceberry (*Amelanchier alnifolia*), alpine currant (*Ribes alpinum*), mountain rose (*Rosa woodsii*), greenleaf manzanita (*Arctostaphylos patula*), and tobacco brush (*Ceanothus velutinus*). In his designs Stille uses this plant community to build the "walls" of the garden, such

as screens, frames for nice views, background for the rest of the garden, and windbreaks to create better microclimates, winter sun, and summer shade.

Although it's near all three communities, Reno is actually located in the second of the native plant communities Stille likes to use, the "Truckee Meadows" community, which is a transition between the Sierra Nevada range and the Great Basin. It features wildflowers and meadows, which Stille interprets, depending on the need at the site, as low-water grasses and wildflowers, or turf. Streambank wheatgrass (*Agropyron riparium*) is a very-low-water-using grass; it may be able to survive on Reno's seven inches of annual precipitation after establishment, though it's more of a coarse, low-maintenance-type grass. Buffalograss and hard fescue are low-water-using grasses, needing only three to seven inches of water above annual natural precipitation. Tall fescue is a moderate-water-use grass (twenty inches plus additional water), and Kentucky bluegrass needs thirty-six inches or more additional water.

Many perennial flowers can provide seasonal color for this zone. Some of the most drought-tolerant ones for a self-sufficient meadow setting include fernleaf yarrow (*Achillea filipendulina*), common yarrow (*A. millefolium*), narrowleaf coreopsis (*Coreopsis lanceolata*), blanket flower (*Gaillardia* spp.), and baby's breath (*Gypsophila paniculata*). Slightly higher-water-using flowers include purple coneflower (*Echinacea purpurea*), iris (*Iris germanica*), and dwarf michaelmas daisy (*Aster novi-belgi* cvs.).

The Great Basin is a high-elevation, mountainous, cold desert. Dominant plant communities, and those most adaptable for very-low-water Xeriscape settings, are the pinyon juniper woodlands and the sagebrush communities common to the foothills of the Basin. Stille's "Great Basin landscape treatment" includes desert shrubs, flowers, and some trees. When water conservation is at a premium, these plants can be used in the same way the "Sierra" plants are, as screens, background, etc., but in general they are used as a dramatic foreground or transition between meadow and "Sierra" plantings, in effect, a "shrub zone."

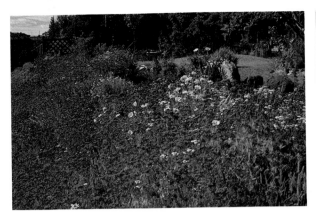

A hillside of easy-to-grow flowers such as Coreopsis lanceolata, *cornflowers* (Centaurea cyanus), *yarrow* (Achillea millefolium), *California poppies* (Eschscholzia californica), *and catchfly* (Silene armeria) *makes an effective ground cover. (Design and photo: Interpretive Gardens, Reno, Nevada)*

Artemisia tridentata (sagebrush) is the key plant of the Great Basin community, but other shrubs used include bitterbrush (*Purshia tridentata*), rabbitbrush (*Chrysothamnus nauseosus*), fernbush (*Chamaebatiaria millefolium*), and apache plume (*Fallugia paradoxa*).

Plant spacing, ground plane cover, and topography show the contrast among the three communities. The Great Basin treatment features wider plant spacing. Mulch is generally scattered quarry rock or coarse decomposed granite with smaller scattered rock (desert pavement). A thick layer of wood chip or pine needle mulch is common in the Sierra Nevada treatment, with a closer spacing of plants, suggesting lushness. This plant community is suitable for existing or created high areas, while the meadow treatment is ideal for flat areas. It features the highest plant density of all, usually covering the ground completely and blocking out any mulch. The Great Basin treatment is suitable for slightly sloping and transition areas, in keeping with its "shrub zone" flavor.

The plants recommended by Stille that appear on the plant list for the whole region are marked. Stille notes that many more plants are suitable for Xeriscape gardening in the Reno area. He says the main drawback for a Xeriscape gardener interested in including native plants is still the limited availability of large-sized native plants. (This is partly because the deep taproots of some of these species, which helps them gather soil moisture, makes it hard for them to live in small containers, or be transplanted easily when large.)

With the substitution of some higher-water-using (if you like) or more appropriate-for-the-area plants, you could use this same type of design thinking across the Great Basin/Rockies/High Plains region. Appropriately enough, Tom Stille was the designer for the Xeriscape Demonstration Garden at the Wichita (Kansas) Botanica Garden that now thrives under the jurisdiction of Don Buma, director of the Botanica.

GREAT PLAINS

Buma has experimented with Xeriscape principles in his own yard, since moving to the area two years ago. He installed tall fescue in his new lawn, which he says is doing well. However, in July and August, hot spells can occur where the temperatures get up to 100 degrees Fahrenheit and higher for several days in a row. Even though he waters twice a week (watering restrictions are in effect in Wichita) for a total of about half an inch, he says the grass struggles through the heat. (This may not seem like much watering until you note that Wichita averages thirty-two inches of rainfall per year, and tall fescue is supposed to be adapted to twenty-five to thirty inches per year; this illustrates how turfgrass water needs are not always clear-cut.) "My advice to people in this part of the Great Plains is to plant mulched shrub and flower beds instead of turf wherever possible, because the heat, combined with the twenty- to thirty-mile-an-hour winds we often have, makes it very difficult to maintain turf without a *lot* of water."

Buma's yard features a beautiful flower garden extending across the front of his home with a small lawn in front. It includes daylilies (*Hemerocallis* spp.), rudbeckia, Shasta daisies (*Chrysanthemum x superbum*), Russian sage (*Perovskia atriplicifolia*), Maximilian's sunflower (*Helianthus maximiliani*), and *Rosa* 'Vonica', a very drought-tolerant shrub rose. (He finds that the Maximilian's sunflower and rudbeckia need a little extra water.) Limber pine (*Pinus flexilis*) and pinyon pine (*P. edulis*) live successfully at the Botanica, although Buma notes that the only evergreen native to Kansas is eastern red cedar (*Juniperuus virginiana*). He says a wide variety of trees and shrubs are available and suitable for Kansas Xeriscape landscapes. One flower tried at the Botanica that he wanted to highlight was *Calamintha nepetoides*, a mint-scented plant. Although he says the flower is a fairly nondescript white blossom, the plant is a noninvasive perennial that gets about eighteen inches high, and that bees and wasps *love*! "They're always buzzing around there."

If you live in the Great Plains/Rockies/Great Basin, look at the annual rainfall and native vegetation near your home. If what you see tells you you are in the more desertlike sections of the region, you might plan your Xeriscape landscape around the Natural Precipitation and Occasional Watering plant palettes. If you live where the precipitation is higher than twenty to twenty-five inches per year and have protected areas out of the wind, you may be able to incorporate some of the plants from the Regular Watering list without having to water as regularly as if you lived in a drier area. A separate plant list for the Prairie Peninsula, which features some of the plants more common in the eastern United States, is included.

The plants in the Natural Rainfall zone should not need watering above normal rainfall amounts of eight to fourteen inches per year after establishment. Many of the perennials and annuals are native to desert regions of the Southwest, but will also grow satisfactorily in more northerly areas. The plants in the Occasional Watering zone may need supplemental irrigation through drought where the rainfall averages less than fourteen to eighteen inches per year. Some of these plants, however, are on the Reno list, too, listed as needing only ten to fourteen inches per year, so they may be more adaptable than we think. The plants in the Regular Watering zone will need roughly eighteen inches or more to survive without regular watering. The hardiness zone references have been included in this list because the regions encompass so many different hardiness zones.

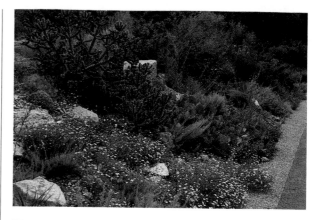

The Xeriscape Demonstration Garden at the Denver Botanic Garden features a montage of native southwestern plants, including cholla (Opuntia imbricata), *prickly pear* (O. phaeacantha), *sand sagebrush* (Artemisia filifolia), *and* Erigeron divergens.

PRAIRIE PENINSULA

Extending into the forests of the eastern United States is a peninsula of prairie that covers Iowa, eastern Nebraska, southeastern South Dakota, southern Minnesota, most of Illinois, and Missouri south to the Ozarks. Once home to glorious tallgrass prairie, it has become part of America's agricultural heartland. The original cover was called oak savannah, meaning that five to fifty percent of the land (depending on local topography and conditions) was oak forest, and the remainder grassland. In the Prairie Peninsula this meant that most of the ground was grassland, with oaks being found in ravines and the occasional forest. After a fire, bur oaks were the first to appear, to be gradually overtaken by northern red oaks and hickories. Maples were part of the vegetation, too, but tend to require moister sites.

The Prairie Peninsula experiences climatic extremes and is characterized by the neutral to alkaline soils typical of prairies and grasslands.

Although Xeriscape gardening is not well known in this area, water is becoming a primary issue, and interest in water-conserving landscaping is on the upswing. After two years of drought in the late 1980s many Iowa lawns were partially killed and are having to be reseeded. Bluegrass is the most common lawn grass, but fescues and buffalograss would make successful substitutes. Dr. Mark Widrlichner of the Plant Introduction Station at Ames, Iowa, says that buffalograss may be more successful in the drier western portions of the region because when buffalograss gets too much moisture (it is adapted to as low as ten- to twelve-inch rainfall sites), it sometimes has trouble competing with weeds and may be difficult to care for.

Some of the most popular and appropriate mulches for the area include shredded bark, straw, grass clippings, and peat moss (especially on flower beds). Dr. Gary Hightshoe, professor of landscape architecture at Iowa State University (also a native plant expert and author), would like to see greater availability of native plants and reconstruction of native woodland habitats. He says there is a good supply of what he calls "the prairie package" and the "wetland package"—that is, those plants and instructions needed to reconstruct a prairie or wetland landscape—but less information about how to reconstruct a woodland, from the dominant over-story plants "right down to the trout lilies." The best list of species and suppliers is available from the University of Minnesota Landscape Arboretum at Chaska (about $40).

According to Hightshoe, the local County Conservation Boards (called Soil Conservation Districts or Natural Resource Commissions in other parts of the country) often maintain lists of sources for local genotypes of plants—that is, plants that are adapted very specifically to your local area. To help preserve local species and to avoid bringing in alien plants that might prove detrimental to native species, Hightshoe recommends that you try to purchase the plants you want from nurseries located within a hundred miles of your home, or else purchase seeds and grow them yourself.

County extension agencies are also valuable sources of appropriate plant information. In some instances the emphasis for the County Conservation Boards is more on prairie or revegetation-type plantings in line with their function as promoters of soil conservation. For $3 you can buy the booklet "Sources of Native Seeds and Plants" from the Soil and Water Conservation Society, 7515 Northeast Ankeny Road, Ankeny, IA 50021.

Though the Prairie Peninsula is part of the Great Plains, most of the plants listed in the Eastern and Northern Forest list (pages 000–00) are adaptable, and often native to the area. A short list of recommended plants (especially wildflowers) is included, and is meant to be read as "in addition to Eastern Forest plants." Of course, many of the Great Plains plants, especially those in the Occasional and Regular Watering categories, can be used in the Prairie Peninsula, and need little supplemental watering because of the area's higher annual rainfall (twenty-four to thirty-five inches). Desert plants may not fare well in this environment.

Xeriscape Plants for the Great Plains/Rockies/Great Basin
Natural Rainfall Zone
(Near-Desert—8–14 inches/year)

BOTANICAL NAME	COMMON NAME(S)	HEIGHT	ZONES
DECIDUOUS TREES			
Chilopsis linearis	Desert willow	25'	7
Elaeagnus angustifolia*/**	Russian olive	15–40'	2
Quercus gambelii	Scrub oak	20'	5
Robinia idahoensis**	Idaho locust	40'	4
EVERGREEN TREES			
Juniperus monosperma	One-seed juniper	20–50'	7–9
Pinus edulis**	Colorado pine	15–40'	4

Xeriscape Plants for the Great Plains/Rockies/Great Basin
Natural Rainfall Zone

BOTANICAL NAME	COMMON NAME(S)	HEIGHT	ZONES
EVERGREEN TREES cont'd			
*Pinus monophylla***	Singleleaf pinyon	10–25'	4
P. ponderosa	Ponderosa pine	60–150'	5
DECIDUOUS SHRUBS			
Caragana microphylla	Littleleaf pea shrub	6'	2
C. pygmaea	Pygmy pea shrub	3'	4
Ceratoides lanata	Winterfat	1–3'	4
*Cercocarpus montanus***	Trueleaf mountain mahogany	3–6'	6
*Chamaebatiaria millefolium***	Fernbush	4'	5
Chrysothamnus nauseosus subsp. *graveolens***	Green rubber rabbitbrush	4'	5
C. n. subsp. *nauseosus*	Blue rubber rabbitbrush	4'	5
C. viscidifolius	Blue rabbitbrush	20–40'	5
*Fallugia paradoxa***	Apache plume	3'	5
Forestiera neomexicana	New Mexico privet	8'	6
Fraxinus anomala	Singleleaf ash	25'	6
Lycium pallidum	Tomatillo	2–3'	6
*Rhus trilobata***	Three-leaf sumac	3–6'	5
Symphoricarpos × *chenaulti*	Chenault coralberry	3–6'	5
EVERGREEN SHRUBS			
Agave utahensis	Utah agave	8'	5
Artemisia filifolia	Threadleaf sage, Sand sage	4'	5
*A. tridentata***	Bigleaf sage	8'	5
A. tridentata spp. *tridentata*	Basin big sagebrush	6'	5
*Atriplex canescens***	Four-wing saltbush	5'	5
Cercocarpus intricatus	Littleleaf mountain mahogany	5'	5
*C. ledifolius***	Curl-leaf mountain mahogany	36'	5
*Cowania mexicana***	Cliff rose	6'	5
Ephedra nevadensis	Mormon tea	3–4'	5
E. torreyana	Torry Mormon tea	2'	5
*E. viridis***	Green Mormon tea	4'	5
Juniperus sabina 'Broadmoor'	Broadmoor juniper	12–18"	4–7
Nolina texana	Texas nolina	3'	5
*Purshia tridentata***	Antelope bitterbrush	4'	6
*Taxus media***	Yew	40'	4
*Yucca baccata***	Banana yucca	3'	6
*Y. elata***	Soaptree yucca	30'	6
GROUND COVERS			
Achillea tomentosa 'Nana'**	Dwarf yarrow, Woolly yarrow	2"	3
Artemisia frigida	Fringed sage, Mountain sage	12–18"	3
*Atriplex gardeneri***	Gardner sage	8–16"	4
Cucurbita foetidissima	Buffalo gourd	6–9"	5
Delosperma cooperi	Purple ice plant	2–3"	6

BOTANICAL NAME	COMMON NAME(S)	HEIGHT	ZONES
GROUND COVERS cont'd			
*Euphorbia myrsinites***	Spurge	3–6"	5
Ipomoea leptophylla	Bush morning glory	3'	5
Oenothera caespitosa	Mexican evening primrose	1'	5
*O. speciosa***	Mexican primrose	6–18"	5
Penstemon pinifolius	Creeping red penstemon, Prairie fire penstemon	12–15"	5–9
Sedum hybridum	Hybrid sedum	4–6"	3
S. spectabilis meteor		12–22"	3
*Sempervivum tectorum**	Hen-and-chicks	1'	4
Sphaeralcea coccinea	Scarlet globe mallow	3'	3
PERENNIALS			
Achillea filipendulina/***	Fernleaf yarrow	3–4'	4
A. millefolium/***	Common yarrow	2'	3
Argemone hispida	Prickly poppy	1–2'	4
Baileya multiradiata	Desert marigold	9"	5
Berlandiera lyrata	Chocolate flower	12–16"	4
Brodiaea hyacinthina	White brodiea	30"	3
B. pulchella	Blue dicks	18–36"	5
*Callirhoe involucrata**	Purple poppy mallow	6–12"	4
Coreopsis lanceolata/***	Lance coreopsis, Tickseed	2–3'	4
Erigeron flagellaris	Whiplash daisy	16"	4
Eriogonum crocatum	Wild buckwheat	10"	6
Eryngium heterophyllum	Button snakeroot, Mexican thistle	18–24"	6
Gaillardia spp.**		8–36"	4
Gypsophila paniculata/***	Perennial baby's breath	3'	4
Linum flavum	Golden perennial flax	1–2'	5
Lupinus argenteus	Silvery lupine	2'	3
Melampodium leucanthum	Blackfoot daisy	1'	7
Mentzelia laevicaulis (biennial)	Blazing star	2–4'	3
Mirabilis multiflora	Colorado four-o'clock	2'	7
Oenothera berlandieri	Mexican evening primrose	8–12"	5
Papaver alpinum	Alpine poppy	6–12"	5
Penstemon barbatus	Beardlip penstemon	2–3'	3–9
P. cardinalis	Cardinal penstemon	3'	5
P. cobaea	White wild snapdragon	12–18"	5
P. cyananthus	Wasatch penstemon	3'	4
P. eatonii	Firecracker penstemon	2'	5
P. jamesii	James penstemon	1'	5
P. palmeri	Palmer's penstemon	2–3'	3–9
P. pseudospectabilis	Desert beardtongue	3–4'	6
P. speciosus	Royal penstemon	2'	5
P. whippleanus	Whipple's penstemon	2'	4
Petalostemon purpureum	Purple prairie clover	2'	3
Potentilla hippiana	Horse cinquefoil	8–12"	4
Psilostrophe tagetina	Paperflower	2'	5
Ratibida columnifera	Prairie coneflower	1–3'	3
Senecio longilobus	Silver groundsel	1–3'	5
Stanleya pinnata	Prince's plume	1–3'	3

Xeriscape Plants for the Great Plains/Rockies/Great Basin
Natural Rainfall Zone

BOTANICAL NAME	COMMON NAME(S)	HEIGHT	ZONES
PERENNIALS cont'd			
Zauschneria arizonica	Fire chalice	1–2'	4
Zinnia grandiflora	Prairie zinnia, Golden paperflower	3–9"	5
ANNUALS			
Abronia villosa	Sand verbena	2'	
Eschscholzia caespitosa	Pastel poppy, Bridal bouquet	1'	
E. mexicana	Mexican gold poppy	1'	
Lesquerella gordonii	Bladderpod	1'	
Lupinus arizonicus	Arizona lupine	1'	
L. sparsiflorus	Arroya lupine	1'	
L. texensis	Texas lupine	1'	
Mentzelia lindleyi	Lindley blazing star	1–4'	
Phacelia campanularia	California bluebells	9"	
Phlox drummondii	Drummond's phlox	6–12"	
Tripterocalyx spp.	Sand verbena	2–15"	
VINE			
Polygonum aubertii	Silver lace vine	20'	4–7

Occasional Watering Zone
(High Plains—14–18 inches/year)

BOTANICAL NAME	COMMON NAME(S)	HEIGHT	ZONES
DECIDUOUS TREES			
Acer grandidentatum	Bigtooth or Wasatch maple	25'	2
Aesculus glabra	Yellow buckeye	35'	4–8
Ailanthus altissima	Tree-of-heaven	75'	5
Catalpa ovata	Chinese catalpa	30'	5
*C. speciosa***	Northern catalpa	45–70'	4–8
Crataegus ambigua	Russian hawthorn	12–20'	4
C. laevigata 'Paul's Scarlet'**		15'	6
C. viridis 'Winter King'		30'	5–7
Fraxinus pennsylvanica 'Marshall Seedless'		36'	3
Malus 'Almey'		12'	4
M. 'Flame'		25'	2
M. sylvestris	Yellow transparent apple	20–25'	3
Morus alba	White mulberry	60'	5–9
Prunus × *blireiana* 'Newport'		12–24'	6
P. cerasus	Montmorency cherry	15–25'	3
P. padus	European bird cherry	40'	4–7
*Quercus robur***	English oak	80'	5–8
Robinia neomexicana	New Mexico locust	25'	5

BOTANICAL NAME	COMMON NAME(S)	HEIGHT	ZONES
EVERGREEN TREES			
Cedrus atlantica var. *glauca***	Blue atlas cedar	40–60'	6–9
Juniperus spp.		30–75'	Vary
*Pinus aristata***	Bristlecone, Foxtail	30–60'	5
P. flexilis	Limber pine	75'	4–7
*P. jeffreyi***	Jeffrey pine	120'	5
*P. nigra***	Austrian pine	60'	4–8
*P. ponderosa***	Ponderosa pine	150'	5
*P. sylvestris***	Scotch pine	90'	3–8
Pseudotsuga taxifolia	Douglas fir	60–130'	
*Sequoiadendron giganteum***	Giant sequoia	250'	7–9 (semihardy, Zone 6)
DECIDUOUS SHRUBS			
Amelanchier alnifolia	Serviceberry	6–12'	5
Amorpha fruticosa	Indigo bush	9'	5
Buddleia alternifolia	Fountain butterfly bush	15'	6–8
Ceanothus fendleri		3'	5
Chaenomeles speciosa	Flowering quince	6–10'	5
*Colutea arborescens***	Common bladder senna	8'	6
*Cotinus coggygria***	Smoke tree	10–15'	5
Cotoneaster acutifolius	Peking cotoneaster	9'	5
C. apiculatus	Cranberry cotoneaster	3'	5
C. divaricatus	Spreading cotoneaster	5'	5
C. multiflorus	Flowering cotoneaster	8'	3
Cytisus × *praecox***	Warminster broom	10'	7
Euonymus alata	Winged euonymus	6'	4
Fendlera rupicola	False mock orange	5'	5
Forsythia × *intermedia*	Forsythia	10'	5
Holodiscus dumosus	Rock spirea	4'	4
Lonicera korolkowii	Blueleaf honeysuckle	10–15'	3
L. tatarica	Tatarian honeysuckle	10'	4
Peraphyllum ramosissimum	Squaw apple	6'	5
*Perovskia atriplicifolia***	Russian sage, Azure sage	5'	6
Philadelphus microphyllus	Littleleaf mock orange	6'	6
Physocarpus monogynus	Mountain ninebark	6'	5
*Prunus besseyi***	Western sand cherry	4–6'	4
P. pensylvanica	Pin cherry	8'	2
P. tomentosa	Nanking cherry	8'	3
P. virginiana var. *demissa*	Western chokecherry	9'	2
Ptelea trifoliata	Water ash	18'	5
Rhamnus cathartica	Common buckthorn	20'	3
R. smithii	Smith buckthorn	9'	3
Ribes aureum	Golden currant	6'	2
R. cereum	Squaw currant	3'	5
R. inerme	Whitestem gooseberry	5'	6
Rosa foetida 'Bicolor'	Austrian copper rose	6'	4
R. f. 'Persiana'	Woods rose	6'	4
R. × *harisonii*	Harison's yellow rose	6'	4
R. rubrifolia	Redleaf rose	6'	2

Xeriscape Plants for the Great Plains/Rockies/Great Basin
Occasional Watering Zone

BOTANICAL NAME	COMMON NAME(S)	HEIGHT	ZONES
DECIDUOUS SHRUBS cont'd			
Rubus deliciosus	Thimbleberry, Boulder raspberry	5'	4
Syringa × chinensis	Chinese lilac	10'	4
S. reflexa	MacFarlane lilac	6'	5
S. villosa	Late lilac	10'	3
Viburnum lantana	Wayfaring tree viburnum	10–15'	4
EVERGREEN SHRUBS			
*Arctostaphylos patula***	Greenleaf manzanita	3–6'	6
Cotoneaster spp.**		3–10"	3
Juniperus chinensis 'Armstrongii'		4'	3
Ligustrum amurense (semievergreen)	Amur privet	10–15'	4
L. regelianum	Regel privet	6'	3
GROUND COVERS			
*Artemisia dracunculus**	Tarragon	1–2'	3
Aster spp.**	Dwarf Michaelmas daisy	12–18"	5
Delosperma nubigenum	Yellow ice plant	2–4"	5
Fragaria americana	Wild strawberry	2–4"	4
*Gypsophila repens**	Creeping baby's breath	4"	4
*Lavandula vera,*** syn. *L. angustifolia*	Lavender	1–3'	5–9
Nepepta spp.*	Catmint	1–2'	3–9
Penstemon strictus 'Bandera'	Rocky Mountain penstemon	2'	4
Potentilla verna var. *nana***	Creeping potentilla	2–6"	3
Sedum spp.*/**	Sedum, Stonecrop	3–8"	
*Sempervivum arachnoideum**	Hen-and-chicks, Cobweb houseleek	4"	3
Symphoricarpos orbiculatus 'Hancock'	Hancock coralberry	18"	3
*Thymus pseudolanuginosus**	Woolly thyme	1–2"	3
*T. vulgaris***	Common thyme	6–12"	3
Zauschneria californica	California fuchsia	1–2'	6
PERENNIALS			
Allium cernuum	Pink nodding onion	1'	3
*Anaphalis margaritacea**	Pearly everlasting	20"	4
*Anemone pulsatilla**	Pasqueflower	1'	5–6
*Armeria pseudarmeria**	Thrift, Sea pink	18–24"	6–7
*Asclepias tuberosa**	Butterfly weed	1–3'	4
*Aster novae-angliae**	New England aster	3–5'	5
A. novi-belgii/**	New York aster, Michaelmas daisy	1–4'	4–9
*Baptisia australis**	False indigo	3–6'	3
Calochortus amoenus	Purple globe tulip	18"	7
C. venustus	Mariposa tulip	1'	7
*Campanula poscharskyana**	Serbian, Polish, or Russian bell-flower	4–6"	4
*C. rotundifolia**	Harebell	1–2'	3

BOTANICAL NAME	COMMON NAME(S)	HEIGHT	ZONES
PERENNIALS cont'd			
*Centaurea montana**	Perennial bachelor's button, Mountain bluet	18–24″	4
*Centranthus ruber**	Red valerian, Jupiter's beard	1–3′	5
*Coreopsis verticillata**	Threadleaf coreopsis	18–30″	4
Dianthus barbatus/***	Sweet William	1–2′	6
*D. plumarius**	Cottage pinks	9–18″	4
Echinacea purpurea/***	Purple coneflower	5′	7
*Echinops ritro**	Globe thistle	3–4′	4
*Epilobium angustifolium**	Fireweed, Willow herb	3–5′	3–9
*Erigeron compositus**	Cutleaf daisy	2–10″	3
Erysimum asperum (biennial)	Western wallflower	30″	3
Goniolimon tataricum, syn. *Limonium tataricum**	Tatarian statice	18″	4
Gutierrezia sarothrae	Snakebroom, Snakeweed	6″–3′	3
*Helianthemum appenninum**	Silver sun rose	12–18″	5
*H. nummularium**	Sun rose	9–12″	6
Helianthus maximiliani	New Mexican sunflower, Maximilian's daisy	5–8′	3
Hemerocallis spp. */***	Daylily	30–42″	4
Iberis sempervirens/***	Evergreen candytuft	1′	4
Iris, bearded*/***		5–30″	4
Lavandula angustifolia/***	Lavender	1–3′	5–6
*Liatris punctata**	Gayfeather	1′	3
*Linum perenne**	Perennial flax	1–2′	5
L. p. var. *lewisii***	Flax	2–3′	5
Lupinus argenteus	Silver lupine	2′	3
*Monarda fistulosa**	Wild bergamot	3–4′	4
Muscari botryoides	Grape hyacinth	4–6″	4
*Oenothera serrulata**	Tooth-leaved evening primrose	6–12″	4
Penstemon alamosensis	Alamo penstemon	2′	6
P. alpinus	Alpine penstemon	3′	3
P. ambiguus	Flat-faced penstemon	2′	6
P. angustifolius	Narrow-leaved penstemon, Whorled penstemon	6–18″	4
P. grandiflorus		4′	4
*P. pinifolius**	Pineleaf penstemon	18″	5
P. secundiflorus	Sidebells penstemon	2′	4
*P. strictus**	Rocky Mountain penstemon	2′	3
P. virgatus	Wand penstemon	2–4′	6
*Potentilla recta**	Sulphur cinquefoil	2′	4
Ratibida columnifera	Mexican hat, Prairie coneflower	1–3′	3
Rudbeckia spp. **	Coneflower	8″–6′	Vary
*Salvia pratensis**	Meadow clary	3′	6
*S. × superba**	Perennial sage, Violet sage, Perennial salvia	18–36″	5
Senecio longilobus	Threadleaf groundsel	1–3′	4
Thelesperma megapotamicum	Cota, Navaho tea	1–3′	4
*Thermopsis montana**	Golden banner	2′	4
Townsendia excapa	Easter daisy	2–12″	4

Xeriscape Plants for the Great Plains/Rockies/Great Basin
Occasional Watering Zone

BOTANICAL NAME	COMMON NAME(S)	HEIGHT	ZONES
PERENNIALS cont'd			
*Tradescantia occidentalis**	Spiderwort	1–3′	3
Viguiera multiflora	Showy goldeneye	1–4′	3
ANNUALS			
Aster bigelovii	Purple aster	3′	
Centaurea cyanus	Mountain bachelor button	20″	
Collinsia heterophylla		1–2′	
Gilia rubra	Red gilia	7′	
Lupinus hartwegii	Hartweg lupine	2–3′	
L. nanus	Sky lupine	20″	
Phacelia grandiflora	Bee phacelia	20–40″	
P. tanacetifolia	Wild heliotrope	1–2′	
Thelesperma filifolia	Showy Navaho tea, Greenthread	1–2′	
Verbesina encelioides	Golden crownbeard	3′	
VINES			
*Campsis radicans***	Common trumpet creeper	30′	4
Clematis ligusticifolia	Western virgin's bower	20′	3
Ipomoea spp.	Morning glory	Varies	Annual
Lonicera japonica 'Halliana'**	Hall's honeysuckle	20–30′	4
Maurandya antirrhiniflora	Snapdragon vine	6′	Annual
Parthenocissus inserta	Virginia creeper, Woodbine	35′	3
*P. quinquefolia***	Virginia creeper	35′	3
P. q. 'Engelmannii'		20–35′	3
Vitis spp.	Grape	Varies	Vary

Regular Watering Zone
(Mountains—18+ inches/year)

BOTANICAL NAME	COMMON NAME(S)	HEIGHT	ZONES
DECIDUOUS TREES			
*Acer platanoides****	Norway maple	90′	3
Aesculus hippocastanum	Horse chestnut	75′	3
Betula pendula 'Gracilis'	Cutleaf weeping birch	18′	2
Cercis canadensis	Eastern redbud	20–35′	5–8
*Crataegus phaenopyrum***	Washington hawthorn	30′	5–9
C. succulenta	Fleshy hawthorn	15′	4
Laburnum × *watereri* var. *vossi***	Golden chain tree	30′	5
Platanus × *acerifolia***	London plane tree	100′	6
P. occidentalis	American sycamore, Buttonwood	75–100′	5
Populus angustifolia	Narrowleaf cottonwood	60′	3

BOTANICAL NAME	COMMON NAME(S)	HEIGHT	ZONES
DECIDUOUS TREES cont'd			
Populus nigra 'Italica'	Lombardy poplar	90'	2
P. sargentii	Plains poplar, Cottonwood	70'	4
P. tremuloides	Quaking aspen	35–50'	2
Pyrus calleryana	Callery pear	30'	4
P. ussuriensis	Ussurian pear	50'	4–6
*Quercus rubra***	Northern red oak	40–100'	4–8
Salix amygdaloides	Peachleaf willow	35–50'	3
*Sorbus aucuparia***	European mountain ash	45'	3–7
Syringa japonica	Japanese tree lilac	30'	4
Tilia cordata	Littleleaf linden	75'	3–8
EVERGREEN TREES			
*Calocedrus decurrens***	Incense cedar	135'	5
Picea pungens	Blue spruce, Colorado spruce	75–100'	3–7
Pinus contorta var. *murrayana***	Lodgepole pine	20–100'	2
Pseudotsuga menziesii	Douglas fir	200'	6–8
DECIDUOUS SHRUBS			
Acer amur	Amur maple	18'	4
A. glabrum	Rocky Mountain maple	24'	4
Alnus tenuifolia	Thinleaf alder	30'	6
Aronia melanocarpa var. *elata***	Glossy black chokeberry	9'	3
Cornus baileyi	Bailey dogwood	7'	5
C. mas	Cornelian cherry	24'	4
C. stolonifera var. *coloradensis*	Colorado red-osier dogwood	6'	3
Euonymus europaea	European euonymus	12'	3
*Hibiscus syriacus***	Althea, Rose of Sharon	5–15'	5
Kolkwitzia amabilis	Beautybush	10'	4
Lonicera maackii	Amur honeysuckle	12–15'	5
Prunus × *cistena*	Purpleleaf cherry	5'	3
Rhamnus frangula 'Tallhedge'	Columnar buckthorn	15–20'	2
Rhus glabra 'Cismontana'	Mountain or Dwarf smooth sumac	3'	2
Ribes alpinum	Alpine currant	5–8'	3
Salix irrorata	Bluestem willow	9'	5
S. purpurea 'Nana'	Dwarf arctic willow	1–3'	5
Sambucus canadensis	American elder	6–10'	4
Spiraea × *bumalda* 'Froebelii'		3'	4
S. nipponica 'Snowmound'		4–6'	4
S. prunifolia 'Plena'			
S. vanhouettei	Vanhoutte spirea	6–8'	4
Syringa persica	Persian lilac	6'	4
Viburnum carlesii	Korean spice viburnum	5'	5
V. dentatum	Arrowwood viburnum	10–15'	3
V. opulus	European cranberrybush viburnum	7–12'	4
EVERGREEN SHRUBS			
*Cotoneaster microphyllus***	Small-leaved cotoneaster	3'	3
Cotoneaster spp.**		1–10'	
Euonymus fortunei 'Sarcoxie'		4'	5

Xeriscape Plants for the Great Plains/Rockies/Great Basin
Regular Watering Zone

BOTANICAL NAME	COMMON NAME(S)	HEIGHT	ZONES
EVERGREEN SHRUBS cont'd			
Euonymus kiautschovica 'Manhattan'		6′	5
*Mahonia aquifolium***	Oregon grape holly	3–6′	
Nandina domestica	Heavenly bamboo	6–8′	7
Picea abies 'Maxwellii'		2–4′	2
Viburnum burkwoodii (semievergreen)	Burkwood viburnum	6′	4
GROUND COVERS			
*Ajuga reptans***		8–10″	4
Ceratostigma plumbaginoides	Plumbago	6–12″	6
*Cotoneaster dammeri***	Bearberry	6″	5
*Dianthus anatolicus**		12–18″	6
D. caesius		3–8″	5
Euonymus fortunei var. *colorata***	Wintercreeper euonymus	6–18″	5–9
*Ranunculus repens**	Creeping buttercup	1′	4–9
*Thymus praecox**	Mother-of-thyme	2–6″	4
Trifolium hybridum	Alsike clover		6
*Vinca minor***	Periwinkle, Myrtle	3–6″	5–9
PERENNIALS			
*Anemone vitifolia**	Japanese anemone	3–4′	7
*Aquilegia caerulea**	Rocky Mountain columbine	2–3′	4
Asclepias speciosa	Showy milkweed	2–4′	3
*Aster alpinus**	Dwarf alpine aster	6–12″	4–9
*Campanula carpatica**	Carpathian harebell	6–12″	4
C. elatines var. *garganica**	Adriatic harebell	6–8″	3
Chrysanthemum maximum	Daisy chrysanthemum	1–3′	5
C. m. 'Little Miss Muffet'		12–14″	5
C. × *morifolium**	Hardy or Garden chrysanthemum	1–4′	5
C. × *superbum*/***	Shasta daisy	1–3′	5
*Clematis integrifolia**	Solitary clematis	2–5′	3–9
*Delphinium elatum**	Candle larkspur	6′	4
*Dianthus deltoides**	Maiden pink	4–12″	4
*D. plumarius**	Cottage or Grass pink	9–18″	4
*Dicentra spectabilis**	Common bleeding heart	1–2′	3–4
*Dictamnus albus**	Gas plant, Dittany	2–3′	4
*Epilobium angustifolium**	Fireweed	2–8′	3
*Erigeron speciosus**	Showy daisy, Mountain aster, Fleabane	12–30″	2
*Geranium sanguineum**	Blood-red geranium, Bloody cranesbill	1′	4
*Geum quellyon**	Sweet avens	2′	5–6
Helenium hoopesii	Orange mountain daisy	3′	3–9
Heliopsis helianthoides var. *scabra**	Heliopsis, False sunflower	5′	4–9
Hemerocallis 'Autumn Red'		3′	3
Iris missouriensis	Western blue flag	2′	3
*I. sibirica**	Siberian iris	2–4′	4
Kniphofia spp.***	Red hot poker	2–4′	5
*Liatrus spicata**	Gayfeather	2–5′	3

BOTANICAL NAME	COMMON NAME(S)	HEIGHT	ZONES
PERENNIALS cont'd			
Lilium spp.*	Garden lily	2–6'	Vary
*Limonium latifolium**	Sea lavender, Statice	2'	3
Lupinus Russell Hybrids*		3–4'	4–9
Monarda menthifolia	Bee balm	3–4'	3
*Myosotis scorpioides**	Dwarf forget-me-not	12–18"	5
Oenothera hookeri	Yellow evening primrose	2–6'	5
*O. tetragona**	Common sundrops	18"	5
Paeonia hybrids*	Garden peony, Chinese peony	3'	5
Papaver nudicaule	Iceland poppy	1–2'	3
*P. orientale***	Oriental poppy	3–4'	5
Pedicularis groenlandica	Elephant head	6–24"	2
*Penstemon hirsutus**	Dwarf hairy beardtongue	1–3'	3–9
*P. perfoliatus**		3'	3
*Physostegia virginiana**	Obedient plant, False dragonhead	4–5'	4
*Platycodon grandiflorus**	Balloon flower	18–30"	4
Rudbeckia fulgida 'Goldsturm'	Orange coneflower, Black-eyed Susan	2–3'	5
Ruta graveolens 'Blue Mound'*	Common rue, Herb-of-grace	2–3'	5
*Saponaria ocymoides**	Rock soapwort	9"	4
*Solidago virgaurea**	European goldenrod	3–4'	4
*Stachys byzantina**	Lamb's ears	18"	5
Thermopsis montana	Golden banner	18"	3
*Veronica prostrata**	Harebell speedwell, Rock speedwell	6"	3
*V. spicata**	Spike speedwell	12–18"	3
ANNUALS			
Cleome serrulata	Rocky Mountain bee plant	3'	
Hymenoxys grandiflora	Alpine sunflower	1'	
Linanthus grandiflorus	Mountain phlox	2'	
VINES			
Akebia quinata	Fiveleaf akebia	30–40'	4
Ampelopsis brevipedunculata	Blueberry climber	25'	4
Aristolochia durior	Dutchman's pipe	30'	4
Celastrus spp.	Bittersweet	20–36'	Vary
*Clematis jackmanii***	Jackman clematis	12'	5
*C. tangutica***	Golden clematis	9'	5
Cobaea scandens	Cup-and-saucer vine	40'	Annual
Euonymus fortunei var. *radicans*	Common wintercreeper	20'	5–9
Hedera helix	English ivy	90'	5
H. h. 'Baltica'		90'	5
Polygonum baldschuanicum	Bukhara fleeceflower	20–30'	4
Wisteria spp.		Varies	Vary

*Did well in a test of several years' duration at Colorado State University.
**Especially well adapted for the Reno, Nevada, area.

**Xeriscape Plants for the Prairie Peninsula
Natural Rainfall Zone**

See Natural Rainfall Zone lists for Eastern and Northern Forests, pages 186–88, plus:

BOTANICAL NAME	COMMON NAME(S)	HEIGHT
EVERGREEN TREES		
Picea rubens	Red spruce	50–70'
DECIDUOUS SHRUBS		
Prunus besseyi	Sand cherry	6
P. hortulana	Hortulan plum	12–20'
Ribes odoratum	Clove currant	9'
Symphoricarpos occidentalis	Western snowberry	3–6'
EVERGREEN SHRUBS		
Juniperus davaurica	Dahurian juniper	30"
J. excelsa (slow-growing)	Spiny Greek juniper	60'
Ligustrum vulgare 'Cheyenne'		10–15'
PERENNIALS		
Anemone caroliniana	Carolina anemone	2–8'
A. cylindrica	Thimbleweed	1–2'
A. patens	Pasqueflower	1'
Baptisia leucantha	White false indigo	3–7'
B. leucophaea		12–32"
Coreopsis palmata	Prairie coreopsis	16–36"
Echinacea angustifolia	Black Sampson	4–20"
Eriogonum crocatum	Wild buckwheat	8"
G. triflorum	Prairie smoke	6–12"
Helianthus maximiliani	Maximilian's sunflower	10'
Liatris punctata	Dotted gayfeather	4–32"
Penstemon cobaea		10–24"
P. cordifolius	Vine penstemon	
P. palmeri	Palmer's penstemon	4'
P. spectabilis	Showy penstemon	4'
ANNUALS		
Argemone hispida	Hedgehog prickly poppy	1–2'
Lupinus hartwegii	Hartweg lupine	2–3'
L. nanus	Sky lupine	20"
VINES		
Campsis radicans	Trumpet creeper	30'
Lonicera × 'Dropmore Scarlet'		15–20'

Occasional Watering Zone

See Occasional Watering Zone lists for Eastern and Northern Forests, pages 188–91, plus:

BOTANICAL NAME	COMMON NAME(S)	HEIGHT
DECIDUOUS TREES		
Zanthoxylum americanum	Prickly-ash	10–35′
EVERGREEN TREES		
Picea pungens	Colorado spruce	75–100′
DECIDUOUS SHRUBS		
Hamamelis vernalis	Vernal witch hazel	6–12′
Rosa palustris	Swamp rose	6′
Salix cotteti	Dwarf willow	1′
S. discolor	Pussy willow	8′
Spiraea japonica	Japanese spirea	4–6′
S. tomentosa	Hardhack spirea	3–6′
Staphylea trifolia	American bladdernut	6–12′
Xanthorhiza simplicissima	Yellow root	3–6′
EVERGREEN SHRUB		
Hypericum spathulatum	Shrubby St.-John's-wort	7–8′
GROUND COVERS		
Cornus canadensis	Bunchberry	3–9″
Hosta spp.	Plantain lily	3′
Lamium maculatum	Dead nettle	6″
PERENNIALS		
Aquilegia canadensis	American columbine	3–4′
Bergenia purpurascens	Saxifrage	10″
Desmodium illinoense	Illinois tick trefoil	2–5′
Dodecatheon amethystinum	Jewel shooting star	1′
D. clevelandii	Cleveland shooting star	10–15″
Mimulus aurantiacus	Bush monkey flower	2–4′
Polemonium reptans	Creeping Jacob's ladder	30″
Silphium laciniatum	Compass plant	2–12′
ANNUALS		
Gilia capitata	Blue thimble flower	1–2′
G. rubra	Red gilia	6′
Phacelia grandiflora	Bee phacelia	1–3′
P. tanacetifolia	Wild heliotrope	1–2′
VINE		
Vitis vulpina	Chicken or River grape	25–35′

Xeriscape Plants for Texas

WILBUR Davis of Austin, Texas, an amateur gardener and small business owner, created a home landscape that was, unbeknownst to him, one of the earliest Texas Xeriscape landscapes. It was discovered one day by Doug Welsh, who happened to drive by and noticed the rare phenomenon (at that time) of native plants in the landscape. Since then the landscape has been much admired and used as a model. Wilbur and his wife, Doris, worked diligently to undo the mauling to which builders subjected their property in constructing their home. (A large, beautiful tree had had its trunk buried under four feet of fill dirt, which trees won't survive. The buried portion had to be excavated by hand and a rock "well" constructed around it.) The large site also featured some difficult grades and drainage problems.

Davis had started with a traditional landscape. The St. Augustinegrass the builders put in had to be watered every other day. Pittosporums were featured as typical foundation plantings. A monumental freeze in 1983 killed virtually all of the Davises' plants, except the natives. At that point Davis made it his intense crusade and hobby to find and establish only native plants in his landscape (a difficult task at that time, because of the scarcity of native plants in nurseries). He tried to find plants that could survive droughts as well as freezes.

He got rid of the St. Augustinegrass by scalping it and digging it out, replacing it with Bermudagrass. He doesn't have an irrigation system for the lawn and doesn't intend to get one. In the hottest part of the season he waters once a week, though the grass could go eight days without watering. In 1990 it went six weeks without being watered, thanks to some timely summer rains.

If your yard is heavily shaded, says Davis, the best choice for Texas yards is St. Augustinegrass, but it is only water-efficient in the shade. Bermudagrass is finer textured and more drought and wear tolerant than St. Augustine, but it won't tolerate shade. (Knowing what he has learned, Davis shakes his head at the fact that a nearby high-dollar subdivision has made it part of the covenants that only St. Augustinegrass be allowed for lawn grass.)

Wandering around the Davis yard is a delight. Large areas of grass have been replaced with meandering raised beds smartly outlined in brick which provide homes for innumerable favorite and experimental native plants.

A depressed pathway along one side of the house doubles cleverly as a drainage swale to collect runoff from a neighbor's steeply sloped lawn, delivering the water to a man-made creek that crosses the back corner of the lot. Davis used shredded cypress bark mulch for the path because it's very soft to walk on, and it doesn't wash away since it knits together slightly.

The Davises' backyard adjoins a greenbelt that has been left to grow naturally, so they started a buffalograss and wildflower meadow in the back section of their lot to tie into this. Closer in are a large play area for their grandchildren and beds for hobby roses.

This model Xeriscape landscape has covered all the seven Xeriscape steps, even maintenance. Doris Davis reports that it takes her husband only an hour every ten days to trim, "weed-eat," and mow the lawn, despite all the meandering flower beds. The lawn still looks lavish and green and the flower beds and array of trees and shrubs provide the Davises with year-round garden color.

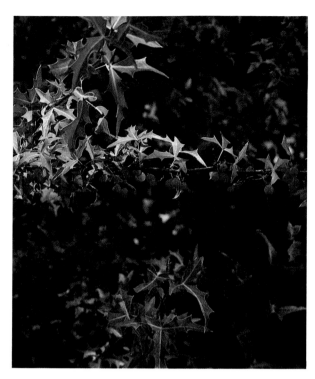

Native to Texas and much of the Southwest, this beautiful little shrub, agarita (Berberis trifoliata), provides year-round interest: fragrant yellow flowers in early spring, red berries from May to July, and hollylike evergreen foliage. (Photo: Wilbur Davis)

Native plants have gotten a lot of press in Texas, beginning years ago when Texas was the first state to pioneer the widespread use of wildflower highway right-of-way plantings. The state Department of Agriculture adopted a resolution promoting the use of natives, and many growers are experimenting with cultivating natives such as oaks, yaupon holly, and magnolia for the nursery trade.

Texas has such a diversity of vegetative areas that it offers an endless variety of models for the Xeriscape gardener who wishes to create a complete or partial native theme. The state has been roughly divided into ten regions with descriptions such as high plains, rolling plains, blackland prairies, post oak savannah, gulf prairies and marshes, and piney woods (moving from west to east across the state). You could do no better than to beg, borrow, or buy a copy of *Texas Native Plants: Landscaping Region by Region* (Sally Wasowski, with Andy Wasowski,

Austin, Texas: Texas Monthly Press, 1984) for a complete description of these natural areas, as well as photos and extensive gardener-friendly information on indigenous native plants.

San Antonio landscape architect Terry Lewis says zoysiagrass is his choice for shady situations in his designs, and Bermudagrass and zoysia are used in sunny areas. The 'Prairie' cultivar developed at Texas A&M seems to create a thicker, fuller grass than the native seed, though it doesn't feature the male flags (seed heads) for which native buffalograss is well known. For mulching he finds that a three-inch depth of shredded bark and hardwood clippings seems to do an adequate job of controlling weeds.

Lewis says Xeriscape gardening is easy to promote in his area. Located on part of the Edwards Aquifer, San Antonio is situated so that when the water in the aquifer lowers to elevation 618, springs will start to dry up. The level has been as low as 620 in recent years. Dry streams in neighboring San Marcos have threatened some wildlife species, and the losses to farmers and those who depend on revenue from water recreation have been enormous. Thus, there's been a tremendous change in the awareness of the public toward more sensitive and sensible watering habits.

The list that follows includes many native wildflowers and shrubs. It was adapted from *Texas Native Plants*, and from the Texas Agricultuural Extension Service's brochure "Landscape Water Conservation . . . Xeriscape." Included are notes where needed about adapted areas. Some plants won't take the heat of south Texas; some need it. Some plants require the higher rainfall or acid soil of east Texas (forty to fifty-five inches), while some will survive on the low rainfall in west Texas (eight to twenty inches). If no specific area is indicated, you can assume it's hardy throughout all of Texas.

Water-use zones are not indicated because of the diverse soils, temperature, and rainfall (ranging from seven to sixty inches per year). Check with your local nursery professional or extension agent for help in determining water use for individual plants in your locale.

BOTANICAL NAME	COMMON NAME(S)	HEIGHT	REGIONS
DECIDUOUS TREES			
Acacia berlandieri	Guajillo	9–15'	WTex
A. constricta	Whitethorn	9–15'	STex
A. farnesiana	Huisache	15–30'	STex
A. rigidula	Blackbrush acacia	10–15'	STex
A. schaffneri var. *bravoensis*	Huisachillo	6–12'	Hardy as far north as Dallas if in protected location
A. wrightii	Wright acacia	6–30'	Hardy through most of Texas except Panhandle
Caesalpinia mexicana	Mexican poinciana	10–20'	Hardy only as far north as Corpus Christi
Carya illinoinensis	Pecan	50–60'	
Celtis laevigata	Hackberry	30–50'	
Cercis canadensis var. *mexicana* (most drought tolerant), *texana*, and *canadensis*	Redbud, Judas tree	10–40'	
Chilopsis linearis	Desert willow	15–25'	Hardy in all but Panhandle
Cordia boisserieri	Wild olive	12–24'	STex
Cotinus obovatus	Texas smoke tree	15–30'	
Diospyros kaki	Japanese persimmon	15–25'	
D. texana	Texas persimmon	10–25'	
Euonymus bungeanas	Pink Lady euonymus	18'	Panhandle only
Eysenhardtia texana	Kidneywood	6–15'	
Fraxinus cuspidata	Fragrant ash	10–25'	Hardy to Dallas
F. texensis	Texas ash	30–45'	
Gymnocladus dioica	Kentucky coffee tree	90'	Panhandle only
Koelreuteria paniculata	Panicled golden raintree	25–35'	S/ETex
Leucaena retusa	Goldenball lead tree	12–25'	Hardy to Midland
Liquidambar styraciflua	Sweet gum	50–60'	ETex
Maclura pomifera 'Fan d'Arc' (male cultivar—no messy fruit)	Osage orange	20–35'	
Malus spp.	Crab apple	20–35'	All but STex
Nyssa sylvatica	Black gum, Sour gum, Tupelo	30–60'	
Parkinsonia texana var. *macrum*, syn. *Cercidium macrum*	Paloverde	9–12'	SWTex
Pinus eldarica	Eldarica pine, Afghan pine, Mondell pine	30–80'	All but ETex
Pistacia chinensis	Chinese pistache	30–50'	
P. texana	Texas pistachio	12–20'	STex
Populus spp.	Cottonwood	40–100'	
Prosopis glandulosa	Honey mesquite	20–30'	
Prunus mexicana	Mexican plum	15–35'	
P. umbellata	Flatwoods plum	12–20'	

BOTANICAL NAME	COMMON NAME(S)	HEIGHT	REGIONS
DECIDUOUS TREES cont'd			
Pyrus calleryana 'Aristocrat'	Aristocrat pear	20–30'	All but STex
P. c. 'Bradford'	Bradford pear	20–30'	All but STex
Quercus glaucoides	Lacey oak	20–30'	
Q. macrocarpa	Bur oak	60–80'	
Q. shumardii	Shumard oak	50'	E/Central Texas
Q. stellata	Post oak	40–50'	
Q. texana	Texas red oak	15–30'	
Rhus lanceolata	Prairie flameleaf sumac	10–20'	
Sapindus drummondii	Soapberry	10–50'	
Sassafras albidum	Eve's necklace	15–30'	
Ulmus crassifolia	Cedar elm	30–60'	
U. parvifolia	Lacebark elm	50'	
Ungnadia speciosa	Mexican buckeye	8–30'	
Viburnum rufidulum	Rusty blackhaw viburnum	12–30'	
EVERGREEN TREES			
Bumelia celastrina	La coma	15–20'	Hardy to at least San Antonio
Cedrus deodara	Deodar cedar	40–60'	
Cercocarpus montanus var. *argenteus* (almost evergreen)	Silverlear mountain mahogany	8–15'	
Condalia hookeri	Brasil	12–15'	STex
Cordia boissieri	Mexican olive	12–15'	Only southernmost Texas
Cupressus arizonica var. *arizonica*	Arizona cypress	30–75'	
Ehretia anacua	Anacua, Sandpaper tree	20–45'	STex
Guaiacum angustifolium	Guayacan	8–20'	Southernmost Texas
Ilex vomitoria	Yaupon holly	12–25'	
Juniperus ashei	Ashe juniper	18'	
J. deppeana var. *deppeana*	Alligator juniper	15–25'	
J. flaccida	Weeping juniper	20–30'	Hardy to Amarillo
J. monosperma	Oneseed juniper	18'	
J. scopulorum	Rocky Mountain juniper	36'	
J. virginiana	Eastern or Canaert red cedar	30–40'	
Magnolia grandiflora	Southern magnolia	50'	ETex
Myrica cerifera	Wax myrtle	6–36'	Needs 25" rainfall or more
Pinus edulis	Colorado pinyon	10–20'	
P. elliottii	Slash pine	80–100'	
P. taeda	Loblolly pine	60–110'	ETex
Pithecellobium flexicaule	Texas ebony	25–30'	
P. pallens	Tenaza	10–15'	Southernmost Texas
Pseudotsuga menziesii var. *glauca*	Blue Douglas fir	15–25'	
Quercus fusiformis	Escarpment live oak	30–40'	
Q. mohriana	Mohr oak	10–20'	
Q. muehlenbergii	Chinquapin oak	40–60'	All but Panhandle

BOTANICAL NAME	COMMON NAME(S)	HEIGHT	REGIONS
EVERGREEN TREES cont'd			
Quercus nigra	Water oak	50–60'	ETex
Q. virginiana	Live oak	40–60'	All but Panhandle
Rhus virens	Evergreen sumac	8–12'	
Sabal mexicana	Texas palm	45'	STex
Sambucus mexicana	Mexican elderberry	10–15'	SWTex
Sophora secundiflora	Texas mountain laurel	6–30'	
Taxodium distichum	Bald cypress	45'	
Vauquelinia angustifolia	Chisos rosewood	9–30'	
DECIDUOUS SHRUBS			
Amorpha fruticosa	Indigobush amorpha	10'	
Anisacanthus quadrifidus var. *wrightii*	Flame acanthus	3–4'	
Baccharis halimifolia	Baccharis, Groundsel	6–8'	
Bouvardia ternifolia	Scarlet bouvardia	2–4'	
Buddleia marrubiifolia	Butterfly bush	3–5'	Tender NTex
Cassia wislizenii	Canyon senna, Dwarf senna	4–10'	
Chaenomeles japonica	Flowering quince	3–5'	
Colubrina texensis	Texas snakewood	4–6'	Tender NTex
Dalea formosa	Feather dalea	2–6'	
D. frutescens	Black dalea	1–3'	
Diospyros texana	Texas persimmon	10–25'	S/Central Texas
Erythrina herbacea	Coralbean	6–15'	Tender NTex
Eupatorium wrightii	White mistflower, White boneset	1–3'	
Forsythia × *intermedia* 'Spectabilis'		6–9'	All but southernmost Texas
Hibiscus syriacus	Althea	6–9'	
Lagerstroemia indica	Crape myrtle	10–25'	All but Panhandle
Lantana horrida	Texas lantana	1½–6'	Dies back in winter north of STex
Mimosa borealis	Fragrant mimosa	2–6'	
Philadelphus texenis	Texas mock orange	3'	Tender NTex
Photinia × *fraseri*	Fraser photinia	6–9'	
Rhus aromatica	Aromatic sumac, Three-leafed sumac, Skunk-bush	3–8'	
R. glabra	Smooth sumac	3–10'	
R. microphylla	Littleleaf sumac	4–15'	
Rosa chinensis	China rose	3–5'	All but Panhandle
R. odorata	Tea rose	3–5'	All but Panhandle
Spiraea cantoniensis, syn. *S. reevesiana*	Bridal wreath spirea	3–5'	
Tecoma stans var. *angustata*	Yellow bells	3–6'	
Viguiera stenoloba	Skeletonleaf goldeneye	1½–4'	
Vitex agnus-castus		10–25'	

BOTANICAL NAME	COMMON NAME(S)	HEIGHT	REGIONS
EVERGREEN SHRUBS			
Abelia grandiflora	Glossy abelia	3–9'	
Artemisia filifolia	Sand sagebrush	3–6'	
Atriplex canescens	Four-wing saltbush	3–8'	
Berberis swaseyi	Texas barberry	3–5'	
B. thunbergii atropurpurea	Barberry	4–6'	
B. trifoliata, syn. *Mahonia trifoliata*	Agarito	3–8'	
Buxus japonica	Japanese boxwood	3–5'	
Choisya dumosa	Starleaf Mexican orange	1–6'	
Chrysactinia mexicana	Damianita	1–2'	
Chrysothamnus nauseosus	Rabbitbrush	2–5'	NTex
Cotoneaster glaucophyllus	Grayleaf cotoneaster	3–5'	All but southernmost Texas
Cupressus arizonica	Arizona cypress	10–25'	All but southernmost Texas
Dasylirion spp.	Sotol	9–15'	Tender NTex
Elaeagnus fruitlandii		6–9'	
Ericameria laricifolia	Larchleaf goldenweed	1–3'	
Euphorbia antisyphilitica	Candelilla	1–3'	Tender NTex
Eurotia lantana	Winterfat	1–3'	
Fallugia paradoxa	Apache plume	2–10'	
Fouquieria splendens	Ocotillo	12–25'	
Hesperaloe parviflora	Red yucca	Leaves 2–3', flower stalks 5'	
Ilex cornuta	Chinese horned holly	6–9'	
I. c. 'Burfordii'	Burford holly	3–5'	
I. c. 'Rotunda'	Dwarf Chinese holly	1–3'	
I. c. 'Rotunda Burfordii'	Dwarf Burford holly	1–3'	
I. decidua	Possumhaw	10–25'	
I. opaca	American holly	10–25'	ETex
I. vomitoria 'Nana'	Dwarf yaupon holly	1–3'	
Jasminum humile	Italian jasmine	6–9'	All but southernmost Texas
Juniperus spp.		3–9'	All but southernmost Texas
Larrea tridentata	Creosotebush	3–10'	
Leucophyllum candidum	Violet silverleaf	2–3'	STex
L. frutescens	Ceniza	4–8'	STex
Leucophyllum spp.	Ceniza, Texas sage	6–9'	W/Central Texas
Lonicera albiflora	White honeysuckle bush	4–10'	
L. fragrantissima	Winter honeysuckle	6–9'	
Nandina domestica		6–9'	
N. d. 'Compacta'	Compact nandina	3–5'	
Nandina 'Harbour Dwarf', 'Gulf Stream', 'Nana'		1–3'	
Nerium oleander	Oleander	10–25'	All but Panhandle
Nolina texana	Sacahuista	1½–2½'	
Opuntia imbricata	Cholla	3–9'	
Opuntia spp.	Prickly pear	1–6'	
Pittosporum tobira	Green pittosporum	6–9'	All but Panhandle
P. t. 'Variegata'	Variegated pittosporum	6–9'	All but Panhandle
P. t. 'Wheeleri'	Dwarf pittosporum	1–3'	S/ETex

BOTANICAL NAME	COMMON NAME(S)	HEIGHT	REGIONS
EVERGREEN SHRUBS cont'd			
Prunus caroliniana	Cherry laurel	10–25'	All but Panhandle
Raphiolepis indica	Indian hawthorn	3–9'	
Rosmarinus officinalis	Rosemary	1–3'	All but Panhandle
Sabal palmetto	Dwarf palmetto	3–5'	All but Panhandle
S. texana	Texas palmetto	10–25'	S/Central Texas
Schaefferia cuneifolia	Desert yaupon	3–6'	
Sophora secundiflora	Texas mountain laurel	10–25'	
Viguiera stenoloba	Skeletonleaf goldeneye	1½–4'	
Washingtonia filifera	California fan palm	10–25'	S/ETex
Wedelia hispida	Zexmenia	1½–3'	Perennial in NTex
Yucca angustifolia	Narrowleaf yucca	Leaves 1–2', flower stalks 2–6'	
Y. rupicola (most winter hardy)	Twisted-leaf yucca	2'	
GROUND COVERS			
Acacia angustissima, syn. *A. hirta* and *A. texensis*	Fern acacia	1–3'	
Ajuga reptans		8–10"	
Artemisia ludoviciana		1–3'	
Berberis repens	Creeping barberry	1–2'	NTex
Calyptocarpus vialis, syn. *Zexmenis hispidula*	Horseherb	8–10"	
Ceanothus americanus	New Jersey tea	1½–5'	
Dalea greggii	Gregg dalea	4–9"	
Dichondra argentea	Silver ponyfoot	2–4"	STex
Hedera helix	English ivy	4–8"	
Liriope muscari		18"	
Oenothera speciosa	Pink evening primrose	1–2'	
Ophiopogon japonicus	Monkey grass	6–8"	
Quincula lobata, syn. *Physalis lobata*	Purple ground cherry	2–6"	
Rosmarinus officinalis	Prostrate rosemary	2–3'	STex
Santolina spp.		1–2'	W/Central Texas
Symphoricarpos orbiculatus	Coralberry, Indian currant	18"–6'	
Trachelospermum asiaticum	Asiatic jasmine	2'	All but Panhandle
T. jasminoides	Confederate jasmine	2'	S/ETex
Tradescantia micrantha	Cherisse	2–6"	
Vinca major	Vinca	2'	
PERENNIALS			
Abronia ameliae	Heart's delight	8"–2'	
Allium stellatum	Prairie onion	1–2'	
Alophia drummondii	Herbetia	4–12"	
Amsonia arenaria	Blue Texas star	12–18"	
Anthericum chandleri	Lila de los llanos	1–3'	
Aquilegia hinckleyana	Hinckley's columbine	18"	

BOTANICAL NAME	COMMON NAME(S)	HEIGHT	REGIONS
PERENNIALS cont'd			
Asclepias tuberosa	Butterfly weed	12–18″	
Aster spp.	Wild blue aster	2–3′	
Berlandiera lyrata	Chocolate daisy, Chocolate flower	1–4′	
B. texana	Green eyes	1–4′	
Callirhoe involucrata	Wine cups	6–12″	
Calylophus spp.		12–18″	
Canna × *generalis*	Garden canna	2–4′	
Cassia roemerana (needs well-drained soil)	Two-leaved senna	1–2′	
Coreopsis grandiflora	Baby sun, Sunray coreopsis	1′	
C. lanceolata	Lanceleaf coreopsis	18–24″	
C. verticillata 'Moonbeam', 'Zagreb'		2–3′	
Cuphea micropetala	Cigar plant	3–4′	E/STex
Echinacea angustifolia	Purple coneflower	18″	
Engelmannia pinnatifida	Cutleaf daisy, Engelmann daisy	18–42″	
Eriogonum wrightii	Perennial buckwheat	12–18″	
Eustylis purpurea	Pinewoods lily	4–12″	
Gaillardia spp.	Indian blanket	18″	
Gutierrezia sarothrae	Snakeweed	12–20″	
Hamelia patens	Firebush	3–5′	S/ETex
Hemerocallis spp.	Daylily	1–3′	
Hibiscus aculeatus	Big thicket hibiscus	2–4′	
Hymenoxys scaposa var. scaposa, syn. *Tetraneuris scaposa*	Four-nerve daisy	1′	
Ipomoea leptophylla	Bush morning glory	18–36″	
Iris fulva × *giganticaeruleu* × *foliosa*	Louisiana iris	3′	
I. xiphioides	Bearded iris	1–3′	
Lantana spp.		1–2′	S/Central Texas
Liatris spp.	Gayfeather	3–6′	
Marshallia caespitosa var. caespitosa	Barbara's buttons	8–18″	
Nemastylis geminiflora	Prairie celestial	4–12″	
Oenothera missourensis	Yellow evening primrose	1′	
Pavonia lasiopetala		3–4′	S/ETex
Penstemon ambiguus	Pink plains penstemon	1–4′	
P. baccharifolius	Rock penstemon	12–18″	
P. cobaea	Wild foxglove	12–18″	
P. harvardii	Harvard penstemon	2–6′	
P. triflorus	Hill Country penstemon	18–24″	
Phlox pilosa	Fragrant phlox	8–12″	
Plumbago auriculata	Blue plumbago	3′	S/ETex
Poliomenta longiflora	Mexican oregano	1–2′	S/Central Texas
Polygala alba	White milkwort	6–12″	

BOTANICAL NAME	COMMON NAME(S)	HEIGHT	REGIONS
PERENNIALS cont'd			
Psilostrophe tagetina	Paperflower	2'	
Ratibida columnaris	Mexican hat	18–36"	
Rudbeckia × 'Goldsturm'		2'	
Salvia coccinea	Scarlet sage	2–3'	
S. engelmannii	Engelmann sage	12–18"	
S. farinacea (tender perennial)	Mealy blue sage	3'	All but Panhandle
S. greggii	Autumn sage	2–3'	W/Central Texas
S. leucantha	Mexican sage	3–4'	S/Central Texas
S. regla	Mountain sage	3–8'	
Sapinaria officinalis	Bouncing bet	1–2'	
Scutellaria wrightii	Shrubby skullcap	6–8"	
Sisyrinchium spp.	Blue-eyed grass	6–12"	
Tephrosia lindheimeri	Tephrosia, Hoary pea	9"	
Teucrium laciniatum	Dwarf germander	3–6"	
Verbena spp.		6–12"	All but Panhandle
Viguiera dentata	Sunflower goldeneye	3–6'	
Viola odorata	Sweet violet	6–8"	
Yucca arkansana	Arkansas yucca	Leaves 1–2', flower stalks 3–4'	
Zephryranthes grandiflora	Pink rain lily	1'	All but Panhandle
ANNUALS			
Amblyolepis setigera	Huisache daisy	1'	
Aphanostephus skirrhobasis	Lazy daisy	12–18"	
Argemone albiflora subsp. *texana*	White prickly poppy	18–24"	
Baileya multiradiata	Desert marigold	9"	
Dithyrea wislizenii (needs sandy soil)	Spectacle pod	18–24"	
Dyssodia setifolia var. *radiata*	Tiny Tim	4–12"	
Eriogonum multiflorum	Wild buckwheat	2'	
Eschscholzia mexicana	Mexican gold poppy	6–12"	
Euphorbia marginata	Snow-on-the-mountain	1–3'	
Eustoma grandiflorum	Texas bluebell, Lisianthus	1'	
Gaillardia pulchella	Indian blanket	1'	
Helenium amarum	Bitterweed	1–2'	
Ipomopsis rubra	Standing cypress	2–4'	
Lepidium montanum (short-lived perennial)	Mountain peppergrass	1–2'	
Linum spp.	Blue flax	1–2'	
Lupinus texensis (four other *Lupinus* spp. are listed, along with this one, as the state flower)	Bluebonnet	1'	
Machaeranthera tanacetifolia	Tahoka daisy	6–12"	
Melampodium leucanthum (perennial south of San Antonio)	Blackfoot daisy	6–12"	

BOTANICAL NAME	COMMON NAME(S)	HEIGHT	REGIONS
ANNUALS cont'd			
Oenothera rhombipetala	Diamond petal primrose	2–3'	
Palafoxia hookerana		2–4'	
Pavonia lasiopetala (perennial in South Texas)		3–4'	
Pectis angustifolia	Limoncillo	9–12"	
Phlox drummondii	Drummond phlox	6–12"	
P. glabriflora	Rio Grande phlox	9–10"	
Psilostrophe tagetina	Paperflower	12–18"	
Rudbeckia hirta (annual or short-lived perennial)	Black-eyed Susan	1–2'	
Sabatia campestris	Meadow pink	9–12"	
Thelesperma filifolium	Greenthread	1'	
Verbena bipinnatifida	Prairie verbena	6–12"	
Xanthisma texanum (needs sandy soil)	Sleepy daisy	12–18"	
VINES			
Antigonon leptopus	Coral vine	40'	All but Panhandle
Bougainvillea spp.		Varies	STex
Campsis radicans	Trumpet vine	30'	
C. r. 'Madame Galen'	Improved trumpet vine	30'	
Ficus pumila	Fig ivy	40'	S/Central Texas
Gelsemium sempervirens	Carolina jessamine	10–20'	ETex
Hedera helix	English ivy	90'	
Lonicera sempervirens	Coral honeysuckle	50'	
Maurandya antirrhiniflora (annual)	Snapdragon vine	6'	
Parthenocissus quinquefolia	Virginia creeper	35'	
P. tricuspidata	Boston ivy	60'	
Polygonum aubertii	Silverlace vine	20–30'	W/Central Texas
Rosa banksiae	Lady Banks' rose	20'	All but Panhandle
R. × bractaeta	Mermaid rose	20'	All but Panhandle
R. setigera	Climbing purple rose	3–6'	
Trachelospermum jasminoides	Confederate jasmine	30'	S/Central Texas
Wisteria spp.		Varies	

Xeriscape Plants for the Southwest

"XERISCAPE landscaping is not just rocks and cactus." This phrase is repeated so often in introductory remarks about Xeriscape gardening that it has almost become a de facto subtitle. I'm hoping that if you've read this far in the book, you already realize the truth of that statement. I've tried to show how lush and green a Xeriscape landscape can be in almost every region.

Now I'll jump to the other side of the fence, and say in the right setting (that is, the desert Southwest), Xeriscape gardening *can* be just rocks and cactus because that's what the land looks like out in the country, in *some* parts of the Southwest. And if it's designed right, a landscape of rocks and cactus can be absolutely stunning. If you doubt me, just visit the Desert Botanical Garden in Phoenix, Arizona (which features over 10,000 varieties of desert flora, including hundreds of different kinds of cacti), and see how mesmerizing it can be.

The point is that even in the desert Southwest, even in the driest part of the country, a Xeriscape landscape can still be green and luxuriant. Whether it be a collection of intriguing cacti, a model of any of the other natural settings in Southwest such as pinyon-juniper mesas, shrubby draws, or piney mountain woods, or even an English-style flower garden, Xeriscape gardening in the Southwest is a lavish affair.

The high desert of New Mexico/southwest Texas, for example, is a lush one. Rabbitbrush (*Chrysothamnus nauseosus*) and creosotebush (*Larrea tridentata*) dot the land as far as the eye can see. It's hard to distinguish much difference between the New Mexican plains and the plains of, say, Wyoming, except that the species of sage and the scurrying animals are different. Where the land is more windswept and barren, cactus and four-wing salt-bush (*Atriplex canescens*) stand firm at regular intervals (evidence of the *very* large root systems some of them send out to mine for water).

As you move from the northeast corner of New Mexico southwest into Arizona and southeastern California, the climate gets warmer and drier (from eighteen inches down to three inches annually in

This striking Albuquerque landscape is designed for low maintenance and low water requirements as well as visual impact. Dry stream beds connect the front and back yards. Near the house desert willows (Chilopsis linearis) preside over grayleaf cotoneaster (Cotoneaster buxifolius), santolina (Santolina chamaecyparissus), and Rocky Mountain penstemon (Penstemon strictus). On the near side of the sidewalk are green santolina (Santolina virens), red yucca (Hesperaloe parviflora), and chamisa (Chrysothamnus nauseosus). (Design: Judith Phillips)

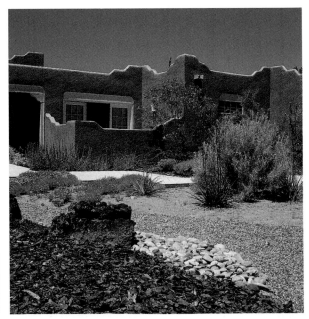

Yuma, Arizona, and in the Coachella Valley/Salton Sea in California). Many small mountain ranges dot New Mexico and Arizona, with typically higher rainfall amounts. In the high mountain areas, especially in New Mexico, general vegetation varies little from that of the characteristic Rockies "look" common from Colorado to Montana.

Because of the diversity of ecosystems in the Southwest, the plant palette for Xeriscape gardens is surprisingly large. There are plants native to the desert, the high plains (or high desert), and the mountains. The differences in "what will grow where" often have more to do with elevation (and therefore minimum temperature during the year) than rainfall. Elevation sets the New Mexican desert apart from the Arizona/Sonoran desert, for instance. Precipitation amounts are similar (about seven or eight inches annually), but because of higher elevation, low winter temperatures average ten to twenty degrees colder in Albuquerque than in Phoenix, so many plants that thrive in Arizona won't survive the "cold" of New Mexico.

Because of the diversity of climates represented, it was impossible to lump the area together into one comprehensive plant list. I have had to content myself with presenting three suggested plant lists, each representative of a typical populated area in the region. The first of the three lists is the most "restrictive." In cold hardiness it is suitable as far north as Albuquerque and, for most of the plants, Santa Fe. (Albuquerque receives an average of eight inches of precipitation annually and experiences a low temperature of about 23 degrees Fahrenheit. In Santa Fe, the numbers are thirteen inches of precipitation and 15 degrees Fahrenheit.) Because elevation plays a part in dictating which plants will be cold hardy in your location, elevation ranges have been included in this list. The list, provided by the New Mexico State University Cooperative Extension Service, was developed by Lynn Ellen Doxon, extension horticulture specialist.

In this list there are three levels of water requirement. The Very-Low-Water Zone corresponds to native and adapted plants in the desert areas of this region, usually receiving an average of ten inches or less annual precipitation. (They will survive on this, but they need a little supplemental watering to keep them looking "ornamental" rather than just gasping along.) The Low-Water Zone corresponds to the high plains areas, which range in annual precipitation from roughly ten to eighteen inches. Plants from the Moderate Zone do best with eighteen inches or more per year (or siting over a high water table). For the true Xeriscape, select plants from the ecological zone you live in. If you choose plants from a higher water zone, realize that you will probably have to continue watering them to some extent for survival even after establishment.

The second list is a smaller one and includes additional drought-tolerant plants usable for landscaping in warmer El Paso (courtesy of John White, county extension agent in horticulture), and the third features some of the plants used in Phoenix for water-efficient landscapes. The fourth list was adapted from the booklet "Lush and Efficient: A Guide to Coachella Valley Landscaping," by the Coachella Valley Water District (P.O. Box 1058, Coachella, CA 92236) and includes plants suitable for Phoenix. Rainfall and/or irrigation allowing, the plants in the first list should grow throughout the desert Southwest, though the reverse is not true, due to cold hardiness.

Because of its cooling effect (both physically and psychologically), turf continues to and probably always will play a part in southwestern landscapes, according to Tucson, Arizona-based landscape architect Mark Novak. Because of the high evapotranspiration rates in the Southwest from most traditional turfgrasses, turf areas are rarely used indiscriminately, or "just for decoration." People will often adopt native or arid vegetation in their front yards and then "create a little visual jewel in the backyard," according to Novak. The turf can do double duty as a play space for small children, or a private area for relaxing and entertaining.

One Albuquerque gardener adopted this strategy. Her front yard features all native vegetation, including scattered flowers and patches of volunteer blue grama grass, and blends very well with the surrounding foothills terrain east of Albuquerque where she lives. A small oval of bluegrass helps cool the north-facing terrace in the back, and runoff from the grass waters a clump of rosebushes just beyond the grass.

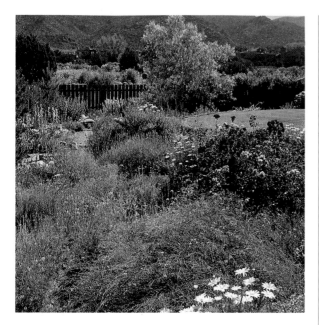

The Xeriscape concept of zoning (grouping plants according to water needs) was put to use in this lavish Albuquerque Xeriscape garden. The small oval of bluegrass cools the owners' back patio, and runoff from the grass waters the roses and Shasta daisies (Chrysanthemum maximum) *adjacent to it. The remaining plants are drought-tolerant New Mexico natives such as blue flax* (Linum lewisii), *prairie coneflower* (Ratibida columnifera), *many* Penstemon *species, and desert willow* (Chilopsis linearis).

A grade change is accomplished with a timber retaining wall, and steps at each end lead down to one of the most beautiful and lavish flower gardens I've ever seen. The dominant flower feature of the garden is a collector-sized variety of penstemons, including showy penstemon (*Penstemon spectabilis*), desert beardtongue (*P. pseudospectabilis*), Rocky Mountain penstemon (*P. strictus*), scarlet bugler (*P. barbatus*), Palmer's penstemon (*P. palmeri*), cardinal penstemon (*P. cardinalis*), pineleaf penstemon (*P. pinifolius*), and narrowleaf penstemon (*P. angustifolia*). Other flowers that have established themselves in her flower garden on a volunteer basis include chocolate flower (*Berlandiera lyrata*), evening primrose (*Oenothera* spp.), and yellow prairie coneflower (*Ratibida columnifera*). Between the flowers and a stunning desert willow tree (*Chilopsis linearis*) that graces the garden, something is in bloom nine or ten months out of the year.

The area receives about nine or ten inches of annual rainfall, and the owner irrigates only the grass lawn (with sprinklers) and the trees and shrubs (with drip emitters). She says the only thing she would change about her landscape is the kind of grass used in the lawn. Because of its high water use and the fact that it must be fertilized, she wishes the bluegrass (the only turfgrass readily available at the time she began her landscape) had been blue grama grass instead. She likes the gray-green color of the grama grass, too, and feels it would have fit in better with the otherwise native theme of her garden. (She would have skipped the roses—which benefit from the runoff from the bluegrass—in that case, or would have installed them in a separate area with drip irrigation.) She says blue grama grass is catching on as a low-maintenance, low-water turfgrass among other new homeowner/landscapers (sometimes needing watering and/or mowing only once a month).

Little or no effort was made to amend the gravelly, sandy soil there with organic matter. After five or six years, some of the perennials have started to "look a little tired," so she's adding organic material to the beds as she refurbishes them. The penstemons, however, thrive in the light, poor soil, and won't grow in a heavy clay soil, so she lets them be.

Lariene Treat installed roughly 2,000 square feet of Xeriscape plants on her "granite rock" site in the Tijaras Canyon east of Albuquerque in May 1990 in response to her severely limited water supply. (The well that serves her home runs dry after less than an hour of drip irrigation.) The only turf area is a fifty-square-foot rim seeded with a buffalograss and blue grama grass mixture around her fish pond. The remainder of the planted area consists of a raised bed and various shrubs, trees, and perennials. The plantings were drip irrigated half an hour a day during the first year, and all are doing extremely well, including volunteer side oats grama, a New Mexico native grass. Other plants included desert willow and golden raintree (*Koelreuteria paniculata*), cherry sage (*Salvia greggii*), big blue sage (*S. azurea*), and Russian sage (*Perovskia atriplicifolia*). Eventually she will fill in the area with a solid mass of color, but even in the second season Treat says her "granite rock is blooming."

These landscapes are good examples of how lush Xeriscape plants can be even in the desert *without* a large investment in water.

A water feature such as a small pond or recirculating fountain can be designed to use very little water. (The water loss from a small fountain may be as low as five gallons per day, which is about the amount of water wasted when someone leaves the water running while shaving or brushing teeth.) The visibility and sound of the water do much to offset the "dry" feeling of an otherwise arid landscape. Water harvesting techniques are especially important here, too. In addition to some of the methods mentioned in the irrigation chapter, you might consider depressing your lawn area two or three inches if you live in an extremely dry area, to make sure that all the rainfall the lawn receives is retained. Be sure to build small berms around trees and shrubs to keep the water they get from running off.

Gravel Mulch

White-rock landscaping seems practically indigenous to the Southwest, even though it doesn't appear anywhere in nature. As you move from New Mexico into Arizona you begin to see gravel on the ground, between plants, but it's usually the same color as the ground (a pinkish gray near Phoenix).

Gravel (or variations or rock mulch) are popular as mulch in the Southwest because they are readily available and because they help stabilize the soil. But gravel has the serious disadvantage of reflecting light and heat back up to any plants growing above it as well as into the adjacent house. It is best used downwind of the house in the prevailing summer wind direction, so that it will not create a heat sink that sends waves of heat into the living area both day and night during the summer. Gravel *can* be installed under deciduous trees upwind of the living area. The trees will block some of the sunlight during the summer, but will allow the rock to store heat during the winter when the branches are bare.

Deciduous vines on trellises can also provide summer cooling while allowing winter heating. Foundation plantings are very useful in desert landscapes because the leaves absorb sunlight, but break it up so it doesn't get reflected back into living areas. Dark-colored plants with small leaves and needles are best at breaking up reflection.

Bark chips are often blown away by the strong winds experienced in some areas. Where wind is a problem, shredded bark is a better choice than chipped bark because the pieces tend to knit themselves together somewhat. An even better alternative is to raise some sort of groundcover planting even if it only gradually replaces the gravel, or to plant windbreak trees or bushes.

Judith Phillips, noted landscape designer, author, and propagator of southwest native plants, often specifies that finely crushed gravel (crusher fines) be used as pathways. She uses bark mulch around plantings, except where water harvesting is being done, and around some mat-forming perennials and ground covers where the mulch may keep the soil surface wet too long and start rot. Examples of these include some *Penstemon* species, ice plant (*Delosperma* spp.), desert zinnia (*Zinnia grandiflora*), and woolly thyme (*Thymus pseudolanuginosus*).

XERISCAPE GARDENING IN THE DRIEST REGIONS

Coachella, California, is located at the western edge of this southwest region near Palm Springs. David Harbison, with the Coachella Valley Water District (he coauthored the booklet mentioned earlier), says the rainfall is so low it's not even considered in figuring watering requirements; all landscape watering is assumed to be irrigation. Harbison cites poor irrigation systems in lawns as the worst water waster. A malfunctioning area in the system leads to a brown patch in the grass, which people then try to green up by overwatering the whole lawn. He recommends Bermudagrass hybrid #328 as being a drought-tolerant cultivar that wears well and doesn't set viable seed. (Common Bermudagrass is invasive even in this desert environment.)

"Lush and Efficient" features a detailed chart of the amount of irrigation water needed to correspond to the plant listings, which has been included with the list. If you live in Phoenix, which does get some summer rains, you can subtract those values out of the table to arrive at a lower water requirement. Harbison noted that the plant list is applicable to the deserts of California, southern Nevada, and Arizona. It features many Sonoran desert plants that tend to be greener than the Mohave desert plants. Southwest natives can provide as much or more color over longer periods than introduced tropical or subtropical plants.

Xeriscape landscaping in the desert is especially challenging because the margin for error is small; if you make a mistake you can pay the price of having to add *large* quantities of water to your plants because the evapotranspiration rate is so high in the heat. Xeriscape gardening is also very rewarding here, too, because a good design will tightly balance the investment in water and plants to provide not only beauty, but also energy savings. Your main concern should be to keep green plants near the home, to take advantage of the cooling effect of the plants as they transpire (using water in the process).

Xeriscape gardening in the desert is very important on the large scale, because of the high cost of importing water. Arizonians in three counties will be helped substantially by the completion of the Central Arizona Project (CAP), which will reach its endpoint about thirty miles south of Tucson in 1992. Phoenix is already using water from this 336-mile-long concrete-lined canal, which imports water from the Colorado River, and water was to be available to Tucson by the end of 1991. Total cost of the project: $3.6 billion.

Tucson is one of the largest cities in the world to be dependent on groundwater. Excessive pumping of groundwater has caused land settling in the valleys north of Tucson, yet the CAP will offset the depletion of groundwater only by sixty percent. The rest will have to be made up by conservation efforts in agricultural and industrial uses, as well as landscaping.

Both Phoenix and Tucson are active in promoting water conservation. For the last ten years Phoenix has requested that all commercial landscaping be at least fifty percent low-water design, and they are attempting to adopt ordinances to that effect. Tucson follows their own suggestions in public landscaping; very little grass is used, for instance, in highway medians, and public buildings are often landscaped in a desert motif. El Paso, Texas, also faces serious water shortages due to groundwater sources not being recharged at the rate they're being depleted, and will have to rely on conservation efforts only. Fortunately, their two-year-old program to promote water conservation in the landscape as well as in other uses had the welcome result of a ten to twelve percent reduction in water demand by mid-1991.

Xeriscape Plants for New Mexico
Very-Low-Water Zone—Desert

BOTANICAL NAME	COMMON NAME(S)	HEIGHT	ELEVATION
DECIDUOUS TREES			
Acacia greggii	Catclaw acacia	20'	to 3,000'
Chilopsis linearis	Desert willow	25'	to 5,000'
Melia azedarach 'Umbraculiformis'	Texas umbrella tree	40'	to 4,000'
Prosopis glandulosa (semideciduous)	Honey mesquite	20'	to 4,500'
DECIDUOUS SHRUBS			
Acacia constricta	Mescat acacia	10–18'	to 6,000'
A. craspedocarpa	Leatherleaf acacia	18'	to 4,000'
Baccharis 'Centennial'		5'	6,500'
B. sarothroides	Desert broom	6–7'	to 6,500'

BOTANICAL NAME	COMMON NAME(S)	HEIGHT	ELEVATION
DECIDUOUS SHRUBS cont'd			
Caesalpinia gilliesii (min. temp. 25°F)	Yellow bird-of-paradise	10'	6,000'
Calliandra spp.	Fairy duster	3'	to 5,000'
Celtis pallida	Desert hackberry	18'	to 5,000'
Chrysothamnus nauseosus	Chamisa, Rabbitbrush	2–5'	2,000–8,000'
Dalea scoparia	Broom dalea	3'	2,000–6,000'
Fallugia paradoxa	Apache plume	2–8'	3,000–8,000'
Fouquieria splendens	Ocotillo	8–25'	to 5,000'
Garrya wrightii	Wright's catclaw	2–8'	3,000–8,000'
Haplopappus laricifolia	Turpentine bush	2–4'	3,000–6,000'
Larrea tridentata	Creosotebush	3–6'	to 6,000'
Parryella filifolia	Dunebroom	2–3'	4,000–6,000'
Parthenium incanum	Mariola	1–3'	2,500–6,000'
Rhus trilobata	Three-leaf sumac	2–6'	3,500–9,000'
R. t. 'Prostrata'	Prostrate sumac	1–3'	3,500–9,000'
EVERGREEN SHRUBS			
Artemisia cana	Silver sage	1½–3'	to 10,000'
A. filifolia	Threadleaf sage, Sand sage	2–5'	to 8,000'
A. tridentata	Bigleaf sage	2–7'	4,500–10,000'
Atriplex canescens	Four-wing saltbush	2–5'	2,500–8,000'
Cowania mexicana	Cliff rose	4–20'	3,000–8,000'
Dasylirion wheeleri	Sotol	3'	to 5,000'
Ephedra viridis	Mormon tea	2–4'	3,000–7,500'
Fallugia paradoxa	Apache plume	3–8'	3,500–8,000'
Leucophyllum fructescens	Texas ranger	5–12'	to 4,000'
Purshia tridentata	Antelope bitterbush	10'	3,500–9,000'
Salvia dorrii	Desert sage	1–3'	to 8,000'
Santolina chamaecyparissus	Lavender cotton, Santolina	1–3'	to 11,000'
S. virens	Green santolina	1–3'	to 11,000'
Vauquelinia californica	Arizona rosewood	20'	2,500–5,000'
Yucca baccata	Datil	3'	4,500–8,000'
Y. elata	Soap tree yucca	6–15'	1,500–6,000'
Y. glauca	Soapweed	4'	to 9,000'
GROUND COVERS			
Anacyclus depressus	Mat daisy	3–12"	3,000–8,000'
Antennaria parvifolia	Pussytoes	6"	7,000–11,000'
Artemisia frigida	Fringed sage	12–18"	4,500–10,000'
Baccharis pilularis 'Twin Peaks'	Dwarf coyotebush	12"	3,000–6,000'
Dalea greggii	Trailing indigo bush	3'	4,000–6,000'
Delosperma nubigenum	Ice plant	1'	3,000–10,000'
Eriogonum umbellatum	Sulphur flower	4–12"	3,000–11,000'
Euphorbia rigida	Spurge	2'	3,000–7,000'
Sedum spurium	Dragon's blood sedum	2–6"	4,000–9,000'
Verbena peruviana		4"	3,000–6,000'
Zinnia grandiflora	Desert zinnia, Rocky Mountain zinnia	8"	3,000–6,000'

Xeriscape Plants for New Mexico
Very-Low-Water Zone—Desert

BOTANICAL NAME	COMMON NAME(S)	HEIGHT	ELEVATION
PERENNIALS			
Amsonia arenaria	Sand stars	2′	4,000–5,000′
Argemone squarrosa	Prickly poppy	32″	3,000–6,500′
Baileya multiradiata	Desert marigold	1–2′	to 6,000′
Berlandiera lyrata	Chocolate flower	16″	4,000–7,000′
Callirhoe involucrata	Poppy mallow	2′	5,000–6,000′
Calylophus spp.	Sundrops	6–20″	4,500–6,000′
Dyssodia acerosa	Needleleaf dogweed	8″	3,500–6,500′
Eustoma grandiflorum, syn. *Lisianthus russellianus* (biennial, sometimes annual)	Tulip gentian	12–18″	4,000–6,500′
Ipomopsis aggregata	Skyrocket gilia	30″	5,000–9,500′
I. longiflora	Blue gilia	2′	4,000–7,000′
I. rubra	Skyrocket	6′	4,000–7,000′
Linum perenne	Blue flax	18″	4,500–9,500′
Lupinus argenteus	Silverstem lupine	8–24″	7,000–10,000′
Machaeranthera bigelovii	Purple aster	5′	4,000–7,000′
Melampodium leucanthum	Blackfoot daisy	6–16″	to 6,500′
Oenothera caespitosa	White evening primrose	10–12″	4,000–7,500′
O. speciosa	Mexican evening primrose	1–2′	3,000–7,000′
Penstemon ambiguus	Bush penstemon	2′	4,000–6,500′
P. cardinalis	Cardinal penstemon	30″	6,000–8,500′
P. crandalii	Crandall's penstemon	10″	6,000–8,000′
P. jamesii	James penstemon	10″	5,000–7,000′
P. palmeri	Palmer penstemon	5′	n/a
P. pseudospectabilis	Desert beardtongue	3′	6,000–7,000′
Psilostrophe tagetina	Paperflower	16″	5,000–7,000′
Ratibida columnifera	Mexican hat	32″	5,000–7,000′
Senecio longilobus	Silver groundsel	18–24″	2,500–7,500′
Sphaeralcea coccinea	Scarlet globe mallow	20″	4,500–8,000′
Talinum calycinum	Flame flower	8″	4,500–7,500′
Townsendia exemia	Easter daisy	1–2′	n/a
Verbena bipinnatifida	Fern verbena	1′	5,000–10,000′
Wyethia scabra	Desert mule's ear	20″	5,000–6,500′
ANNUALS			
Abronia villosa	Sand verbena	2′	
Aster bigelovii (or biennial)	Purple aster	3′	
Linum grandiflorum rubrum	Scarlet flax	12–18″	
Lupinus arizonicus	Arizona lupine	3′	
L. sparsiflorus	Arroya lupine	8–12″	
Sanvitalia procumbens	Creeping verbena	4–6″	
VINE			
Macfadyena unguis-cati	Cat's-claw vine	25–30′	3,000–6,000′

Moderate-Water Zone—High Plains

BOTANICAL NAME	COMMON NAME(S)	HEIGHT	ELEVATION
DECIDUOUS TREES			
Albizia julibrissin var. *rosea*	Mimosa	20′	to 5,500′
Amorpha fruticosa	False indigo	20′	to 6,000′
Catalpa speciosa		80′	to 10,000′
Celtis occidentalis	Hackberry	90′	to 7,000′
C. reticulata	Western hackberry	20–30′	1,500–6,000′
Cercis occidentalis	Western redbud	16′	to 6,000′
Chilopsis catalpa	Catalpa	25′	n/a
Cotinus coggygria	Smoke tree	30′	to 6,000′
Forestiera neomexicana	Desert olive, New Mexico olive	20′	3,000–7,000′
Fraxinus greggii	Littleleaf ash	20′	to 4,000′
Gymnocladus dioica	Kentucky coffee tree	80′	to 8,000′
Koelreuteria paniculata	Golden raintree	20–35′	to 8,000′
Maclura pomifera	Osage orange	50′	to 8,000′
Pistacia chinensis	Chinese pistache	60′	to 6,000′
Prunus virginiana var. melanocarpa	Chokecherry	20′	to 8,000′
Ptelea trifoliata	Hop tree	20′	to 8,500′
Quercus gambelii	Gambel oak, Encino	20–70′	4,000–8,500′
Q. macrocarpa	Bur oak	50–80′	to 8,000′
Robinia ambigua 'Idahoensis', 'Purple Robe'		40–50′	to 7,000′
R. neomexicana	Rose locust	25′	4,000–8,500′
R. pseudoacacia	Black locust	40–80′	to 8,000′
Sapindus drummondii	Soapberry	20–40′	to 6,000′
Sophora secundiflora	Mescal bean	5–20′	to 6,500′
Ulmus parvifolia	Chinese elm	50′	to 8,000′
Ungnadia speciosa	Mexican buckeye	25′	to 5,000′
Vitex agnus-castus	Chaste tree	25′	to 6,000′
Ziziphus jujuba	Chinese jujube	20–30′	to 5,000′
EVERGREEN TREES			
Cupressocyparis leylandii	Leyland cypress	100′	to 6,000′
Cupressus arizonica	Arizona cypress	70′	to 3,500′
Juniperus chinensis 'Columnaris', 'Hetzii', 'Keteleeri', 'Robusta Green', 'Spartan', 'Torulosa'		Varies	to 10,000′
J. scopulorum 'Cologreen', 'Gray Gleam', 'Wichita Blue'	Rocky Mountain juniper	20–50′	5,000–9,000′
J. virginiana 'Hillspire', 'Manhattan Blue', 'Sky Rocket'	Eastern red cedar	40–60′	to 10,000′
Pinus edulis	Pinyon pine	35′	4,000–8,000′
P. eldarica	Afghan pine	100′	to 5,000′
P. ponderosa	Ponderosa pine	60–130′	3,500–9,500′
P. sylvestris	Scotch pine	70′	to 10,000′
Quercus turbinella	Shrub live oak, Encino	5–15′	4,000–8,000′

Xeriscape Plants for New Mexico
Moderate-Water Zone—High Plains

BOTANICAL NAME	COMMON NAME(S)	HEIGHT	ELEVATION
DECIDUOUS SHRUBS			
Amelanchier utahensis	Utah serviceberry	6–15′	4,000–10,000′
Amorpha fruticosa	Indigo bush	4–10′	2,500–6,000′
Anisacanthus wrightii	Hummingbird trumpet	3–5′	to 6,500′
Buddleia davidii var. nanhoensis	Dwarf butterfly bush	3–5′	to 11,000′
Caragana spp.	Peashrub	20′	to 11,000′
Caryopteris clandonensis	Blue mist	2′	to 11,000′
Ceanothus fendleri		3′	5,000–10,000′
Ceratoides lanata	Winterfat	1–2′	to 10,000′
Cercocarpus ledifolius	Curl-leaf mountain mahogany	15–30′	4,000–10,000′
C. montanus	Mountain mahogany	4–12′	3,000–9,500′
Chamaebatiaria millefolium	Fernbush	2–5′	4,000–7,000′
Cotoneaster horizontalis	Rockspray cotoneaster	2–3′	to 11,000′
Fendlera rupicola	Cliff fendlerbrush	6′	3,000–7,000′
Hippophae rhamnoides	Sea buckthorn	30′	to 11,000′
Holodiscus dumosus	Rock spirea	3–6′	5,500–10,000′
Jasminum nudiflorum	Winter jasmine	10–15′	5,000–7,000′
Rhus glabra var. *cismontana*	Cutleaf sumac	3–4′	5,000–7,000′
R. microphylla	Littleleaf sumac	3–6′	2,000–7,000′
Rosa woodsii	Woods rose	4′	5,000–7,500′
Salvia greggii	Cherry sage	3′	5,000–7,000′
Shepherdia argentea	Silver buffaloberry	10–15′	3,000–5,000′
Symphoricarpos albus	Snowberry	2–6′	4,000–10,000′
S. orbiculatus	Coralberry	2–6′	4,000–10,000′
EVERGREEN SHRUBS			
Arctostaphylos pungens	Pointleaf manzanita	3–6′	3,000–8,000′
Berberis thunbergii	Barberry	18″–6′	to 10,000′
Cotoneaster buxifolius	Grayleaf cotoneaster	1–6′	to 7,000′
C. lacteus	Red clusterberry, Parney cotoneaster	6–8′	to 7,000′
C. salicifolius	Willowleaf cotoneaster	15′	to 8,000′
Elaeagnus pungens	Silverberry	6–15′	to 7,000′
Hesperaloe parviflora (min. temp. 25°F)	Red yucca	3–4′	to 7,000′
Rhus glabra	Smooth sumac	20′	to 5,000–7,000′
R. trilobata	Three-leaf sumac	2–6′	to 3,500–9,000′
Sophora secundiflora	Texas mountain laurel	5–20′	to 6,500′
Spartium junceum	Spanish broom	6–10′	to 6,500′
Xylosma congestum (min. temp. 15°F)		8–10′	to 5,000′
GROUND COVERS			
Anthemis nobilis	Chamomile	3–12″	3,000–8,000′
Berberis repens	Creeping mahonia	3–9″	5,500–10,000′

BOTANICAL NAME	COMMON NAME(S)	HEIGHT	ELEVATION
GROUND COVERS cont'd			
Cotoneaster dammeri 'Coral Beauty', 'Eichholz', 'Lowfast'		3–6"	to 10,000'
C. salicifolius var. *repens*	Dwarf willowleaf cotoneaster	6"	to 8,000'
Cytisus decumbens	Creeping broom	8"	3,000–6,500'
Euphorbia cyparissias	Cypress spurge	1'	4,000–9,000'
E. epithymoides	Cushion spurge	12–18"	4,000–10,000'
Gypsophila repens	Creeping baby's breath	4–8"	4,000–11,000'
Juniperus chinensis 'Ames', 'Armstrongii', 'Blue Point', 'Fruitlandii', 'Gold Coast', 'Hetzii', 'Glauca', 'Mint Julep', 'Old Gold', 'Pfitzer', 'Sargent', 'Sea Green'		Varies	to 11,000'
J. horizontalis 'Andorra', 'Bar Harbor', 'Blue Chip', 'Cover-all', 'Emerald Spreader', 'Hughes', 'Prince of Wales', 'Turquoise Spreader', 'Youngstown'		Varies	to 11,000'
J. sabina 'Arcadia', 'Broadmoor', 'Buffalo', 'Scandia', 'Tam'		Varies	to 11,000'
Penstemon caespitosus	Mat penstemon	4"	5,000–11,000'
PERENNIALS			
Allium cernuum	Pink nodding onion	1–2'	2,000–11,000'
Anacyclus depressus	Mat daisy	3–6"	3,000–8,000'
Anemopsis californica	Yerba de Mansa	4–20"	3,500–4,500'
Coreopsis lanceolata	Lanceleaf coreopsis	10–36"	3,000–8,000'
Delosperma nubigenum	Yellow ice plant	1"	3,000–10,000'
Eriogonum umbellatum	Sulphur buckwheat	4–12"	5,000–11,000'
Erysimum asperum	Western wallflower	30"	n/a
Gaillardia grandiflora	Firewheel	2–4'	4,000–6,500'
Gaura lindheimeri		2–4'	3,500–7,500'
Helianthus maximiliani	New Mexican sunflower, Maximilian's daisy	10'	3,000–10,000'
Ipomoea leptophylla	Bush morning glory	3'	to 4,500'
Liatris punctata	Gayfeather	1–3'	5,000–8,000'
Mirabilis multiflora	Four-o'clock	18"	to 8,000'
Oenothera pallida	Pale evening primrose	12–18"	4,000–7,500'
Penstemon alpinus	Alpine penstemon	3'	n/a
P. eatonii	Firecracker penstemon	2'	6,000–7,000'
P. strictus	Rocky Mountain penstemon	2'	8,000–9,500'
Petalostemon purpureum	Purple prairie clover	3'	5,000–7,000'
Phyla nodiflora	Creeping lippia	3'	3,000–5,000'
Potentilla anserina	Silver cinquefoil	2"	6,500–9,500'
Rudbeckia hirta var. *pulcherrima*	Black-eyed Susan	3'	6,500–9,000'
R. laciniata var. *hortensia* 'Golden Glow'		6–9'	6,500–9,000'

Xeriscape Plants for New Mexico
Moderate-Water Zone—High Plains

BOTANICAL NAME	COMMON NAME(S)	HEIGHT	ELEVATION
PERENNIALS cont'd			
Salvia azurea var. *grandiflora*	Pitcher sage	3–4'	3,000–7,000'
S. officinalis	Garden sage	2'	3,000–10,000'
Saponaria ocymoides	Soapwort	6–9"	5,000–10,000'
Silene laciniata	Mexican campion	8–24'	6,500–10,000'
Sisyrinchium bellum	Blue-eyed grass	4–12"	6,000–9,000'
Tagetes lemmonii	Mountain marigold	3'	3,000–5,000'
Tanacetum vulgare	Tansy	3'	3,000–10,000'
Thelesperma megapotamicum	Cota or Navaho tea	32"	4,500–7,500'
Thermopsis montana	Mountain golden pea	1–2'	7,000–10,000'
T. pinetorum	Golden banner	1–2'	7,000–10,000'
Viguiera multiflora	Showy goldeneye	3'	Unknown
Zauschneria californica	Hummingbird plant, California fuchsia	1–2'	to 6,000'
ANNUALS			
Castilleja indivisa	Texas paintbrush	6–12"	
Cleome serrulata	Rocky Mountain bee plant	3'	
Linanthus grandiflorus	Mountain phlox	15"	
Lupinus arizonicus	Arizona lupine	3'	
L. sparsiflorus	Arroyo lupine	1'	
VINES			
Campsis radicans	Trumpet vine	30'	3,000–10,000'
Clematis ligusticifolia	Western virgin's bower	20'	4,000–8,500'
Maurandya antirrhiniflora (annual)	Snapdragon vine	6'	
Parthenocissus inserta	Woodbine	35'	3,000–10,000'
P. quinquefolia	Virginia creeper	35'	3,000–10,000'
P. tricuspidata	Boston ivy	60'	3,000–10,000'
Periploca graeca	Silk vine	40'	3,000–8,000'
Polygonum aubertii	Silver lacevine	20–30'	3,000–8,000'

Regular Watering—Mountains

BOTANICAL NAME	COMMON NAME(S)	HEIGHT	ELEVATION
DECIDUOUS TREES			
Carya illinoinensis	Pecan	100'	to 7,000'
Cercis canadensis	Redbud, Judas tree	40'	to 8,000'
Fraxinus oxycarpa 'Raywood'		35'	to 7,000'
F. pennsylvanica 'Marshall', Summit'		60'	to 10,000'

BOTANICAL NAME	COMMON NAME(S)	HEIGHT	ELEVATION
DECIDUOUS TREES cont'd			
F. velutina 'Fan-Tex', 'Rio Grande', 'Modesto'		40′	2,000–7,000′
Juglans major	Arizona walnut	30–50′	2,000–7,000′
Platanus wrightii	Arizona sycamore	40–80′	to 6,000′
Populus fremontii	Cottonwood	40–80′	to 6,500′
Prunus americana	American plum	30′	to 6,000′
Quercus emoryi	Emory oak	60′	4,000–7,000′
Rhamnus cathartica	Buckthorn	20′	4,000–10,000′
Vitex agnus-castus	Chaste tree	6–25′	2,000–6,000′
EVERGREEN TREES			
Cedrus atlantica	Atlas cedar	80′	to 6,000′
Pinus aristata	Bristlecone pine	20–50′	7,500–11,000′
Pseudotsuga menziesii	Douglas fir	80–200′	4,000–11,000′
DECIDUOUS SHRUBS			
Amelanchier alnifolia	Serviceberry	30′	to 10,000′
Chaenomeles japonica	Flowering quince	2–6′	to 11,000′
Genista lydia	Summer broom	2′	to 4,000′
Potentilla fruticosa	Shrubby cinquefoil	1–3′	7,000–11,500′
Prunus besseyi	Western sand cherry	2–3′	6,000–11,500′
Punica granatum	Pomegranate	20–30′	to 6,000′
Rhamnus frangula 'Columnaris'	Tallhedge buckthorn	12–15′	to 11,000′
Rhus glabra	Smooth sumac	20′	5,000–7,000′
Ribes aureum	Golden currant	2–6′	3,500–8,000′
Rosa foetida 'Austrian Copper', 'Persian Willow'		5–10′	3,000–9,000′
R. rugosa	Rugosa rose	3–8′	3,000–11,000′
Syringa vulgaris	Common lilac	20′	4,000–11,000′
EVERGREEN SHRUBS			
Pinus mugo var. *mugo*	Dwarf mugo pine	2–10′	to 11,000′
Tecoma stans	Yellow bell	20′	to 4,000′
GROUND COVERS			
Convallaria majalis	Lily-of-the-valley	1′	4,500–11,000′
Euonymus fortunei var. *colorata*	Purpleleaf wintercreeper	10″	3,000–11,000′
Galium odoratum	Sweet woodruff	6–12″	4,000–10,000′
Lamium maculatum	Spotted nettle	6″	4,000–8,000′
Paxistima myrsinites	Oregon boxwood	30′	5,000–11,000′
Vinca minor	Periwinkle	6–12″	4,000–10,000′
PERENNIALS			
Achillea millefolium	Yarrow	1–3′	2,000–11,000′
A. taygetea	Moonshine yarrow	1–2′	2,000–11,000′
Agastache cana	Giant hyssop	2′	7,000–10,000′

Xeriscape Plants for New Mexico
Regular Watering—Mountains

BOTANICAL NAME	COMMON NAME(S)	HEIGHT	ELEVATION
PERENNIALS cont'd			
Anthemis tinctoria	Marguerite	2–3'	5,000–10,000'
Aquilegia spp.	Columbine	1–4'	7,000–12,000'
Aster novae-angliae	New England aster	1–4'	3,000–8,000'
Bellis perennis	English daisy	3–6"	3,000–10,000'
Campanula medium	Canterbury bells	3'	4,000–8,000'
Coreopsis lanceolata		10–36"	3,000–8,000'
Delphinium hybrids		15–96"	4,000–11,000'
Dicentra spectabilis	Bleeding heart	18–24"	3,000–11,000'
Echinacea purpurea	Purple coneflower	4–5'	3,000–10,000'
Geum ciliatum	Prairie smoke	4–24"	4,000–6,500'
Helianthus maximiliani	Maximilian sunflower	10'	3,000–10,000'
Heuchera sanguinea	Coralbells	15–30"	3,000–10,000'
Iberis sempervirens	Candytuft	9–12"	3,000–10,000'
Lupinus perennis	Sundial lupine	2'	3,000–10,000'
Mondara spp.	Bergamot	2–4'	3,000–8,000'
Oenothera hookeri	Evening primrose	2–6'	3,000–7,000'
Paeonia officinalis	Peony	2–4'	4,500–11,000'
Solidago hybrids		1–3'	3,000–10,000'
Veronica spicata		10–36"	3,000–10,000'
Viola spp.		4–12"	3,000–7,500'
ANNUALS			
Clarkia unguiculata		1–3'	
Consolida ambigua	Larkspur	1–5'	
Helianthus annus	Sunflower	10'	
Lupinus texensis	Texas bluebonnet	1'	
Nemophila menziesii	Baby blue-eyes	6–10"	
Tagetes spp.	Marigold	6–36"	
VINES			
Clematis jackmanii		12'	3,000–10,000'
C. tangutica	Golden lanterns	9'	4,000–10,000'
Rosa banksiae	Lady Banks' rose	20'	3,000–6,500'

Xeriscape Plants for El Paso, Texas

BOTANICAL NAME	COMMON NAME(S)	HEIGHT
DECIDUOUS TREES		
Cercis canadensis var. *mexicana*	Mexican redbud	10–40'
C. c. var. *texensis*	Texas redbud	10–40'
Chilopsis linearis	Desert willow	25'
Parkinsonia aculeata (semideciduous)	Retama, Mexican paloverde	15–25'
Prosopis glandulosa (semideciduous)	Mesquite	20–30'
P. pubescens	Screw-bean mesquite, Tornillo	10–15'

BOTANICAL NAME	COMMON NAME(S)	HEIGHT
DECIDUOUS TREES cont'd		
Sambucus mexicana (semideciduous)	Mexican elder	10–15'
Sapindus drummondii	Soapberry	10–50'
EVERGREEN TREES		
Juniperus deppeana	Alligator juniper	15–20'
Sophora secundiflora	Texas mountain laurel	6–12'
DECIDUOUS SHRUBS		
Acacia constricta	White thorn	9–15'
Artemisia filifolia (semideciduous)	Sand sagebrush	3–6'
Cassia wislizenii	Canyon senna	4–6'
Choisya dumosa	Starleaf Mexican orange	1–3'
Dalea formosa	Feather dalea	2–3'
Fallugia paradoxa (semideciduous)	Apache plume	2–8'
Quercus turbinella (semideciduous)	Scrub oak	10–20'
Rhus aromatica	Aromatic sumac	3–8'
R. microphylla	Littleleaf sumac	8–20'
Ungnadia speciosa	Mexican buckeye	10–30'
EVERGREEN SHRUBS		
Atriplex canescens	Four-wing saltbush	3–8'
Berberis trifoliata	Agarito, Algerita	3–6'
Dasylirion wheeleri	Sotol	18–42"
Ephedra antisyphilitica	Mormon tea, Joint fir	3–6'
Ericameria larcifolia	Larchleaf goldenweed	1–3'
Fouquieria splendens	Ocotillo	12–25'
Larrea tridentata	Creosote	3–5'
Leucophyllum frutescens	Texas sage, Ceniza	4–5'
Rhus virens	Evergreen sumac	8–12"
Yucca eluta		30'
GROUND COVERS		
Coldenia gregii	Gregg coldenia	1–2'
Commelina spp.	Widow's tears	1–2'
Dicondra brachypoda	Ponyfoot dicondra	2–4"
Gutierrezia sarothrae	Broom snakeweed	12–20"
Hesperaloe parviflora	Red yucca	Leaves 2–3', flower stalks 5'
Pectis angustifolia	Limoncillo	8"
Pennisetum villosum	Hueco mountain grass	1–2'
Trichloris crinita	Three-flowered trichloris	2–3'
Verbena bipinnatifida	Prairie verbena	6–12"
V. canescens	Sweet William verbena	6–18"
PERENNIALS		
Abronia ameliae	Heart's delight	8"–2'
A. angustifolia	Sand verbena	8"–2'
Baileya multiradiata (short-lived perennial)	Desert marigold	9"

Xeriscape Plants for El Paso, Texas

BOTANICAL NAME	COMMON NAME(S)	HEIGHT
PERENNIALS cont'd		
Berlandiera lyrata	Chocolate daisy	1–4'
Liatris punctata	Dwarf gayfeather	1–2'
Melampodium leucanthum	Blackfoot daisy	1'
Oenothera speciosa	White evening primrose	1–2'
Penstemon ambiguus	Pink plains penstemon	1–4'
Polygala alba	White milkwort	6–12"
Psilostrophe tagetina	Paperflower	2'
Ratibida columnaris	Mexican hat	18–36"
Viguiera stenoloba	Goldeneye skeletonleaf	18–24"
Zinnia grandiflora	Plains zinnia	3–9"
ANNUALS		
Eschscholzia mexicana	Mexican golden poppy	1'

Xeriscape Plants for Phoenix/Coachella Valley
Low-Water Zone

BOTANICAL NAME	COMMON NAME(S)	HEIGHT	MINIMUM TEMPERATURE (FAHRENHEIT)
DECIDUOUS TREES			
Acacia penatula (semideciduous)	Sierra Madre acacia	15–20'	20°
Cercidium floridum (semideciduous)	Blue paloverde	25'	
C. praecox (semideciduous)	Sonoran paloverde	20–30'	
Dalea spinosa	Smoke tree	12–20'	20°
Ficus carica	Fruiting fig	15–25'	18°–25°
Jacaranda mimosifolia (semideciduous)		30–60'	20°–25°
Lagerstroemia indica	Crape myrtle	15–25'	
Parkinsonia aculeata (semideciduous)	Ironwood	15–25'	20°
Prosopis chilensis (semideciduous)	Chilean mesquite	25–40'	
P. juliflora var. *velutina*	Velvet mesquite	20–30'	
Vitex agnus-castus	Chaste tree	15–25'	
EVERGREEN TREES			
Acacia craspedocarpa	Leatherleaf acacia	10–15'	18°
A. smallii (evergreen to semideciduous)	Sweet acacia	20–25'	20°
A. stenophylla	Shoestring acacia	25–30'	0°
Ceratonia siliqua	Carob tree	30–40'	22°
Cupressus glabra	Arizona cypress	25'	

BOTANICAL NAME	COMMON NAME(S)	HEIGHT	MINIMUM TEMPERATURE (FAHRENHEIT)
EVERGREEN TREES cont'd			
Eucalyptus camaldulensis	Red gum	60–80'	15°
E. microtheca		30–40'	10°
E. spathulata	Swamp mallee	15–30'	24°
Nerium oleander		12–20'	24°
Olea europaea	Olive	30–40'	18°
Pinus pinea	Italian stone pine	30–50'	20°
Pithecellobium flexicaule	Texas ebony	20–30'	15°
Pittosporum phillyraeoides	Willow pittosporum	15–25'	15°
Prosopis alba (almost evergreen)	Argentine mesquite	25–40'	
Quercus ilex	Holly oak	30–40'	
Q. suber	Cork oak	30–40'	5°
Rhus lancea	African sumac	30–40'	15°
Schinus molle	California pepper	30–35'	20°
PALMS			
Brahea armata	Mexican blue fan palm	20–30'	18°
B. edulis	Guadalupe palm	30'	20°
Butia capitata	Pindo palm	10–20'	
Chamaerops humilis	Dwarf fan palm	10–15'	18°
DECIDUOUS SHRUBS			
Caesalpinia cacalaca	Mexican bird-of-paradise	15'	25°
C. pulcherrima	Red bird-of-paradise	5–8'	25°
Cassia wislizenii	Shrubby senna	3–5'	
Justicia californica (semideciduous)	Chuparosa	2–5'	20°
Tecoma stans var. *augustata* (semideciduous)	Yellow bells	6–8'	24°
EVERGREEN SHRUBS			
Baccharis sarothroides	Desert broom	6–9'	
Bougainvillea spp.	La Jolla bougainvillea	3–4'	32°
Calliandra eriophylla	Fairy duster	3–5'	20°
Carissa grandiflora	Natal plum	5–7'	32°
Cassia artemisioides	Feathery cassia	6–20'	20°
C. nemophila	Bushy senna	4–5'	23°
C. phyllodinea	Desert cassia	3–5'	20°
Dalea pulchra	Indigo bush	3–4'	20°
Dodonaea viscosa	Green hop bush	8–10'	20°
Encelia farinosa	Brittle bush	2–3'	25°
Lantana camara	Bush lantana	2–4'	30°
Larrea tridentata	Creosotebush	5–12'	
Leucophyllum candidum 'Silver Cloud'		3'	5°

Xeriscape Plants for Phoenix/Coachella Valley
Low-Water Zone

BOTANICAL NAME	COMMON NAME(S)	HEIGHT	MINIMUM TEMPERATURE (FAHRENHEIT)
EVERGREEN SHRUBS cont'd			
Leucophyllum frutescens 'Green Cloud', 'White Cloud'		4–6'	5°
L. zygophyllum	Blue ranger	4'	
Muhlenbergia dumosa	Giant mullee	2–3'	24°
M. rigens	Dwarf mullee	18"	24°
Nerium oleander 'Petite'	Dwarf oleander	3–4'	28°
Rhus ovata	Sugarbush	8–12'	20°
Rosmarinus officinalis	Rosemary	3–4'	
Ruellia peninsularis	Blue ruellia	2'	
Salvia greggii	Red salvia	3'	20°
Simmondsia chinensis	Jojoba	3–4'	20°
Tecoma stans	Yellow bells	8–12'	28°
Yucca pendula	Pendulous yucca	6–10'	
GROUND COVERS			
Acacia redolens var. *prostrata*	Prostrate acacia	3–4'	20°
Baccharis sarothroides 'Centennial'		2–3'	
Cerastium tomentosum	Snow-in-summer	6"	
Lantana montevidensis	Purple trailing lantana	18–36"	30°
Oenothera berlandieri	Mexican evening primrose	8–12"	
Rosmarinus officinalis var. *prostratus*	Prostrate rosemary	18–24"	
Verbena tenuisecta	Moss verbena	6–8"	
PERENNIALS			
Baileya multiradiata	Desert marigold	12–20"	
Eschscholzia californica (perennial in this area)	California poppy	1'	
ANNUALS			
Dimorphotheca aurantiaca	African daisy	4–6"	
Lasthenia glabrata	Goldfield	6–12"	
Linum glabrata 'Rubrum'	Scarlet flax	12–18"	
Lupinus odoratus	Lupine	1–2'	
Orthocarpus purpurascens	Owl's clover	6–12"	
VINES			
Antigonon leptopus	Rosa de montana	40'	30°
Bougainvillea spp.		Varies	32°
Ficus pumila	Creeping fig	40'	20°
Macfadyena unguis-cati	Cat's claw	25–30'	

Moderate-Water Zone

BOTANICAL NAME	COMMON NAME(S)	HEIGHT	MINIMUM TEMPERATURE (FAHRENHEIT)
DECIDUOUS TREES			
Bauhinia spp. (semideciduous)	Orchid tree	20′	28°
Lysiloma thornberi (semideciduous)	Feather bush	15–25′	26°
Prunus vesuvious 'Krauteri'	Purple plum	15–35′	
EVERGREEN TREES			
Acacia saligna	Willow acacia	15–25′	20°
Brachychiton populneus	Bottle tree	30–50′	18°
Callistemon viminalis	Bottlebrush tree	15–20′	25°
Citrus spp.		20–30′	28°
Geijera parviflora	Australian willow	15–20′	24°
Grevillea robusta	Silk oak	40–60′	24°
Pinus canariensis	Canary Island pine	30–50′	20°
P. roxburghii	Chir pine	30–40′	20°
Schinus terebinthifolius	Brazilian pepper	25–35′	25°
Vaquelina californica	Arizona rosewood	10–20′	20°–25°
PALM			
Cycas revoluta	Sago plum	4–8′	15°
EVERGREEN SHRUBS			
Asparagus densiflorus	Asparagus	12–18″	30°
Euphorbia milii	Crown-of-thorns	3–4′	32°
Ilex vomitoria	Stokes holly	18–24″	
Juniperus 'Prostrata'	Prostrate juniper	18–24″	
J. sabina 'Tamariscifolia'	Tam juniper	18–36″	
J. 'Seagreen'		4–6′	
Nandina domestica	Heavenly bamboo	5–8′	10°
Philodendron selloum		3–5′	30°
Pittosporum tobira	Wheeler's dwarf	24–30″	20°
Pyracantha spp.	Firethorn		
Thevetia peruviana	Yellow oleander	6–15′	30°
GROUND COVERS			
Fragaria chiloensis	Ornamental strawberry	3–4″	
Gazania spp.		6–12″	28°
Lippia repens		4–6″	
Polygonum capitatum	Pink clover blossom	4–6″	32°
Potentilla verna	Spring cinquefoil	6–12″	
PERENNIALS			
Aquilegia caerulea	Rocky Mountain columbine	3′	
Penstemon eatonii	Eaton's penstemon	4–5′	

Xeriscape Plants for Phoenix/Coachella Valley
Moderate-Water Zone

BOTANICAL NAME	COMMON NAME(S)	HEIGHT	MINIMUM TEMPERATURE (FAHRENHEIT)
VINES			
Bignonia violacea	Violet trumpet vine	8–20′	20°
Gelsemium sempervirens	Carolina jessamine	10–20′	15°
Lonicera japonica 'Halliana'	Hall's honeysuckle	20–30′	
Parthenocissus tricuspidata	Boston ivy	10–20′	
Rosa banksiae	Lady Banks' rose	10–25′	
Tecomaria capensis	Cape honeysuckle	10–20′	30°
Trachelospermum jasminoides	Star jasmine	10–15′	20°
Vitis pomifera	Grape	10–20′	
Wisteria sinensis	Chinese wisteria	10–30′	

High-Water Zone

BOTANICAL NAME	COMMON NAME(S)	HEIGHT	MINIMUM TEMPERATURE (FAHRENHEIT)
DECIDUOUS TREES			
Platanus wrightii	Arizona sycamore	30–40′	10°
Populus alba	Poplar	40–60′	
P. fremontii	Fremont cottonwood	50–100′	15°
EVERGREEN TREE			
Fraxinus uhdei	Majestic beauty ash	25–40′	
PALMS			
Phoenix dactylifera	Date palm	40–50′	20°
Washingtonia filifera	California fan palm	20–50′	15°
W. robusta	Mexican fan palm	50–80′	20°
DECIDUOUS SHRUB			
Rosa spp.	Rose	2–5′	
EVERGREEN SHRUBS			
Euryops virides	Green euryops	3–4′	28°
Raphiolepis indica	Indian hawthorn	4–6′	24°
GROUND COVERS			
Liriope japonica	Giant lilyturf	18″	24°
Ophiopogon japonicus	Mondo grass	6–8″	

Coachella Valley Tree and Shrub Irrigation Guide

For plants identified as high-, medium-, or low-water users in the plant guide.

MONTH	Gallons per day for 18-foot-tall evergreen trees			Gallons per day for 3½-foot-diameter evergreen shrubs			Irrigations per week
	HIGH	MED.	LOW	HIGH	MED.	LOW	
January	7.8	5.3	3.7	0.6	0.4	0.25	1
February	11.3	7.9	5.6	0.9	0.6	0.4	2
March	16.1	11.2	7.9	1.3	0.9	0.5	2
April	22.1	15.4	10.8	1.8	1.2	0.7	3
May	26.8	18.7	13.1	2.1	1.5	0.9	4
June	31.5	22.0	15.4	2.5	1.8	1.1	4
July	31.5	22.0	15.4	2.5	1.8	1.1	4
August	26.1	18.3	12.8	2.1	1.5	0.9	4
September	23.6	16.5	11.6	1.9	1.3	0.8	3
October	16.1	11.2	7.9	1.3	0.9	0.5	2
November	10.1	7.1	4.9	0.9	0.6	0.3	2
December	6.3	4.4	3.1	0.5	0.4	0.2	1

Xeriscape Plants for California

XERISCAPE gardening in California has an urgency shared by few other areas of the country. Although mild and balmy, much of California's climate is technically arid or semiarid. San Francisco, San Diego, and Los Angeles receive only one to two inches of their annual precipitation totals of nine to twenty inches during the May through September months. Landscape plantings through the 1940s reflected that situation, with the use of many native and dry-adapted plants. But the advent of large-scale water projects, which involved much purchasing of water from other western states, turned many of the populated areas of California into lush, water-guzzling oases. The climate, especially in the San Diego area, is so mild year-round (average minimum and maximum temperatures are 47 and 77 degrees Fahrenheit, respectively) that nearly any plant that doesn't need cold can survive there, given enough water.

But population pressure finally outstripped water supplies in the late 1970s and 1980s, with the result that some communities, notably Santa Barbara and San Francisco, were forced to put into effect near-total bans on landscape watering in 1990. Water shortages are particularly acute along the coast of California because some of these communities deliberately didn't join the large-scale state water projects in an effort to control growth. In 1991 some communities were faced with possible restrictions to 300 gallons per day per household, which is just barely enough to cover inside water use for the average family. Virtually none was left over for landscape use.

The result of all this is that Xeriscape gardening is very dynamic in California now; a great deal of experimentation is going on to define the limits of drought tolerance in the landscape plants used

there. The climate and soil are very similar to those of the Mediterranean, so plants from that area and from South Africa, New Zealand, and Australia are among those being tested. San Diego Xeriscape promoters hesitate to commit to one Xeriscape plant list because there are so many variables that figure in, such as amount of sun, soil type, and exposure to wind. Many nurseries are now tagging plants as being water-conserving, and are finding from experience that a large proportion of the plants they carried already fit the bill; they were sometimes just being watered too much.

There are so many Xeriscape demonstration areas in California that it's worth contacting your water department about whether they have one available. Even if you don't live in one of the major cities, there's very likely one nearby.

Steven Davis, a 1990 Xeriscape award recipient in San Diego, found great satisfaction in planning his acre-and-a-half homesite to withstand potential future restrictions in watering. (The area has already been subject to voluntary restrictions.) In his yard, an excellent example of how a large site can be adapted to Xeriscape gardening, Davis made strong use of the concept of zoning. His landscape moves gradually from the local chapparal-type vegetation native to this area eighteen miles inland in the foothills of the Cuyamaca Mountains to small, intensely and scaped areas just adjacent to his house used for entertaining and play.

He carefully studied the coloring, disease resistance, and heights of drought-tolerant cedars and junipers, moving from bluish gray and gray-green tones on the outskirts of the property to brighter greens near the house. Deodar cedar, Atlantic white cedar, Pfitzer junipers, Blue Haven junipers, and Broadmoor junipers were among those used. Bar

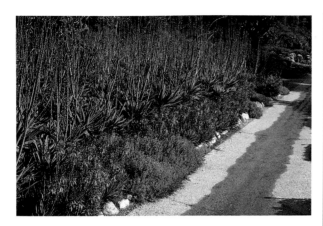

Although the idea of cactus and yuccas are often shunned by Xeriscape enthusiasts, red yucca (Hesperaloe parviflora), with its striking blooms and coarse foliage, offers interest in Xeriscape gardens from California to Texas to Florida. (Photo: Doug Welsh)

Harbor juniper didn't do well for him and the Broadmoor juniper was greener than he liked, but in general these species have fared well.

By using these extremely drought-tolerant evergreen species Davis attempted to create a "piney mountain look," and thus the appearance of having more water around than there really was. Several huge boulders that were on the site originally were left to enhance that effect. Since his site is in the foothills rather than a valley area, Davis used the area around Taos, New Mexico, as a model. Taos is located in a foothills area, too, at the edge of a high desert, with pine forests nearby.

To balance the grayish stone and beige shingles used on his house's exterior, Davis selected plants with more vividly colored flowers as well as foliage near his house. Plants such as bougainvillea ('San Diego Red'), statice (purple), *Raphiolepis indica* 'Clara Springtime' (pink), New Zealand tea tree (*Leptospermum scoparium*) (pink to red), rosea ice plant (*Drosanthemum floribundum*) (red and purple), and knife acacia (*Acacia cultriformis*) (yellow) were used to create a "Gorman painting," modeled after Davis's favorite painter, R. C. Gorman, a southwestern artist whose representational works in the 1980s featured strong pastel colors leaning toward fuchsias, purples, and reds.

Other plants used in Davis's landscape included Dwarf coyote brush (*Baccharis pilularis*), prostrate

acacia (*Acacia redolens*), *Eucalyptus sideroxylon*, *Melaleuca liniafolia* (white), Bailey acacia (*Acacia baileyana*), and ice plant (*Delosperma* 'Hollywood White'; a fire-resistant ground cover). He estimates that five to eight percent of his landscape is in fescue turf. Bermudagrass is a more drought-tolerant choice for San Diego, but the Davises do considerable entertaining, and Davis chose fescue over Bermudagrass because he wanted the year-round green. Bermudagrass goes dormant and turns brown for a while in the winter in San Diego.

A "pre-amended" soil was brought into the site for the plantings farther away from the house as the native soil is very alkaline and rather poor. Amendments included sawdust and gypsum to loosen the soil. Wood chips were used for mulch.

The drought of 1977 left an indelible memory on water districts around San Francisco. As a result, the San Francisco Bay area is now a hotbed of Xeriscape gardening, too. Coastal California is one area of the country where large lawns of traditional thirsty turfgrasses are inappropriate. To publicize this the North Marin Water District, which serves Novato, California (north of San Francisco), offered a $310 rebate to new homeowners who installed no more than 800 square feet of grass or no more than twenty percent of the total "softscape area" (that is, exclusive of patios, walks, decks, and driveways), whichever was less. This was a temporary program in force in the late 1980s, which the district is attempting to reinstate.

Ali Davidson, landscape architect and water conservation consultant located in Petaluma, California, uses water-thrifty plants as the structure, or "bones of the garden," in her designs. She selects low-water trees, shrubs, and vines to serve as the "walls" for the outdoor "rooms," and accents them with a mosaic of richly textured flowering perennials. She designs with bee- and butterfly-attracting salvias (especially the apricot-colored *Salvia brenthurst*, and the rich blues and greens of *S. guaranitica* and *S. superba* 'East Friesland'). Lavatera (*Lavatera thuringiaca*), Matilija poppy (*Romneya coulteri*), and Mediterranean-type plantings such as lavender (*Lavandula* spp.), yarrow (*Achillea* spp.), iris, and thyme (*Thymus* spp.) are drought-tolerant herb-garden favorites. Mexican tulip poppy (*Hunnemannia fulariifolia*) and monkey flower (*Mimulus*

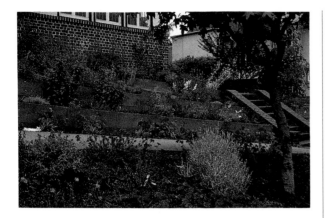

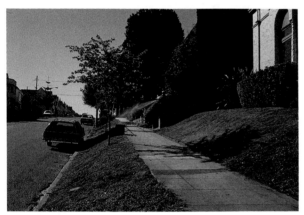

Ali Davidson, landscape architect and water conservation consultant in Petaluma, California, designed these beautiful "Eighth Avenue gardens" for a San Francisco client. Three adjacent homeowners pooled resources to replace threadbare slopes of near-dead grass with these exuberant flowered terraces. The plants were installed in early April 1990 and received only drip irrigation (photographed in July of that year). The second photo of a neighboring yard (with the homeowner hand-watering the dying grass after a summer-long ban on sprinkler irrigation) shows what the yard looked like previously. (Design and photo: Ali Davidson Associates)

spp.) are prized for children's gardens. Arctostaphylos is her favorite native plant, especially 'Dr. Hurd,' an elegant eight-foot-tall tree with nodding snow white bells and red sculpted wood. She favors the native *Prunus lyonii*, a polished green shrub reaching ten to twelve feet in height, for formal hedges, and the brilliantly gold flannel bush (*Fremontodendron* spp.) as an espaliered accent against a warm wall. Davidson likes to combine potato vine (*Solanum jasminoides*), which is evergreen in west-

evergreen in western California, and wisteria for an airy, scented effect. She recommends buying a tree wisteria for trellis and arbor planting in a seven-gallon container, rather than starting smaller, because it will take too long to achieve the desired height.

In California and other arid climates smaller trees are a common element in the landscape because dwarfing is a natural response to drought. Because of the small size of many trees, the distinction between trees and shrubs is very blurred sometimes, and in some cases they may be used interchangeably in the landscape.

California has one of the most diverse sets of climates and vegetation ranges of any state, ranging from desert to moist, cool seaside areas, and montane regions. Fortunately, many of the plants that have been identified as drought tolerant are able to thrive in several regions. The plants on this list are generally adaptable (assuming soil and shade needs have been met) to areas west of the mountains in northern and southern California. This general list is followed by additional plants suited for the southern coastal area around Los Angeles and San Diego, the northern coastal area around San Francisco, and two inland areas that cover roughly the northern half of the San Joaquin Valley (including the cities of Sacramento, Stockton, Modesto, and Merced), and the southern half of the San Joaquin Valley (Fresno, Visalia, and Bakersfield). Plants for the colder, high desert regions east of the Sierra Nevada

Large areas of drought-tolerant perennial flowers are an effective way to reduce watering needs. This bed of gazanias (Gazania rigens) is at the Los Angeles Arboretum. (Photo: Doug Welsh)

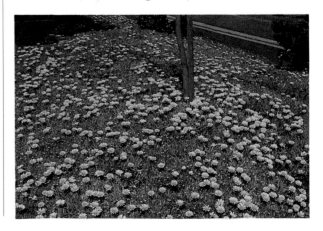

Mountains are included in the Great Plains/Rocky Mountain/Great Basin list, and those for the Mohave Desert (southeastern California) are in the Southwest section.

The southern coastal region corresponds roughly to *Sunset Western Garden Book* Zones 21 through 24, and the northern coastal region to Zones 14 to 17. Inland areas include Zones 7 to 9. The differences in what plants grow where have to do with the temperatures and available moisture of the areas. The southern inland area, for instance, has average annual precipitation of six to ten inches, while the potential evapotranspiration, or ET, is

fifty-two to fifty-six inches per year. The northern inland area receives sixteen to twenty inches of precipitation compared to forty-eight to fifty-two inches of potential ET. These values are at the extreme end. As you move out of the valleys into surrounding foothills, the rainfall amounts rise and the ET stress falls.

Around the San Francisco Bay area rainfall can range from twenty to forty inches per year, while the ET rate is thirty-two to forty inches, so the gap is much smaller. In the southern coastal area rainfall is twelve to twenty inches, and the ET is forty to forty-eight inches per year.

Xeriscape Plants for Western California
Natural Rainfall or Occasional Watering Zone

BOTANICAL NAME	COMMON NAME(S)	HEIGHT
DECIDUOUS TREES		
Ailanthus altissima (almost a "weed" tree, will grow in the harshest site)	Tree-of-heaven	30–50'
Albizia julibrissin	Silk tree	20–35'
Alnus cordata	Italian alder	40'
Fraxinus 'Moraine'	Moraine ash	30–60'
F. oxycarpa 'Raywood'	Raywood ash	40'
Ginkgo biloba cvs.	Maidenhair tree	30–80'
Koelreuteria bipinnata	Chinese flame tree	20–40'
Platanus acerifolia	London plane tree	50'
Prunus spp.		10–45'
Punica granatum	Pomegranate	6–10'
Robinia umbigua 'Idahoensis'	Idaho locust	40'
R. pseudoacacia	Black locust	40–70'
Sambucus spp.	Elderberry	10–18'
Sapium sebiferum	Chinese tallow tree	30'
Sophora japonica	Chinese scholar tree	15–40'
Zelkova serrata	Sawleaf zelkova	40–60'
EVERGREEN TREES		
Acacia baileyana	Bailey acacia	20–30'
A. decurrens	Green wattle	30–50'
A. d. var. *dealbata*	Silver wattle	30–50'
A. longifolia	Sydney golden wattle	20'
A. melanoxylon	Blackwood acacia	30–50'
Brachychiton populneus	Bottle tree	40'
Callistemon citrinus	Lemon bottlebrush	15–25'
Casuarina cunninghamiana	Australian pine	50–70'
C. equisetifolia	Horsetail tree	50'
C. stricta	Beefwood, She-oak	25'

Xeriscape Plants for Western California
Natural Rainfall or Occasional Watering Zone

BOTANICAL NAME	COMMON NAME(S)	HEIGHT
EVERGREEN TREES cont'd		
Cedrus atlantica	Atlas cedar	30–50'
C. deodara	Deodar cedar	40–80'
Ceratonia siliqua	Carob tree	25–40'
Cupressocyparis leylandii	Leyland cypress	20–30'
Cupressus glabra	Smooth Arizona cypress	30–60'
Eriobotrya deflexa	Bronze loquat	15–25'
Eucalyptus globulus 'Compacta'	Dwarf blue gum	25–50'
E. gunnii	Cider gum	40–75'
E. leucoxylon	White ironbark	30–60'
E. microtheca	Coolibah tree	30–40'
E. polyanthemos	Silver dollar gum	30–80'
E. pulverulenta	Silver mountain gum	15–35'
E. rudis	Desert gum	15–30'
E. sideroxylon	Red ironbark	30–50'
E. viminalis	Manna gum	80–150'
Feijoa sellowiana	Pineapple guava	10–20'
Grevillea robusta	Silk oak	50–80'
Laurus nobilis	Sweet bay	15–35'
L. 'Saratoga'	Hybrid laurel	25'
Melaleuca quinquenervia	Cajeput tree	40'
Nerium oleander	Oleander	20'
Olea europaea	Olive	25–35'
Photinia fraseri		8–12'
Pinus canariensis	Canary Island pine	60–80'
P. eldarica	Eldarica pine	40'
P. halepensis	Aleppo pine	25–50'
P. pinea	Italian stone pine	30–60'
P. thunbergiana	Japanese black pine	20–30'
Podocarpus gracilior	African fern pine	40'
Prunus lyonii	Catalina cherry	30'
Quercus ilex	Holly oak	25–40'
Rhamnus alaternus	Italian buckthorn	10–20'
Rhus lancea	African sumac	25'
Schinus molle	California pepper tree	20–40'
S. terebinthifolius	Brazilian pepper tree	15–30'
Sequoia sempervirens	Coast redwood	50–100'
DECIDUOUS SHRUBS		
Buddleia davidii	Butterfly bush	10–12'
Punica granatum	Pomegranate	10–12'
Xylosma congestum	Shiny xylosma	8–15'
X. c. 'Compacta'		3'
EVERGREEN SHRUBS		
Acacia baileyana	Bailey acacia	20'
Arbutus unedo 'Compacta'	Dwarf strawberry tree	6'

BOTANICAL NAME	COMMON NAME(S)	HEIGHT
EVERGREEN SHRUBS cont'd		
Atriplex lentiformis	Quail bush	3–9'
Callistemon citrinus	Lemon bottlebrush	12'
C. rigidus	Stiff bottlebrush	10'
Cassia spp.	Senna	3–5'
Cistus spp.	Rock rose	2–10'
Cotoneaster buxifolius	Bright bead cotoneaster	4–6'
C. congestus		3'
C. lacteus	Red clusterberry	6–10'
Dodonaea viscosa	Hopseed bush	12–16'
Elaeagnus pungens	Silverberry	6–12'
Eriogonum arborescens	Santa Cruz buckwheat	3–4'
E. giganteum	St. Catherine's lace	3–8'
Escallonia exoniensis		5–10'
Eucalyptus macrocarpa	Desert mallee	6–12'
Euryops pectinatus	Golden shrub daisy	3–6'
Feijoa sellowiana	Pineapple guava	10–20'
Grevillea 'Aromas'		5–8'
G. 'Noellii'		3–5'
G. rosmarinifolia	Rosemary grevillea	3–6'
G. thelemanniana	Hummingbird bush	4–8'
Hakea suaveolens	Sweet hakea	10–18'
Hypericum beanii		3–5'
Isomeris arborea	Bladderpod	3–6'
Juniperus chinensis 'Mint Julep'		3'
Lantana camara	Bush lantana, Common lantana	3–6'
Laurus nobilis	Sweet bay	15–35'
Lavandula spp.	Lavender	2–4'
Leonotis leonurus	Lion's tail	6'
Leptospermum frutescens, L. f. 'Compactum'	Texas ranger	5–10'
L. scoparium	New Zealand tea tree	6–8'
Mahonia higginsae		8–12'
M. pinnata	California holly grape	4–5'
M. repens	Creeping mahonia	1–3'
Myrsine africanam	African box	5–8'
Myrtus communis	Myrtle	5–8'
Nandina domestica	Heavenly bamboo	8'
Phlomis fruticosa	Jerusalem sage	3'
Plumbago auriculata	Cape plumbago	5–6'
Podocarpus macrophyllus	Yew pine	10'
Prostanthera rotundifolia	Mint bush	4–6'
Psidium guajava	Guava	15–30'
Pyracantha spp.	Firethorn	10–15'
Raphiolepis indica	Indian hawthorn	3–14'
Rhamnus alaternus	Italian buckthorn	10–20'
R. californica	California coffeeberry	8–12'
Ribes viburnifolium	Evergreen currant	3'
Salvia clevelandii	Cleveland sage	1–3'
S. leucantha	Mexican bush sage	2–3'
S. mellifera	Black sage	2–5'

Xeriscape Plants for Western California
Natural Rainfall or Occasional Watering Zone

BOTANICAL NAME	COMMON NAME(S)	HEIGHT
EVERGREEN SHRUBS cont'd		
Sarcococca ruscifolia	Fragrant sarcococca	4–6'
Tecomaria capensis	Cape honeysuckle	8–12'
Trichostema lanatum	Woolly blue curls	3–5'
GROUND COVERS		
Acacia redolens	Prostrate acacia	24–30"
Armeria maritima (sandy soil)	Sea thrift	8"
Centaurea cineraria	Dusty miller	18"
Ceratostigma plumbaginoides	Dwarf plumbago	6–12"
Chamaemelum nobile	Chamomile	3"
Coprosma kirkii	Creeping coprosma	2–3'
Cotoneaster buxifolius	Bright bead cotoneaster	5'
C. congestus		3'
Gazania spp.		6"
Juniperus chinensis 'Parsonii'	Prostrata juniper	1–2'
J. virginiana 'Silver Spreader'		18"
Lampranthus spectabilis		1'
Lantana montevidensis	Trailing lantana	1'
Oenothera berlandieri (can be invasive if overwatered)	Mexican evening primrose	8–12"
Osteospermum spp.	African daisy	6"–3'
Pyracantha 'Santa Cruz Prostrata'	Firethorn	3'
Sedum acre	Golden moss sedum	¾"
S. sieboldii		6"
Thymus spp.	Thyme	1–12"
Viola odorata (can be invasive)	Sweet violet	6"
PERENNIALS		
Achillea spp.	Yarrow	3–4'
Aster frikartii 'Monch', 'Wonder of Staffa'		2'
Aurinia saxatilis	Perennial alyssum	8–12"
Centranthus ruber	Jupiter's beard	18–24"
Chrysanthemum parthenium	Feverfew	18"
Coreopsis auriculata 'Nana'	Tickseed	3–4"
Crocosmia crocosmiiflora	Montebretia	3'
Erysimum hieraciifolium	Siberian wallflower	18"
Freesia tecolote hybrids		1'
Gaillardia grandiflora	Blanket flower	6"–4'
Geranium sanguineum	Trailing geranium	18"
Hunnemannia fumariifolia	Mexican tulip poppy	2'
Hemerocallis spp.	Daylily	18–24"
Iris douglasiana and hybrids	Douglas iris	12–18"
I. foetidissima	Gladwin iris	18"
Iris hybrids	Bearded iris	2–4'
Lavandula angustifolia	English lavender	3'
L. dentata	French lavender	3'

BOTANICAL NAME	COMMON NAME(S)	HEIGHT
PERENNIALS cont'd		
Lavandula stoechas	Spanish lavender	3'
Lotus scoparius	Deerweed	18"–4'
Mimulus spp.	Monkey flower	1–4'
Nepeta faassenii	Catmint	2'
Origanum dictamnus	Dittany of Crete	1'
Osteospermum spp.	African daisy	2–4'
Penstemon centranthifolius	Scarlet bugler	1–4'
P. heterophyllus	Blue penstemon	1–4'
P. h. var. *purdyi*	Beardtongue	8–24"
P. hybridus	Hybrid penstemon	2–4'
P. spectabilis	Showy penstemon	4'
Rudbeckia hirta	Gloriosa daisy	3–4'
Ruta graveolens	Common rue	2'
Scabiosa columbaria var. *anthemifolia*	Pincushion flower	30"
Tagetes lemmonii	Bush marigold	4'
Tulipa clusiana	Lady tulip	9"
Verbena spp.		1'
Watsonia pyramidata		3'
Zantedeschia althiopica	Calla lily	18"
ANNUALS		
Cleome spinosa	Spider flower	4–6'
Tithonia speciosa	Torch flower	4'

Southern Coastal

See Western California list of plants, pages 243–47, plus:

BOTANICAL NAME	COMMON NAME(S)	HEIGHT
DECIDUOUS TREES		
Koelreuteria paniculata	Goldenrain tree	15–30'
Ziziphus jujuba	Chinese jujube	20–30'
EVERGREEN TREES		
Acacia cyanophylla	Blueleaf wattle	30'
A. pendula	Weeping acacia	20'
A. podalyriifolia	Pearl acacia	25'
Agonis flexuosa	Peppermint tree	40'
Arbutus unedo	Strawberry tree	10–25'
Ceanothus arboreus	Feltleaf ceanothus	25'
C. 'Ray Hartman'		8–16'
Escallonia bifida	White escallonia	15–25'
Eucalyptus calophylla		35–50'
E. camaldulensis	Red gum	60–140'
E. erythrocorys	Red cap gum	15–30'
E. ficifolia	Red flowering gum	40'

Southern Coastal

BOTANICAL NAME	COMMON NAME(S)	HEIGHT
EVERGREEN TREES cont'd		
Eucalyptus lehmannii	Bushy yate	15–25'
Fraxinus uhdei	Evergreen ash	80'
Geijera parviflora	Australian willow	25'
Hakea laurina	Sea urchin	30'
Heteromeles arbutifolia	Toyon	15–25'
Lavatera thuringiaca		10–15'
Leptospermum laevigatum	Australian tea tree	15'
Lyonothamnus spp.	Catalina ironwood	15–45'
Melaleuca armillaris	Drooping melaleuca	10–25'
M. elliptica		8–16'
M. nesophylla	Pink melaleuca	30'
Metrosideros excelsus	New Zealand Christmas tree	20–30'
Myoporum laetum		25–30'
Pinus radiata	Monterrey pine	70–100'
P. sylvestris	Scot's pine	70'
P. torreyana	Torrey pine	20–60'
Pittosporum crassifolium	Karo tree	8–12'
P. phillyraeoides	Willow pittosporum	18'
P. rhombifolium	Queensland pittosporum	15–30'
P. undulatum	Victorian box	35–40'
P. viridiflorum	Cape pittosporum	15–25'
Prunus caroliniana	Carolina cherry laurel	20–40'
P. lyonii	Catalina cherry	15–45'
Psidium littorale	Strawberry guava	15–30'
Quercus agrifolia	Coast live oak	30–60'
Rhus integrifolia	Lemonadeberry	15'
R. ovata	Sugarbush	5–12'
Tristania conferta	Brisbane box	40–70'

DECIDUOUS SHRUBS
See list of Northern Inland deciduous shrubs, page 253.

EVERGREEN SHRUBS
See list of Northern Inland evergreen shrubs, pages 254–55, plus:

Acacia baileyana 'Purpurea'	Purpleleaf acacia	20'
A. cyclopis		10–15'
A. pycnantha	Golden wattle	15–20'
A. redolens		2–4'
A. saligna	Willow acacia	15–20'
A. verticillata	Star acacia	15'
Alyogne huegelii	Blue hibiscus	4'
Arctostaphylos densiflora 'James West'		3–4'
A. franciscana		3'
A. 'Greensphere'		4'
A. hookeri	Monterey manzanita	2–4'
A. pumila	Sandmat manzanita	2–4'

BOTANICAL NAME	COMMON NAME(S)	HEIGHT
EVERGREEN SHRUBS cont'd		
Atriplex nummularia		6–9'
Berberis darwinii	Darwin's barberry	5–7'
Bougainvillea spp.		Varies
Callistemon rigidus	Stiff bottlebrush	10'
C. viminalis	Weeping bottlebrush	15–30'
Cassia spp.	Senna	3–5'
Ceanothus cyaneus	San Diego ceanothus	12'
Cistus corbariensis	White rock rose	2–5'
Dendromecon rigida	Bush poppy	3–8'
Echium fastuosum	Pride-of-Madeira	3–6'
Encelia californica	California encelia	2–4'
Eriogonum arborescens	Santa Cruz buckwheat	3–4'
E. cinereum	Ashyleaf buckwheat	3–6'
E. fasciculatum	Common buckwheat	1–4'
E. giganteum	St. Catherine's lace	3–8'
E. latifolium var. *rubescens*	Red buckwheat	1'
Escallonia exoniensis		5–10'
Grevillea 'Aromas'		5–8'
G. banksii	Crimson coneflower	15'
G. lanigera	Woolly grevillea	3–5'
Isomeris arborea	Bladderpod	3–6'
Leonotis leonurus	Lion's tail	6'
Mahonia higginsiae		8–12'
M. repens	Creeping mahonia	1–3'
Rhamnus californica	California coffeeberry	8–12'
Rhus laurina	Laurel sumac	6–15'
R. ovata	Sugarbush	2.5–10'
Ribes viburnifolium	Evergreen currant	3'
Romneya coulteri	Matalija poppy	4–8'
Salvia clevelandii (southern coastal only)	Cleveland sage	1–3'
GROUND COVERS		
Arctostaphylos edmundsii	Little Sur manzanita	2–3'
A. e. 'Carmel Sur'		9–10"
A. e. 'Danville'		12–15"
A. e. 'Little Sur'		10"
A. 'Emerald Carpet'		10–18"
A. hookeri 'Monterey Carpet'		1'
A. h. 'Wayside'		2–3'
A. 'Indian Hill'		6–10"
A. 'Sea Spray'		10–15"
A. uva-ursi	Bearberry	6–12"
A. u. 'Point Reyes'		18"
A. u. 'Radiant'		6–8"
A. 'Winterglow'		10–15"
Artemisia pycnocephala	Coast sagebrush	1–2'
Atriplex glauca		5–10"
Ceanothus gloriosus	Point Reyes ceanothus	6–24"
C. g. var. *exaltatus* 'Emily Brown'		2–3'

Southern Coastal

BOTANICAL NAME	COMMON NAME(S)	HEIGHT
GROUND COVERS cont'd		
Ceanthus gloriosus var. *porrectus*		18″
C. griseus var. *horizontalis*	Carmel creeper	2–3′
C. g. var. *h.* 'Yankee Point'		2–3′
C. hearstiorum	Hearst ceanothus	6″
C. maritimus	Maritime ceanothus	2–3′
C. rigidus 'Snowball'		3–5′
Ceratostigma plumbaginoides	Dwarf plumbago	6–12″
Cistus salviifolius	Sageleaf rock rose	1–2′
Delosperma alba	White trailing ice plant	6″
Drosanthemum floribundum	Rosea ice plant	6″
Eriogonum crocatum		18″
Hypericum calycinum	Aaron's beard	1′
Lampranthus aurantiacus	Ice plant	1′
L. spectabilis		1′
Lippia canescens		2–3″
Lupinus nanus	Annual lupine	6–24″
Mahonia repens	Creeping mahonia	1–3′
Maleophora crocea	Ice plant (reddish yellow flowers)	
Myoporum debile		12–15″
M. parvifolium		3–12″
Ribes viburnifolium	Evergreen currant	3′
Salvia sonomensis	Creeping sage	6–12″
Trifolium frageriferum 'O'Connor's' (southern coastal only)		6–15″
Zauschneria californica	California fuchsia	1–2′

PERENNIALS

See Low- and Average-Water-Use lists of perennials in the Appendix, plus:

Amaryllis belladonna	Naked lady lily	2–3′
Dietes vegeta	Fortnight lily	2–4′
Diplacus hybrids	Monkey flower	30″
Echium fastuosum	Pride-of-Madeira	4–8′
Erigeron karvinskianus	Fleabane	10–20″
Eriogonum spp.	Buckwheat	1–5′
Euphorbia characias var. *wulfenii*	Spurge	30–36″
Limonium perezii	Sea lavender	18–24″
Pelargonium hortorum (hardy to 26°F)	Common geranium	3′
Romneya coulteri	Matilija poppy	6–8′
Salvia clevelandii	Cleveland sage	4′
S. leucantha	Mexican sage	3–4′
Scilla peruviana	Peruvian scilla	1′
Tulbaghia violacea	Society garlic	18″
Zephyranthes candida	Zephyr flower	1′

ANNUALS

See Low- and Average-Water-Use lists of annuals in the Appendix.

Northern Coastal

BOTANICAL NAME	COMMON NAME(S)	HEIGHT
DECIDUOUS TREES		
Carpinus betulus var. *fastigiata*	Upright European hornbeam	40'
Crataegus phaenopyrum	Washington hawthorn	20'
Koelreuteria paniculata	Goldenrain tree	15–30'
Malus 'Robinson'	Robinson crab apple	25'
Prunus cerasifera cvs.	Purpleleaf plum	25–30'
Pyrus calleryana cvs.	Flowering pear	40'
EVERGREEN TREES		
Acacia cyanophylla	Blueleaf wattle	30'
A. pendula	Weeping acacia	20'
A. podulyriifolia	Pearl acacia	25'
Agonis flexuosa	Peppermint tree	40'
Arbutus unedo	Strawberry tree	10–25'
Brachychiton acerifolius	Flame tree	50'
Ceanothus arboreus	Feltleaf ceanothus	25'
C. 'Ray Hartman'		8–16'
Comarostaphylis diversifolia	Summer holly	6–15'
Escallonia bifida	White escallonia	15–25'
Eucalyptus calophylla		35–50'
E. camaldulensis	Red gum	60–140'
E. erythrocorys	Red cap gum	15–30'
E. ficifolia	Red flowering gum	40'
E. lehmannii	Bushy yate	15–25'
E. leucoxylon var. *rosea*		25'
Fraxinus uhdei	Evergreen ash	80'
Geijera parviflora	Australian willow	25'
Hakea laurina	Sea urchin	30'
Heteromeles arbutifolia	Toyon	15–25'
Lavatera assurgentiflora	Tree mallow	10–15'
Leptospermum laevigatum	Australian tea tree	15'
Lithocarpus densiflorus	Tanbark oak	40–80'
Lyonothamnus spp.	Catalina ironwood	15–45'
Melaleuca armillaris	Drooping melaleuca	10–25'
M. elliptica		8–16'
M. nesophylla	Pink melaleuca	10'
Metrosideros excelsus	New Zealand Christmas tree	20–30'
Myoporum laetum		25–30'
Pinus eldarica	Eldarica pine	40'
P. radiata	Monterey pine	70–100'
P. sylvestris	Scot's pine	70'
P. torreyana	Torrey pine	20–60'
Pittosporum crassifolium	Karo tree	8–12'
P. phillyraeoides	Willow pittosporum	18'
P. rhombifolium	Queensland pittosporum	15–30'
P. undulatum	Victorian box	35–40'
P. viridiflorum	Cape pittosporum	15–25'
Prunus caroliniana	Carolina cherry laurel	20–40'

Northern Coastal

BOTANICAL NAME	COMMON NAME(S)	HEIGHT
EVERGREEN TREES cont'd		
Prunus lyonii	Catalina cherry	15–45'
Psidium littorale	Strawberry guava	15–30'
Quercus agrifolia	Coast live oak	30–60'
Rhus integrifolia	Lemonadeberry	15'
R. ovata	Sugarbush	5–12'
Tristania conferta	Brisbane box	40–70'

DECIDUOUS SHRUBS
See Northern Inland list of deciduous shrubs, page 254, plus:

Eriophyllum staechadifolium	Lizard tail	1–5'

EVERGREEN SHRUBS
See Northern Inland and Southern Coastal lists of evergreen shrubs, pages 254–55 and 248–49, plus:

Berberis thunbergii	Japanese barberry	4–6'
Cytisus praecox 'Warminster'		3–5'
Escallonia exoniensis 'Frades'		6'
Viburnum tinus	Laurustinus	3–20'

GROUND COVERS
See Southern Coastal list of ground covers, pages 249–50.

PERENNIALS
See Western California list of perennials, pages 246–47, and Low- and Average-Water-Use lists of perennials in the Appendix, plus:

Cyclamen hederifolium		6–8"

ANNUALS
See Western California list of annuals, page 247, and Low- and Average-Water-Use lists of annuals in the Appendix.

Southern Inland

See Western California list of plants, pages 243–47, plus:

BOTANICAL NAME	COMMON NAME(S)	HEIGHT
DECIDUOUS TREES		
Carpinus betulus var. *fastigiata*	Upright European hornbeam	40'
Celtis sinensis	Chinese hackberry	30–50'
Dalea spinosa	Smoke tree	15–25'
Elaeagnus angustifolia	Russian olive	15–20'
Juglans spp.	Walnut	20–35'
Lagerstroemia indica	Crape myrtle	10–25'
Malus 'Robinson'	Robinson crab apple	25'
Prunus cerasifera cvs.	Purpleleaf plum	25–30'

BOTANICAL NAME	COMMON NAME(S)	HEIGHT
EVERGREEN TREES		
Eucalyptus niphophila	Snow gum	15–20'
Quercus suber	Cork oak	40–60'
EVERGREEN SHRUBS		
Acacia baileyana 'Purpurea' (all but northern coastal)	Purpleleaf acacia	20'
A. farnesiana	Sweet acacia	15–20'
A. greggii	Catclaw acacia	10'
Calliandra tweedii	Trinidad flamebush	8–12'

PERENNIALS

See Low- and Average-Water-Use lists of perennials in the Appendix.

ANNUALS

See Low- and Average-Water-Use lists of annuals in the Appendix.

Northern Inland

See Western California list of plants, pages 243–47, plus:

BOTANICAL NAME	COMMON NAME(S)	HEIGHT
DECIDUOUS TREES		
Carpinus betulus var. *fastigiata*	Upright European hornbeam	40'
Celtis sinensis	Chinese hackberry	30–50'
Crataegus phaenopyrum	Washington hawthorn	20'
Dalea spinosa	Smoke tree	15–25'
Elaeagnus angustifolia	Russian olive	15–20'
Juglans spp.	Walnut	20–35'
Koelreuteria paniculata	Goldenrain tree	15–30'
Lagerstroemia indica	Crape myrtle	10–25'
Malus 'Robinson'	Robinson crab apple	25'
Pistacia chinensis	Chinese pistache	30–40'
P. vera	Pistachio nut	18–30'
Prunus cerasifera cvs.	Purpleleaf plum	25–30'
Quercus engelmannii	Mesa oak	30–50'
Q. lobata	Valley oak	60–75'
Ziziphus jujuba	Chinese jujube	20–30'
EVERGREEN TREES		
Arbutus unedo	Strawberry tree	10–25'
Ceanothus arboreus	Feltleaf ceanothus	25'
C. 'Ray Hartman'		8–16'
Comarostaphylis diversifolia	Summer holly	6–15'
Eucalyptus calophylla		35–50'
E. camaldulensis	Red gum	60–140'
E. niphophila	Snow gum	15–20'
Geijera parviflora	Australian willow	25'

Northern Inland

BOTANICAL NAME	COMMON NAME(S)	HEIGHT
EVERGREEN TREES cont'd		
Heteromeles arbutifolia	Toyon	15–25'
Pinus thunbergiana	Japanese black pine	20–30'
P. torreyana	Torrey pine	20–60'
Pittosporum phillyraeoides	Willow pittosporum	18'
P. undulatum	Victorian box	35–40'
Prunus caroliniana	Carolina cherry laurel	20–40'
P. lyonii	Catalina cherry	15–45'
Quercus agrifolia	Coast live oak	30–60'
Q. chrysolepis	Canyon live oak	30–40'
Q. suber	Cork oak	40–60'
DECIDUOUS SHRUBS		
Cercis occidentalis	Western redbud	6–16'
Chaenomeles cvs. (northern inland and coastal only)	Flowering quince	2–8'
Cytisus spp.	Broom	1–15'
Lupinus albifrons	Silver lupine	2–6'
L. arboreus	Tree lupine	2–8'
L. chamissonis	Dune lupine	1–4'
Philadelphus virginalis (northern inland and coastal only)	Mock orange	5–9'
Ribes aureum (northern inland only)	Golden currant	3–8'
R. speciosum	Fuchsia-flowering gooseberry	3–6'
Sambucus spp.	Elderberry	10–18'
EVERGREEN SHRUBS		
Acacia baileyana 'Purpurea' (all but northern coastal)	Purpleleaf acacia	20'
A. cultriformis	Knife acacia	10–15'
A. farnesiana (inland only)	Sweet acacia	15–20'
A. greggii (inland only)	Catclaw acacia	10'
Arctostaphylos densiflora 'Harmony'		3–9'
A. d. 'Howard McKim'		5–7'
A. d. 'Sentinel'		6–8'
Artemisia californica	California sagebrush	3–6'
Bougainvillea spp. (vine)		Varies
Calliandra tweedii (inland only)	Trinidad flamebush	8–12'
Ceanothus 'Blue Cushion'		3–5'
C. 'Concha'		6–10'
C. 'Frosty Blue'		16'
C. griseus	Carmel ceanothus	6–8'
C. g. var. *horizontalis* 'Santa Ana'		3–6'
C. g. var. *h.* 'Louis Edmunds'		6–12'
C. impressus	Santa Barbara ceanothus	6–10'
C. 'Joyce Coulter'		3–5'

BOTANICAL NAME	COMMON NAME(S)	HEIGHT
EVERGREEN SHRUBS cont'd		
Ceanothus 'Julia Phelps'		6'
C. 'Mountain Haze'		6–8'
C. purpureus	Hollyleaf ceanothus	2–4'
C. rigidus 'Snowball'		3–5'
C. 'Sierra Blue'		8–12'
Chamelaucium uncinatum	Geraldton waxflower	5–7'
Convolvulus cneorum	Bush morning glory	2–4'
Dendromecon harfordii	Island bush poppy	6–20'
Eucalyptus macrocarpa (all but southern coastal)	Desert mallee	6–12'
Hakea suaveolens	Sweet hakea	10–18'
Leonotis leonurus	Lion's tail	6'
Leptospermum scoparium	New Zealand tea tree	6–8'
Mahonia aquifolium	Oregon grape holly	5–8'
M. 'Golden Abundance'		5–8'
M. pinnata	California holly grape	4–5'
Pittosporum tobira 'Wheeleri'	Wheeler's dwarf pittosporum	1–3'
Plumbago auriculata	Cape plumbago	5–6'
Psidium guajava	Guava	15–30'
Salvia leucantha	Mexican bush sage	2–3'
S. mellifera	Black sage	2–5'
Trichostema lanatum	Woolly blue curls	3–5'
GROUND COVERS		
Atriplex glauca		5–10"
Lupinus nanus	Annual lupine	20"
Mahonia repens	Creeping mahonia	3'
Zauschneria californica	California fuchsia	1–2'

PERENNIALS

See Low- and Average-Water-Use lists of perennials in the Appendix.

ANNUALS

See Low- and Average-Water-Use lists of annuals in the Appendix.

Xeriscape Plants for the Pacific Northwest

THE AREA in Washington and Oregon west of the Cascade Mountains and extending to the Pacific Ocean receives thirty-two to one hundred inches of precipitation each year. Yet, according to Dan Borroff, landscape contractor and low-water plant enthusiast in Seattle, only six to ten of Seattle's thirty-nine inches per year falls as summer rain from May 1 to October 1. This creates a unique situation for prospective Xeriscape gardeners because many of the plants that will survive contentedly with only this moderate amount of summer rain will not tolerate the soggy soils that predominate during the winter months. They often suffer when water around the crown of plants (at the ground line) freezes, causing damage in the plant's tissues.

A drought-tolerant plant list for the Pacific Northwest includes many nonnatives, particularly from the Mediterranean, largely because the natives that are ornamental normally grow along streams and need lots of additional water in a landscape. Incorporation of organic material into the soil is usually essential in the Seattle area because soils tend to be sterile glacial sand, although clayey soils are present, too. Soils are often moderately acid because of the high rainfall rate, so lime is needed to modify the pH for turfgrasses. Borroff often uses grass mixtures for lawns because the weather is too cool for many of the fine-bladed cool-season grasses, and the ones that are drought tolerant are broad-bladed. Perennial ryegrass is successful as a turfgrass, but is only moderately drought tolerant.

Borroff would like to see much more information about Xeriscape landscaping disseminated in his area, but is frustrated by the fact that even though King County (Seattle) has a population of roughly one and a half million, it has only one part-time county extension agent, and even that service may be cut. (He asked us to include the telephone number for the county agent and to urge readers with questions on Xeriscape gardening to call, because the funding for that office is based on the number and subject of the questions it receives. The number is 206-296-3900, or you can write to them at King County Cooperative Extension, 612 Smith Tower, 506 2nd Avenue, Seattle, WA 98104.)

Seattle is expected to grow in population by 300,000 in the next ten years, and there are no additional sources of water available. One reservoir that supplies water could be enlarged, but there is a great deal of opposition to that project. Moderate water rationing has already been experienced. Several islands in Puget Sound draw water from wells on aquifers, which are even now showing saltwater intrusion.

The Seattle Water Department has demonstration gardens with information on Xeriscape gardening. Seattle Tilth, a nonprofit organization dedicated to promoting environmentally responsible gardening and composting, has created several demonstration beds of drought-tolerant plants, including one edible-plant garden.

Gil Schieber, a horticulturist who maintains the demonstration beds on the grounds of the Seattle Tilth headquarters, also collects seeds and experiments on a continuing basis with plants suitable for Xeriscape gardening in the Pacific Northwest. He finds that many traditional Mediterranean plants work well in the Zones 7 to 8 climate typical of the area west of the Cascades. Every few years, though, in Seattle, plant hardiness is tested when the tem-

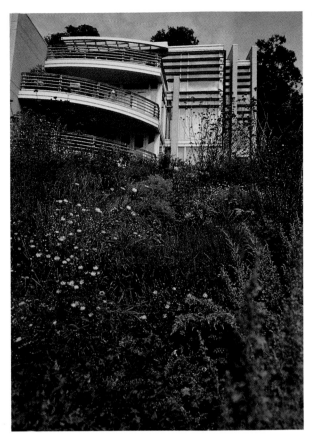

The richly varied texture of this hillside of flowers forms a perfect foil for the ultra-modern lines of this Seattle area residence. (Design and photo: Dan Borroff Landscape)

perature drops down to five to ten degrees above zero (Zone 6). To counteract potential freezing damage during wet winter months Schieber recommends ensuring that the Mediterranean plants, which are not accustomed to wet winters, have "perfect drainage," by installing them in a sandy, or even gravelly, soil base.

Because of his interest in horticulture, Schieber got rid of all the grass in his medium-sized residential lot (seventy-five by one hundred feet) in his first year of experimenting with Xeriscape gardening, replacing it with wood chips and numerous planting beds and areas for testing drought-tolerant plants. He adds that Seattle residents really have no choice but to water their lawns in July and August (at a cost of roughly $3.50/thousand gallons). Expected rainfall amounts for those months are only

an inch each month, and in recent years have averaged one-third of an inch per month.

Rainfall rates for December and January average ten and six inches, respectively. To take advantage of this, Schieber recommends planting perennials and deciduous plants in the fall during the wet season, though evergreens are still planted in early spring.

Schieber's yard is a showcase for drought-tolerant plants, ornamentals, and edible plants. A local hardy plant society comes through on tours, and he participates in semiannual Garden Open Days, a new fund-raising tradition in Seattle similar to those popular in England.

Of the dozens of ornamental grasses and turfgrasses he has tested, Schieber found that *Stipa, Miscanthus, Calamagrostis* (feather reed grass), and fescues, both red and creeping fescue, did well, through *Bouteloua* (blue grama grass) did not. *Bouteloua*, along with many other drought-tolerant plants native to the Southwest, didn't thrive because they need more heat. With summer temperatures reaching only 75 to 85 degrees Fahrenheit, Seattle experiences roughly 2,000 "degree-days" per year (a measure of the total number of hours in a year that the temperature is above a minimal growing temperature of 55 degrees). By contrast, southern California or Arizona might typically have 3,000 to 3,500 degree-days per year. The result is that though many of these plants survive, they just don't grow.

Many of the landscape plants commercially available in Seattle are drought tolerant, although the diversity is limited because growers tend to raise and sell plants that grow quickly. Many other suitable plants are not grown because they are too slow-growing and/or have long taproots that make them hard to transplant. Mail order provides some variety, but for the most part Schieber grows many of the plants he wants to try himself from seeds and cuttings.

He uses a microspray system for irrigation, similar to that used for agricultural and commercial greenhouse purposes, which he turns on every ten days or so. He admits this creates some problems with splashing plants and watering mulch instead of plants, but has found it works better for him than drip irrigation. Water from drip emitters tends to drop straight down through the extremely sandy soil he has, rather than spread out; in sandy soil many more emitters are needed to give good coverage of planting areas and the result is a too-cumbersome and complicated system.

Schieber favors the use of local materials for mulch and soil amendment, and what's plentifully available in the Northwest is shredded tree chips and bark. He says little stone is used for mulch because of the difficulty in keeping stone beds clean and weed-free. The "weeds" he has to pull from his wood chip mulch beds are usually the self-seedlings from his cultivated plants such as moss, thyme, violets, and sage.

Schieber found a unique source of free paving material when his neighbor had a driveway broken up and replaced. He caught the dump truck before it drove away and asked them to leave the fifteen yards of broken concrete pieces with him instead. Schieber set the chunks, which are four inches thick and roughly one and one half feet wide each way (weighing thirty to forty pounds) in a mosaic next to the street to provide a landing area for people getting out of cars. He says they acquire a patina of moss in Seattle's climate and provide a home for plants that grow well in cracks. When constructing a walkway from the pieces, Schieber placed three to five pieces across with the largest in the middle. (Broken concrete pieces can be obtained from street departments or contractors when sidewalks or driveways are being replaced. They should be laid on a bed of sand or gravel to minimize settling and heaving.)

Seattle residents have an excellent resource for gardening made possible by the city's pioneering efforts to promote the recycling of household waste. They have launched several programs for curbside recycling, education of citizens on the joys and how-tos of composting yard waste, and a municipal project to compost the yard waste of those who don't want to compost at home. (Yard waste accounts for a staggering ten to twenty-five percent of landfill volume.) In the first year of operation the composting facility shredded 260,000 cubic yards of raw yard waste and produced 50,000 cubic yards of rich black compost that residents and landscapers can purchase for soil improvement and mulch. This stellar effort at reusing resources (at undoubtedly substantial expense) pointedly highlights what we thoughtlessly throw away when we bag up yard waste to be hauled off to the dump.

ALASKA

Although Alaska's precipitation ranges from 150 inches per year in some narrow areas along its southern coast to near-desert conditions (in terms of precipitation, which is as low as 4.4 inches per year) above the Arctic Circle, most of the state receives precipitation ranging from twelve to thirty inches. Anchorage receives fourteen to eighteen inches each year.

According to Cathy Wright, horticulturist at the Plant Materials Center (Alaska Department of Agriculture) near Anchorage, drought or water short-

Though the colors of some drought-tolerant plants may be subtle, by focusing on shape and size contrasts you can still create an exciting composition. Lamb's ears (Stachys byzantina) *echoes the sweeping curves of spider flower* (Cleome hasslerana) *in the background, and contrasts with the tidy shape of threadleaf coreopsis* (Coreopsis verticillata). *(Design: Post Landscape)*

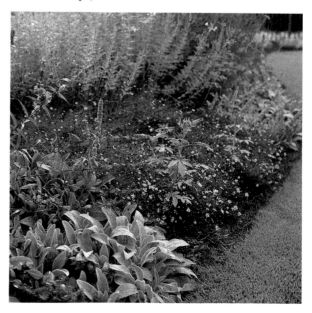

age is not usually a problem for Alaskan gardeners. More of a problem is frost damage, which can occur during extreme short-term fluctuations in temperature. The temperature may rise thirty degrees, for instance, in a few hours, melting snow mulch and bringing plants out of cold dormancy long enough to start moving fluids through their tissues. Then when the temperature drops again, ice crystals form in the plants, damaging them.

When selecting plants, home landscapers are advised to buy native plants adapted to these extreme conditions or to purchase plants from sources located as far north as possible. Mugo pine (*Pinus mugo* var. *mugo*), lilacs (*Syringa* spp.), cinquefoil (*Potentilla* spp.), and natives such as spruce (*Picea* spp.), birch (*Betula* spp.), and lodgepole pine (*Pinus contorta*) do well in that environment. Many gardeners, according to Wright, start plants early in greenhouses because of the very short growing season, bed them out in June, and then go on to grow spectacularly large vegetables and flowers because of the extra sunlight afforded by twenty plus hours of daylight each day.

A tree and shrub list provided by Wright appears at the end of the chapter and is intended primarily for the Anchorage area, which has a different climate than some other areas of Alaska. Summer there is characterized by long periods of drought. Little moisture falls from mid-May through July. Rainfall and increased cloud cover appear in August and September. Newly planted trees and shrubs virtually always need additional watering. In the winter plants are subject to long periods of cold and darkness; temperatures may drop to thirty to forty below zero in some areas. Root systems freeze in October or November, remaining frozen till sometime in April. Because of the harsh climate home landscapers are advised not to try to transplant large native trees, especially white spruce (*Picea glauca*), because the mortality rate is very high.

Xeriscape Plants for the Pacific Northwest

BOTANICAL NAME	COMMON NAME(S)	HEIGHT
DECIDUOUS TREES		
Acer campestre	Hedge maple	25′
A. glabrum	Rocky Mountain maple	24′
A. grandidentatum	Bigtooth maple	18–25′
A. saccharinum	Silver maple	100′
Aesculus californica	California buckeye	15–30′
Ailanthus altissima	Tree-of-heaven	60′
Albizia julibrissin	Silk tree	36′
Aralia elata	Japanese angelica tree	45′
Broussonetia papyrifera	Paper mulberry	48′
Castanea mollissima	Chinese chestnut	60′
Catalpa speciosa	Western catalpa	90′
Celtis australis	European hackberry	75′
C. reticulata	Western hackberry	30′
C. sinensis	Chinese hackberry	60′
Cercis occidentalis	Western redbud	30–40′
Cornus nuttallii	Western dogwood, Pacific dogwood	75′
Cotinus obovatus	American smoke tree	30′
Crataegus spp.	Hawthorn	15–30′
Fraxinus oxycarpa 'Raywood'	Raywood ash, Claret ash	40′
Ginkgo biloba		120′
Juglans hindsii	California black walnut, Hinds black walnut	50′
Maclura pomifera	Osage orange	60′

BOTANICAL NAME	COMMON NAME(S)	HEIGHT
DECIDUOUS TREES cont'd		
Malus sargentii	Sargent's crab apple	25'
Morus alba	White mulberry	45'
M. nigra	Black mulberry	50'
Phellodendron amurense	Amur cork tree	30'
Platanus × acerifolia	London plane tree	100'
Quercus alba	White oak	70–90'
Q. coccinea	Scarlet oak	60–80'
Q. garryana	Garry oak	90'
Q. kelloggii	California black oak	90'
Q. lobata	Valley oak	60–75'
Sambucus caerulea	Blue elderberry	45'
Sorbus spp.	Mountain ash	15–60'
Taxodium distichum	Bald cypress	150'
Tilia tomentosa	Silver linden	90'
Zelkova serrata	Japanese zelkova	90'
EVERGREEN TREES		
Abies concolor	White fir	120'
Acacia baileyana	Bailey acacia	30'
Arbutus menziesii	Madrone	75'
A. unedo	Strawberry tree	10–30'
Calocedrus decurrens	Incense cedar	135'
Cedrus atlantica	Atlas cedar	120'
C. deodara	Deodar cedar	150'
Cercocarpus betuloides	Birchleaf mountain mahogany	5–12'
C. ledifolius	Curl-leaf mountain mahogany	20–30'
Cupressocyparis × leylandii	Leyland cypress	100'
Cupressus arizonica	Arizona cypress	70'
C. glabra	Smooth-barked Arizona cypress	70'
Eucalyptus niphophila	Snow gum	20'
Ficus carica	Common fig	30'
Ilex aquifolium	English holly	70'
Laurus nobilis	Mediterranean laurel	30'
Ligustrum lucidum	Glossy privet	30'
Lithocarpus densiflorus	Tan oak	75'
Photinia serrulata	Chinese photinia	36'
Pinus spp.		30–180'
Prunus laurocerasus 'Otto Luyken'	Otto Luyken cherry laurel	18'
P. lusitanica	Portuguese laurel	6–60'
Pseudotsuga menziesii	Douglas fir	300'
Quercus chrysolepis	Canyon live oak	60'
Q. ilex	Holly oak	60'
Sequoiadendron giganteum	Giant sequoia	300'
Thuja plicata	Western red cedar, Giant arborvitae	80'
Umbellularia californica	Oregon myrtle	75'

BOTANICAL NAME	COMMON NAME(S)	HEIGHT
DECIDUOUS SHRUBS		
Amelanchier alnifolia	Western serviceberry	24'
Aronia arbutifolia	Red chokeberry	4–8'
A. prunifolia	Purple chokeberry	4'
Buddleia alternifolia	Fountain butterfly bush	10–20'
Callicarpa spp.	Beautyberry	2–6'
Calycanthus occidentalis	Western spicebush	4–12'
Ceanothus spp.		2–12'
Chaenomeles spp. and cvs.	Flowering quince	3–10'
Colutea arborescens	Bladder senna	8'
Corylus spp. and cvs.	Filbert	10–20'
Cotinus coggygria	European smoke tree	25'
Cytisus spp.	Broom	1–15'
(*Cytisus scoparius*—Scotch broom— is invasive in southern California)		
Deutzia spp.		5–8'
Elaeagnus spp.	Russian olive	6–20'
Forsythia spp.		2–10'
Genista spp.	Broom	2–20'
Hamamelis spp.	Witch hazel	8–15'
Holodiscus discolor	Ocean spray, Cream bush	3–20'
Kerria japonica	Japanese kerria	4–6'
Kolkwitzia amabilis	Beautybush	10–12'
Lavandula spica	English lavender	1–3'
Ligustrum spp.	Privet	5–15'
Philadelphus lewisii	Western mock orange	4–10'
Photinia × *fraseri*	Fraser photina	10'
P. glabra	Japanese photinia	6–10'
Rhamnus frangula	Alder buckthorn	15–18'
Rhodotypos scandens	Jet bead	4–6'
Ribes aureum	Golden currant	3–6'
R. sanguineum	Red flowering currant	4–12'
R. speciosum	Fuchsia flowering gooseberry	3–6'
Robinia hispida	Rose acacia	6–8'
Rosa eglanteria	Eglantine rose	8–12'
R. harisonii	Harison's yellow rose	6–8'
R. multiflora (considered invasive in some areas)	Multiflora rose	8–10'
Shepherdia spp.	Buffaloberry	6–18'
Spartium junceum (invasive in southern California)	Spanish broom	12'
Vaccinium parvifolium	Red huckleberry	4–12'
Viburnum spp.		4–20'
EVERGREEN SHRUBS		
Aucuba japonica	Japanese aucuba	6–8'
Berberis stenophylla	Rosemary barberry	3–9'
B. verruculosa	Warty barberry	3–4'
Buxus microphylla var. *japonica*	Japanese boxwood	3–4'
Carpenteria californica	Bush anemone	3–6'

BOTANICAL NAME	COMMON NAME(S)	HEIGHT
EVERGREEN SHRUBS cont'd		
Cistus spp. and cvs.	Rock rose	2–5′
Cotoneaster spp.		1–10′
Escallonia spp.		10–15′
Euonymus spp.		6–15′
Garrya elliptica	Coast silk tassel	8–15′
Gaultheria shallon	Salal	2–10′
Halimium ocymoides		2–3′
Ligustrum spp.	Privet	7–12′
Lonicera nitida	Shrubby honeysuckle	6′
Lupinus arboreus	Tree lupine	5–8′
Mahonia pinnata	California holly grape	2′
Nandina domestica	Heavenly bamboo	6–8′
Osmanthus spp.	Osmanthus	10–30′
Paxistima myrsinites	Oregon box	5–10′
Phillyrea latifolia	Mock privet	15–30′
Photinia spp.		6–12′
Phygelius capensis	Cape figwort	3′
Pittosporum spp.		3–10′
Quercus vacciniifolia	Huckleberry oak	2′
Raphiolepis umbellata	Yedda buckthorn	4–6′
Rhamnus alaternus	Italian buckthorn	12–20′
R. californica	California coffeeberry	3–15′
Rhododendron impeditum		1′
Stranvaesia davidiana		6–20′
Taxus spp.	Yew	2–45′
Vaccinium ovatum	Evergreen huckleberry	3–10′
GROUND COVERS		
Ajuga reptans	Carpet bugle	8–10″
Armeria maritima	Common thrift, Sea pink	6″
Calluna vulgaris	Scotch heather	3–4″
Campanula spp.	Bellflower	4–12′
Ceanothus griseus var. *horizontalis* 'Yankee Point'		18–30″
Erica carnea	Heath	16″
E. herbacea		16″
Euonymus fortunei	Wintercreeper	6–18″
Geranium incanum	Cranesbill	6–10″
Hedera helix	English ivy	6–12″
Houttuynia cordata		9″
Myoporum parvifolium		3–6″
Nepeta faassenii	Catmint	12–18″
Osteospermum fruticosum	Trailing African daisy	6–12″
Pyracantha spp.	Firethorn	18″
Rosa spp.		Varies
Rubus calycinoides		3–5″

BOTANICAL NAME	COMMON NAME(S)	HEIGHT
GROUND COVERS cont'd		
Sarcococca hookerana var. *humilis*		18″
Saxifraga stolonifera	Saxifrage, Strawberry geranium	2′
Vinca minor	Periwinkle	6–8″
PERENNIALS		
Aethionema spp.		12″
Allium moly		20″
Amaryllis belladonna	Belladonna lily	18–24″
Brodiaea spp.		10–30″
Calamintha nepetoides		12–15″
Cyclamen neapolitanum		4″
Cynoglossum spp.	Hound's tongue	2′
Dicentra eximia	Fringed bleeding heart	12–15″
Erigeron glaucus	Beach aster	18–30″
Eryngium tripartitum		2–3′
Erysimum spp.	Wallflower	3′
Iris foetidissima	Gladwin iris	18–24″
Lithodora diffusa		6–12″
Phlomis fruticosa	Jerusalem sage	4′
Tallima grandiflora		18–24″
VINES		
Campsis radicans	Trumpet creeper	30′
Clematis armandii	Evergreen clematis	15′
Polygonum aubertii	Silver lace vine	20–30′
Vitis spp.	Grape	Varies
Wisteria spp.		Varies
FERN		
Dryopteris filix-mas	Male fern	6′

Recommended Trees and Shrubs for Anchorage, Alaska

(Listed for cold hardiness rather than drought tolerance)

BOTANICAL NAME	COMMON NAME(S)	HEIGHT
DECIDUOUS TREES		
Alnus crispa	Green alder	2–30′
A. sinuata		2–30′
A. tenuifolia (transplantable only if young plants used)	Mountain alder	2–30′
Betula papyrifera (native varieties more adaptable than those grown commercially)	White paper birch	20–80′
B. pendula var. *gracilis*	White paper birch	60′

Recommended Trees and Shrubs for Anchorage, Alaska

BOTANICAL NAME	COMMON NAME(S)	HEIGHT
DECIDUOUS TREES cont'd		
Malus 'Almey', 'Antonovka', 'Dolgo', 'Hopa', 'Radiant', 'Red Splendor', 'Royalty' (susceptible to sun scald, not salt tolerant, use in protected areas)	Crab apple	20–30′
M. baccata (exceptional winter hardiness)	Siberian crab apple	32′
Prunus maackii (fast growing, very hardy, attractive winter effect; new tree in mass cultivation)	Amur chokecherry	40–50′
P. padus var. *commutata* (very hardy, fast growing)	European bird cherry, May Day tree	40′
P. virginiana (not as attractive and symmetrical as *P. padus*)	Common chokecherry	35′
P. v. 'Schubert' (hardy, fast growing, should be an excellent street tree; easily overwatered, is salt tolerant)	Canada red cherry	20–25′
Sorbus aucuparia	European mountain ash	45′
S. decora	Showy mountain ash	20′
EVERGREEN TREES		
Picea glauca (very hardy)	White spruce	90′
P. g. var. *densata*	Black Hills spruce	40′
P. pungens	Colorado green spruce	80–150′
P. p. var. *glauca* and vars.	Colorado blue spruce	80–150′
Pinus aristata (very slow growing; plant in protected area)	Bristlecone pine	8–10′
P. contorta var. *latifolia*	Lodgepole pine	75′
P. flexilis	Limber pine	80′
DECIDUOUS SHRUBS		
Acer ginnala (very hardy, fast growing)	Amur maple	20′
Amelanchier alnifolia	Saskatoon serviceberry	6–12′
A. canadensis	Shadblow serviceberry, Juneberry	20–30′
A. florida	Pacific serviceberry	6–18′
Betula nana (slow growing)	Dwarf Arctic birch	3′
Caragana arborescens (very hardy)	Siberian peashrub	6–18′
Cornus sericea, syn. *C. stolonifera* (very hardy)	Red-osier dogwood, Red twig dogwood	5–7′
Cotoneaster acutifolius (very hardy)	Peking cotoneaster	5–7′
Elaeagnus commutata	Silverberry	3–12′
Lonicera tatarica	Tatarian honeysuckle	5–10′
Myrica gale (likes peat soil)	Sweet gale	1–4′
Potentilla fruticosa	Potentilla, Cinquefoil	3–5′
Prunus besseyi (foundation planting; marginally hardy)	Western sand cherry	5–6′
P. tomentosa (very hardy)	Nanking cherry	12′
P. triloba	Flowering plum, Rose-tree-of-China	5–6′

BOTANICAL NAME	COMMON NAME(S)	HEIGHT
DECIDUOUS SHRUBS cont'd		
Ribes alpinum (excellent as specimen or hedge plant)	Alpine currant	3–6'
R. grossularia 'Pixwell'		3–4'
R. laxiflorum	Trailing black currant	2–5'
R. nigrum	Black currant	4–6'
R. odoratum	Yellow-flowering clove currant	5–6'
R. sativum 'Red Lake'	Common garden currant	3–5'
R. uva-crispa (very hardy)	Cultivated gooseberry	3–4'
Rosa 'Nutkana' and 'Woodsii'		3–4'
R. rubrifolia (good foliage accent plant)	Red-leaved rose	5–6'
R. 'Terese Bugnet'		5–6'
Rubus idaeus 'Boyne', 'Latham' (annual cleanup necessary)	Raspberry	2–4'
Sambucus racemosa 'Callicarpa'	Red elderberry	4–12'
Shepherdia canadensis	Soapberry	7'
Sorbaria sorbifolia (very hardy)	Ural false spirea, Ashleaf spirea	5–6'
Sorbus scopulina	Greene's mountain ash	15'
Spiraea beauverdiana	Beauverd spirea, Alaska spirea	3'
Syringa chinensis (very hardy)	Chinese lilac	10–12'
S. meyeri (very hardy)	Korean lilac	3–4'
S. oblata var. *dilatata*	Korean early lilac	10–12'
S. patula 'Miss Kim' (may need winter protection)		3–4'
S. persica (very hardy)	Persian lilac	6'
S. prestoniae 'James MacFarlane', 'Pocahontas' (very hardy)		9'
S. vulgaris hybrids (very hardy)	Common lilac	20'
Viburnum edule (very hardy)	Highbush cranberry	8'
EVERGREEN SHRUBS		
Juniperus communis var. *nana* (very hardy)	Common juniper	6–8'
J. horizontalis 'Andorra', 'Bar Harbor', 'Wiltonii', 'Yukon Belle' (specimen planting only, not recommended for mass plantings; subject to winter burn; needs good drainage)	Creeping juniper	1'
J. sabina 'Broadmoor', 'Buffalo' (should not be planted under overhangs; needs snow cover)	Savin juniper	2'
Ledum groenlandicum (does best in peat soil)	Labrador tea	3'
Picea abies var. *nidiformis* (slow growing; subject to winter burn)	Bird's nest spruce	3–4'
Pinus mugo var. *mugo* (slow growing in early years)	Mugo pine	6–8'
P. m. var. *pumilio* (slow growing in early years)	Dwarf mugo pine	2–3'

Xeriscape Plants for Hawaii

XERISCAPE gardening in Hawaii is in an experimental stage, made fascinating by the extreme diversity of rainfall ranges within a relatively small total area. The average annual rainfall on the islands (total area 6,424 square miles, equivalent to a square about eighty miles on a side) ranges from less than ten inches per year (desert) to well over three hundred inches per year (tropical rain forest). On the island of Kauai, Mount Waialeale has received as much as 460 inches in a year, the forty-year mean world record.

Says Chester Lao, hydrogeologist for the Honolulu Board of Water Supply (HBWS), "When I say Honolulu's average rainfall is thirty-five inches per year, it's because that's what it is in downtown Honolulu. But if you go half a mile west [toward the coast] it drops to twenty inches per year!" The phenomenon that occurs in the southwestern United States mainland is similar. Only a small portion of the rainfall generated from ocean evaporation falls on the southern California coastal area. More falls on the mountains of California farther inland, and most of the remaining moisture falls on the Rocky Mountains. In Hawaii this process is telescoped into a distance you could drive in less than half an hour.

The favorite story of Paul Weissich (Xeriscape consultant for the HBWS) about Hawaii's amazing rainfall gradient concerns a botanic garden on the windward (rainiest) side of Oahu for which he was in charge of choosing plants. The 400-acre tract (about two-thirds of a square mile) had a forty-inch difference in average annual rainfall rate from one side to the other (a distance of about four city blocks). The difficulty lay in choosing plants that wouldn't get rained out if they were planted too close to the wet side!

This makes it difficult for water conservation promoters to create meaningful guidelines in terms of plant lists. They are developing a list of plants for annual rainfall ranges of, for instance, ten to thirty inches, thirty to sixty inches, sixty to eighty inches, etc., but haven't yet completed the project.

Weissich notes that Oahu (the third largest Hawaiian island and home of the greatest population concentration) is not currently suffering from any water shortage. "We are simply trying to plan ahead. Population projections for the next ten years show that if present demand per person remains the same, we will begin to have water supply problems. If we can cut back thirty percent on the per capita consumption now, we should be able to supply the future population."

All of the water on Oahu is furnished by groundwater. Because it's lighter, fresh water floats on top of salt water in an inverted "lens" several hundred feet thick beneath the island. The lens is recharged by the massive rainfall generated by the prevailing trade winds. On the island of Hawaii some of the water is supplied by surface reservoirs that occasionally dwindle if rainfall is lower than normal. A few homes on the island of Hawaii have no water service, actually depending on rooftop catchment systems for their supply, and these homes suffer water shortage during low rainfall periods on rare occasions.

Part of Honolulu is classified as a "tropical desert" because it receives forty-five inches or less of rainfall a year, while the evapotranspiration rate may be as high as seventy-five inches per year because of solar radiation. Under these conditions, Lao notes, "without irrigation only xeriphytes [dry-soil-adapted plants] and phreatophytes [plants with their roots in the water table] can survive." (Note: The term "tropical desert" is only a meteorological one, not really reflective of the appearance of the plant cover.)

Fortunately, many excellent native plants fill this bill. Promoters of Xeriscape gardening are making a concerted effort to encourage the use of native plants, for several reasons. For one thing, notes Weissich, they are "the obvious solution" to the landscaping/water supply problem. For another, their use is a "step toward their conservation."

According to Denise DeCosta, information officer at HBWS, Hawaii is "the endangered species capital of the world." Although Hawaii constitutes less than 0.02 of the total U.S. landmass, it contains almost half of the nation's threatened and endangered species. Propagation of natives (not removal from the wild) is encouraged to help reverse that trend. Although the use of native plants in landscaping is still somewhat limited, people are becoming more aware of their value. DeCosta notes that newcomers try to incorporate more of the "island" plants, especially orchids, bromeliads ("plants that look like they're from outer space"), and succulents. Says DeCosta, "Exotics that are not invasive are acceptable." Some of the exotics are also very high-water-requiring plants, so people are encouraged to "zone" those plants together in small areas, and use plants adapted to the natural rainfall for most of the landscape.

"Our biggest challenge," says DeCosta, "is convincing people that the xeriphytes don't need to be heavily watered. We have people even in the high rainfall areas who seem to want to make sure their plants get the most irrigation they possibly can!"

The HBWS maintains an extensive Xeriscape demonstration garden called the Halawa Xeriscape Garden. Hundreds of plants from many parts of the world are being tested there for drought tolerance, how they respond to the intense climate in terms of reaching their ultimate size (sometimes growing *much* larger than in other environments), and their potential for invasiveness. Says DeCosta, "Our initial list of suggested plants for Xeriscape gardens included many that were recommended in other states, especially southern California. But now we

are trying to replace that list slowly with appropriate natives and other tropical plants that do well in our experimental garden." The garden was shown to over 10,000 people in 1990, and a free class offered once a month through the University of Hawaii Cooperative Extension Service is well attended.

Bermudagrass and zoysiagrass are commonly used for lawns, though they may require lots of water (because of the high evapotranspiration rate). St. Augustinegrass, as well as certain drought-tolerant cultivars of Bermudagrass and zoysiagrass, is less needy of moisture. In the "drier" parts of the state (less than sixty to seventy inches of rainfall per year), the best strategy for a Xeriscape landscape may be to replace grass areas with mulch and xeriphytic plants wherever practical. These can include ground covers, for a "green look," and any of the hundreds of striking specimen plants available to Hawaiians. Organic mulches include bark chips or bagasse (plant residue from sugarcane harvest). The use of peat moss or Hawaiian tree fern fiber is strongly discouraged because their use requires the destruction of the plant (while bark chips and bagasse are byproducts of an already-processed plant). Inorganic mulches might be rock or various gravel products. Mulch depth is two to three inches; less for small gravel.

The plant list is taken almost entirely from the list of plants grown at the Halawa Xeriscape Garden, with a few added native plants recommended by Paul Weissich (who has worked with Hawaiian plants since 1957). He stresses that the relative drought tolerance of the plants is variable according to soil type, amount of insolation (sunshine), elevation, etc. Of course, the usual precautions apply: plants will need supplemental watering until established.

Weissich echoes DeCosta's thought that the list of Xeriscape plants for Hawaii will undoubtedly change as the experimental garden continues for a few more years. "Some of the species in the garden are derived from the Pacific Southwest and have already or are in the process of failing in our continuously warm and humid climate."

Natural Rainfall Zone

BOTANICAL NAME	COMMON NAME(S)	HEIGHT
TREES		
Acacia koa, syn. *A. koaia* (better away from dry coasts)	Koaia	100'
Bauhinia blakeana	Hong Kong orchid tree	25'
Beaucarnea recurvata	Ponytail, Bottle palm	30'
Cassia fistula × *javanica*	Rainbow shower	40–50'
Ceratonia siliqua	Carob tree	30'
Clusia rosea	Autograph tree	35'
Delonix regia	Royal poinciana	40'
Dodonaea viscosa	Aalii	25'
Enterolobium cyclocarpum	Earpod tree	100'
Eriobotrya japonica	Loquat	30'
Erythrina sandwicensis	Wiliwili	45'
Feijoa sellowiana	Pineapple guava	25'
Ficus aspera var. *parcelli*	Mosaic fig	25–30'
F. benjamina	Benjamin banyan	50–100'
F. buxifolia, syn. *F. lingua*	Boxwood ficus	90–100'
F. carica	Fig	10–12'
Guaiacum officinale	Lignum vitae	20'
Heritiera littoralis	Looking-glass tree	40–50'
Laurus nobilis	Bay laurel	50–60'
Melia spp.		30'
Olea europaea	Olive tree	25–30'
Samanea saman	Monkey pod	80'
Sapindus oahuensis	Oahu, Soapberry	45'
S. saponaria	Ae, Soapberry	75'
Schinus molle	California pepper tree	25'
S. terebinthifolius	Christmas berry tree	15–30'
Tamarix aphylla	Desert athel	30–50'
SHRUBS		
Abutilon menziesii	Kooloaula	6'
Achyranthes splendens	Hinahina	3–6'
Adenium obesum	Desert rose	6'
Agave attenuata		6'
Anisacanthus thurberi	Desert honeysuckle	3–5'
Caesalpinia pulcherrima	Ohaialii	15'
Carissa grandiflora	Carissa	20'
Clerodendrum inerme	Sorcerer's flower	6'
Clusia spp.	Small-leaf clusia	6–8'
Coprosma repens, syn. *C. baueri*, 'Variegata'	Variegated mirror plant	20' (in Calif.)
Dasylirion longissimum	Bear grass	4–6'
D. wheeleri	Spoonflower	6'
Euphorbia cotinifolia	Hierba mala	15'
Furcraea spp.	Variegated furcraea	10'
Gardenia brighamii	Nanu	15'
G. volkensii	Volken's gardenia	20'
Grewia occidentalis	Lavender star	10'

BOTANICAL NAME	COMMON NAME(S)	HEIGHT
SHRUBS cont'd		
Heliotropium arborescens	Heliotrope	4′
Hibiscus brackenridgei	Mao hau hele	9′
Juniperus chinensis 'Pfitzerana'	Japanese garden juniper	1–2′
Kalanchoe spp.		12′
Lantana camara 'Radiation'		3–5′
L. montevidensis		2′
Malvaviscus arboreus var. *mexicanus*	Miniature Turk's-cap	10–12′
Pittosporum tobira 'Wheeleri'	Wheeler's dwarf pittosporum	20′
Plumbago zeylanica	Iliee	6′
Portulacaria afra	Miniature jade	12′
Punica granatum 'Nana'	Dwarf pomegranate	12–15″
Raphiolepis indica	Dwarf Indian hawthorn	4′
Sansevieria spp.	Bowstring hemp	6′
Serissa japonica		6′
Sesbania tomentosa (does well in coastal salt areas)	Ohai	2–3′
Strelitzia reginae var. *juncea*	Bird-of-paradise	5′
Tradescantia spathacea	Oyster plant	10–12″
Wikstroemia uva-ursi	Akia	3′
Yucca aloifolia	Spanish bayonet	15–20′
GROUND COVERS		
Aptenia cordifolia	Hearts-and-flowers	4–6″
Asparagus densiflorus 'Myers'	Foxtail asparagus	2′
A. d. 'Sprengeri'	Sprenger asparagus	2′
Boerhavia diffusa (good on coastal dunes)	Alena	3–6″
Bougainvillea 'Crimson Jewel'		Vine
Carissa grandiflora var. *prostrata*	Creeping natal palm	1′
Carpobrotus edulis	Giant ice plant	2–3′
Heliotropium anamalum (good on coastal dunes)	Hinahina	2–4″
Hibiscus calyphyllus, syn. *H. rockii*	Rock's hibiscus	2′
H. 'Carnation'	Carnation hibiscus	6–9′
Jacquemontia ovalifolia subsp. *sandwicensis* (good on coastal dunes)	Pau-o-hiiaka	1″
Jasminum sambac 'Grand Duke of Tuscany'	Giant pikake	4′
Juniperus chinensis 'Procumbens'	Japanese garden juniper	1–2′
Kalanchoe 'Cinnabar'		
Lantana 'Gold Mound'		2′
Lipochaeta integrifolia (good on coastal dunes)	Nehe	3–6″
Lippia graveolens	Mexican oregano	2–3′
Origanum vulgare	Wild marjoram	30″
Plectranthus amboinicus	Wheeler's dwarf	1–2′
Punica granatum 'Nana'	Dwarf pomegranate	6′
Rosmarinus officinalis var. *prostratus*	Creeping rosemary	1–2′
Sedum spp.		3–18″
Sida fallax	Ilima papa	2″
Stapelia nobilis	Giant carrion flower	10″

Xeriscape Plants for Hawaii
Natural Rainfall Zone

BOTANICAL NAME	COMMON NAME(S)	HEIGHT
GROUND COVERS cont'd		
Tecoma capensis	Cape honeysuckle	3–4'
Tradescantia spathacea	Oyster plant	10–12"
PERENNIALS		
Agapanthus africanus	Lily-of-the-Nile	20"
Crassula argentea	Jade plant	6'
Epidendrum spp.		3–4'
Euphorbia milii	Crown-of-thorns	1–3'
VINES		
Antigonon leptopus	Mexican creeper	40'
Bauhinia punctata	Red bauhinia	10'
Bougainvillea 'Jamaica White'		10–13'
B. 'Rosenka'		10–13'
Lonicera japonica	Japanese honeysuckle	20–30'
L. j. 'Purpurea'	Purple honeysuckle	20–30'
Macfadyena unguis-cati	Cat's-claw climber	25–30'
Podranea ricasoliana	Pink trumpet vine	20'
Vitis labrusca	Fox grape	35'
V. vinifera	Wine grape	6–13'

Occasional Watering Zone

BOTANICAL NAME	COMMON NAME(S)	HEIGHT
TREES		
Aleurites moluccana	Kukui	40'
Brexia madagascariensis	Brexia	30'
Caesalpinia ferrea	Brazilian ironwood	50'
Cordia subcordata	Kou	30'
Erythrina variegata 'Tropic of Coral'	Tropic coral wiliwili	40–50'
E. v. var. *orientalis*	Coral tree	30'
Hibiscus waimae (needs 50–60" of rainfall)	Koki o ke oke o	30'
Metrosiderous polymorphus (best with 50 +" of rainfall, but will survive on less)	Ohi a lehua	100'
Murraya koenigii	Curry tree	12–15'
Plumeria hybrids		40'
Pseudobombax ellipticum	Shaving brush tree	35'
Tabebuia chrysantha	Trumpet tree	60–90'
Terminalia bursarina	Bendee	20–25'

BOTANICAL NAME	COMMON NAME(S)	HEIGHT
SHRUBS		
Calliandra spp.	Haole lehua	6–15′
Cuphea hyssopifolia	False heather	1–2′
C. micropetala, syn. *C. salvadorensis* and *C. subuligera*	Cigar flower	3′
Cycas revoluta	Sago palm	10′
Ficus deltoidea	Mistletoe fig	6′
F. microcarpa var. *crassifolia*	Taiwan ficus	10′
Hibiscus arnottianus subsp. *immaculatus* (needs 50–60″ of rainfall)		12′
H. kokio (needs 50–60″ of rainfall)	Kokioula	10′
H. schizopetalus 'Pagoda'	Coral hibiscus	12′
Nandina domestica	Heavenly bamboo	10′
N. d. var. *compacta nana*	Dwarf nandina	1–3′
Plumbago auriculata	Cape leadwort	6′
Turnera ulmifolia	Yellow alder	1–3′
GROUND COVERS		
Aspidistra elatior 'Variegata'	Variegated cast iron plant	1′
Gardenia jasminoides 'Prostrata'	Creeping gardenia	2′
Ophiopogon japonicus	Mondo grass	1′
Psilotum nudum	Moa	1′
Russelia equisetiformis	Coral plant	4′
PERENNIALS		
Crinum amabile	Spider lily	6′
C. asiaticum		2–6′
Hibiscus schizopetalus	Pagoda hibiscus	8–12′
VINES		
Bougainvillea 'Temple Fire'		6′
Pyrostegia venusta	Flame vine	6′
Schefflera arboricola compacta 'Hawaiian Elf'		10′
Tristellateia australasiae	Bagnit	6–10′

APPENDIXES

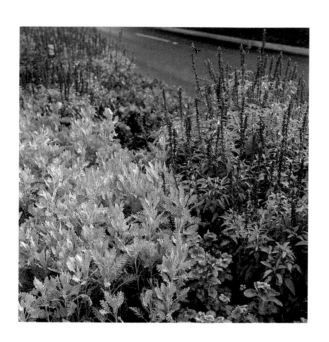

Annuals for Xeriscape Landscaping

Low to Very Low Water Use or Dry Soil

COOL SEASON ANNUALS

BOTANICAL NAME	COMMON NAME(S)	COLOR(S)	HEIGHT
Abronia umbellata	Sand verbena	Pink	6–24″
Baileya multiradiata	Desert marigold	Yellow	20″
Brachycome iberidifolia	Swan River daisy	Blue, white, rose	8–18″
Calandrinia umbellata	Rock purslane	Pink	6″
Centaurium erythraea	Centaury	Pink	20″
Collinsia grandiflora	Blue-lips	White, purple	8–15″
C. heterophyllya		White, rose, purple	1–2′
Consolida ambigua	Rocket larkspur	Violet, rose, pink, blue, white	1–2′
Cynoglossum amabile 'Blanche Burpee'		Blue	18–24″
Dianthus armeria	Deptford pink	Pink	16″
Dimorphotheca pluvialis	Cape marigold	White	16″
D. sinuata		White	1′
Dyssodia tenuiloba	Dahlberg daisy	Yellow	8–12″
Echium lycopsis	Viper's bugloss	Blue, white, lavender, purple, rose	2′
Emilia javanica	Tassel flower	Red	1–2′
Erodium cicutarium	Pin-clover, Alfilaria, Filaree	Pink	18″
Erysimum linifolium	Alpine wallflower	Pink, lilac, mauve, yellow	6–18″
E. perofskianum		Yellow	2′
Eschscholzia californica	California poppy	Yellow	8–12″
Felicia amelloides	Blue marguerite	Blue, purple	1–3′
F. bergerana	Kingfisher daisy	Blue	4–8″
Lavatera trimestris		Pink	2–3′
Matricaria recutita	German camomile	White	12–30″
Mesembryanthemum crystallinum	Ice plant	Pink, white	6″
Monarda citriodora	Horsemint, Lemonmint	Purple	12–18″
Myosotis sylvatica	Forget-me-not	Blue, pink, white	6–18″
Nemophila maculata	Five spot	White, blue	1′
N. menziesii	Baby blue-eyes	Blue	1′

Low to Very Low Water Use or Dry Soil

COOL SEASON ANNUALS (cont'd)

BOTANICAL NAME	COMMON NAME(S)	COLOR(S)	HEIGHT
Papaver nudicaule	Iceland poppy	Red, yellow, orange, white	1′
P. rhoeas	Corn poppy, Flanders poppy	Red	3′
P. somniferum	Opium poppy	Red	3–4′
Phacelia campanularia	California bluebell	Blue	8″
Venidium fastuosum	Cape daisy	Yellow	2–3′
Xanthisma texana	Sleepy daisy, Star-of-Texas	Yellow	2–4′

WARM SEASON ANNUALS

BOTANICAL NAME	COMMON NAME(S)	COLOR(S)	HEIGHT
Actinotus helianthi	Flannelflower	White	2′
Cassia fasciculata	Partridge pea	Yellow	18″
Cleome hasslerana	Spider flower	Pink, rose-purple, white	4–5′
Cosmos bipinnatus	Garden cosmos	Pink	4–6′
C. sulphureus 'Bright Lights'		Orange, yellow	2–6′
Dorotheanthus bellidiformis	Livingstone daisy	Pink, red, yellow	3″
Gaillardia pulchella	Blanket flower, Indian blanket	Yellow, red-yellow	1–2′
Gazania rigens	Treasure flower	Yellow	16″
Helianthus annuus	Common sunflower	Yellow, white	12′
Helichrysum bracteatum	Strawflower	Yellow, red, orange, purple, white	2–3′
Hunnemannia fumariifolia	Mexican tulip poppy	Yellow	1–2′
Oenothera deltoides	Desert evening primrose	White	2–10″
Osteospermum hyoseroides		Yellow-violet, yellow-orange	2′
Portulaca grandiflora	Moss rose	White, pink, yellow, red, purple	10″
P. oleracea	Purslane	Yellow	10″
P. pilosa		Reddish purple	4–6″
Rudbeckia hirta	Black-eyed Susan	Yellow	1–3′
Satureja hortensis	Summer savory	White	18″

Low to Moderate Water Use or Average Soil (in Dryness)

COOL SEASON ANNUALS

BOTANICAL NAME	COMMON NAME(S)	COLOR(S)	HEIGHT
Agrostemma githago	Corn cockle	Pink	1–3'
Alonsoa warscewiczii	Mask flower	Red	1–3'
Anagallis arvensis	Scarlet pimpernel	White, red	18"
Anchusa capensis	Cape forget-me-not, Bugloss	Blue, pink, white	18"
Androsace lactiflora		White	1'
A. septentrionalis		White	8"
Anethum graveolans	Common dill	Yellow	30"
Arctotis stoechadifolia	Blue-eyed African daisy	Violet-white, red-yellow	30–48"
Barbarea verna	Early wintercress	Yellow	12–18"
B. vulgaris	Wintercress	Yellow	2–3'
Calendula officinalis	Pot marigold	Orange	12–18"
Campanula medium	Canterbury bells	Violet	2–4'
Carum carvi	Caraway	White	1–2'
Centaurea americana	Basketflower	Pink	4–6'
C. cyanus	Bachelor's button, Cornflower	Purple, blue, pink, white	20"
Cerinthe major	Honeywort	Yellow	20"
Cheiranthus cheiri	Wallflower	Yellow	30"
Chrysanthemum carinatum	Tricolor chrysanthemum	Orange-red-yellow, white-yellow, red-yellow	2–3'
C. coronarium	Crown daisy	Yellow	4'
Cirsium japonicum	Plumed thistle	Red	30"
Clarkia amoena	Farewell-to-spring	Pink	1–3'
C. purpurea		Pink	3'
C. unguiculata		Pink	18–36"
Coriandrum sativum	Coriander	Pink	3'
Crepis rubra	Hawk's-beard	Pink	8–18"
Cynoglossum officinale		Pink	2'
Dianthus barbatus	Sweet William	Pink	1–2'
D. chinensis	China pink, Indian pink	Red, white, lilac	12–18"
Diascia barberae	Twinspur	Pink	8–15"
Digitalis purpurea 'Campanulata'		Pink	4'
Fragaria vesca 'Alpine'	Alpine strawberry	White	9–12"
Glaucium corniculatum	Horned poppy	Orange, red	18"
G. flavum	Sea poppy, Horned poppy	Yellow	2–3'
Gypsophila elegans 'Golden Garden Market'		White	10–18"
Hedysarum coronarium	French honeysuckle	Red	2–4'
Hyoscyamus niger	Henbane, Stinking nightshade	White	1–2'
Iberis amara	Rocket candytuft	White	1'
I. pinnata		White	1'
I. umbellata	Globe candytuft	Pink	8–16"
Ionopsidium acaule	Diamond flower	Pink	3'
Ipomopsis aggregata	Skyrocket	White	2'

Low to Moderate Water Use or Average Soil (in Dryness)
COOL SEASON ANNUALS (cont'd)

BOTANICAL NAME	COMMON NAME(S)	COLOR(S)	HEIGHT
Ipomopsis rubra	Standing cypress	Red-yellow	2–3'
Lathyrus odoratus	Sweet pea	Pink	4–6' (vine-like)
Lavatera arborea	Tree mallow	Pink	4–10"
Layia platyglossa	Tidy tips	Yellow	1–2'
Linaria maroccana	Toadflax	Pink	18"
Linum grandiflorum	Flowering flax	Pink	1–2'
L. usitatissimum	Common flax	Blue, white	3–4'
Lobelia erinus	Edging lobelia	Blue	3–8"
Lobularia maritima	Sweet alyssum, Snowdrift	Pink, white	1'
Lonas annua	African daisy, Yellow ageratum	Yellow	1'
Lunaria annua	Honesty, Moonwort	Pink	18–36"
Lupinus subcarnosus	Bluebonnet	Blue	8–10"
L. texensis	Texas bluebonnet	Blue	1'
Machaeranthera tanacetifolia	Tahoka daisy	Lavender-blue	1–2'
Malcolmia maritima	Virginia stock	Pink	6–12"
Malope trifida		Pink	2–3'
Malva verticillata var. *crispa*	Curled mallow	White	1'
Matthiola incana 'Annua'		Pink	12–30"
M. longipetala	Evening stock	Pink	18"
Mentzelia lindleyi	Blazing star	Yellow	1–2'
Myosotis sylvatica	Forget-me-not	Blue, pink, white	6–18"
Nigella damascena	Love-in-a-mist	Blue, white, pink, purple	12–18"
Oxypetalum caeruleum	Southern star	Blue	3'
Penstemon gloxinioides		White, crimson, blue	2–3'
Phlox drummondii	Annual phlox, Drummond phlox	White, red, purple	18"
Pimpinella anisum	Anise	Yellow	2'
Reseda alba	White mignonette	White	3'
R. lutea	Wild mignonette	Yellow	30"
R. odorata	Common mignonette	Yellow	1'
Salpiglossis sinuata	Painted tongue	Gold, red, pink, blue	3'
Saxifraga cymbalaria		Yellow	18"
Senecio elegans	Purple ragwort	Pink	2'
Silybum marianum	Holy thistle	Pink	4'
Trachelium caeruleum	Throatwort	Blue, white	1–4'
Trachymene coerulea	Blue laceflower	Blue, lavender	18–30"
Tropaeolum majus	Garden nasturtium	Yellow, orange	1'
T. peregrinum	Canary-bird flower	Yellow, orange, red	8' (vine)
Ursinia anthemoides 'Sunshine Blend'		Yellow	18"
Viola rafinesquii	Field pansy	White	3–8"
V. tricolor	Johnny-jump-up	Purple-white-yellow	1'
Xeranthemum annuum	Immortelle, Everlasting	Pink	2–3'

WARM SEASON ANNUALS

BOTANICAL NAME	COMMON NAME(S)	COLOR(S)	HEIGHT
Abelmoschus esculentus	Okra	Yellow	2–6'
Abutilon hybridum	Chinese lantern, Flowering maple	Red, pink, purple, yellow, white	1–3'
Ageratum houstonianum	Common garden ageratum	White, blue, pink	14"
Alcea rosea	Garden hollyhock	White, red, pink	5–9'
Amaranthus caudatus	Love-lies-bleeding	Red	3–5'
A. hybridus var. *erythrostachys*	Prince's feather	Red, brownish red	3–4'
Ammobium alatum 'Chelsea Physic'	Winged everlasting	White	3'
Anagallis monellii linifolia	Flaxleaf pimpernel	Scarlet, white, blue	8–18"
Arachis hypogaea	Peanut	Yellow	12–18"
Argemone mexicana	Mexican poppy	Yellow	3'
A. munita	Prickly poppy	White	2–5'
Asclepias curassavica	Blood flower	Orange-red	2–4'
Borago officinalis	Borage, Talewort	Blue	2'
Callistephus chinensis 'Early Charm Choice'		Pink	9–24"
Cassia fasciculata	Partridge pea	Yellow	18"
Catananche caerulea	Cupid's dart, Blue succory	Blue	2'
Catharanthus roseus	Madagascar periwinkle	Pink, white	2'
Celosia cristata	Plumed celosia	Orange, red, yellow	1–2'
Chrysanthemum parthenium	Feverfew	White, yellow	2–3'
Convolvulus tricolor	Dwarf morning glory	Blue	1'
Coreopsis tinctoria	Golden coreopsis	Yellow-mahogany	2–3'
Cuphea ignea 'Hidcote'		Red	8–15"
Datura inoxia	Angel's trumpet	White	3'
Emilia javanica	Tassel flower	Red	1–2'
Gaura lindheimeri		White	4'
Helianthus annuus	Common sunflower	White, yellow, orange, maroon, bicolored	12'
Heliotropium arborescens	Common heliotrope	Purple, violet, white	2–4'
Hibiscus moscheutos	Rose mallow, Swamp mallow	White, pink	5'
Ipomoea alba	Moonflower	White	8–10' (vine)
I. coccinea	Star impomoea	Scarlet	10' (vine)
I. × multifida	Cardinal climber	Red	8–10' (vine)
I. quamoclit	Cypress-vine	Scarlet	20' (vine)
Lantana camara	Yellow sage, Red sage	Yellow, pink, red, white, lavender	4'
L. montevidensis	Weeping lantana	Pink	3'
Limonium sinuatum	Statice	Blue, lavender, red, salmon, yellow, white	12–30"
Lychnis coeli-rosa 'Love'		Pink	12–20"
Martynia annua		White	6'
Mimosa pudica	Sensitive plant, Humble plant	Rose-purple, lavender	3'
Mirabilis jalapa	Four-o'clock	Pink	18–36"

Low to Moderate Water Use or Average Soil (in Dryness)
WARM SEASON ANNUALS (cont'd)

BOTANICAL NAME	COMMON NAME(S)	COLOR(S)	HEIGHT
Nicandra physalodes	Apple of Peru	Blue, violet, white	4–8′
Nicotiana alata	Flowering tobacco	Pink, white, purple, red, green	5′
N. tabacum	Tobacco	Pink	6′
Nierembergia hippomanica var. *violacea*	Cupflower	Violet-blue	6–15″
Oenothera biennis	Evening primrose	Yellow, turning gold	3–6′
O. erythrosepala	Evening primrose	Yellow, turning orange or red	2–8′
O. laciniata	Evening primrose	Yellow, turning red	6–24″
O. missourensis	Missouri evening primrose	Yellow, turning red	15″
O. primiveris	Evening primrose	Yellow, turning orange	6–9″
O. speciosa	Showy evening primrose	White, turning pink	1–2′
Orthocarpus purpurascens	Owl's clover	Pink	1′
Osteospermum 'Buttermilk'		White	12–18″
O. hyoseroides		Yellow-violet, yellow-orange	2′
Pelargonium × domesticum	Martha Washington geranium	White, pink, red	18″
P. × hortorum	Zonal geranium, Fish geranium	Red, pink, peach, white, coral	1–3′
P. peltatum	Ivy geranium	White, rose	3′
Petunia × hybrida	Common garden petunia	Pink, white, blue, purple, yellow	8–18″
Phaseolus coccineus	Scarlet runner bean	Red, white	6–8′
Polygonum capitatum	Knotweed	Pink	6′
P. orientale	Kiss-me-over-the-garden-gate	Pink	6′
Ricinus communis	Castor bean	Red	4–15′
Salvia farinacea	Mealy-cup sage	Blue	3′
S. patens	Gentian sage	Blue	3′
S. sclarea	Clary, Clear-eye	Pink	3′
S. splendens	Scarlet sage	Red	3′
S. viridis		White, rose, purple	18″
Sanvitalia procumbens	Creeping zinnia	Yellow	6″
Scabiosa atropurpurea	Sweet scabiosa, Mourning bride	Pink	2–3′
S. stellata		Pink	18″
Silene armeria	Sweet William catchfly	Pink	18″
Tagetes erecta	African marigold	Orange, yellow	18–36″
T. patula	French marigold	Yellow-red	18″
T. tenuifolia	Dwarf marigold, Signet marigold	Yellow, orange	1′
Thelesperma burridgeanum		Yellow-brown	12–18″
Thunbergia alata	Black-eyed Susan vine	White, orange-yellow	6′
Tolpis barbata	Yellow hawkweed	Yellow-red-brown	8–12″
Trachelium caeruleum	Throatwort	Blue	1–4′

BOTANICAL NAME	COMMON NAME(S)	COLOR(S)	HEIGHT
Verbena × hybrida	Garden verbena	Pink, red, purple, yellow, white	1′
V. peruviana		Red	1–2′
Zinnia elegans	Common zinnia	Pink, purple, white, yellow, green, orange	3′
Z. haageana	Mexican zinnia	Yellow-red, orange-red	2′

Moderate to High Water Use or Moist Soil

This list of flowers is included for information in grouping plants according to water needs only. If you live in a fairly dry climate you may want to avoid using these plants, or realize you'll have to water them very regularly. Otherwise, they might be used in areas of your landscape that naturally get extra moisture, such as a hollow or a pocket of soil more clayey than the rest of the yard.

COOL SEASON ANNUALS

BOTANICAL NAME	COMMON NAME(S)	COLOR(S)	HEIGHT
Antirrhinum majus	Common snapdragon	Red, yellow, orange, white, pink	3′
Bellis perennis	English daisy	Red, white, pink	6″
Calceolaria crenatiflora	Pocketbook plant	Yellow	1–2′
C. integrifolia		Yellow	2–5′
C. mexicana		Yellow	18″
Limnanthes douglasii	Meadow foam, Marsh flower	Yellow, white	4–12″
Lunaria annua	Honesty, Moonwort	Purple, white	18–36″
Mimulus guttatus	Monkey flower	Yellow	2′
M. × hybridus	Monkey flower	Red, red-yellow	12–14″
Nemesia strumosa		White, yellow, pink, red, orange, purple	2′
Platystemon californicus	Creamcups	Yellow, cream-colored	6–12″
Primula malacoides	Fairy primrose	Rose, white, lilac, pink	4–18″
P. obconica	German primrose	Lilac, pink, red, white	1′
P. × polyantha	Polyanthus primrose	Purple, blue, rose, white, red, yellow	1′
Sabatia angularis	Rose pink	Pink	3′
Schizanthus pinnatus	Butterfly flower	Pink, rose, purple, white	4′
S. × wisetonensis		White, blue, pink, yellow, red, multicolored	1–2′
Senecio × hybridus	Cineraria	White, pink, blue, purple	1–3′
Ursinia anthemoides		Yellow, orange	18″
Viola cornuta	Horned violet, Bedding pansy	Purple, red, orange, white	8″
V. × wittrockiana	Pansy	Purple, blue, red, orange, white	9″

Moderate to High Water Use or Moist Soil
WARM SEASON ANNUALS

BOTANICAL NAME	COMMON NAME(S)	COLOR(S)	HEIGHT
Abutilon hybridum	Chinese lantern, Flowering maple	Red, pink, purple, yellow, white	1–3′
Asperula orientalis	Woodruff	Blue	1′
Begonia × semperflorens-cultorum	Wax begonia	White, pink, red	8–12″
Browallia speciosa		Purple, blue, white	8–12″
B. viscosa		Blue, white	12–20″
Daturia inoxia	Angel's trumpet	White	3′
D. metel	Horn-of-plenty	Yellow, blue, white, purple, red	5′
Eustoma grandiflorum, syn. *Lisianthus russellianus*	Prairie gentian, Bluebell	Purple	2–3′
Exacum affine	Persian violet	Blue, mauve	1–2′
Hibiscus moscheutos	Rose, mallow, Swamp mallow	White, pink	3–8′
Impatiens 'New Guinea'		Red, purple	1–2′
I. wallerana	Busy Lizzy, Patient Lucy	Red, pink, orange, salmon, purple, white, multicolored	1–2′
Lopezia hirsuta	Mosquito flower	White, pink, red	1–3′
Omphalodes linifolia	Navelwort	White	1′
Torenia fournieri	Wishbone flower	Blue-yellow, white-yellow, pink-yellow	10–12″

Perennials for Xeriscape Landscaping
Low to Very Low Water Use or Dry Soil

BOTANICAL NAME	COMMON NAME(S)	COLOR(S)	HEIGHT	ZONES
Acanthus mollis	Bear's-breech	Foliage important	3–4′	8–10
A. spinosus	Shiny bear's-breech	White	3–4′	5–6
Achillea 'Moonshine'		Yellow	2′	4–10
A. ptarmica 'The Pearl'		White	18–24″	4–10
Arabis procurrens	Rock cress	White	1′	4–10
Armeria maritima	Plantain thrift	Pink	6–10″	4–10
Asclepias tuberosa	Butterfly weed	Orange	1–3′	4–10
Aster × frikartii	Aster	Blue	2–3′	6–10
A. tataricus	Tatarian aster	Blue	6–8′	4–10
Astilbe chinensis 'Pumila'		Pink	8–12″	5–10
Baptisia perfoliata		Foliage important	2′	8–10
Callirhoe involucrata	Poppy mallow, Wine cups	Pink	6–12″	4–10
Catananche caerulea	Cupid's dart	Blue	2′	5–10
Centaurea hypoleuca 'John Coutts'		Pink	18–24″	4–10
C. macrocephala	Globe centaurea	Yellow	3′	3–4

BOTANICAL NAME	COMMON NAME(S)	COLOR(S)	HEIGHT	ZONES
Coreopsis lanceolata	Lance coreopsis	Yellow	2–3′	4–10
C. verticillata	Threadleaf coreopsis	Yellow	18–30″	4–10
Eriophyllum lanatum	Woolly eriophyllum	Yellow	2′	5–10
Eryngium bourgatii	Mediterranean eryngo	White	2′	5–10
E. × zabelii	Zabel eryngo	Blue	24–30″	5–10
Euphorbia characias		Yellow	3–4′	8–10
E. corollata	Flowering spurge	White	18–36″	4–10
E. cyparissias	Cypress spurge	Yellow	8–12″	4–10
E. epithymoides	Cushion spurge	Yellow	3–6″	5–10
E. myrsinites	Myrtle euphorbia	Yellow	3–6″	5–10
Filipendula vulgaris	Dropwort	White	2–3′	4–10
Gaillardia grandiflora	Blanketflower	Red-yellow	8–36″	4–10
Gaura lindheimeri	White gaura	White	5′	6–10
Geum coccineum		Red	6–8″	5–6
Goniolimon tataricum	Tatarian statice	Pink	18″	4–10
Helianthemum nummularium 'Fire Dragon'		Yellow	9–12″	6–10
Helichrysum hybridum 'Sulfur Light'		Yellow	18″	5–10
Iris 'Pacific Coast'		White	9–18″	4–10
Lavandula angustifolia	Lavender	Purple	1–3′	5–6
Leontopodium alpinum	Edelweiss	White	6–12″	4–10
Linum perenne	Perennial flax	Blue	1–2′	5–10
Malva alcea	Hollyhock mallow	Pink, white	2–4′	4–10
M. moschata	Musk mallow	White, pink	1–3′	4–10
Marrubium incanum	Silver horehound	Foliage important	2–3′	4–10
Monarda fistulosa	Wild bergamot	Pink	3–4′	4–10
Oenothera missourensis	Missouri evening primrose	Yellow	3–6″	5–10
O. tetragona	Common sundrop	Yellow	18″	5–10
Opuntia humifusa	Prickly pear	Yellow	2–6″	5–6
Potentilla nepalensis	Nepal cinquefoil	Red	2′	5–10
P. recta 'Macrantha'	Sulphur cinquefoil	Yellow	2′	4–10
P. tabernaemontani	Spring cinquefoil	Yellow	3″	5–10
P. × tonguei	Staghorn cinquefoil	Yellow	8–12″	5–10
Sedum spectabile	Showy stonecrop	Pink	2′	4–10
S. spurium	Two-row stonecrop	Red, pink	6″	4–10

Low to Moderate Water Use or Average Soil

BOTANICAL NAME	COMMON NAME(S)	COLOR(S)	HEIGHT	ZONES
Achillea filipendulina	Fernleaf yarrow	Yellow	3–4′	4–10
A. millefolium	Common yarrow	Pink, yellow, white	2′	3–10
Adenophora confusa	Ladybells	Purple	3′	4–10
Ajuga reptans 'Burgundy Glow'		Foliage important	3–6″	3–10
Alchemilla conjuncta		Foliage important	4–6″	4–10

Low to Moderate Water Use or Average Soil (cont'd)

BOTANICAL NAME	COMMON NAME(S)	COLOR(S)	HEIGHT	ZONES
Alchemilla mollis	Lady's-mantle	Yellow	15″	4–10
Alstroemeria ligtu	Peruvian lily	Red	2′	8–10
Amsonia tabernaemontana	Blue star, Willow amsonia	White, blue	2′	4–10
Anchusa azurea	Italian bugloss	Blue	42–60″	4–10
Anemone pulsatilla	Pasqueflower	Purple, blue	1′	5–6
Anaphalis margaritacea	Pearly everlasting	White	20″	4–10
A. triplinervis	Pearly everlasting	White	12–18″	4–10
Anigozanthos flavidus	Kangaroo paw	Red	3–4′	9–10
Anthemis sanctijohannis	St. John's camomile	Orange	1–3′	4–10
A. tinctoria	Golden marguerite	Yellow	3′	4–10
Aquilegia caerulea	Rocky Mountain columbine	Blue	2–3′	4–10
A. canadensis	Common columbine	Yellow	1–2′	4–10
A. hybrids		Pink, yellow, white	1–3′	5–10
Arctotheca calendula	Capeweed	Yellow	1′	9–10
Armeria pseudarmeria	Plantain thrift	White, pink	18–24″	6–7
Asphodeline lutea	Asphodela king's spear	Yellow	2–3′	6–10
Aster novae-angliae	New England aster	Purple, pink	3–5′	5–10
Aubrieta deltoidea	False rock cress	Purple	6″	5–10
Belamcanda chinensis	Blackberry lily, Leopard flower	Yellow-red	2–4′	5–10
Boltonia asteroides 'Snowbank'	White boltonia	White, violet, purple	3–5′	4–10
Buphthalum salicifolium	Yellow oxeye daisy	Yellow	1–2′	4–10
Campanula carpatica	Carpathian harebell	Blue, white	6–12″	4–10
C. garganica		Blue	6″	6–10
C. glomerata	Danesblood bellflower	Blue, white	1–3′	3–4
C. portenschlagiana	Dalmatian bellflower	Bluish purple	6–8″	5–10
C. poscharskyana	Serbian bellflower	Lilac	4–6″	4–10
C. rotundifolia	Bluebell	Blue	1–2′	3–10
Centaurea montana		Blue	18–24″	3–4
Centranthus ruber	Red valerian, Jupiter's beard	Red, white	1–3′	5–10
Cerastium biebersteinii	Taurus cerastrium	White	6″	4–10
Ceratostigma plumbaginoides	Leadwort	Blue	12″	6–10
Chrysanthemum frutescens, syn. *Argyranthemum frutescens*	Marguerite daisy	White, yellow, pink	2–3′	9–10
C. leucanthemum, syn. *Leucanthemum vulgare*	Oxeye daisy	White	2′	3–10
C. nipponicum, syn. *Nipponanthemum nipponicum*	Nippon chrysanthemum	White	18–24″	5–6
C. × superbum		White	1–3′	5–10
C. zawadskii, syn. *Dendranthema zawadskii*		Yellow, white, pink	18″	5–10
Chrysogonum virginianum	Golden star, Green-and-gold	Yellow	2–3′	9–10

BOTANICAL NAME	COMMON NAME(S)	COLOR(S)	HEIGHT	ZONES
Chrysopsis mariana	Maryland golden aster	Yellow	1–3′	5–10
Corydalis lutea	Yellow corydalis	Yellow	1′	5–10
Crambe cordifolia	Heartleaf crambe	White	6′	6–10
Crocosmia masoniorum		Orange	3′	6–10
Cynoglossum nervosum	Great hound's tongue	Blue	2′	5–10
Dianthus × allwoodii	Allwood pink	Red, pink, white	12–18″	4–10
D. barbatus	Sweet William	Red, purple, white, multicolored	1–2′	6–10
D. deltoides	Maiden pink	Red, pink	4–12″	4–10
D. gratianopolitanus	Cheddar pink	Pink, red	6–8″	5–10
D. plumarius	Grass pink	Pink, purple, white, multicolored	9–18″	4–10
Dietes vegeta	African iris	White	2′	8–10
Digitalis grandiflora	Yellow foxglove	Yellow	3′	4–10
Draba densiflora	Rock cress draba	Yellow	2–3″	4–10
Echinacea purpurea	Purple coneflower	Pink, white	5′	7–10
Echinops ritro	Globe thistle	Blue	3–4′	4–10
Elsholtzia stauntonii	Staunton elsholtzia	Lavender	5′	7–10
Eremurus stenophyllus	Foxtail lily	Orange	2–5′	7–10
Erigeron hybrids	Fleabane	Pink, purple	1–2′	5–10
Eupatorium coelestinum	Mist flower, Hardy ageratum	Violet-blue	2′	5–10
Filipendula vulgaris	Dropwort	White	2–3′	4–10
Foeniculum vulgare	Common fennel	Foliage important	3–5′	4–10
Fragaria chiloensis	Chiloe strawberry	White	6–8″	5–10
Galega officinalis	Goat's rue	Pink, white, purple	2–3′	5–10
Geranium dalmaticum		Rose	6″	5–10
G. himalayense	Lilac cranesbill	Blue	8–15″	4–10
G. 'Johnson's Blue'		Blue	1′	4–10
G. macrorrhizum	Bigroot cranesbill	Pink, magenta	12–18″	5–10
G. maculatum	Wild geranium	Lilac	12–20″	5–10
G. sanguineum var. *lancastriense*	Blood red cranesbill	Reddish purple, pink	12–18″	4–10
Gypsophila paniculata	Baby's-breath	White, pink	3′	4–10
Heliopsis helianthoides var. *scabra*	False sunflower	Orange-yellow	3–4′	5–10
Hemerocallis spp.	Daylily	Yellow, red, orange, maroon	30–42″	4–10
Indigofera incarnata	Chinese indigo	Rose	12–18″	8–10
Inula ensifolia	Swordleaf inula	Yellow	1′	4–10
Iris, bearded		Wide range of colors	5–30″	4–10
Iris pallida var. *dalmatica* 'Variegata'		Foliage important	3′	6–10
I. pumila	Dwarf bearded iris	Yellow, lilac	4–8″	4–10
I. tectorum	Roof iris	Purple, blue	8–12″	5–6
Kniphofia uvaria	Red hot poker, Torch lily	Red-yellow	2–4′	5–10
Lamiastrum galeobdolon 'Herman's Pride'		Foliage important	1–2′	4–10
Liatris aspera		Purple, white	3′	4–10

Low to Moderate Water Use or Average Soil (cont'd)

BOTANICAL NAME	COMMON NAME(S)	COLOR(S)	HEIGHT	ZONES
Linaria purpurea	Purple toadflax	Purple	2–3′	5–10
Linum flavum	Golden flax	Yellow	1–2′	4–10
Macleaya cordata	Plume-poppy	White	6–10′	4–10
Monarda didyma	Bee balm, Oswego tea	Scarlet	2–3′	4–10
Nepeta mussinii	Mauve catmint	Blue	1′	4–10
Oenothera speciosa	Showy primrose	Pink, white	6–18″	5–10
Omphalodes cappadocica	Navelwort	Blue	6–10″	6–10
Origanum vulgare 'Aureum'		Foliage important	30″	4–10
Paeonia mlokosewitschii	Caucasian peony	Yellow	18–24″	5–10
P. suffruticosa	Japanese tree peony	Red, white	4–7′	5–10
P. tenuifolia	Fernleaf peony	Purple, red	2′	5–10
Papaver orientale	Oriental poppy	Scarlet, blue	3–4′	5–10
Penstemon barbatus	Beardlip penstemon	Red	2–3′	4–10
P. × gloxinioides	Gloxinia penstemon	White, crimson, blue	2–3′	9–10
P. hirsutus		Blue	2–3′	5–10
Perovskia atriplicifolia	Azure salvia	Blue	3–5′	5–6
Petrorhagia saxifrage	Tunic flower	White, pink	6–10″	5–10
Phlomis russeliana	Sticky Jerusalem-sage	Yellow	3′	6–10
Physalis alkekengi	Chinese lantern plant	Blue, yellow	2′	5–10
Potentilla atrosanguinea	Ruby cinquefoil	Red	12–18″	5–10
Prunella grandiflora	Self heal	Blue, pink	12″	5–10
Romneya coulteri	California tree poppy	White	8′	7–10
Roscoea humeana	Hume roscoea	Violet	8–12″	4–10
Rudbeckia fulgida	Orange coneflower	Orange-yellow	2–3′	6–10
R. nitida 'Herbstsonne'		Yellow	4–7′	4–10
Ruta graveolens	Common rue	Yellow	2–3′	5–10
Salvia argentea	Silver sage	Foliage important	2′	5–10
S. azurea var. *grandiflora*	Pitcher's sage	Blue, white	4–5′	6–10
S. farinacea	Mealy-cup sage	Blue	3′	8–10
S. officinalis		Foliage important	2′	5–10
S. pratensis	Meadow clary	Blue	3′	6–10
S. × superba	Violet sage	Purple	18–36″	5–10
Saponaria officinalis	Bouncing bet	White	1–3′	4–10
Sedum aizoon	Aizoon stonecrop	Yellow	12–18″	4–10
S. 'Autumn Joy'		Pink, rusty red	2′	4–10
S. kamtschaticum	Orange stonecrop	Orange-yellow	6–12″	4–10
S. maximum	Great stonecrop	Pink, purple	1–2′	4–10
S. 'Ruby Glow'		Red	6–8″	4–10
S. sieboldii	October daphne	Pink	6–9″	4–10
Sidalcea malviflora	Checker bloom, Prairie mallow	Pink	30″	5–10
Sisyrinchium striatum	Argentine blue-eyed grass	Yellow	12–18″	7–8
Smilacina racemosa	False Solomon's seal	White	8–12″	5–10
Stachys macrantha	Big betony	Purple, pink	12–18″	4–10
Symphytum grandiflorum	Ground-cover comfrey	White, pink, blue	8–12″	5–10
S. × rubrum	Comfrey	Red	18″	5–10

BOTANICAL NAME	COMMON NAME(S)	COLOR(S)	HEIGHT	ZONES
S. × uplandicum	Russian comfrey	Blue	2–3′	5–10
Tanacetum argentum, syn. *Chrysanthemum coccineum*	Pyrethrum, Painted daisy	Red, pink, lilac, white	1–3′	4–10
T. vulgare, syn. *Chrysanthemum parthenium*	Feverfew	White	2–3′	4–5
T. vulgare var. *crispum*	Tansy	Yellow	2–3′	4–10
Thermopsis caroliniana	Carolina thermopsis	Yellow	3–5′	3–10
Tradescantia × andersoniana	Common spiderwort	Pink, blue	24–30″	5–10
T. hirsuticaulis		Blue	1′	6–10
Verbascum chaixii	Chaix mullein	Yellow, white	3′	5–10
Verbena peruviana		Red	3–4″	5–10
V. rigida	Vervain	Blue	1–2′	4–10
Veronica grandis var. *holophylla*		Blue	2–3′	5–10
V. latifolium	Hungarian speedwell	Blue	12–18″	4–10
V. spicata	Speedwell	Blue	12–18″	4–10
V. virginica	Culver's root, Blackroot	White	2–6′	4–10

Moderate to High Water Use or Moist Soil

(See note about moist soil flowers, page 281.)

BOTANICAL NAME	COMMON NAME(S)	COLOR(S)	HEIGHT	ZONES
Aconitum × bicolor	Hybrid monkshood	White, violet, blue	3–4′	5–10
A. carmichaelii	Azure monkshood	Blue	6′	3–4
A. napellus	Common monkshood	Blue	4′	5–10
Actaea rubra (red berries)	Red baneberry	White	18–24″	4–10
Alcea rosea	Garden hollyhock	White, pink, purple, red, yellow	5–9′	4–10
Anemone × hybrida	Japanese anemone	Pink, white	1–5′	6–10
A. vitifolia 'Robustissima'		Pink	2–3′	5–10
Anthericum liliago	St. Bernard's lily	White	3′	5–10
Arenaria verna var. *caespitosa**	Irish moss	White	2″	5–10
Arisaema triphyllum	Jack-in-the-pulpit	White	1–3′	4–10
Artemisia lactiflora	Ghost plant	White	5′	4–10
Arum italicum 'Pictum' (takes dry shade)		Foliage important	12–16″	5–6
Aruncus dioicus	Goatsbeard	White	4–6′	4–10
Asarum canadense	Wild ginger	Foliage important	6–8″	4–10
A. europaeum	European wild ginger	Foliage important	5″	5–10
Astilbe × arendsii	False spirea	Red, white, pink	2–4′	5–10
A. tacquetii 'Superba'		Magenta, purple	3–4′	5–10
Begonia grandis	Hardy begonia	Pink	3–4′	5–10
Bergenia cordifolia	Heartleaf bergenia	Pink	12–18″	3–10

Moderate to High Water Use or Moist Soil (cont'd)

BOTANICAL NAME	COMMON NAME(S)	COLOR(S)	HEIGHT	ZONES
Bergenia hybrids		Pink, purple, white, red	3–4′	5–10
Brunnera macrophylla	Siberian bugloss	Blue	12–18″	4–10
Calceolaria 'John Innes'		Yellow	1–2′	4–10
*Caltha palustris**	Cowslip, Marsh marigold	Yellow	1–2′	4–10
Campanula lactiflora	Milky bellflower	White, blue	4′	4–10
C. latifolia	Great bellflower	Blue	2–4′	4–10
C. persicifolia	Peach-leaved bellflower	White, blue	2–3′	4–10
Chelone lyonii	Pink turtlehead	Rose-purple	3′	4–10
Chrysanthemum × *morifolium*	Florist's chrysanthemum	Pink, white, yellow, orange, purple	4′	5–10
Cimicifuga racemosa	Black snakeroot, Black cohosh	White	3–4′	4–10
C. simplex	Kamchatka bugbane	White	3–4′	4–10
Clematis heracleifolia var. *davidiana*	Tube clematis	Blue	3–4′	4–10
C. recta	Ground clematis	White	2–5′	4–10
Convallaria majalis	Lily-of-the-valley	White	6–12″	4–10
Coreopsis auriculata 'Nana'		Yellow	12–18″	4–10
Delphinium elatum	Candle larkspur	Blue, white, pink, purple	6′	4–10
Dicentra cucullaria	Dutchman's breeches	White	5–8″	4–10
D. 'Luxuriant'		White, yellow	12–18″	4–10
D. spectabilis	Common bleedingheart	Rose-red	1–2′	3–4
Dictamnus albus (must have sun)	Gasplant	Purple, white, red	2–3′	3–4
Digitalis × *mertonensis*		Pink	3′	5–10
Disporum sessile 'Variegatum'	Variegated Japanese fairy-bells	White	15–24″	4–10
Doronicum cordatum	Leopard's bane	Yellow	12–30″	4–10
Epimedium grandiflorum	Longspur epimedium	Pink	1′	5–10
E. × *rubrum*	Red epimedium	Pink	1′	5–10
E. × *versicolor*	Persian epimedium	Yellow	1′	5–10
E. × *warleyense*	Warly epimedium	Orange	9–12″	5–10
E. × *youngianum* 'Niveum'	Snowy epimedium	White	8–10″	5–10
Euphorbia griffithii	Fire glow euphorbia	Orange	3′	5–10
Filipendula palmata	Meadowsweet	Pink	6″	4–10
F. rubra	Queen-of-the-prairie	Pink	4–7′	3–10
F. ulmaria	Queen-of-the-meadow	White	3–5′	4–10
Galax urceolata	Galaxy	White	30″	5–10
Galium odoratum	Sweet woodruff	White	1′	5–10
Galtonia candicans	Giant summer hyacinth	White	3–4′	5–10
Gentiana asclepiadea	Willow gentian	Blue	2′	6–7
Geranium dalmaticum		Pink	6″	5–10
G. endressii	Pyrenean cranesbill	Pink	12–18″	4–10
G. psilostemon	Armenian cranesbill	Magenta	2′	4–10
Geum quellyon	Chilean avens	Orange, red, yellow	2′	5–6
Gillenia trifoliata	Bowman's root	White	2–3′	5–10

BOTANICAL NAME	COMMON NAME(S)	COLOR(S)	HEIGHT	ZONES
Helenium autumnale	False sunflower	Yellow, orange, mahogany	5′	4–10
Helianthus angustifolius	Swamp sunflower	Yellow	5′	6–7
H. × multiflorus	Perennial sunflower	Yellow	6′	6–7
Helleborus foetidus	Stinking hellebore	Green	12–18″	6–7
H. lividus	Corsican hellebore	Greenish yellow	2′	8–10
H. niger	Christmas rose	White	1′	4–10
H. orientalis	Lenten rose	Pink	18″	5–10
Hesperis matronalis	Dane's-rocket	Purple, mauve	2–3′	4–10
Heuchera sanguinea	Coralbells	Red	1–2′	4–10
Heucherella tiarelloides		Pink	18″	4–10
Hibiscus coccineus	Scarlet rose mallow	Scarlet	6–8′	6–10
H. moscheutos	Rose mallow, Swamp mallow	White, pink, red	3–8′	5–10
Hosta fortunei 'Aureo-marginata'		Foliage important	2′	4–10
H. 'Krossa Regal'		Foliage important	3′	4–10
H. lancifolia	Narrowleaf plantain lily	Foliage important	2′	4–10
H. sieboldiana	Siebold plantain lily	Foliage important	30″	4–10
H. undulata	Wavyleaf plantain lily	Foliage important	3′	4–10
Houttuynia cordata 'Variegata'		Foliage important	1′	5–10
Incarvillea delavayi	Hardy gloxinia	Purple	1′	6–10
Iris cristata	Crested iris	White, blue	4–6″	4–10
I. enstata	Japanese iris	White	2–3″	5–9
I. laevigata 'Variegata'	Variegated rabbit-ear iris	Purple	18–24″	5–10
I. 'Louisiana'*	Louisiana iris	Many colors	3–4′	5–10
I. pseudacorus 'Variegata'*	Yellow flag	Yellow	5′	5–6
I. sibirica	Siberian iris	White, lilac, purple	2–4′	4–10
Kirengeshoma palmata		Yellow	4′	5–10
Lamium maculatum	Dead nettle	Purple	18″	4–10
Liatris spicata	Gayfeather	Purple	2–5′	3–10
Ligularia dentata	Bigleaf goldenray	Foliage important	4′	4–10
L. przewalskii 'The Rocket'		Yellow	4–6′	4–10
L. tussilaginea 'Aureo-maculata'		Foliage important	2′	6–7
Limonium latifolium	Sea lavender	Purple	4–6′	4–10
Liriope muscari 'John Birch'		Foliage important	18″	6–10
Lobelia cardinalis	Cardinal flower	Scarlet	3–6′	3–10
Lupinus Russell hybrids		White, red, pink, blue	2–3′	5–10
Lychnis chalcedonica	Maltese cross	Scarlet	18–30″	4–10
L. coronaria	Rose campion	Pink	18–36″	4–10
L. viscaria	German catchfly	White, pink	12–18″	4–10
Meconopsis cambrica	Welsh poppy	Yellow, orange	2′	6–10
Mertensia virginica	Virginia bluebells	Purple, blue, white	2′	4–10

Moderate to High Water Use or Moist Soil (cont'd)

BOTANICAL NAME	COMMON NAME(S)	COLOR(S)	HEIGHT	ZONES
Mimulus guttatus	Common monkey flower	Yellow	2′	9–10
M. lewisii	Lewis's monkey flower	Rose-purple	30″	9–10
Myosotis scorpioides var. *semperflorens*	True forget-me-not	Blue	12–18″	5–10
Omphalodes cappadocica	Navelwort	Blue	6–10″	6–10
Paeonia lactiflora	Chinese peony	White, red, yellow	30–36″	5–10
P. officinalis	Common peony		3′	5–9
Phlox carolina	Carolina phlox	Purple, rose, white	18″	4–10
P. divaricata	Wild sweet William	Mauve	18″	4–10
P. paniculata	Garden phlox, Perennial phlox	Purple, white, red, blue	3–4′	4–10
P. stolonifera	Creeping phlox	Purple	1′	4–10
Phormium tenax 'Variegatum'	Variegated New Zealand flax	Foliage important	8–15′	9–10
Physostegia virginiana	False dragonhead, Obedient plant	Red, pink, lilac	4–5′	4–10
Platycodon grandiflorus	Balloon flower	Blue, white, purple	18–30″	4–10
Polemonium caeruleum	Jacob's ladder	Purple	3′	4–10
P. foliossimum	Leafy polemonium	Violet	24–30″	4–10
P. reptans	Creeping polemonium	Blue	8–12″	4–10
Polygonatum odoratum var. *thunbergii*	Solomon's seal	White	42″	5–10
P. stolonifera	Creeping phlox	Purple	1′	4–10
Polygonum affine	Himalayan fleeceflower	Pink	18″	4–10
P. bistorta 'Superbum'	European bistort	Pink	18″	4–10
*Primula helodoxa**	Amber primrose	Yellow	18–36″	6–10
*P. japonica**	Japanese primrose	Pink, purple, white	8–16″	6–10
P. sieboldii	Japanese star primrose	Pink, purple	1′	5–10
P. veris	Cowslip primrose	Yellow-orange	6–8″	5–6
P. vulgaris	English primrose	Yellow	6″	5–10
Prunella grandiflora	Self heal	Pink, blue	1′	5–10
Pulmonaria angustifolia	Blue lungwort	Blue	6–12″	4–10
P. longifolia		Blue	1′	5–10
P. saccharata	Bethlehem sage	White, purple	8–14″	4–10
Ranunculus repens	Creeping buttercup	Yellow	1–2′	4–10
Rhexia mariana	Maryland meadow beauty	Purple	1–2′	6–10
R. virginica	Deer grass	Purple	9–18″	6–10
Rodgersia aesculifolia	Fingerleaf rodgersflower	White	4′	5–6
R. podophylla	Bronzeleaf rodgersflower	Yellowish white	5′	5–6
Sanguisorba canadensis	Great burnet, American burnet	White	3–6′	4–10
Saxifraga stolonifera	Strawberry geranium	White	2′	6–10
S. × urbium	London pride saxifrage	Pink	1′	7–10
Scabiosa caucasica	Pincushion flower	Blue, white	30″	4–10
Shortia galicifolia	Oconee bells	White	8″	5–10
Silene schafta	Moss campion	Pink, purple	6″	5–6
Solidago 'Gold Dwarf'		Yellow	1′	4–10
Stokesia laevis	Stokes's aster	Blue	6″	5–6
Stylophorum diphyllum	Celandine poppy	Yellow	18″	6–10

BOTANICAL NAME	COMMON NAME(S)	COLOR(S)	HEIGHT	ZONES
Thalictrum aquilegifolium	Columbine meadowrue	Lavender	2–3'	5–6
T. rochebrunianum	Lavender mist meadowrue	Purple, pink	3–5'	5–6
T. speciosissimum	Dusty meadowrue	Yellow	3–5'	5–6
Tricyrtis hirta	Toadlily	Purple	3'	6–10
Trillium grandiflorum	Snow trillium	White	12–18"	5–10
Trollius europaeus	Common globeflower	Yellow	2'	5–6
T. ledebourii	Ledebour globeflower	Orange, yellow	2–3'	5–6
Uvularia grandiflora	Big merrybells	Yellow	30"	5–10
Valeriana officinalis	Common valerian	Pink, white, lavender	2–4'	5–10
Veratum viride	American white hellebore	Foliage important	3–7'	5–6
Viola cornuta	Horned violet	Violet, white, orange, yellow, red	5–8"	5–10
V. odorata	Sweet violet	Purple, white	6–8"	5–10
V. striata	Striped violet	White-purple	4–16"	5–10
Zantedeschia aethiopica	Calla lily	White	1–3'	7–10

**Wildflowers for Xeriscape Landscaping
For Sunny, Dry Exposures**
(under 15" rainfall/irrigation per year)

ANNUALS

BOTANICAL NAME	COMMON NAME(S)	COLOR(S)	HEIGHT
*Centaurea cyanus**	Cornflower	Blue	20"
Coreopsis tinctoria	Plains coreopsis	Yellow-maroon	2–3'
*Cosmos bipinnatus**	Cosmos	Pink, white, red	4–6'
Eschscholzia californica (tender perennial, often acts as annual)	California poppy	Yellow-orange	8–12"
Gaillardia pulchella	Annual gaillardia	Yellow-red	1–2'
Gilia tricolor	Bird's eyes	Lavender, white	42"
Gypsophila elegans	Baby's breath	White	10–18"
*Helianthus annuus**	Sunflower	Yellow	12'
Linanthus grandiflorus	Mountain phlox	White, lavender	2'
Linaria maroccana	Spurred snapdragon, Toadflax	Pink, yellow, violet	18"
*Lobularia maritima** (tender perennial, often acts as annual, reseeding readily)	Sweet alyssum	White, lavender	1'
Oenothera missourensis	Dwarf evening primrose	Yellow	15"
Papaver rhoeas	Corn poppy	White, pink, red	3'
Sanvitalia procumbens	Creeping zinnia	Yellow	6"
Silene armeria (sometimes a biennial)	Sweet William catchfly	Pink	18"

For Sunny, Dry Exposures (cont'd)
(under 15″ rainfall/irrigation per year)

PERENNIALS

BOTANICAL NAME	COMMON NAME(S)	COLOR(S)	HEIGHT	ZONES
*Achillea filipendula**	Gold yarrow	Yellow	3–4′	4–10
*A. millefolium**	White yarrow	White	2′	3–10
Anthemis tinctoria (sometimes a biennial)	Yellow marguerite	Yellow	3′	4–10
*Cerastium tomentosum**	Snow-in-summer	White	6″	4–10
Dianthus barbatus	Sweet William	Pink, white, red	1–2′	6–10
Erigeron speciosus	Fleabane daisy	Violet	42″	4–10
Gaillardia aristata	Perennial gaillardia	Orange-red	2–3′	3–9
Linum perenne var. *lewisii*	Blue flax	Blue	2–3′	5–10
Lychnis chalcedonica	Maltese cross	Scarlet	18–30″	4–10
Penstemon strictus	Prairie penstemon	Blue	42″	4–10
Ratibida columnifera	Prairie coneflower	Yellow-red	1–3′	3–10
Saponaria ocymoides	Soapwort	Pink	9″	2–10

For Sunny to Partly Shaded, Moist Exposures
(over 15″ rainfall/irrigation per year)

ANNUALS

BOTANICAL NAME	COMMON NAME(S)	COLOR(S)	HEIGHT
Chrysanthemum multicaule	Yellow daisy	Yellow	1′
Clarkia unguicultata		Pink, lavender	18–36″
Delphinium ajacis	Larkspur	White, pink, violet	1–2′
*Iberis umbellata***	Annual candytuft	Pink, white	8–16″
Linum grandiflorum var. *rubrum*	Scarlet flax	Scarlet	1–2′
Lupinus texensis	Texas bluebonnet	Blue	1′
*Mimulus tigrinus***	Monkeyflower	Yellow-red-cream	6–10″
Mirabilis jalapa (tender perennial, often acts as an annual)	Four-o'clock	Red, pink, white	18–36″
*Myosotis sylvatica***	Forget-me-not	Blue	6–18″
*Nemophila menziesii***	Baby blue-eyes	Blue	1′

PERENNIALS

BOTANICAL NAME	COMMON NAME(S)	COLOR(S)	HEIGHT	ZONES
Anthemis nobilis	Roman camomile	White	1′	3–8
Aquilegia spp.***	Columbine	Yellow, red, blue	1–3′	Vary
Aster novae-angliae	New England aster	Violet	3–5′	5–10
Bellis perennis (sometimes a biennial—invasive in the Northwest)	English daisy	White, rose	6–8″	3–10

BOTANICAL NAME	COMMON NAME(S)	COLOR(S)	HEIGHT	ZONES
Chrysanthemum leucanthemum, * syn. *Leucanthemum vulgare*	Oxeye daisy	White	2'	3–10
Coreopsis lanceolata	Lanceleaf coreopsis	Yellow	2–3'	4–10
Dianthus deltoides	Maiden pink	Pink	4–12"	4–10
*Dicentra eximia***	Bleeding heart	Pink	2'	3–10
Echinacea purpurea	Purple coneflower	Purple	5'	7–10
Erysimum asperum	Wallflower	Orange	3'	4–10
*Hesperis matronalis***	Dame's rocket	Violet	2–3'	4–10
Liatris spicata	Gayfeather	Purple	1'	6–10
Lupinus perennis	Perennial lupine	Blue	2'	3–10
Papaver nudicaule	Iceland poppy	White, red, yellow, orange	1–2'	3–10
*Rudbeckia hirta** (grown as an annual)	Black-eyed Susan	Yellow	1–3'	
Viola kitaibeliana	Johnny-jump-up	Purple-yellow	2'	8–10

*Can be very aggressive and may eventually dominate a planting.
**Can be grown satisfactorily in shaded spots such as beneath tree or shrub canopies, provided there is some filtered sunlight.

Source: Adapted from Colorado State University Cooperative Extension Bulletin No. 7.233, "Wildflowers for Colorado Landscapes."

Ornamental Grasses for Xeriscape Landscaping
Dry Soil or Very Low Water Use

BOTANICAL NAME	COMMON NAME(S)	HEIGHT	ZONES
Agrostis nebulosa	Cloud grass	8–20"	Annual
Andropogon spp.	Bluestem, Beardgrass	Varies	4–9
Arrhenatherum elatius var. *bulbosum*	Tuber oat grass	8–18"	4–9
Bouteloua gracilis	Blue grama grass, Mosquito grass	1–2'	3–10
Briza maxima	Big quaking grass	2–3'	Annual
B. media	Quaking grass	6–18"	5–9
Calamagrostis epigens	Reed grass	3–4'	3–6
Cortaderia selloana	Pampas grass	14'	8–10
Elymus glaucus	Lyme grass, Wild rye	2'	4–9
Eragrostis trichodes	Sand love grass	4'	Annual
Festuca amethystina	Large blue fescue	12"	4–8
F. mairei	Maires fescue	2'	5–9
F. muelleri	Mueller's fescue	6–12"	5–9
F. ovina var. *glauca*	Blue fescue	6–12"	4–9
Helictotrichon sempervirens	Blue oat grass	18–30"	4–8
Hordeum jubatum	Squirrel-tail grass, Foxtail barley	24–30"	3–9
Koeleria glauca	Blue hair grass	1'	3–9

Dry Soil or Very Low Water Use (cont'd)

BOTANICAL NAME	COMMON NAME(S)	HEIGHT	ZONES
Lamarckia aurea	Goldentop	18–24″	Annual
Melica ciliata	Silky-spike melic grass	1–2′	6–8
Panicum virgatum	Switch grass	4–6′	5–9
Phalaris arundinacea var. *picta*	Ribbon grass	1–3′	4–8
P. canariensis	Canary grass	2–3′	Annual
Phormium tenax	New Zealand flax	3–4′	9–10
Schizachyrium scoparium, syn. *Andropogon scoparius*	Little bluestem grass	3–4′	4–9
Sorghastrum nutans, syn. *Chrysopogon nutans*	Indian grass	8–18″	6–10
Spartina pectinata	Cord grass	8′	5–9
Stipa calamagrostis		3–4′	3–4
S. pennata	Feather grass	2–3′	5–9
Triticum turgidum	Bearded wheat	2–4′	Annual

Average Soil or Water Use

BOTANICAL NAME	COMMON NAME(S)	HEIGHT	ZONES
Agrostis nebulosa	Cloud grass	8–20″	Annual
Andropogon gerardii	Big bluestem grass	4–6′	4–9
Arrhenatherum elatius var. *bulbosum*	Tuber oat grass	8–18″	4–9
Avena fatua	Wild oats	3–4′	Annual
A. sterilis	Animated oats	3–4′	Annual
Bromus macrostachys	Bromegrass	18–24″	Annual
Calamagrostis acutiflora var. *stricta*	Feather reed grass	5′	5–9
C. arundinacea var. *brachytricha*	Foxtail grass, Korean feather reed	30–36″	5–9
C. epigens	Reed grass	3–4′	3–6
Cortaderia selloana	Pampas grass	14′	8–10
Dactylis glomerata	Variegated orchard grass	1–2′	4–9
Elymus glaucus	Lyme grass, Wild rye	2′	4–9
Eragrostis curvula	Weeping love grass	3–4′	8–9
E. spectabilis	Purple love grass	18–24″	5–9
E. tef	Love grass	18–24″	7–10
Erianthus ravennae	Ravenna grass, Plume grass	14′	5–10
Festuca spp.	Fescue	Varies	Varies
Glyceria maxima 'Variegata'	Variegated manna grass	2′	4–8
Hakonechloa macra 'Aureola'		12–24″	4–9
Helictotrichon sempervirens	Blue oat grass	18–30″	4–8
Koeleria glauca	Blue hair grass	1′	3–9
Lagurus ovatus	Hare's tail grass	18–24″	Annual

BOTANICAL NAME	COMMON NAME(S)	HEIGHT	ZONES
Luzula nivea	Snowy woodrush	2'	4–8
L. sylvatica	Greater woodrush	1'	5–9
Miscanthus floridulus	Giant miscanthus	10'	6–9
M. sinensis 'Gracillimus'	Maiden grass	6–8'	6–9
M. s. 'Silver Feather'	Silver feather grass	6–7'	6–9
M. s. 'Variegatus'	Striped eulalia grass	4–6'	6–9
M. s. 'Zebrinus'	Zebra grass	6–8'	6–9
Panicum virgatum	Switch grass	3–6'	3–9
Pennisetum alopecuroides	Australian fountain grass	3–4'	6–9
P. setaceum	Crimson fountain grass	2–3'	7–10
P. villosum	Feathertop	2–3'	5–10
Phalaris arundinacea var. picta	Ribbon grass	1–3'	4–8
P. canariensis	Canary grass	2–3'	Annual
Phormium tenax	New Zealand flax	3–4'	9–10
Rhynchelytrum repens	Champagne grass	3–4'	7–10
Setaria italica	Foxtail millet	2–4'	Annual
S. lutescens, syn. *S. glauca*	Foxtail grass	18–24"	Annual
Sorghum bicolor	Black sorghum	4–6'	Annual
Spartina pectinata	Cord grass	3–7'	5–9
Stipa gigantea	Giant feather grass	6'	7–9
Triticum aestivum	Wheat	3–4'	Annual
T. turgidum	Bearded wheat	2–4'	Annual

Moist Soil or Moderate Water Use

BOTANICAL NAME	COMMON NAME(S)	HEIGHT	ZONES
Aira elegans	Hair grass	12–18"	Annual
Alopecurus pratensis var. *aureus*	Yellow foxtail grass	1'	4–6
Arundinaria pygmaea	Pygmy bamboo	16"	8–10
A. viridistriata		30–36"	7–10
Arundo donax	Giant reed	15'	7–10
Calamagrostis acutiflora var. stricta	Feather reed grass	5'	5–9
C. arundinacea var. brachytricha	Foxtail grass, Korean feather reed	30–36"	3–6
C. epigens	Reed grass	3–4'	3–9
Carex buchananii	Leatherleaf sedge grass	18–24"	6–9
C. conica 'Variegata'		2–4"	7–9
C. grayi	Gray's sedge	24–30"	2–9
C. morrowii 'Aureo-variegata'	Japanese sedge grass	12–18"	6–9
C. pendula	Common sedge grass	30"	5–9
Coix lacryma-jobi	Job's tears	3–4'	Annual
Cortaderia selloana	Pampas grass	14'	8–10
Cyperus alternifolius	Umbrella plant	3'	8–10
C. papyrus	Papyrus, Egyptian paper reed	10'	10
Deschampsia caespitosa	Tufted hair grass	1–2'	4–9

Moist Soil or Moderate Water Use (cont'd)

BOTANICAL NAME	COMMON NAME(S)	HEIGHT	ZONES
Erianthus ravennae	Ravenna grass	14'	5–10
Glyceria maxima 'Variegata'	Manna grass	2'	4–8
Holcus mollis 'Albo-variegatus'	Velvet grass	4"	4–7
Hystrix patula	Bottlebrush grass	2–4'	4–9
Imperata cylindrica var. rubra	Japanese blood grass	12–18"	7–9
Juncus effusus	Common rush	1–3'	4–8
Luzula nivea	Snowy woodrush	2'	4–8
Milium effusum 'Aureum'	Golden grass	15"	6–9
Miscanthus floridulus	Giant miscanthus	10'	6–9
M. sacchariflorus	Silver banner grass	5'	5–9
M. sinensis 'Gracillimus'	Maiden grass	6–8'	6–9
M. s. 'Silver Feather'		6–7'	6–9
M. s. 'Variegatus'	Striped eulalia grass	4–6'	6–9
M. s. 'Zebrinus'	Zebra grass	6–8'	6–9
Molinia caerulea	Moor grass	18–24"	4–8
Nandina domestica	Heavenly bamboo	8'	6–10
Phalaris arundinacea var. picta	Ribbon grass	1–3'	4–8
Phragmites australis	Reed grass	15'	5–10
Phyllostachys aurea	Yellow grove bamboo	12'	7–8
P. aureosulcata	Yellow grove bamboo	30'	6–7
Pseudosasa japonica	Arrow bamboo, Metake	20'	6–7
Sasa palmata		7½'	6–10
S. veitchii	Kuma bamboo grass	5'	7–10
Shibataea kumasaca		8'	6–7
Spartina pectinata	Cord grass	3–7'	5–9
Zizania aquatica	Wild rice	6–8'	Annual

Prairie Grasses for Xeriscape Landscaping
Low-Water Zone
(12 + " annual precipitation)

BOTANICAL NAME	COMMON NAME(S)	HEIGHT	ZONES
Agropyron smithii	Western wheatgrass	2–4'	3–9
Andropogon gerardii	Big bluestem grass	4–6'	3–9
A. hallii	Sand bluestem	2–5'	3–9
A. virginicus	Broom sedge	2–4'	4–10
Bouteloua curtipendula	Side-oats grama	2–3'	3–10
B. gracilis	Blue grama grass	1–2'	3–10
B. hirsuta	Hairy grama grass	6–24"	3–9
Bromus kalmi		2–4'	3–8
Buchloe dactyloides	Buffalograss	6–12"	3–10
Calamagrostis canadensis	Bluejoint	2–5'	3–7
Calamovilfa longifolia	Prairie sand reed	2–6'	3–6
Elymus canadensis	Canada wild rye	2–5'	3–8
E. virginicus	Virginia wild rye	2–4'	3–9
Eragrostis spectabilis	Purple love grass	18–24"	5–9
E. trichodes	Sand love grass	2–4'	5–9

BOTANICAL NAME	COMMON NAME(S)	HEIGHT	ZONES
Festuca ovina	Sheep fescue	1–2'	3–9
Hordeum jubatum	Squirrel-tail grass, Foxtail barley	1–2'	4–9
Koeleria cristata	Junegrass	1–2'	3–9
Panicum scribnerianum		1–2'	3–9
P. virgatum	Switch grass	3–6'	4–9
Phalaris arundinacea	Reed canary grass	2–5'	4–8
Poa glaucifolia		1–2'	3–9
P. interior	Inland bluegrass	1–2'	3–9
Schizachyrium scoparium, syn. *Andropogon scoparius*	Little bluestem grass	2–5'	4–9
Sorghastrum nutans	Yellow Indian grass	3–7'	6–10
Sporobolus asper		2–4'	3–9
S. heterolepis	Prairie dropseed	1–3'	3–9
Stipa comata	Needle-and-thread	1–2'	4–9
S. spartea	Porcupine grass	2–3'	3–6
Tridens flavus	Purpletop	3–5'	4–10

Moderate Water Zone
(20 + " annual precipitation)

BOTANICAL NAME	COMMON NAME(S)	HEIGHT	ZONES
Festuca rubra	Red fescue	2–3'	5–8
Hystrix patula	Bottlebrush grass	2–4'	4–9
Phragmites communis	Common reed grass	6–8'	3–10
Spartina pectinata	Cord grass	3–7'	5–9

Drought-Tolerant Ground Covers

BOTANICAL NAME	COMMON NAME(S)	HEIGHT	ZONES
Abronia umbellata (often grown as an annual)	Prostrate sand verbena	2"	8–10
Achillea tomentosa	Woolly yarrow	6–24"	4–10
Aegopodium podagraria 'Variegatum'	Goutweed	1'	4–10
Antennaria dioica var. *rosea*	Pussytoes	4–12"	4–8
Arabis alpina	Rock cress	6–8"	6–9
A. caucasica	Wall cress	12"	4–8
Arctostaphylos uva-ursi	Bearberry, Kinnikinnick	1'	3–10 (West) 3–7 (East)
Arctotheca calendula	Cape weed	1'	9
Artemisia absinthium	Common wormwood	30–48"	4–9
A. caucasica	Silver spreader	6"	5–9
A. ludoviciana	Western sage	2–3'	5–9
A. schmidtiana 'Silver Mound'		4–12"	4–9
A. s. 'Nana'		4–12"	4–9
A. stellerana	Beach wormwood	30"	3–9
Atriplex semibaccata	Australian saltbush	1'	8–10

BOTANICAL NAME	COMMON NAME(S)	HEIGHT	ZONES
Aurinia saxatile 'Citrina'		6–12"	4–10
Baccharis pilularis	Dwarf coyote brush	8–24"	8–10
Bergenia cordifolia		10–24"	3–10
B. crassifolia		10–24"	3–10

(Bergenia plantings look best with regular watering in good soil, but will survive poor soil and little supplemental watering in cool summer areas)

Ceanothus gloriosus	Point Reyes ceanothus	12–18"	8–10
Cephalophyllum 'Red Spike'		3–5"	9–10
Cerastium tomentosum	Snow-in-summer	6"	4–10
Cistus salviifolius	Sageleaf rock rose	2'	9–10
Cotoneaster adpressus	Creeping cotoneaster	18"	4–10
C. dammeri, syn. *C. humifusus*	Bearberry cotoneaster	6"	5–10
C. horizontalis	Rock cotoneaster	3'	4–10
Dalea greggii	Trailing indigo bush	4–9"	9–10
Delosperma spp.	Ice plant	1–6"	Varies
Duchesnea indica	Indian mock strawberry	6"	3–10
Erigeron karvinskianus	Mexican daisy, Santa Barbara daisy	10–20"	9–10
Eriogonum umbellatum	Sulphur flower	1'	9–10
Euphorbia marginata	Snow-on-the-mountain	2'	Annual
E. mysinites	Myrtle euphorbia	3–6"	5–10
Festuca ovina glauca	Blue fescue	4–10"	3–10
Genista hispanica	Spanish broom	1–2'	6–9
G. lydia, syn. *Cytisus lydia*		2'	7–9
G. pilosa		18"	6–9
Grevillea lanigera		4'	9–10

(Genista and grevillea do well in coastal areas and where summers are hot and dry—except desert)

Helianthemum nummularium 'Wisley Pink'		6–12"	6–10
Hemerocallis spp.	Daylily	4'	4–10
Hypericum calycinum	Aaronsbeard, Creeping St. John's-wort	1'	6–10

(Drought-tolerant, but looks better with some watering)

Iberis sempervirens	Candytuft	1'	4–10
Juniperus chinensis 'Pfitzerana', 'Hetzii'	Chinese juniper	3'	4–10
J. c. var. *procumbens* 'Nana'		1'	4–10
J. communis var. *saxatilis*		1'	2–9
J. conferta 'Blue Pacific', 'Emerald Sea'		1'	5–10
J. horizontalis 'Bar Harbor', 'Blue Mat'		1'	5–10
J. h. 'Douglasii'		1'	4–10
J. h. 'Plumosa'		18"	4–10
J. h. 'Wiltonii'		4"	2–10
J. sabina var. *tamariscifolia*	Tamarix Savin juniper	2'	4–10
J. squamata 'Blue Carpet'		1'	4–10

BOTANICAL NAME	COMMON NAME(S)	HEIGHT	ZONES
Kochia scoparia var. *trichophylla* 'Childsii'		2–3'	Annual
Lantana spp. (invasive in the Gulf states)		1½'	9–10
Leontopodium alpinum	Edelweiss	4–12"	4–10
Liriope spicata	Creeping lilyturf	8–10"	5–10
Mahonia aquifolium 'Compacta'	Compact Oregon grape	2–3'	5–9 (West) 5–8 (East)
M. nervosa	Longleaf mahonia	2'	(same)
M. repens	Creeping mahonia	3'	(same)
(Mahonia needs light or partial shade in desert gardens)			
Phlox subulata 'Sampson'		6"	4–10
Polygonum affine 'Superbum'		18"	4–7
P. cuspidatum var. *compactum*	Knotweed, Reynoutria fleeceflower	10–24"	4–10
Potentilla tridentata	Cinquefoil	9"	3–10
Ribes viburnifolium	Catalina perfume, Evergreen currant	3'	9–10
Rosmarinus officinalis	Rosemary	2–3'	7–10
R. o. var. *prostratus*	Trailing rosemary	6–24"	7–10
Santolina chamaecyparissus	Lavender cotton	1–2'	6–10
S. virens	Green lavender cotton	10–18"	6–10
Saponaria ocymoides	Rock soapwort	4–8"	4–9
Scaevola 'Mauve Clusters'		12"	9–10
Sedum spp.	Stonecrop	3–18"	Varies
Sempervivum spp.	Houseleek, Hen-and-chicks	4–6"	4–10
Stachys byzantina	Lamb's ears	18"	5–10
Teucrium chamaedrys	Wall germander	6"	6–10
Thymus serpyllum	Creeping thyme	4"	4–10

Drought-Tolerant Trees and Shrubs

BOTANICAL NAME	COMMON NAME(S)	HEIGHT	ZONES
DECIDUOUS TREES			
Acer ginnala	Ginnala maple, Amur maple	20'	2–10
Carya glabra	Pignut hickory	75–100'	5–10
Celtis occidentalis	Hackberry	40–60'	3–10
Fraxinus pennsylvanica var. *lanceolata*	Green ash	60'	2–10
Gleditsia triacanthos var. *inermis*	Thornless honey locust	80'	4–10
Gymnocladus dioica	Kentucky coffee tree	90'	5–10
Koelreuteria paniculata	Goldenrain tree	30–40'	5–10
Prunus americana	American plum	8–35'	3–10
P. serotina (subject to tent caterpillars in the East)	Black cherry	90'	3–10
P. virginiana	Chokecherry	35–50'	2–10

BOTANICAL NAME	COMMON NAME(S)	HEIGHT	ZONES
DECIDUOUS TREES cont'd			
Quercus macrocarpa	Bur oak	70–80'	2–10
Robinia pseudoacacia (invasive in the Midwest)	Black locust	75'	3–10
Sophora japonica	Chinese scholar tree, Japanese pagoda tree	50–75'	4–10
Sorbus aucuparia	European mountain ash, Rowan tree	45'	3–10
Ulmus alata	Winged elm	15–70'	6–10
U. parvifolia	Lacebark elm, Chinese elm	50'	5–10
U. pumila (can be invasive)	Siberian elm	10–30'	3–9
Viburnum lentago	Nannyberry viburnum	20–35'	2–10
V. prunifolium	Black haw	20–35'	3–10
EVERGREEN TREES			
Juniperus scopulorum	Rocky Mountain juniper	30–40'	4–9
J. virginiana	Eastern red cedar	40'	3–9
DECIDUOUS SHRUBS			
Acanthopanax sieboldianus*	Fiveleaf aralia	5–8'	7–10
Amorpha canescens	Lead plant	3–6'	3–10
Aronia melanocarpa	Black chokeberry	3–6'	3–10
Berberis × mentorensis	Mentor barberry	5–7'	4–8
B. thunbergii (invasive in the Northeast and Midwest)	Japanese barberry	7'	4–10
B. t. 'Crimson Pygmy'		2'	4–10
Buddleia davidii	Orange-eye butterfly bush	6–10'	5–9
Caragana arborescens	Siberian pea shrub	7–9'	2–7
Caryopteris × clandonensis	Blue-mist shrub, Blue spirea	2'	5–10
Ceanothus americanus*	New Jersey tea	5'	3–10
Comptonia peregrina	Sweet fern	5'	3–10
Cornus racemosa	Gray dogwood, Panicled dogwood	8–15'	4–10
Corylus americana	American filbert	3–10'	5–10
Cytisus × praecox (many *Cytisus* spp. are invasive in the Southwest)	Warminster broom	10'	7–10
Diervilla lonicera*	Dwarf bush honeysuckle	3'	3–10
Elaeagnus commutata	Silverberry	6–12'	2–10
Hippophae rhamnoides	Sea buckthorn	10–25'	4–10
Lagerstroemia indica	Crape myrtle	21'	7–10
Physocarpus opulifolius	Common ninebark	6–12'	2–10
Potentilla fruticosa	Longacre potentilla, Shrubby cinquefoil	3–4'	2–10
Rhus aromatica	Fragrant sumac	12–20'	3–10
R. copallina	Shining sumac, Flaming sumac	8–30'	4–10
R. glabra	Smooth sumac	8–30'	2–10
R. typhina	Staghorn sumac	30'	3–10
Ribes alpinum	Alpine currant	7'	2–10

BOTANICAL NAME	COMMON NAME(S)	HEIGHT	ZONES
DECIDUOUS SHRUBS cont'd			
Rosa rugosa	Rugosa rose	6'	2–10
Shepherdia argentea	Silver buffaloberry	6–12'	2–10
Symphoricarpos albus	Snowberry	3–6'	3–10
S. orbiculata	Coralberry, Indian currant	3–6'	2–10
Syringa vulgaris	Common lilac	20'	3–10
Vitex agnus-castus	Chaste tree	7–20'	6–7
EVERGREEN SHRUBS			
Abelia × *grandiflora* (semi-evergreen)	Glossy abelia	5'	5–10
Juniperus communis	Common juniper	3–9'	2–10
J. squamata 'Blue Star'		1'	4–10
J. virginiana 'Grey Owl'		10'	3–9
Mahonia aquifolium	Oregon grape holly	3–6'	7–10
M. bealei	Leatherleaf mahonia	12'	7–10
Myrica pensylvanica	Northern bayberry	3–10'	3–10
Pinus mugo	Mugo pine	8'	2–10
Pyracantha coccinea	Scarlet firethorn	6'	6–10
Yucca filamentosa	Adam's needle	3'	4–10
Y. glauca	Soapweed	3'	5–10

*More common in the eastern United States.

Drought-Tolerant Vines

BOTANICAL NAME	COMMON NAME(S)	HEIGHT	ZONES
Bougainvillea spp.		Varies	10
Campsis radicans	Trumpet creeper	30'	4–10
Cissus antarctica	Kangaroo ivy	Varies	10
Clematis ligusticifolia	Western virgin's bower	20'	3–10
Cobaea scandens	Cup-and-saucer vine, Cathedral bells	40'	Annual
Convolvulus mauritanicus	Ground morning glory	6'	8–10 (or annual)
Euonymus fortunei var. *radicans*	Common wintercreeper	20'	5–9
Ipomoea tricolor	Morning glory	10'	Annual
Lathyrus latifolius	Perennial sweet pea	9'	5–10
Lonicera japonica 'Halliana' (grows only in drier areas; in the eastern United States it's considered a pest)	Hall's honeysuckle	20–30'	4–10
L. sempervirens	Trumpet honeysuckle	50'	3–10
Macfadyena unguis-cati	Cat's-claw vine, Yellow trumpet vine	25–30'	9–10
Maurandya antirrhiniflora	Snapdragon vine	6'	Annual
Parthenocissus quinquefolia	Virginia creeper	35'	3–10

Drought-Tolerant Vines (cont'd)

BOTANICAL NAME	COMMON NAME(S)	HEIGHT	ZONES
Parthenocissus tricuspidata	Boston ivy	60'	4–10
Polygonum aubertii	Silver-lace vine	20–30'	4–7
Rosa banksiae	Lady Banks' rose	20'	5–10
Solanum jasminoides	Potato vine	15'	7–9
Tecomaria capensis	Cape honeysuckle	6'	9–10
Thunbergia alata	Black-eyed Susan vine	6'	Annual
Vitis spp.	Grape	Varies	Vary
Wisteria sinensis	Chinese wisteria	25'	5–10

NOTE: One vine strictly to avoid, especially if you live in the Southeast, is the kudzu vine (*Pueraria lobata*). Although it appears in some vine botanies, it is appropriately called "the vine that ate the South." Originally from South America, it may grow as much as sixty feet per year and has taken over fields and forests in the Southeast, literally covering everything in sight.

Plants for Dry Shade

BOTANICAL NAME	COMMON NAME(S)	HEIGHT	ZONES
DECIDUOUS TREES			
Aesculus glabra	Ohio buckeye	30'	3–10
A. octandra	Yellow buckeye	50–75'	4–10
Catalpa speciosa	Northern catalpa	90'	4–10
Crataegus spp.	Hawthorn	10–50'	Vary
Fraxinus americana	White ash	120'	3–10
F. pennsylvanica var. lanceolata	Green ash	50–75'	2–10
Gleditsia triacanthos var. inermis	Thornless honey locust	80'	4–10
Gymnocladus dioca	Kentucky coffee tree	90'	4–10
Koelreuteria paniculata	Golden raintree	30–40'	5–10
Morus alba	White mulberry	45'	4–10
Prunus americana	American plum	20–35'	3–10
P. padus	European bird cherry	45'	3–10
Quercus gambelii	Gambel oak, Scrub oak	20–65'	4–10
Q. macrocarpa	Bur oak	70–80'	2–10
Robinia pseudoacacia	Black locust	75'	3–10
DECIDUOUS SHRUBS			
Buddleia alternifolia	Fountain butterfly bush	10–20'	6–8
B. davidii	Orange-eye butterfly bush	6–10'	5–9
Caragana microphylla	Littleleaf peashrub	5'	2–10
Cercocarpus ledifolius	Curl-leaf mahogany	20–30'	4–10
C. montanus	Mountain mahogany	5–10'	6–10
Chaenomeles speciosa	Flowering quince	6–10'	5–10
Colutea arborescens	Common bladder senna	5–8'	6–9
Cotoneaster apiculatus	Cranberry cotoneaster	2–3'	4–10
C. horizontalis	Small-leaved cotoneaster, Rockspray cotoneaster	2–3'	5–9

BOTANICAL NAME	COMMON NAME(S)	HEIGHT	ZONES
DECIDUOUS SHRUBS cont'd			
Cotoneaster multiflorus	Flowering cotoneaster	5–6'	5–10
Cytisus × praecox	Warminster broom	6–10'	7–10
Elaeagnus commutata	Silverberry	8–12'	1–7
E. umbellata	Autumn olive	12–15'	3–8
Euonymus alata	Winged euonymus, Burning bush	8–12'	4–7
Fendlera rupicola	False mock orange	5–6'	6–10
Forestiera neomexicana	New Mexican privet	10'	5–10
Kerria japonica	Japanese kerria	6–8'	5–8
Ligustrum amurense	Amur privet	8	4–10
L. regelianum	Regel privet	4–5'	4–10
Lonicera korolkowi	Blueleaf honeysuckle	12–15'	5–9
L. tatarica	Tatarian honeysuckle	12'	3–9
Physocarpus monogynus	Mountain ninebark	6'	3–8
P. opulifolius	Common ninebark	5–10'	3–8
Potentilla fruticosa	Bush cinquefoil	2–4'	2–9
Rhamnus cathartica	Common buckthorn	20'	6–10
R. frangula	Alder buckthorn	10–18'	3–9
Rhus glabra	Smooth sumac	8–20'	3–10
R. typhina	Staghorn sumac	10–30'	3–10
Rosa × harisonii	Harison's yellow rose	5–8'	4–10
R. hugonis	Father Hugo rose	6–8'	5–10
R. rubrifolia	Redleaf rose	10–30'	3–10
R. rugosa	Shrub rose, Rugosa rose	4–6'	3–10
Rubus deliciosus	Thimbleberry, Boulder raspberry	3–5'	6–10
Sarcococca ruscifolia	Fragrant sarcococca	3–6'	7–10
Shepherdia argentea	Silver buffaloberry	6–12'	2–10
Symphoricarpos orbiculatus	Indian currant coralberry	3–5'	3–10
S. o. 'Hancock'	Hancock coralberry	18"	3–10
Syringa × chinensis	Chinese lilac	10–15'	4–8
S. meyeri	Meyer's lilac	4–8'	4–8
S. × persica	Persian lilac	5–6'	4–8
S. reflexa	MacFarlane lilac	16'	5–10
S. villosa	Late lilac	8–10'	2–7
S. vulgaris	Common lilac	8–15'	3–7
Viburnum lantana	Wayfaring-tree viburnum	10–15'	4–8
V. lentago	Nannyberry viburnum	15–20'	2–9
EVERGREEN SHRUBS			
Aucuba japonica		6–10'	7–9
Berberis thunbergii	Japanese barberry	4–7'	4–8
B. thunbergii 'Crimson Pygmy'	Crimson Pygmy barberry	2'	4–8
Fallugia paradoxa	Apache plume	3–7'	5–10
Juniperus chinensis 'Pfitzerana'	Pfitzer juniper	8'	4–10
Mahonia aquifolium	Oregon grape holly	3–5'	5–10

BOTANICAL NAME	COMMON NAME(S)	HEIGHT	ZONES
GROUND COVERS			
Aegopodium podagraria	Variegated bishop's gout-weed	6–14″	4–9
Ajuga reptans	Bugleweed	6″	4–10
Cerastium tomentosum	Snow-in-summer	6″	4–10
Duchesnea indica	Mock strawberry	2–3″	4–10
Euonymus fortunei	Wintercreeper	6″–2′	5–8
Festuca ovina var. *glauca*	Blue fescue	4–10″	4–9
Fragaria chiloensis	Wild strawberry	6–10″	5–10
Iris pumila	Dwarf bearded iris	4–8″	4–10
Juniperus communis var. *saxatalis*	Mountain common creeper	1′	2–9
Lavandula vera	Lavender	18″	5–10
Mahonia repens	Creeping mahonia	1′	5–9
Polygonatum commutatum	Great Solomon's seal	7″	4–10
Potentilla verna var. *nana*	Creeping potentilla	2–6″	4–8
Sedum spp.	Stonecrop	6–12″	Vary
Sepervivum arachnoideum	Hen-and-chicks, Cobweb houseleek	4″–2′	5–10
Veronica repens	Creeping veronica	1′	6–11 (West) 6–7 (East)
PERENNIALS			
Acanthus mollis	Bear's-breech	3–4′	8–10
Bergenia cordifolia		12–16′	2–10
Chrysanthemum maximum	Shasta daisy	1–2′	4–5
Corydalis lutea	Yellow corydalis	1′	5–10
Hemerocallis spp.	Daylily	3–4′	3–10
Penstemon strictus 'Bandera'	Rocky Mountain penstemon	1–2′	4–9
Tradescantia virginiana	Common spiderwort	18–26″	4–10
ANNUALS			
Abronia umbellata	Sand verbena	6–24′	
Centaurium erythraea	Centaury	20″	
Cleome hasslerana	Spiderflower	4–5′	
Collinsia grandiflora	Blue lips	8–15″	
Consolida ambigua	Rocket larkspur	1–2′	
Cosmos bipinnatus		4–6′	
Dyssodia tenuiloba	Dahlberg daisy	8–12″	
Erysimum perofskianum		2′	
Eschscholzia californica	California poppy	8–12″	
Gaillardia pulchella	Blanket flower, Indian blanket	1–2′	
Helianthus annuus 'Italian White'		12′	
Myosotis sylvatica	Forget-me-not	6–18″	
Nemophila maculata	Five spot	1′	
N. menziesii	Baby blue-eyes	1′	
Nierembergia hippomanica	Cup flower	6–8″	

BOTANICAL NAME	COMMON NAME(S)	HEIGHT	ZONES
ANNUALS cont'd			
Oenothera deltoides	Desert evening primrose	2–10″	
Phacelia campanularia	California bluebell	8″	
VINES			
Clematis ligusticifolia	Western virgin's bower	20′	3–10
Lonicera japonica 'Halliana'	Hall's honeysuckle	20–30′	4–10
Parthenocissus inserta	Hiedra, Thicket creeper	35′	3–10
P. quinquefolia, P. q. 'Engelmannii'	Virginia creeper	20–35′	3–10
Tropaeolum majus	Indian cress	8–12′	Annual
FERN			
Dennstaedtia punctilobula	Hay-scented fern	1′	3–8

Drought-Tolerant Trees and Shrubs for Seaside Gardens

BOTANICAL NAME	COMMON NAME(S)	HEIGHT	ZONES
DECIDUOUS TREES			
Ailanthus altissima (invasive in the eastern U.S.)	Tree-of-heaven	60′	4–10
Fraxinus velutina	Velvet ash	20–45′	5–10
Populus alba	White poplar	90′	3–10
Quercus marilandica	Blackjack oak	35–50′	6–10
Robinia pseudoacacia (invasive in Midwest)	Black locust	40–75′	3–10
Schinus molle	California pepper tree	40′	9–10
Ulmus pumila (can be invasive)	Dwarf elm	10–30′	3–9
EVERGREEN TREES			
Cupressus macrocarpa	Monterey cypress	75′	7–10
Eucalyptus spp. (some species invasive in the Southwest)		15–200′	Vary
Juniperus excelsa 'Stricta'	Greek juniper	60′	7–10
J. lucayana	West Indies juniper	50′	9–10
J. virginiana	Eastern red cedar	40′	3–9
Malaleuca leucadendron (M. quinquenervia is invasive in Florida)	Cajeput tree	40′	10
Olea europaea	Common olive	25′	9–10
Pinus rigida	Pitch pine	75′	4–10
DECIDUOUS SHRUBS			
Baccharis halimifolia		12′	5–10
Comptonia peregrina	Sweet fern	5′	3–10
Cytisus spp. (some are invasive in the Southwest and Northwest)	Broom	8″–6′	Vary

BOTANICAL NAME	COMMON NAME(S)	HEIGHT	ZONES
DECIDUOUS SHRUBS cont'd			
Elaeagnus angustifolia	Russian olive	20′	2–10
Ligustrum amurense	Amur privet	15′	3–10
Potentilla spp.		6″–4′	2–10
Prunus maritima	Beach plum	6′	3–10
Rhamnus spp.	Buckthorn	10–20′	Vary
Rhus spp.	Sumac	8–30′	Vary
Rosa rugosa	Rugosa rose	6′	2–10
R. spinosissima	Scotch rose	3′	4–10
R. virginiana	Virginia rose	6′	3–10
Shepherdia canadensis	Russet buffaloberry	6–12′	2–10
Tamarix spp. (invasive in the Southwest)	Tamarisk	4–15′	Vary
EVERGREEN SHRUBS			
Arctostaphylos uva-ursi	Bearberry, Kinnikinick	1′	3–10 (West) 3–7 (East)
Atriplex spp.	Saltbush	4′	5–7
Euonymus japonica	Evergreen euonymus	15′	8
Juniperus communis	Common juniper	6″–36′	2–10
J. conferta	Shore juniper	1′	5–10
J. horizontalis	Creeping juniper	4–18″	Vary
Ligustrum ovalifolium	California privet	15′	5–10
Myrica pensylvanica	Northern bayberry	3–10′	3–10
Nerium oleander		12′	7–9
Pittosporum tobira	Japanese pittosporum	2–10′	
Raphiolepis umbellata	Yedda hawthorn	6′	7–10
Ruscus aculeatus	Butcher's broom	18″–4′	7–10

Drought-Tolerant Bulbs
Spring-Flowering Bulbs

(Water only if spring season is dry. Plants are dormant during the summer and require no special watering.)

BOTANICAL NAME	COMMON NAME(S)	COLOR(S)	HEIGHT	ZONES
Anemone blanda	Greek anemone	Purple, pink, red, white	4–6″	6–10
Crocus spp.		Purple, white, yellow	2–6″	3–10
Eremurus spp.	Foxtail lily	White, pink, yellow, orange, peach, cream	3–9′	5–9
Erianthus spp.	Winter aconite	Yellow	2–4″	4–9
Erythronium spp.		White, yellow, purple	6–24″	3–9

BOTANICAL NAME	COMMON NAME(S)	COLOR(S)	HEIGHT	ZONES
Fritillaria imperialis	Crown imperial	Orange, red, yellow	2–4'	5–10
F. meleagris	Guinea hen flower	Purple-white (checkered pattern), white	1'	5–10
F. michailovskyi	Michael's flower	Bronze-maroon	8–12"	5–10
Galanthus spp.	Snowdrop	White	3–8"	3–9
Hyacinthoides (Scilla) hispanica	Spanish bluebell	Blue, white, pink	1'	4–10
Hyacinthus orientalis		Blue, purple, red, white, pink, yellow, cream, apricot	8–12"	4–10
Ipheion uniflorum	Spring starflower	White	6"	6–10
Iris reticulata		Blue, lavender, purple	6"	3–8
Leucojum spp.	Snowflake	White	9"	4–10
Muscari spp.	Grape hyacinth	Blue, white	4–12"	2–10
Narcissus spp.	Daffodil	White, yellow, gold, orange, apricot	3–24"	4–10
N. bulbocodium	Miniature daffodil	Yellow, orange, white	6–14"	4–10
Ornithogalum umbellatum	Star-of-Bethlehem	White-green stripes	1–2'	4–10
Scilla siberica		Blue, pink, white	6"	1–8
Tulipa spp.		Red, salmon, orange, yellow, gold, cream	6–20"	3–10
T. (Dutch)		Every color except blue	18–30"	3–7

Summer-Flowering Bulbs

(Water only during prolonged summer drought.)

BOTANICAL NAME	COMMON NAME(S)	COLOR(S)	HEIGHT	ZONES
Acidanthera bicolor	Abyssinian gladiolus, Peacock orchid	White	18–24"	7–10
Crocosmia, syn. *Montbretia*		Yellow, orange, scarlet	2–4'	8–10
Gladiolus spp.		All colors	1–5'	8–10
Ranunculus asiaticus (requires dry soil in summer)	Buttercup	All colors but green and blue	18"	8–10
Sparaxis spp.	Harlequin flower	Red, yellow, blue, purple, white	12–18"	9
Zephyranthes spp.	Rain lily, Fairy lily, Zephyr lily	White, pink, yellow, apricot	6–8"	7

Bibliography

Design

Ball, Ken, with members of AWAA Water Conservation Committee. *Xeriscape Programs for Water Utilities*. Denver, Colo.: American Water Works Association, 1990.

Burke, Ken, and A. Cort Sinnes. *Shade Gardening*. San Francisco: Ortho Books, 1982.

Chatto, Beth. *The Dry Garden*. London: J. M. Dent & Sons, Ltd., 1978.

————. *The Green Tapestry*. New York: Simon & Schuster, 1989.

Creasey, Rosalind. *Earthly Delights*. San Francisco: Sierra Club Books, 1985.

————. *The Complete Book of Edible Landscaping*. San Francisco: Sierra Club Books, 1982.

Damrosch, Barbara. *Theme Gardens*. New York: Workman Publishing, 1982.

Feldman, Fran, and Cornelia Fogle, et al., eds. *Waterwise Gardening*. Menlo Park, Calif.: Lane Publishing Co., 1990.

Hobhouse, Penelope. *Color in Your Garden*. Boston: Little, Brown, 1985.

Robinette, Gary O. *Water Conservation in Landscape Management*. New York: Van Nostrand Reinhold, 1984.

Sunset Books and *Sunset* Magazine, editors of. *Waterwise Gardening: Beautiful Gardens with Less Water*. Menlo Park, Calif.: Lane Publishing, 1989.

Thorpe, Pamela. *The American Weekend Gardener*. New York: Random House, 1988.

Wheatly, Margaret Tipton. *Successful Gardening with Limited Water*. Santa Barbara, Calif.: Woodbridge Press, 1978.

Soils

Brady, Nyle C. *The Nature and Properties of Soils, 8th edition*. New York: Macmillan, 1974.

Campbell, Stu. *Let It Rot*. Pownal, Vt.: Storey Communications, 1975.

Feucht, James R., and Jack D. Butler. *Landscape Management*. New York: Van Nostrand Reinhold, 1988.

Logsdon, Gene. *The Gardener's Guide to Better Soil*. Emmaus, Pa.: Rodale Press, 1975.

Lawns

Beard, Dr. James B. *How to Have a Beautiful Lawn*. Kansas City, Mo.: Intertic Publishing, 1975.

Crockett, James Underwood, et al. *Lawns and Ground Covers*. New York: Time-Life Books, 1971.

Franklin, Stuart. *Building a Healthy Lawn*. Pownal, Vt.: Storey Communications, 1988.

Schultz, Warren. *The Chemical-Free Lawn*. Emmaus, Pa.: Rodale Press, 1989.

General Plants

Allen, Oliver E., and the editors of Time-Life Books. *The Time-Life Book of Shade Gardening*. New York: Henry Holt, 1979.

Heriteau, Jacqueline, and Dr. Marc Cathey. *The National Arboretum Book of Outstanding Garden Plants*. New York: Simon & Schuster, 1990.

Hogan, Elizabeth. *Sunset Western Garden Book*. Menlo Park, Calif.: Lane Publishing Co., 1988.

L. H. Bailey Hortorium Staff. *Hortus Third*. New York: Macmillan, 1976.

Smith, Richard M. *Wild Plants of America*. New York: Wiley, 1989.

Taylor's Guide to Water-Saving Gardening. Boston: Houghton Mifflin, 1990.

Trees, Shrubs, Vines

Appleton, Bonnie Lee. *Landscape Rejuvenation.* Pownal, Vt.: Storey Communications, 1988.

Brimer, John Burton. *The Home Gardener's Guide to Trees and Shrubs.* New York: Hawthorn Books, 1976.

Cravens, Richard. *Vines.* Alexandria, Va.: Time-Life Books, 1979.

Crockett, James Underwood. *Evergreens.* New York: Time-Life Books, 1971.

Davis, Brian. *The Gardener's Illustrated Encyclopedia of Trees and Shrubs.* Emmaus, Pa.: Rodale Press, 1987.

DeWolf, Gordon, Jr., Ph.D., and Gordon E. Jones, et al. *Taylor's Guide to Shrubs.* Boston: Houghton Mifflin, 1986.

DeWolf, Gordon, Jr., and Norman Taylor. *Taylor's Guide to Trees.* Boston: Houghton Mifflin Company, 1988.

Hightshoe, Gary L. *Native Trees, Shrubs, and Vines for Urban and Rural America.* New York: Van Nostrand Reinhold, 1988.

Preston, Richard J. *North American Trees.* Ames, Iowa: Iowa State University Press, 1968.

Snyder, Leon C. *Trees and Shrubs for Northern Gardens.* Minneapolis: University of Minnesota Press, 1980.

Wilson, William H. *Landscaping with Wildflowers and Native Plants.* San Francisco: Ortho Books, 1984.

Wyman, Donald. *Shrubs and Vines for American Gardens.* London: The Macmillan Company/Collier-Macmillan, 1969.

————. *Trees for American Gardens.* New York: Macmillan, 1990.

Flowers

Art, Henry. *A Garden of Wildflowers: 101 Native Species and How to Grow Them.* Pownal, Vt.: Storey Communications, 1986.

Bartholomew, Mel. *Square Foot Gardening.* Emmaus, Pa.: Rodale Press, 1981.

Clausen, Ruth Rogers. *Perennials for American Gardens.* New York: Random House, 1989.

Crockett, James Underwood, and Oliver E. Allen. *Wildflower Gardening.* Alexandria, Va.: Time-Life Books, 1977.

————. *Annuals.* New York: Time-Life Books, 1971.

DeWolf, Gordon, Jr., Ph.D., and Pamela Harper, et al. *Taylor's Guide to Perennials.* Boston: Houghton Mifflin, 1986.

————. *Taylor's Guide to Annuals.* Boston: Houghton Mifflin, 1986.

James, Theodore, Jr. *Flowering Bulbs.* New York: Macmillan, 1991.

Jelitto, Leo, and Wilhelm Schacht. *Hardy Herbaceous Perennials* (2 vols.). Portland, Oreg.: Timber Press, 1985.

Miles, Bebe. *Wildflower Perennials for Your Garden.* New York: Hawthorn Books, 1976.

Orr, Robert T., and Margaret C. Orr. *Wildflowers of Western America.* New York: Galahad Books, 1974.

Snyder, Leon C. *Flowers for Northern Gardens.* Minneapolis: University of Minnesota Press, 1983.

Venning, Frank D. *A Guide to Field Identification: Wildflowers of North America.* New York: Golden Press, 1984.

Ground Covers, Ornamental Grasses

Brown, Lauren. *Grasses: An Identification Guide.* Boston: Houghton Mifflin, 1979.

DeWolf, Gordon, Jr., ed. *Taylor's Guide to Ground Covers, Vines and Grasses.* New York: Houghton Mifflin, 1987.

Grounds, Roger. *Ornamental Grasses.* New York: Van Nostrand Reinhold, 1981.

Hitchcock, A. S., and Agnes Chase. *Manual of the Grasses of the United States.* New York: Dover, 1971.

Loewer, Peter. *The Annual Garden: Flowers, Foliage, Fruits and Grasses for One Summer Season.* Emmaus, Pa.: Rodale Press, 1988.

————. *Growing and Decorating with Grasses.* New York: Walker and Company, 1977.

Mackenzie, David S. *Complete Manual of Perennial Ground Covers.* Englewood Cliffs, N.J.: Prentice-Hall, 1989.

Oakes, A. J. *Ornamental Grasses and Grasslike Plants.* New York: Van Nostrand Reinhold, 1990.

Ottesen, Carole. *Ornamental Grasses.* New York: McGraw-Hill, 1989.

Reinhardt, Thomas A., Martina Reinhardt, and Mark Moskowitz. *Ornamental Grass Gardening.* Los Angeles: HP Books, Michael Friedman Publishing Group, Inc., 1989.

Maintenance

Burke, Ken, ed. *Easy Maintenance Gardening.* San Francisco: Ortho Books, 1982.

Roth, Susan A., ed. *All About Pruning.* San Ramon, Calif.: Ortho Books, 1989.

Central and Eastern United States

Gates, Frank C. *Annotated List of the Plants of Kansas: Ferns and Flowering Plants.* Manhattan, Kans.: Kansas State and College of Agriculture and Applied Science, 1940.

Huddleston, Sam, and Michael Hussey. *Grow Native: Landscaping with Native and Apt Plants of the Rocky Mountains.* Columbus, Nebr.: Apple Tree Image Publishers, 1975.

Knopf, Jim. *The Xeriscape Flower Gardener.* Boulder, Colo.: Johnson Books, 1991.

Landscaping for Water Conservation: Xeriscape! Aurora, Colo.: City of Aurora, Colorado, Utilities Department, 1989.

McGregor, Ronald L., et al. *Flora of the Great Plains.* Lawrence, Kans.: University Press of Kansas, 1986.

Roberts, Rhoda, and Ruth Ashton Nelson. *Mountain Wild Flowers of Colorado.* Denver, Colo.: Denver Museum of Natural History, 1957.

Wasowski, Sally, with Andy Wasowski. *Native Texas Plants: Landscaping Region by Region.* Austin: Texas Monthly Press, 1988.

Weaver, J. E. *Native Vegetation of Nebraska.* Lincoln, Nebr.: University of Nebraska Press, 1965.

West

Coate, Barry, et al. *Water Conserving Plants and Landscapes for the Bay Area.* Oakland, Calif.: East Bay Municipal Utility District, 1990.

Coates, Margaret Klipstein. *Perennials for the Western Garden.* Boulder, Colo.: Pruett Publishing Company, 1976.

Crocker, Cedric, ed. *Gardening in Dry Climates.* San Ramon, Calif.: Ortho Books, 1989.

Desert Botanical Garden Staff. *Arizona Highways Presents Desert Wildflowers.* Phoenix: Arizona Department of Transportation, State of Arizona, 1988.

Duffield, Mary Rose, and Warren D. Jones. *Plants for Dry Climates.* Tucson: HP Books, 1981.

Perry, Bob. *Trees and Shrubs for Dry California Landscapes: Plants for Water Conservation.* San Dimas, Calif.: Land Design Publishing, 1981.

Phillips, Judith. *Southwest Landscaping with Native Plants.* Santa Fe: Museum of New Mexico Press, 1987.

Rabkin, Richard, and Jacob Rabkin. *Nature in the West: A Handbook of Habitats.* New York: Holt, Rinehart and Winston, 1981.

Index

Page numbers in *italic* indicate illustrations.